Glutamine

Biochemistry, Physiology, and Clinical Applications

Glutamine

Glutamine

Biochemistry, Physiology, and Clinical Applications

Edited by
Dominique Meynial-Denis

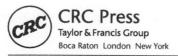

CRC Press
Taylor & Francis Group
Boca Raton London New York

CRC Press is an imprint of the
Taylor & Francis Group, an **informa** business

CRC Press
Taylor & Francis Group
6000 Broken Sound Parkway NW, Suite 300
Boca Raton, FL 33487-2742

First issued in paperback 2021

© 2017 by Taylor & Francis Group, LLC
CRC Press is an imprint of Taylor & Francis Group, an Informa business

No claim to original U.S. Government works

ISBN 13: 978-1-03-209704-6 (pbk)
ISBN 13: 978-1-4822-3429-9 (hbk)

Visit the Taylor & Francis Web site at
http://www.taylorandfrancis.com

and the CRC Press Web site at
http://www.crcpress.com

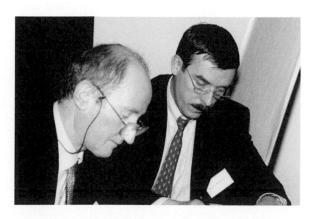

This book is dedicated to the memory of Dr. Maurice Arnal and Professor Bernard Beaufrère. Gifted with imagination and vision and exemplars of scientific rigor, both were renowned scientists in the field of amino acid and protein metabolism, to which they made outstanding contributions. In spirit they were humanists and at all times retained a sense of humility. In 1992, Dr. Arnal created the Human Nutrition Research Center in Clermont-Ferrand, which is now one of the most active in France. Professor Bernard Beaufrère joined Dr. Arnal's project to become assistant director and then director until his untimely death in 2002.

For me, it was a privilege and a pleasure to work with two men of such exceptional qualities and throughout my career as a scientist I have attempted to apply their high standards to all areas of my work.

Contents

SECTION I   Basics of Glutamine Metabolism

SECTION II   New Data on the Biochemistry of Glutamine

SECTION III   Molecular and Cellular Aspects
of Glutamine Metabolism

SECTION IV   Glutamine, the Brain and Neurological Diseases

SECTION V   Glutamine and the Intestinal Tract

SECTION VI   Glutamine and the Catabolic State: Role of Glutamine in Critical Illness During Childhood

SECTION VII   Glutamine and the Catabolic State: Role of Glutamine in Critical Illness from Adulthood

SECTION VIII   Glutamine and the Catabolic State: Role of Glutamine in Cancer

SECTION IX   Glutamine, Immunity, and Exercise

SECTION X   Glutamine and Aging

SECTION XI   Conclusion

Preface

This book gathers advanced expertise on the most significant aspects of glutamine metabolism and its health implications. Its aim is to present fully up-to-date coverage of research in this field.

This book is didactically orientated and addressed to nutritionists with a research interest in amino acids, glutamine, or catabolic states; graduate students in nutrition; medical students and postdoctoral researchers in nutrition, biology, and medicine; dieticians and pharmacists looking for a comprehensive update on glutamine; and clinicians with an interest in catabolic states and/ or artificial nutrition. Readers will be interested in finding out about experimental research in the most advanced areas of glutamine metabolism, and in its designation as conditionally essential, as a regulator of cellular function, as a therapeutic nutrient to improve mucosal recovery in the intestine during certain diseases or aging, as a potential adjuvant in patient therapy, and as a potential metabolic target in cancer therapy and imaging.

Such a book can only come into being through the efforts of many people. I would like to acknowledge the efforts of the contributors who enthusiastically accepted to participate in this project and for their understanding and willing cooperation during the preparation of this book. I must also thank Morey Haymond for readily agreeing to write the introduction. I am deeply grateful to Maurice Arnal, without whose initial efforts and foresight, this book would never have gotten off the ground. His help and support throughout my career and up to his death in 2000 was invaluable. I am greatly indebted to Bernard Beaufrère who believed in me and gave me the confidence to take up research. My thanks go to Philip Calder, a firm supporter who was instrumental in turning my thoughts on glutamine metabolism into a book. I would like to thank Kevin Brindle for critically reading the manuscript and providing valuable comments to improve the relevance of the chapter on the use of hyperpolarized ^{15}N glutamine as a new therapeutic target in cancer. I would like also to thank Marc Ferrara, director of the Human Nutrition Unit to which I belong, who allowed me to embark on this project. I am grateful to Blandine Tamboise, for secretarial assistance in the preparation of this book. Finally, I would like to thank my husband, Christian, and my daughters, Audrey-Marie and Marie-Anaïs, for their total support and their patience during the hours I spent at my computer and not with them.

Dominique Meynial-Denis
Clermont-Ferrand, France

Editor

Dominique Meynial-Denis studied biochemistry and molecular biology at the University Paul Sabatier of Toulouse, France and earned her PhD on intermolecular interactions between drug and plasma proteins using magnetic resonance spectroscopy (MRS) at the same University in 1985. Since 1986, she has worked as a scientist at the National Institute of Agricultural Research (INRA) in Clermont-Ferrand in the Department of Human Nutrition. She began specialist research into sarcopenia and aging in 1994. She applied MRS in work on metabolic pathways of amino acids in muscle during aging. Meynial-Denis earned a second PhD in 1998 on amino acid fluxes throughout skeletal muscle during aging. More recently, her main interest has been the effect of glutamine supplementation in advanced age. She is a member of the Société de Gérontologie et de Gériatrie (SFGG), of the International Association of Gerontology and Geriatrics (IAGG), of the Société Française de Nutrition Entérale et Parentérale (SFNEP), of the Société Européenne de Nutrition Clinique et Métabolisme (ESPEN), and of the Société Française de Nutrition (SFN). She is a regular referee for different international nutrition journals. As an editor of books that give an overview of latest scientific findings from recognized international experts she aims to enhance the status of research in the field.

Contributors

Naji N. Abumrad
Division of General Surgery
Vanderbilt University Medical Center
Nashville, Tennessee

Jan Albrecht
Department of Neurotoxicology
Mossakowski Medical Research Centre
Polish Academy of Sciences
Warsaw, Poland

Mireille Andriamihaja
INRA/AgroParisTech
Nutrition Physiology and Ingestive Behavior
Paris, France

Chantal Bemeur
CRCHUM
and
Département de nutrition
Université de Montréal
Montréal, Canada

Guy Bielicki
NMR Platform
INRA Clermont-Ferrand/Theix
Saint Genes Champanelle, France

François Blachier
INRA/AgroParisTech
Nutrition Physiology and Ingestive Behavior
Paris, France

Barrie P. Bode
Department of Biological Sciences and the
    Center for Biochemical and Biophysical
    Studies
Northern Illinois University
DeKalb, Illinois

Alice Bonanni
Nephrology, Dialysis and Transplant
    Division
Department of Internal Medicine
University of Genoa and IRCCS AOU
    San Martino-IST
Genova, Italy

Jan Böttger
Institut für Biochemie, Lehrstuhl Allgemeine
    Biochemie
der Medizinischen Fakultät der Universität
    Leipzig
Leipzig, Germany

Roger F. Butterworth
Département de médecine
Université de Montréal
Montréal, Canada

Philip C. Calder
Human Development & Health Academic Unit
University of Southampton
Southampton, United Kingdom

Lindy Castell
Green Templeton College
University of Oxford
Oxford, United Kingdom

Carine Chassain
CHU Clermont-Ferrand
Clermont-Ferrand, France

Moïse Coëffier
Nutrition, Inflammation and Dysfunction of
    Gut-Brain Axis
and
Institute for Innovation and Biomedical Research
University of Rouen
and
Nutrition Department
Rouen University Hospital
Rouen, France

Vinicius Fernandes Cruzat
School of Biomedical Sciences, CHIRI
    Biosciences
Curtin University
Perth, Western Australia, Australia

Norman P. Curthoys
Department of Biochemistry and Molecular
    Biology
Colorado State University
Fort Collins, Colorado

Pierre Déchelotte
Nutrition, Inflammation and Dysfunction of
    Gut-Brain Axis
and
Institute for Innovation and Biomedical Research
University of Rouen
and
Nutrition Department
Rouen University Hospital
Rouen, France

Giacomo Deferrari
Nephrology, Dialysis and Transplant Division
Department of Internal Medicine
University of Genova and IRCCS AOU San
    Martino-IST
Genova, Italy

Ronaldo Vagner Thomatieli dos Santos
Department of Bioscience
University Federal of São Paulo
Santos, Brazil

Franck Durif
CHU Clermont-Ferrand
and
Auvergne University
Clermont-Ferrand, France

Gaewyn Ellison
School of Biomedical Sciences, CHIRI
    Biosciences
Curtin University
Perth, Western Australia, Australia

Giacomo Garibotto
Nephrology, Dialysis and Transplant Division
Department of Internal Medicine
University of Genova and IRCCS AOU San
    Martino-IST
Genova, Italy

Rolf Gebhardt
Institut für Biochemie, Lehrstuhl Allgemeine
    Biochemie
der Medizinischen Fakultät der Universität
    Leipzig
Leipzig, Germany

Theodorus B. M. Hakvoort
Tytgat Institute for Liver and Intestinal Research
Academic Medical Center
University of Amsterdam Meibergdreef
Amsterdam, The Netherlands

Morey W. Haymond
Department of Pediatrics
Children's Nutrition Research Center
Baylor College of Medicine
Houston, Texas

Youji He
Tytgat Institute for Liver and Intestinal Research
Academic Medical Center
University of Amsterdam Meibergdreef
Amsterdam, the Netherlands

Essam Imseis
Division of Gastroenterology and Hepatology
Department of Pediatrics
University of Texas Medical School at Houston
Houston, Texas

Farook Jahoor
Children's Nutrition Research Center
Baylor College of Medicine
Houston, Texas

Christina C. Kao
Children's Nutrition Research Center
Baylor College of Medicine
Houston, Texas

Xiangfeng Kong
Institute of Subtropical Agriculture, Chinese
    Academy of Sciences
Changsha, China

Wouter H. Lamers
Tytgat Institute for Liver and Intestinal Research
Academic Medical Center
University of Amsterdam Meibergdreef
Amsterdam, The Netherlands

Antonio Lancha Jr.
Laboratory of Applied Nutrition and
    Metabolism
University of Sao Paulo
Brazil

Nan Li
Department of Pediatrics
University of Florida
Gainesville, Florida

Yuying Liu
Division of Gastroenterology and Hepatology
Department of Pediatrics
University of Texas Medical School at Houston
Houston, Texas

Liya Ma
Department of Pediatrics
University of Florida
Gainesville, Florida

Cyril Mamotte
School of Biomedical Sciences, CHIRI
    Biosciences
Curtin University
Perth, Western Australia, Australia

Luise V. Marino
Department of Nutrition and Dietetics
University Hospital Southampton NHS
    Foundation Trust
Southampton, United Kingdom

Madlen Matz-Soja
Institut für Biochemie, Lehrstuhl Allgemeine
    Biochemie
der Medizinischen Fakultät der Universität
    Leipzig
Leipzig, Germany

Addison K. May
Division of Trauma and Surgical Critical Care
Vanderbilt University Medical Center
Nashville, Tennessee

Dominique Meynial-Denis
Human Nutrition Unit
INRA, CRNH Auvergne
Clermont-Ferrand, France

Chunlong Mu
Laboratory of Gastrointestinal Microbiology
Nanjing Agricultural University
Nanjing, China

Kaushik Mukherjee
Division of Trauma and Surgical Critical Care
Vanderbilt University Medical Center
Nashville, Tennessee

Josef Neu
Department of Pediatrics
University of Florida
Gainesville, Florida

Philip Newsholme
School of Biomedical Sciences, CHIRI
    Biosciences
Curtin University
Perth, Western Australia, Australia

Natalie Redgrave
Green Templeton College
University of Oxford
Oxford, United Kingdom

Jean-Pierre Renou
Mission Imagerie INRA Clermont-FD/Theix
St. Genes-Champanelle
Champanelle, France

J. Marc Rhoads
Division of Gastroenterology and Hepatology
Department of Pediatrics
University of Texas Medical School at Houston
Houston, Texas

Marcelo Macedo Rogero
Department of Nutrition, School of Public
    Health
University of Sao Paulo
Sao Paulo, Brazil

Jan M. Ruijter
Tytgat Institute for Liver and Intestinal Research
Academic Medical Center
University of Amsterdam Meibergdreef
Amsterdam, The Netherlands

Marie Smedberg
Department of Aneastesiology and Intensive
    Care Medicine
Karolinska University Hospital Huddinge and
    CLINTEC Karolinska Institutet
Stockholm, Sweden

Monika Szeliga
Department of Neurotoxicology
Mossakowski Medical Research Centre
Polish Academy of Sciences
Warsaw, Poland

Daniel Tomé
INRA/AgroParisTech
Nutrition Physiology and Ingestive Behavior
Paris, France

Irene van Herk
Tytgat Institute for Liver and Intestinal Research
Academic Medical Center
University of Amsterdam Meibergdreef
Amsterdam, The Netherlands

Jacqueline L.M. Vermeulen
Tytgat Institute for Liver and Intestinal Research
Academic Medical Center
University of Amsterdam Meibergdreef
Amsterdam, The Netherlands

Daniela Verzola
Nephrology, Dialysis and Transplant Division
Department of Internal Medicine
University of Genova and IRCCS AOU San
    Martino-IST
Genova, Italy

Jan Wernerman
Department of Aneastesiology and Intensive
    Care Medicine
Karolinska University Hospital Huddinge and
    CLINTEC Karolinska Institutet
Stockholm, Sweden

Paul Wischmeyer
Department of Anesthesiology
University of Colorado Denver
Aurora, Colorado

Guoyao Wu
Department of Animal Science
Texas A&M University
College Station, Texas

Hongyu Xue
Department of Anesthesiology
University of Colorado Denver
Aurora, Colorado

Yuxiang Yang
Laboratory of Gastrointestinal
    Microbiology
Nanjing Agricultural University
Nanjing, China

Yulong Yin
Institute of Subtropical Agriculture, Chinese
    Academy of Sciences
Changsha, China

Wei-Yun Zhu
Laboratory of Gastrointestinal Microbiology
Nanjing Agricultural University
Nanjing, China

Magdalena Zielińska
Department of Neurotoxicology
Mossakowski Medical Research Centre
Polish Academy of Sciences
Warsaw, Poland

Introduction: The Magic of a Marvelous Amino Acid—Glutamine

Morey W. Haymond

This book is a truly unique contribution to the science of amino acid metabolism and particularly the role of glutamine in a wide variety of processes within the human body. Dominique Meynial-Denis is to be congratulated for her identifying this as an important need in the scientific literature at this time. She has gathered the collective experience and wisdom of some of the most prominent investigators from all over the broad scientific world today. Each of these individuals has made unique and important contributions to our understanding of the role of glutamine in human and animal physiology. These authors collectively provide the reader with the current state of knowledge of the clinical science and medicine today. This is both a superb and timely compendium of glutamine's role and effects as well as identifying future avenues for exploration.

Glutamine holds a distinct position in our understanding of physiologic and pathophysiological processes. As a 4 carbon molecule containing both an amino and an amide nitrogen, glutamine is a very unique nonessential amino acid. It serves in much the same way as other nonessential amino acids in providing substrate for protein synthesis. However, in contrast to most other amino acids, glutamine is pivotally involved in a variety of biological systems and is central to a number of specific regulatory homeostatic mechanisms in mammals and most likely other life forms. In this introduction, I have attempted to highlight a number of these effects. None are treated with the depth that each of the contributing authors have in their chapters. By reviewing a little of the history and the variety of research surrounding the role of glutamine in mammalian metabolism, you will be equally intrigued as to the importance and uniqueness of this single structure.

Glutamine is the most abundant free amino acid circulating in the human body. Its plasma concentrations are 3–200 times those of any other amino acid (Stein et al. 1954). As you will read, this amino acid serves as an important intermediary in a large number of vital functions in the human body. The history of glutamine and the discovery of its multiple roles in mammals traverse over 130 years of scientific investigation. Schulze and Boshard first identified glutamine in 1883 when they isolated it from beet juice (Meister 1956). This was a unique observation and discovery considering the analytical techniques available to scientists of that time. As glutamine spontaneously deaminates to glutamate *in vitro*, it has been one of the most difficult amino acids to quantitate accurately. It was not until 1935 that Krebs (Krebs 1935) reported the enzymatic synthesis of glutamine from glutamate and ammonia using guinea pig and the rat kidney, thus establishing that glutamine was most likely ubiquitously present in mammalian tissues. As you will read, there is ongoing and tremendous interest in glutamine and its potential therapeutic utility to this day.

ROLE OF GLUTAMINE IN MUSCLE

Since the early studies of Cahill, G.F., Jr. and coworkers, it is recognized that muscle releases alanine and glutamine in excess to their content in the muscle itself (Pozefsky et al. 1969; Marliss et al. 1971). It continues to be thought that these amino acids provide a nontoxic form to transport ammonia from one tissue to another for subsequent reuse or disposal. Although no absolutes can be stated, it has been stated that alanine is transported for the disposal of the nitrogen as urea in the liver and glutamine to the kidney where the nitrogen is disposed of as ammonium. However, it is clear that both substrates are catabolized in both liver and kidney. In both organs, the carbon skeletons of alanine and glutamine serve as potential gluconeogenic substrates with one entering as pyruvate and the other as α-ketoglutarate. Although it has been speculated that glutamine may provide some direct or indirect stimulation of muscle protein synthesis, this may not be the case (Wilkinson et al. 2006). Although there is evidence that glutamine may affect mTOR and protein synthesis in tumor cells (see below), there is no evidence of this in muscle. Thus, glutamine's primary role is muscle is as an amino acid for protein synthesis and as a vehicle to transport carbon and nitrogen for other organ functions.

GUT METABOLISM

Glutamine has been investigated extensively as a potential nutrient source and/or growth factor for the human gut. The classic papers of Windmueller and Spaeth provide the first description of the uptake of glutamine by the gut with the release of a number of urea-cycle intermediates (Windmueller and Spaeth 1974; Windmueller and Spaeth 1975). This led to speculation about the role of this amino acid in gut nutrition and nitrogen flux, at least in the rat gut. Glutamine has been subsequently tested in a number of well-designed clinical trials as an agent that might stimulate gut growth. In subjects with short-gut syndrome, glutamine enteral treatment (with or without growth hormone) demonstrated no clear beneficial effect. Additional studies continue to explore the utility of glutamine supplementation in situations of gut injury such as radiation-induced intestinal damage. In this condition, it has been demonstrated to decrease gut permeability and inflammation but was not superior to standard nutrition in maintaining weight (Yao et al. 2015). Finally it appears that glutamine supplementation reverses the effect of aging on the gut mucosa in a rodent model (Beaufrère et al. 2014).

CANCER AND GLUTAMINE

In certain neoplasms, glutamine appears to affect the proliferation of these tumors (Chen and Cui 2015). A potential mechanism for this appears to be through mTOR. As tumor growth involves protein anabolism, it is not clear why this effect appears to be restricted to these specific neoplastic tissues as there is no clear evidence of a protein anabolic effect of glutamine in other tissues (Marwood and Bowtell 2008). This does not mean that glutamine may not be having an effect(s) but that other mechanisms may be offsetting any anabolic effect on mTOR (Yuan et al. 2015). This is clearly an area in need of and receiving new investigative scrutiny in both normal and neoplastic tissues as you will find in the chapters by Dr. Bode and Dr. Meynial-Denis in this monograph.

RENAL ACID–BASE METABOLISM AND GLUCONEOGENESIS

One of the well-established roles of glutamine in daily physiology is its central role in the maintenance of pH homeostasis via its metabolism in the kidney. Under conditions of acidosis (whether metabolic or respiratory), the kidney plays a primary counter-regulatory role, which has been referred to as the acid or pH switch (Goodman et al. 1966). Glutamine is taken up by the kidney and ammonia released from both the amide and amino nitrogens. This ammonia is secreted into the lumen of the renal tubule and combines with filtered H^+ ions forming ammonium, which is excreted in the urine, and thus removing a mole for mole of H^+ with each mole of ammonia secreted. Several of the more common physiologic causes of mild and severe metabolic acidosis are fasting ketosis and diabetic ketoacidosis, respectively. The kidney is one of three tissues that contain all of the enzymatic capability to produce glucose via gluconeogenesis, the others being the gastrointestinal tract and the liver. The role of this enzyme in the gut is unclear in humans and in other animal models (Newsholme and Carrié 1994; Kim et al. 2015). As the nitrogen groups in glutamine are utilized for hydrogen excretion, the carbon from the glutamine is directed to renal gluconeogenesis.

Under more prolonged fasting or diabetic ketoacidosis, ketone bodies are produced from the partial oxidation of fatty acids in the liver. Both β-hydroxybutyrate and acetoacetate are produced as free acids. The ketone bodies, but not fatty acids, can cross the blood–brain barrier and be oxidized, thus displacing to a considerable proportion the dependence of the CNS on glucose per se. With progressive fasting, hepatic glycogen stores are depleted and glucose production decreases, as does the plasma glucose resulting in a decrease in insulin secretion in normal health, or in the absence of an effective plasma insulin concentration in diabetes, fasting promotes fatty acid mobilization and ketogenesis. In addition to decreasing brain glucose utilization, the acidosis induced by ketosis results in an increase in the net production of glucose from the kidney via gluconeogenesis. During prolonged fasting it has been estimated that as much as 40% of glucose production is derived via renal gluconeogenesis but other substrates such as lactate, alanine, pyruvate, and α-ketoglutarate also contribute (Owen et al. 1969). Thus, one can appreciate the interrelationships among brain glucose utilization, hepatic and renal gluconeogenesis, and maintenance of acid–base balance—all of which relate back to an important role of glutamine in this latter process. It is of interest that despite the central role of the kidney in glutamine catabolism the plasma glutamine concentrations are not recognized to be elevated in renal failure.

ANTIOXIDANT AND GLUTAMINE METABOLISM

Chapters by Drs. Jahoor, Abumrad, Smedberg, and Coeffier provide current and erudite discussion of the roles amino acid supplementation and glutamine may play in stress with aging, critical illness, obesity, and disease. A number of studies have reported lower glutamine concentrations in critically ill children, which is associated with a greater degree of organ failure (Elmark et al. 2015). Whether this is a cause and effect or an association is not clear, but studies are underway to determine whether glutamine supplementation will impact biomarkers or true outcomes (Wernerman 2014). As more evidence is accumulated in the pathophysiology of the metabolic syndrome, it is increasingly clear that the generation of intracellular free radical may play a significant part in the complications recognized with this disorder(s) (Elmark et al. 2015). In humans, the plasma and red blood cell glutathione are used as surrogate makers for abnormalities in the intracellular oxidative stress (Wernerman 2014). The potential of utilizing specific oral amino acids, one of which is glutamine, to alter this oxidative stress has been demonstrated in short-term studies that provide the impetuous for longer-term interventional trials to determine whether these have a therapeutic effect. This will be an important area to follow, and understanding the role that amino acid supplementation may have on oxidative stress may lead to new avenues of research and potentially simple therapeutic interventions in humans.

CENTRAL NERVOUS SYSTEM AND GLUTAMINE METABOLISM

Plasma glutamine concentrations are quite stable under both feeding and fasting conditions. Even under more prolonged fasting conditions, plasma glutamine concentrations may decrease by only 20%–30%. In contrast, in conditions such as urea cycle inborn errors of metabolism or in hepatic failure, the plasma concentrations of glutamine can be exceedingly elevated. These conditions are frequently associated with hyperammonemic encephalopathy. Under these conditions, one might speculate that the glutamine pool extensively expanded because of the increased availability of ammonia. The observation that glutamine supplementation in a subject with a previously unknown partial defect in the urea cycle led to transient encephalopathy is concerning but demonstrates the close relationship among glutamine, ammonia, the urea cycle, and brain function (Ramadan et al. 2013; Zielinska et al. 2014). The precise role of glutamine in brain metabolism remains to be clarified, but as glutamine is deamidated by glutaminase to glutamate and that glutamate is a potent neurotransmitter, it would not be surprising to find a clear link.

MICROBIOME

The role of the microbiome in human health and disease is currently under intense study in broad areas of medicine and health. Our symbiotic relationship with our individually larger biomass of bacteria is an interesting and potentially powerful new tool to be used in human disease identification, understanding a pathophysiology role, if any, and in disease prevention. It has been demonstrated that the administration of glutamine can alter the human microbiome (Van Zwol et al. 2010; de Souza et al. 2015). It remains to be determined whether changes in the human microbiome are a cause or an effect and will only be determined by research currently underway that may lead to new hypotheses to be tested. At this point in time it is unclear what beneficial role, if any, that glutamine may have in this exciting new area of clinical research.

SUMMARY

The above offering is only intended to entice the readers to delve deeply into this literature by promoting not only a deeper understanding of glutamine metabolism and its complexity and interactions with other systems and pathways but also to stimulate new thoughts and ideas about the importance and role of glutamine in human physiology.

REFERENCES

Beaufrère AM, Neveux N, Patureau M et al. Long-term intermittent glutamine supplementation repairs intestinal damage (structure and functional mass) with advanced age: Assessment with plasma citrulline in a rodent model. *J Nutr Health Aging*. 2014 Nov;18(9):814–9.

Chen L, Cui H. Targeting glutamine induces apoptosis: A cancer therapy approach. *Int J Mol Sci*. 2015 Sep 22;16(9):22830–55.

de Souza AZ, Zambom AZ, Abboud KY et al. Oral supplementation with L-glutamine alters gut microbiota of obese and overweight adults: A pilot study. *Nutrition*. 2015 Jun;31(6):884–9.

Ekmark L, Rooyackers O, Wernerman J et al. Plasma glutamine deficiency is associated with multiple organ failure in critically ill children. *Amino Acids*. 2015 Mar;47(3):535–42. PMID: 25500971.

Goodman AD, Fuisz RE, Cahill GF Jr. Renal gluconeogenesis in acidosis, alkalosis, and potassium deficiency: Its possible role in regulation of renal ammonia production. *J Clin Invest*. 1966 Apr;45(4):612–9.

Kim M, Son YG, Kang YN et al. Changes in glucose transporters, gluconeogenesis, and circadian clock after duodenal-jejunal bypass surgery. *Obes Surg*. 2015 Apr;25(4):635–41.

Krebs HA. Metabolism of amino-acids: The synthesis of glutamine from glutamic acid and ammonia, and the enzymic hydrolysis of glutamine in animal tissues. *Biochem J*. 1935 Aug;29(8):1951–69.

Marliss EB, Aoki TT, Pozefsky T et al. Muscle and splanchnic glutamine and glutamate metabolism in postabsorptinve and starved man. *J Clin Invest*. 1971 Apr;50(4):814–7.

Marwood S, Bowtell J. No effect of glutamine supplementation and hyperoxia on oxidative metabolism and performance during high-intensity exercise. *J Sports Sci*. 2008 Aug;26(10):1081–90.

Meister A. Metabolism of glutamine. *Physiol Rev*. 1956 Jan;36:103–127. PMID: 13297549.

Newsholme EA1, Carrié AL. Quantitative aspects of glucose and glutamine metabolism by intestinal cells. *Gut*. 1994 Jan;35(1 Suppl):S13–7.

Owen OE, Felig P, Morgan AP et al. Liver and kidney metabolism during prolonged starvation. *J Clin Invest*. 1969 Mar;48(3):574–83.

Pozefsky T, Felig P, Tobin JD et al. Amino acid balance across tissues of the forearm in postabsorptive man. Effects of insulin at two dose levels. *J Clin Invest*. 1969 Dec;48(12):2273–82.

Ramadan S, Lin A, Stanwell P. Glutamate and glutamine: A review of *in vivo* MRS in the human brain. *NMR Biomed*. 2013 Dec;26(12):1630–46.

Stein WH, Bearn AG, Moore S. The amino acid content of the blood and urine in Wilson's disease. *J Clin Invest*. 1954 Mar;33(3):410–9.

Van Zwol A, Van Den Berg A, Knol J et al. Intestinal microbiota in allergic and nonallergic 1-year-old very low birth weight infants after neonatal glutamine supplementation. *Acta Paediatr*. 2010 Dec;99(12):1868–74.

Wernerman J. Glutamine supplementation to critically ill patients? *Crit Care*. 2014 Mar 18;18(2):214.

Wilkinson SB1, Kim PL, Armstrong D et al. Addition of glutamine to essential amino acids and carbohydrate does not enhance anabolism in young human males following exercise. *Appl Physiol Nutr Metab.* 2006 Oct;31(5):518–29.

Windmueller HG, Spaeth AE. Intestinal metabolism of glutamine and glutamate from the lumen as compared from blood. *Arch Biochem Biophys.* 1975 Dec;171(2):662–72.

Windmueller HG, Spaeth AE. Uptake and metabolism of plasma glutamine by the small intestine. *J Biol Chem.* 1974 Aug 25;249(16):5070–9.

Yao D, Zheng L, Wang J et al. Perioperative alanyl-glutamine-supplemented parenteral nutrition in chronic radiation enteritis patients with surgical intestinal obstruction: A prospective, randomized, controlled study. *Nutr Clin Pract.* 2015 Jun 15. pii: 0884533615591601. [Epub ahead of print] PMID: 26078286.

Yuan L, Sheng X, Willson AK et al. Glutamine promotes ovarian cancer cell proliferation through the mTOR/S6 pathway. *Endocr Relat Cancer.* 2015 Aug;22(4):577–91.

Zielińska M, Popek M, Albrecht J. Roles of changes in active glutamine transport in brain edema development during hepatic encephalopathy: An emerging concept. *Neurochem Res.* 2014 Sep;39(3):599–604.

Section I

Basics of Glutamine Metabolism

1 An Introduction to Glutamine Metabolism

Vinicius Fernandes Cruzat and Philip Newsholme

CONTENTS

1.1 INTRODUCTION

Hlaziwetz and Habermann first described glutamine as a molecule with biologically important properties in 1873. They suggested that the presence of ammonia (as NH_4^+), detected following hydrolysis of proteins, arose by degradation linked to amide groups from glutamine and asparagine (Mora 2012). About 10 years later, Schulze and Bosshard isolated glutamine from a natural source (beet juice), and Damodaran and his collaborators contributed to the first description of glutamine metabolism. However, the number of studies investigating glutamine metabolism and links to intermediary metabolism increased following the early work of Sir Hans Adolf Krebs (1900–1981), who was responsible for some of the most important discoveries in metabolic biochemistry and physiology in the twentieth century (Nobel Prize in Physiology or Medicine in 1953).

Sir Hans Krebs published the first significant paper on glutamine metabolism in the *Biochemical Journal* in 1935. He determined that glutamine synthesis is an energy-requiring process and also described two different isoforms of glutaminase (GLS, EC 3.5.1.2), an enzyme responsible for glutamine hydrolysis to glutamate and NH_4^+ (Krebs 1935). The description of glutamine synthesis utilizing NH_4^+ and glutamate through an endergonic process was confirmed by the discovery of glutamine synthetase (GS, EC 6.3.1.2), which utilizes ATP to drive the reaction (Brosnan 2001). The degradation of glutamine by glutaminase remains one of the most important effect in the intermediary metabolism of amino acids, occurring in multiple organs, tissues, and cells.

After World War II, studies showed that glutamine was essential for cell function and growth (Curi et al. 2005a; Eagle et al. 1956). In culture, cells utilize glutamine in a greater amount than any other amino acid (Curi et al. 2005a; Eagle et al. 1956). Eagle and colleagues observed structural degeneration followed by cell death in isolated mouse fibroblasts cultivated in the absence of glutamine (Eagle 1959). Throughout the 1960s, 1970s, and 1980s, the University of Oxford was the location for several of the key researchers who have shaped our current understanding of the regulation of energy and amino acid metabolism in healthy states and in diseases (e.g., diabetes, inflammatory diseases, and cancer). Hans Krebs, Philip Randle, Derek Williamson, and Eric Newsholme all worked on metabolic regulation utilizing different research models, from isolated cells *in vitro*, to human and *in vivo* experiments. Studies with various cells types, such as HeLa cells (Eagle 1959), lymphocytes (Ardawi and Newsholme 1982), macrophages (Newsholme et al. 1987), and enterocytes (Yamauchi et al. 2002) demonstrated the importance of glutamine for cell division, function, and maintenance of intermediary metabolism. Glutamine can lead to the production of

3

ATP, NADPH, CO_2, and donate nitrogen atoms for macromolecular synthesis, including purines, pyrimidines, and amino sugars (Newsholme et al. 2003b). As glutamine is the body's most abundant and versatile amino acid, it is understandable that the survival, maintenance, and proliferation of cells cannot occur without this molecule.

Since the organism can synthesize and release glutamine from tissues such as skeletal muscle, the amino acid is classified as nutritionally dispensable (nonessential). However, in some conditions, such as sepsis, recovery from burns, or surgery, glutamine availability can be compromised due to the increased requirements triggered by catabolic processes and/or elevated inflammatory and oxidative stress profiles in both human (Rodas et al. 2012) and animal models (Cruzat et al. 2010). Hence, in various conditions, glutamine can become a conditionally essential amino acid (Newsholme et al. 2011b). To improve L-glutamine availability during physiological stress, many research scientists and clinical investigators have attempted exogenous replacement therapy and determined outcomes in healthy individuals and patients recovering from disease. This chapter highlights key aspects of glutamine biochemistry and metabolism, its importance for the whole-body health, as well as the increased interest in nutritional supplementation.

1.2 GLUTAMINE BIOCHEMISTRY AND METABOLISM

L-glutamine ($C_5H_{10}N_2O_3$) deserves special attention compared to other amino acids. Biochemically, glutamine is an L-α-amino acid with a molecular weight of 146.15 kDa and is synthesized by several tissues in the body, of which the most important is the skeletal muscle. Its chemical composition is as follows: carbon (41.09%), oxygen (32.84%), nitrogen (19.17%), and hydrogen (6.90%). At physiological pH, the carboxyl group of glutamine carries a negative charge, whereas the amino group is protonated, resulting in a molecule carrying with a net charge of 0, thus placing it in the classification "neutral amino acids." The side-chain amide group is easily removed by various enzymatic reactions and even by spontaneous hydrolysis at room temperature. These particular biochemical characteristics confer to L-glutamine the ability to be hydrophilic and a preferred substrate for cells requiring a source of L-glutamate and/or NH_3 for physiological purposes (Young and Ajami 2001).

Healthy humans, weighing approximately 70 kg, are associated with 70–80 g of glutamine distributed in a number of body tissues, since the endogenous production of glutamine as estimated by isotopic techniques is 40–80 g/24 h (Wernerman 2008). A similar result was obtained when using pharmacokinetic techniques (Berg et al. 2007). Both techniques may underestimate the actual *de novo* synthesis of glutamine because the distribution volume of glutamine is large and, therefore, the equilibration time is also long (Wernerman 2008). In blood, the normal glutamine concentration is between 500 and 700 μmol/L (D'Souza and Powell-Tuck 2004) (Newsholme et al. 2011b). This may fall to critically low levels of below 400 μmol/L during periods of inflammation and recovery from major surgery or burns (Newsholme 2001). Glutamine synthesis appears to be essential for the functioning of some critical organs such as the brain. Regarding hydrolysis, NH_3 liberation-form glutamine plays a key role in acid–base balance (Newsholme et al. 2003a).

There are many enzymes involved in glutamine metabolism, starting from glutamate, and, depending on ATP availability, glutamine synthetase (GS) promotes glutamine synthesis from glutamate. Glutamate in turn is synthesized from 2-oxoglutarate and an ammonium ion (NH_4^+). Hence, the synthesis of glutamine provides an efficient mechanism for nitrogen export and transport and also NH_3 removal. Glutamine hydrolysis occurs by means of the glutaminase (GLS) enzyme, releasing NH_4^+ (Newsholme et al. 2003a) (Figure 1.1).

Glutamine and the related amino acid glutamate are 5-carbon amino acids (Figure 1.1). Glutamate is a molecule in which the amide nitrogen of glutamine is replaced by a carboxyl group, conferring to it a net negative charge. This biochemical difference partially accounts for the transport of these two amino compounds across the cell membranes through different transport systems, at very different rates, and, therefore, impacting on cell function in markedly different ways (Newsholme et al. 2003b).

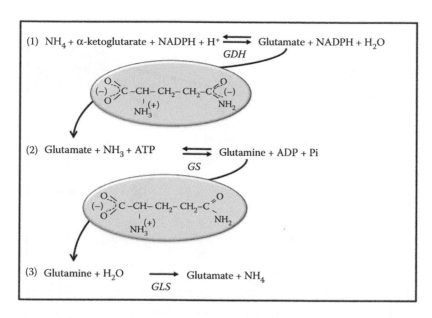

FIGURE 1.1 (1) Chemical structure of glutamate and its synthesis through glutamate dehydrogenase (GDH). (2) Chemical structure of glutamine and its synthesis through glutamine synthetase (GS). (3) Degradation of glutamine through glutaminase (GLS).

Several organs can express and operate both GLS and GS activities; however, the overall effect depends on multiple factors, including metabolic and energy status. Some cell types and tissues, such as cells of the immune system, kidney, and intestine, are considered predominantly glutamine-consuming tissues (van de Poll et al. 2004). GLS can be one of the two major isoforms termed the *liver* and the *kidney isoforms*. The kidney form appears to be the most common and is also found in brain, leucocytes, fetal rat liver, and the intestinal tract (Neu et al. 1996). Both isoforms can be found associated with the inner membrane of the mitochondrial matrix. The liver GLS exhibits a lower affinity for glutamine than does kidney-type GLS. In response to starvation or high-protein diet or even high catabolic situations/diseases, such as sepsis and uncontrolled diabetes, GLS activity increases, since under these situations there is a heightened catabolism of amino acids, whether derived from muscle stores or from dietary sources (Cruzat et al. 2014b; Labow et al. 2001).

The purposes of this upregulation of GLS expression and increased GLN catabolism are partly to support increased gluconeogenesis, which requires precursors derived from the carbon skeleton of GLN, and to deliver additional nitrogen to the urea cycle for disposal. On the other hand, skeletal muscles, lungs, liver, and brain exhibit a higher capacity for glutamine synthesis by means of GS and, therefore, may be considered predominantly glutamine-synthesizing tissues (Figure 1.2a) (Antonio and Street 1999; Frayn et al. 1991). As a whole, all tissues are important to glutamine metabolism and homeostasis; however, liver and skeletal muscle play key roles in the maintenance of glutamine availability. Glutamine concentration can be altered in catabolic situations, such as sepsis (Cruzat et al. 2014b; Newsholme 2001), infections (Rogero et al. 2008), surgery (Rodas et al. 2012), trauma (Flaring et al. 2003), and intense and prolonged physical exercise (Cruzat and Tirapegui 2009; Newsholme et al. 2011b), as shown in Figure 1.2b.

The liver is the central site for nitrogen metabolism in the body and is the tissue that exhibits the highest capacity for glutamine synthesis. Liver glutamine is an important vehicle for the nontoxic transport of NH_3 from the intermediary metabolism of amino acids between tissues (Curi et al. 2007; Newsholme et al. 2003b). Glutamine-associated nitrogen is transported to the central organs in addition to that transported as alanine. Of these two amino acids, which are released by skeletal muscle and account for up to 60% of the overall amino acid load in the blood (Cunningham et al.

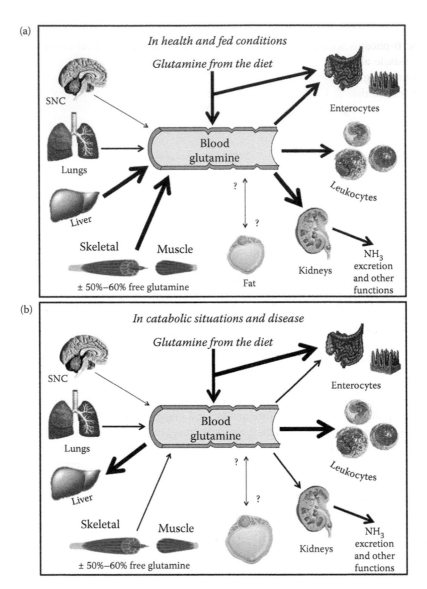

FIGURE 1.2 Predominance (thick arrows) in the synthesis and degradation of glutamine by various tissues and organs in health or fed state (a) and catabolic situations or disease (b). Abbreviations: central nervous system (CNS), ammonia (NH_3), glutamine (GLN). (Modified from Rowbottom DG, Keast D and Morton AR. 1996. *Sports Med* 21, 80–97.)

2005; Newsholme et al. 2011a), glutamine is considered the most versatile and available amino acid (Neu et al. 1996).

In the hepatocyte, after the action of GLS, glutamate is formed from glutamine and, subsequently, may promote carbamoyl-phosphate synthesis by mitochondrial carbamoyl-phosphate synthetase I (CPS I) or CPS II in the cytosol. The enzyme is allosterically activated by N-acetylglutamate and may thus be indirectly regulated by glutamate concentration. Carbamoyl phosphate may combine with ornithine in the urea cycle to produce citrulline, which is subsequently converted to arginosuccinate and then arginine. Arginine is subsequently cleaved by arginase to produce urea and ornithine (Newsholme et al. 2003b; Oliveira-Yamashita et al. 2009). The utilization of the amide nitrogen atom of glutamine, catalyzed by the glutamine amidotransferases, leads to the synthesis of such important biological compounds as the pyridine nucleotide coenzymes, purines, pyrimidines, glucosamine-6-phosphate, and asparagine (Figure 1.3).

Skeletal muscle also plays an important role in glutamine metabolism, since quantitatively it is the main tissue for glutamine *de novo* synthesis, storage, and release. This is not due to a high GS activity per se, but due to the increased availability of the branched-chain amino acids (BCAA), which contribute to glutamine synthesis (Shimomura et al. 2004). Skeletal muscle tissue represents up to 40% of the total body mass (Neu et al. 1996). The BCAA (L-valine, L-leucine, and L-isoleucine) are predominantly metabolized in skeletal muscle tissue, following protein ingestion through the diet (Shimomura et al. 2006). Glutamine synthesis is ultimately dependent on BCAA metabolism via BCAA aminotransferase (Hiscock and Pedersen 2002). Studies demonstrate that BCAA can be transaminated, releasing α-ketoglutarate and glutamate, which can donate its amino group to pyruvate, generating alanine or incorporate free NH_3, for *de novo* synthesis of glutamine (Nicastro et al. 2012; Rutten et al. 2005).

The glutamine synthesis over degradation ratio in the skeletal muscle is approximately 50 mmol/h, higher than any other amino acid (Newsholme et al. 2003b). In catabolic situations (Flaring et al.

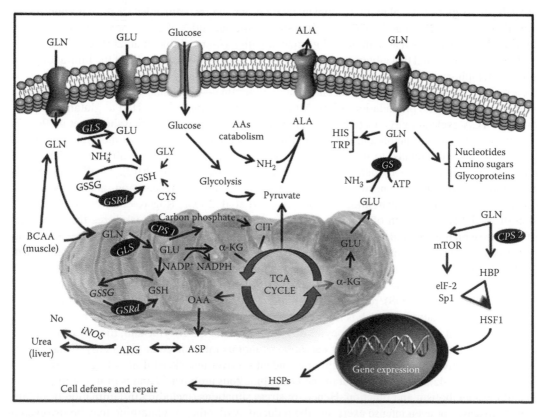

FIGURE 1.3 General overview of glutamine metabolism. From glutamine, glutamate is produced through glutaminase activity (GLS), releasing ammonium ion (NH_4^+). Inside the mitochondria or in the cytosol, glutamine, and glutamate are important precursors for the synthesis of the intermediate metabolism of amino acids, such as alanine (ALA); antioxidant defenses, such as glutathione (GSH); and cell homeostasis, such as heat-shock proteins (HSP) via mammalian target of rapamicin (mTOR) and hexosamine biosynthetic pathway (HBP). Cells, especially muscle cells, can synthesize glutamine through glutamine synthetase (GS), using glutamate, ATP, and ammonia (NH_3). Other abbreviations: alpha ketoglutarate, α-KG; arginine, ARG; asparagine, ASP; carbamoyl phosphate synthetase I and II, CPS 1 and 2, respectively; citrulline, CIT; cysteine, CYS; eukaryotic initiation factor 2, eIF-2; glycine, GLY; heat-shock factor 1, HSF1; histidine, HIS; inducible nitric oxide synthase, iNOS; oxaloacetate, OAA; oxidized GSH, GSSG; tryptophan, TRP.

2003), intense muscle proteolysis is observed, and a number of tissues begin to depend on the ability of the skeletal muscle to supply glutamine (Neu et al. 1996; Petry et al. 2014). This effect can contribute to the disequilibrium of the intermediary metabolism, with the loss of homeostasis in the kidneys, intestine, and lymphoid organs as glutamine synthesis and degradation capacity become dysregulated (Newsholme et al. 2003a).

Whereas in plasma the glutamine concentration is about 20% of the total free amino acids concentration, in skeletal muscle this is about 40%–60%. Depending on the muscle under study, when the *de novo* synthesis of glutamine is inhibited experimentally, the intramuscular storages can be depleted in about 7 h. Glutamate is responsible for 40% of glutamine synthesis, and, compared to other amino acids, is the most abundant intracellular amino acid (reported concentrations vary between 2 and 20 mM), and glutamine is the most abundant extracellular amino acid *in vivo* (0.7 mM compared to an approximate L-glutamate concentration of 20 μM) (Manso Filho et al. 2009; Newsholme et al. 2003a). L-glutamate cannot readily cross the plasma membrane of skeletal muscles because it has an overall charge of −1 at pH 7.4, and the amino acid transporter transporting glutamate into the cell does so at relatively low rates due to a low density of the transporter in the plasma membrane (Newsholme et al. 2003a). Hence, to increase glutamine concentration in skeletal muscles and the availability of glutamate, glutamine supplementation may be recommended. It is also important to note that in the skeletal muscle of mammalian species the quantities of amino acids other than glutamine and glutamate, such as alanine and glycine, are high (Manso Filho et al. 2009).

It is widely accepted that glutamine is utilized at high rates by isolated cells of the immune system such as lymphocytes, macrophages, and neutrophils (Newsholme 2001). Although the activity of the first enzyme responsible for the metabolism of glutamine—phosphate-dependent GLS—is high in these cells, the rate of oxidation is low. Much of the glutamine is converted to glutamate, aspartate (via TCA cycle activity), lactate, and under conditions at rest, CO_2 (Newsholme et al. 2003b). The process of inflammation and infection stimulates immune cells to consume high amounts of glutamine, which is related to the demand for immune cell survival and proliferation, leading to an imbalance of whole-body defenses (Newsholme 2001; Rodas et al. 2012). T-cell proliferation, B-lymphocyte differentiation, macrophage phagocytosis, antigen presentation, and cytokine production are dependent on glutamine availability (Curi et al. 2005b; Rogero et al. 2010). The provision of NADPH, via action of $NADP^+$-dependent malic enzyme, which catalyzes the conversion of malate (which is derived from glutamate via formation of 2-oxoglutarate, succinate, and fumarate) to pyruvate is an example of glutamine participation in intracellular intermediary metabolism. NADPH is required for biosynthetic reactions such as fatty acid synthesis or for production of free radicals such as superoxide anion (O_2^-) or nitric oxide (NO) by the NADPH oxidase and inducible nitric oxide synthase (iNOS), respectively (Figure 1.3). Moreover, NADPH is also required for glutathione reductase activity, which is important for antioxidant systems (Newsholme et al. 2003a).

It is important to convey that leukocytes do not possess the GS enzyme and, therefore, are unable to synthesize glutamine. Hence, under catabolic situations immune cells, especially T and B lymphocytes (adaptive immunity), are highly dependent on liver and skeletal muscle glutamine stores (Cruzat et al. 2014a). As a whole, glutamine is an ubiquitous amino acid and is of major importance in cellular metabolism and function. Hence, in stress situations (including inflammation or inflammatory diseases or even intense exercise), the reduced availability of glutamine may be involved in the acceleration of adverse metabolic outcomes.

1.3 EMERGING ROLE OF GLUTAMINE FOR CELL DEFENSE

In the past 20–30 years, many studies have reported the critical importance of glutamine to the body's defenses, especially to cells of both the innate and adaptive immune system. However, based on results from both *in vitro* and *in vivo* studies no clear-cut trends were found with respect to cytokine secretory profiles, levels of activation, and physiological outcomes. For example, when incubated *in vitro* in the presence of lower levels of glutamine, identical to the lowest plasma glutamine concentration measured after some heavy sessions of exercise training (300–400 μM), lymphocytes will function normally (Newsholme 2001) as compared to lymphocytes incubated at the accepted physiological concentration (600 μM) (Hiscock and Pedersen 2002). Hence, glutamine-dependent deficiencies occur only in situations characterized by severely depressed glutamine availability, such as observed in a high-intensity sport environment (Hiscock and Pedersen 2002) or severe catabolic illnesses (Wernerman 2008).

In response to several forms of stress, cells rapidly increase glucose uptake and utilization, which may be related to the capacity to defend and respond appropriately (Moley and Mueckler 2000). Experimental evidence suggests that inhibition of both glycolysis and the hexosamine biosynthetic pathway (HBP) results in decreased cell survival (Zachara et al. 2004). HBP are vital components for maintaining integrity and function of mucosal surfaces, and under stress situations they appear to be part of an early cellular protective response. It appears that depletion of ATP is an important stimulus and signal to initiate a response to stress (Newsholme et al. 2014). However, low intracellular ATP levels do not necessarily explain dysregulation of cell function, as ATP turnover may increase in such situations, satisfying cellular demands. The source of fuel required to maintain elevated ATP turnover can be modulated to elevate glucose, amino acid, and fatty acid input, as required.

Glutamine and its metabolites are important for the production and optimal activity of HBP. Furthermore, glutamine stimulates the expression of argininosuccinate synthetase (ASS) gene via O-glycosylation of Sp1 (Hamiel et al. 2009; Zachara and Hart 2006), a key transcription factor required for the most basic mechanisms of cellular protection, namely, heat-shock proteins (HSP) response (Heck et al. 2011). Glutamine availability was also identified as a limiting step for the activation of the mammalian target of rapamycin (mTOR) (Nicklin et al. 2009). Many initiation factor complexes (e.g., eIF2, eIF4F) that are assembled from multiple subunits are sensitive to activation by the mTOR cascade (Sartorelli and Fulco 2004), which results in coordinated protein synthesis and degradation (Newsholme et al. 2014).

It is not only the key intracellular proteins and transcription factors, which are HBP O-glycosylated following stress or injury, such as Sp1 (Hamiel et al. 2009; Zachara and Hart 2006) but the phosphorylation of the eIF2 (Dokladny et al. 2013b) also promotes the activation of the main thermal shock eukaryotic factor (Heat Shock Factor [HSF-1]), leading to the expression of HSPs (Xue et al. 2012) (Figure 1.3). HSPs are a family of polypeptides clustered according to molecular weight, which are increased in amount in response to an increase in intracellular denatured proteins. Some examples of HSP include HSP110, HSP100, HSP90, HSP70, and HSP27. The HSP response can be triggered by variations in body temperature, inflammation, and oxidative stress. Early studies documented novel protein responses in the salivary gland cells of *Drosophila buskii* after heat shock by Ritossa in 1962 (Heck et al. 2011). At lower temperatures, less heat-shock protein expression occurs. Thus, these proteins were described as temperature sensitive; in other words, thermal or heat-shock proteins (Heck et al. 2011).

HSP can be considered as stress-sensitive proteins, as further studies by Ritossa demonstrated that a number of agents or metabolic stressors could stimulate HSP levels. Various events such as exposition to heavy metals, UV radiation, amino acid analogs, bacterial or viral infections, inflammation, cyclooxygenase inhibitors (including acetylsalicylic acid), oxidative stress, cytostatic drugs (anticancer), growth factors, and cell development and differentiation can induce the expression of HSP (Heck et al. 2011; Wischmeyer 2002). All these factors strongly activate HSF-1, leading to the expression of HSP (Xue et al. 2012).

Although the connection between glutamine availability and the HSP response is not clear and may need further investigation, the reduction of body's glutamine concentration may contribute to cell death (Cruzat et al. 2014a; Lightfoot et al. 2009). Recent studies have demonstrated that glutamine-induced HSP70 response may modulate autophagy by regulating the mTOR/Akt pathway (Dokladny et al. 2013a) and block signaling pathways associated with protein degradation (Singleton and Wischmeyer 2007). However, it is unlikely that glutamine supplementation can be used as an enhancer of muscle performance or muscle mass gain and strength under normal situations (Candow et al. 2001; Gleeson 2008). Glutamine supplements may be useful in replenishing previously depleted body glutamine stores (e.g., by high-throughput exercise and inflammatory diseases).

The role of amino acids, especially glutamine, has been recognized in cell defense mechanisms, through impact on antioxidant properties. Made up of three amino acid residues—cysteine, glutamate, and glycine—glutathione (γ-L-glutamyl-L-cysteinylglycine, GSH) is found in high concentrations in cells and can directly react with ROS in non-enzymatic reactions as well as acting as an electron donor in peroxide reduction, catalyzed by glutathione peroxidase enzyme (GPx) (Cruzat and Tirapegui 2009; Newsholme et al. 2011b). During the 1960s and 1970s, Sir Hans Krebs, Hems, and Vina in the Metabolic Research Laboratory, University of Oxford, made key findings in relation to GSH, especially in mammalian cells (Valencia et al. 2001). In 1978 they described the regulation of hepatic GSH and its maintenance in isolated hepatocytes (Vina et al. 1978). Subsequently, different groups around the world have demonstrated through studies that GSH levels are reduced in stress in animals and humans (Cruzat and Tirapegui 2009; Meister 1983; Newsholme et al. 2011b; Rodas et al. 2012). GSH is the most important and more concentrated non-enzymatic antioxidant in cells (Cruzat and Tirapegui 2009; Flaring et al. 2003). Decreased glutamine concentrations, especially in liver and skeletal muscles, may compromise *de novo* synthesis of GSH, since glutamine is the immediate precursor of glutamate, even if cysteine and glycine were maintained at relatively constant levels (Rutten et al. 2005).

During catabolic states, elevated oxidative stress can be observed associated with an increase in the intracellular redox state, as indicated by the ratio between the intracellular concentration of glutathione disulfide (GSSG) and GSH, that is, [GSSG]/[GSH], resulting in a reduction of GSH and an increase in the amounts of GSSG (Galley 2011). The redox state of cells is consequently related to GSH concentration, which is influenced by the availability of amino acids. A higher glutamine/glutamate ratio reinforces substrate availability for GSH (Cruzat et al. 2014a).

Quantitatively, the liver is the main organ for *de novo* synthesis of GSH, being responsible for nearly 90% of the circulating GSH in physiological conditions. The elevated concentration of hepatic GSH is mainly due to the high activity of glutathione reductase in this tissue. Methods to directly increase the GSH concentration through supplementation, or even addition of glutamate, are not effective and can be toxic, sometimes accelerating the cell senescence process (Finkel and Holbrook 2000). A number of studies demonstrate that glutamine supplementation can be an effective option to increase the availability of GSH in the organism if required (Cruzat et al. 2007; Cruzat and Tirapegui 2009). Furthermore, it is important to note that gradual stimuli, such as physical activity, stimulates per se the *hormesis* and adaptation of the organism, stimulating antioxidant mechanisms (Finkel and Holbrook 2000; Lamb and Westerblad 2011).

1.4 CONSIDERATIONS ABOUT THE EXOGENOUS REPLACEMENT OF GLUTAMINE

In vitro studies with various cell types, such as muscle cells, intestinal mucosa, cells of the immune system, specific neurons of the central nervous system, hepatocytes, pancreatic β-cells, and others, have demonstrated that L-glutamine is required in the incubation medium for growth and normal function (Curi et al. 2007; Newsholme et al. 1999, 2003b; Rogero et al. 2009). Glutamine can supply carbon and nitrogen to essential biosynthetic pathways and as such can be considered a key macronutrient (Figure 1.3).

It is known that the skeletal muscle concentration of glutamine in athletes can reach 20 mM (60% of the intramuscular pool) (Newsholme et al. 2011b). However, exhaustive exercise (i.e., high-intensity and long-term strenuous exercises) leads to a catabolic situation that promotes a decrease in the whole-body L-glutamine pool with a concomitantly transient immune depression and may contribute to overtraining syndrome (Cruzat et al. 2010; Rowbottom et al. 1996; Santos et al. 2007).

TABLE 1.1

Glutamine Balance in Postoperative Trauma Based on the Calculations for a Patient Weighing 70 kg

Intestinal glutamine utilization	10–14 g/d
Kidney glutamine uptake	4 g/d
Immune cells uptake	2–4 g/d*
Glutamine efflux from muscle	8–10 g/d
Balance	−12 g/d

Source: Adapted from Furst P, Alteheld B and Stehle P. 2004. *Clin Nutr* 1, 3–15; * Newsholme F. et al. 1999. *J Nutr Biochem* 10, 316–324.

Thus, in a healthy context, glutamine is considered a nonessential amino acid commonly supplied to the blood by synthesis from precursors in the skeletal muscle. However, under stress situations, glutamine availability can be compromised (Figure 1.2b). Table 1.1 shows the glutamine balance in the postoperative trauma, according to Furst et al. (2004) and Newsholme et al. (1999). Hence, strategies to correct potential glutamine deficiency have included exogenous replacement with L-glutamine, through oral supplementation. In some severe catabolic and uncontrolled inflammatory response (e.g., sepsis), low plasma glutamine concentration is associated with poor clinical outcomes and increased risk of mortality (Rodas et al. 2012). Indeed, immune function including lymphocyte proliferation is dependent on extracellular glutamine concentration (Figure 1.4).

Different preparations of L-glutamine supplementation can be used for nutritional supplementation, and the application partially depends on the patient catabolic situation. Given parenterally, by itself or as part of a total parenteral nutrition (TPN) formulation, L-glutamine supplementation results in the normalization of the availability of total body glutamine (Flaring et al. 2003; Mondello et al. 2010; Weitzel and Wischmeyer 2010). The results of studies of clearance and distribution

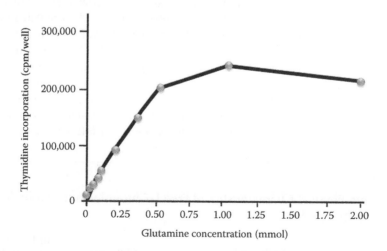

FIGURE 1.4 Lymphocyte proliferation is dependent on extracellular glutamine concentration. Lymphocytes obtained from rat spleens were incubated *in vitro* in RPMI medium containing antibiotics. They were exposed to the T-cell mitogen concanavalin A at the start of the incubation in medium containing extracellular glutamine in various concentrations. Proliferation is expressed as increase in radioactively labeled thymidine incorporation into DNA during the last 18 h of a 66-h incubation. (For more, see Newsholme P. 2001. *J Nutr* 131, 2515S–2522S; discussion 2523S–2514S.)

kinetics may vary according to renal flux and other tissue uptake (Berg et al. 2007); therefore, the dosage of glutamine may be guided by regular measurement of plasma concentration. Most of the studies with postoperative patients show that a daily i.v. or TPN L-glutamine dosage (20–30 g) or 0.3–0.5 g/kg body weight can reduce the rate of decrease in blood glutamine and also glutamine in tissues such as liver and skeletal muscle (Roth 2008; Weitzel and Wischmeyer 2010).

Free L-glutamine has limited solubility in water and is an unstable amino acid in aqueous solution (hydrolysis will degrade glutamine by approximately 5% per day at 37°C). Moreover, amino acid cannot be heat-sterilized, as it will be rapidly hydrolyzed to glutamate and NH_3. Thus, L-glutamine in its free form is not included in the crystalline amino acid solutions for parenteral use until the dipeptide forms were introduced in the 1990s (Furst et al. 2004; Wernerman 2008). The L-glutamine dipeptides are stable during heat sterilization and are highly soluble and, therefore, suitable constituents of liquid nutrition preparations. In fact, current industrial production levels of L-glutamine dipeptides has allowed their routine use in clinical nutrition.

The glutamine-containing dipeptides (Table 1.2) can be formed from L-glycine (L-glycyl-L-glutamine), L-alanine (L-alanyl-L-glutamine), and, as witnessed recently, with L-arginine (L-arginyl-L-glutamine). Several clinical and experimental studies have shown that glutamine-containing dipeptides added to parenteral formulas improve the clinical conditions of individuals with transplanted bone marrow (Ziegler et al. 1992), attenuating reduction in GSH (Flaring et al. 2003), diminishing muscular atrophy during the metabolic stress following surgery, reducing the rate of hospital infection (Grau et al. 2011), promoting immune function (Exner et al. 2003), and improving the nitrogen balance (Mondello et al. 2010), thereby lowering overall hospital costs (Dechelotte et al. 2006), length of stay, and mortality (Klassen et al. 2000; Rodas et al. 2012; Weitzel and Wischmeyer 2010).

Administered in a peripheral vein as a dipeptide, L-alanyl-L-glutamine (Ala-Gln) is the most prevalent supplement form for L-glutamine and can be found in commercial products in a concentration of 200 g/L (20 g/100 mL flask), with an osmolality <900 mOsm (Table 1.2). L-glycyl-L-glutamine (Gly-Gln) also can be found in clinical nutrition field, commonly added in amino acid solutions at 30.27 g/L. Some studies have shown different immunological effects comparing the administration of Ala-Gln and L-glycyl-L-glutamine (Gly-Gln). Exner et al. (2003) observed that both supplements restored plasma glutamine concentration 48 h after major abdominal surgery; however, only Gly-Gln administration resulted in a higher *ex vivo* LPS-stimulated tumor necrosis factor (TNF)-α release. According to the authors, the presence of glycine might enhance glutamine uptake by human monocytes, which would lead to an enhancement of TNF-α secretion. In another study, it was found that the infusion of both dipeptides caused an elevation of the postoperative glutamine plasma levels and, nonetheless, the Ala-Gln infusion attained a higher increase compared to Gly-Gln (Spittler et al. 2001). This effect is possibly related to the fact that the plasma half-life of intravenously injected Gly-Gln is considerably higher than that of Ala-Gln. However, only Gly-Gln supplementation reduced the development of immunosuppression following surgery, when using

TABLE 1.2

Chemical and Physical Characteristics of Free L-Glutamine and Synthetic L-Glutamine Dipeptides

Compound	Solubility (g/L H₂O at 20°C)	Stability	[Glutamine] (g/20 g Dipeptide)	Share of Other Amino Acid Bounded (g/20 g Dipeptide)
Glutamine	36.0	No	20	–
L-alanyl-L-glutamine	568.0	Yes	13.46	8.2
L-glycyl-L-glutamine	154.0	Yes	13.2	6.8
L-arginyl-L-glutamine	N/A	Yes	N/A	N/A

the expression of HLA-DR, a gene product of the major histocompatibility complex (MHC) class II antigen in monocytes, as a marker of immune state (Spittler et al. 2001).

Despite immunological recovery differences, a meta-analysis (Wang et al. 2010) and a review (Roth 2008) revealed that most of the effects cited above, including that of the Ala-Gln supplement, were associated with lower infections and complications in patients with severe catabolic conditions. Gly-Gln is possibly less effective, perhaps because there were not enough trials with the Gly-Gln subgroup. Hence, further studies are needed to determine the different physiological effects of supplementation and impact on clinical outcomes.

On the other hand, i.v. or TPN solutions are very invasive and may expose the patient to enhanced risk of infections so that, as far as possible, enteral alternatives should be considered preferentially. Furthermore, enteral routes are much more physiological and provide the physiological generation of other amino acid derivatives (e.g., citrulline and arginine), which can only be accounted for if L-glutamine is given via this route (Krause and de Bittencourt 2008).

The greater efficiency rendered by enteral L-glutamine dipeptides is a result of its differentiated membrane transport by enterocytes through the glycopeptide transport protein-1 (PepT-1). PepT1 was cloned by Fei et al. (1994) and is a carrier-mediated mechanism for the uptake of small peptides across the brush-border membrane of the enterocyte in the jejunum, followed by the ileum (Nässl et al. 2011). Although transporters of free amino acids exhibit substrate specificity, PepT1 can potentially transport up to common 400 di- and tri-peptides and some peptidomimetic compounds that result from combining the 20 different dietary amino acids (Gilbert et al. 2008). An interesting characteristic of this transport protein is that 2 or 3 amino acids di- or tri- peptides can be transported into the cell by PepT1 for the same energy expenditure required to transport a single free amino acid (Gilbert et al. 2008).

Enteral nutritional solutions with L-glutamine supplementation (dipeptide vs. free amino acids) are important to tissues other than the gut. Results from pancreatic β-cells (which are also dependent on alanine and glutamine metabolism) shed light on a possible mechanism. L-alanine oxidation is important for boosting glucose-stimulated insulin secretion and causes an increase in intracellular glutamate concentration (Newsholme et al. 2003b), while glutamine is important for β-cell viability and function (Cunningham et al. 2005; Newsholme et al. 2005). Furthermore, alanine may protect these cells from apoptosis induced by proinflammatory cytokines, by enhancing antioxidant defenses (Cunningham et al. 2005). Active and healthy skeletal muscle releases alanine and glutamine into the circulation (60% of the overall amino acid delivery), but alanyl-glutamine delivery via enteral or parenteral routes may be important for cell defense and survival during periods of catabolic stress, when skeletal muscle function may be compromised.

1.5 CONCLUSION AND FUTURE PERSPECTIVES

Glutamine plays a critical role in amino acid, protein, and nitrogen metabolism; it is required as a building block of proteins and also provides a nitrogen source for biosynthesis. For healthy populations, L-glutamine synthesized and released from the skeletal muscle is sufficient to maintain glutamine availability and homeostasis. On the other hand, in severe catabolic situations, insufficient glutamine availability in the body may be observed, and exogenous supply is now required. Physicians and nutritionists may use glutamine i.v. or TPN solutions containing glutamine in dipeptide form, and the efficacy of this nutritional intervention is clearly important for the metabolism of amino acids and the recovery of the patient. In oral or enteral nutrition, L-glutamine dipeptides or more complex free amino acid solutions containing L-alanine, L-glycine, or even L-arginine, have been identified for possible supplementation therapy. Despite this, the exact frequency and optimal dosage according to the disease or extreme exercise need to be determined.

It is important to note that L-glutamine supplementation may not prevent inflammation, damage, disease, or even enhance performance but may help the recovery of cells under severe catabolic situations, enhancing cell defenses, attenuating apoptosis and uncontrolled inflammatory response.

If the condition is diagnosed early and managed appropriately, providing optimal supplementation and nutritional support, patient outcomes can be improved.

REFERENCES

Antonio, J. and C. Street. 1999. Glutamine: A potentially useful supplement for athletes. *Can J Appl Physiol* 24, 1–14.

Ardawi, M.S. and E.A. Newsholme. 1982. Maximum activities of some enzymes of glycolysis, the tricarboxylic acid cycle and ketone-body and glutamine utilization pathways in lymphocytes of the rat. *Biochem J* 208, 743–748.

Berg, A., A. Norberg, C.R. Martling, L. Gamrin, O. Rooyackers, and J. Wernerman. 2007. Glutamine kinetics during intravenous glutamine supplementation in ICU patients on continuous renal replacement therapy. *Intensive Care Med* 33, 660–666.

Brosnan, J.T. 2001. Amino acids, then and now—A reflection on Sir Hans Krebs' contribution to nitrogen metabolism. *IUBMB Life* 52, 265–270.

Candow, D.G., P.D. Chilibeck, D.G. Burke, K.S. Davison, and T. Smith-Palmer. 2001. Effect of glutamine supplementation combined with resistance training in young adults. *Eur J Appl Physiol* 86, 142–149.

Cruzat, V.F., A. Bittencourt, S.P. Scomazzon, J.S. Leite, P.I. de Bittencourt, Jr., and J. Tirapegui. 2014a. Oral free and dipeptide forms of glutamine supplementation attenuate oxidative stress and inflammation induced by endotoxemia. *Nutrition* 30, 602–611.

Cruzat, V.F., L.C. Pantaleao, J. Donato, Jr., P.I. de Bittencourt, Jr., and J. Tirapegui. 2014b. Oral supplementations with free and dipeptide forms of L-glutamine in endotoxemic mice: Effects on muscle glutamine-glutathione axis and heat shock proteins. *J Nutr Biochem* 25, 345–352.

Cruzat, V.F., M.M. Rogero, A.K. Ou, I.S.O. Pires, and J. Tirapegui. 2007. Effect of alanyl-glutamine supplementation on muscle damage in rats submitted to exhaustive exercise. *Ann Nutr Metab* 51, 386–387.

Cruzat, V.F., M.M. Rogero, and J. Tirapegui. 2010. Effects of supplementation with free glutamine and the dipeptide alanyl-glutamine on parameters of muscle damage and inflammation in rats submitted to prolonged exercise. *Cell Biochem Funct* 28, 24–30.

Cruzat, V.F. and J. Tirapegui. 2009. Effects of oral supplementation with glutamine and alanyl-glutamine on glutamine, glutamate, and glutathione status in trained rats and subjected to long-duration exercise. *Nutrition* 25, 428–435.

Cunningham, G.A., N.H. McClenaghan, P.R. Flatt, and P. Newsholme. 2005. L-Alanine induces changes in metabolic and signal transduction gene expression in a clonal rat pancreatic beta-cell line and protects from pro-inflammatory cytokine-induced apoptosis. *Clin Sci (Lond)* 109, 447–455.

Curi, R., C.J. Lagranha, S.Q. Doi, D.F. Sellitti, J. Procopio, and T.C. Pithon-Curi. 2005a. Glutamine-dependent changes in gene expression and protein activity. *Cell Biochem Funct* 23, 77–84.

Curi, R., C.J. Lagranha, S.Q. Doi, D.F. Sellitti, J. Procopio, T.C. Pithon-Curi, M. Corless, and P. Newsholme. 2005b. Molecular mechanisms of glutamine action. *J Cell Physiol* 204, 392–401.

Curi, R., P. Newsholme, J. Procopio, C. Lagranha, R. Gorjao, and T.C. Pithon-Curi. 2007. Glutamine, gene expression, and cell function. *Front Biosci* 12, 344–357.

D'Souza, R. and J. Powell-Tuck. 2004. Glutamine supplements in the critically ill. *J Royal Soc Med* 97, 425–427.

Dechelotte, P., M. Hasselmann, L. Cynober, B. Allaouchiche, M. Coeffier, B. Hecketsweiler, V. Merle et al. 2006. L-alanyl-L-glutamine dipeptide-supplemented total parenteral nutrition reduces infectious complications and glucose intolerance in critically ill patients: The French controlled, randomized, double-blind, multicenter study. *Crit Care Med* 34, 598–604.

Dokladny, K., M.N. Zuhl, M. Mandell, D. Bhattacharya, S. Schneider, V. Deretic, and P.L. Moseley. 2013a. Regulatory coordination between two major intracellular homeostatic systems: Heat shock response and autophagy. *J Biol Chem* 288, 14959–14972.

Dokladny, K., M.N. Zuhl, M. Mandell, D. Bhattacharya, S. Schneider, V. Deretic., and P.L. Moseley. 2013b. Regulatory coordination between two major intracellular homeostatic systems: Heat shock response and autophagy. *J Biol Chem* 288, 14959–14972.

Eagle, H. 1959. Amino acid metabolism in mammalian cell cultures. *Science* 130, 432–437.

Eagle, H., V.I. Oyama, M. Levy, C.L. Horton, and R. Fleischman. 1956. Growth response of mammalian cells in tissue culture to L-glutamine and L-glutamic acid. *J Biol Chem* 218, 607–616.

Exner, R., D. Tamandl, P. Goetzinger, M. Mittlboeck, R. Fuegger, T. Sautner, A. Spittler, and E. Roth. 2003. Perioperative GLY-GLN infusion diminishes the surgery-induced period of immunosuppression: Accelerated restoration of the lipopolysaccharide-stimulated tumor necrosis factor-alpha response. *Ann Surg* 237, 110–115.

Fei, Y.J., Y. Kanai, S. Nussberger, V. Ganapathy, F.H. Leibach, M.F. Romero, S.K. Singh, W.F. Boron, and M.A. Hediger. 1994. Expression cloning of a mammalian proton-coupled oligopeptide transporter. *Nature* 368, 563–566.

Finkel, T. and N.J. Holbrook. 2000. Oxidants, oxidative stress and the biology of ageing. *Nature* 408, 239–247.

Flaring, U.B., O.E. Rooyackers, J. Wernerman, and F. Hammarqvist. 2003. Glutamine attenuates post-traumatic glutathione depletion in human muscle. *Clin Sci (Lond)* 104, 275–282.

Frayn, K.N., K. Khan, S.W. Coppack, and M. Elia. 1991. Amino acid metabolism in human subcutaneous adipose tissue *in vivo*. *Clin Sci (Lond)* 80, 471–474.

Furst, P., B. Alteheld, and P. Stehle. 2004. Why should a single nutrient—glutamine—improve outcome? The remarkable story of glutamine dipeptides. *Clin Nutr* 1, 3–15.

Galley, H.F. 2011. Oxidative stress and mitochondrial dysfunction in sepsis. *Br J Anaesth* 107, 57–64.

Gilbert, E.R., E.A. Wong, and K.E. Webb., Jr. 2008. Board-invited review: Peptide absorption and utilization: Implications for animal nutrition and health. *J Anim Sci* 86, 2135–2155.

Gleeson, M. 2008. Dosing and efficacy of glutamine supplementation in human exercise and sport training. *J Nutr* 138, 2045S–2049S.

Grau, T., A. Bonet, E. Minambres, L. Pineiro, J.A. Irles, A. Robles, J. Acosta et al. 2011. The effect of L-alanyl-L-glutamine dipeptide supplemented total parenteral nutrition on infectious morbidity and insulin sensitivity in critically ill patients. *Crit Care Med* 39, 1263–1268.

Hamiel, C.R., S. Pinto, A. Hau, and P.E. Wischmeyer. 2009. Glutamine enhances heat shock protein 70 expression via increased hexosamine biosynthetic pathway activity. *Am J Physiol Cell Physiol* 297, C1509–C1519.

Heck, T.G., C.M. Scholer, and P.I. de Bittencourt. 2011. HSP70 expression: Does it a novel fatigue signalling factor from immune system to the brain? *Cell Biochem Funct* 29, 215–226.

Hiscock, N. and B.K. Pedersen. 2002. Exercise-induced immunodepression—plasma glutamine is not the link. *J Appl Physiol* 93, 813–822.

Klassen, P., M. Mazariegos, N.W. Solomons, and P. Furst. 2000. The pharmacokinetic responses of humans to 20 g of alanyl-glutamine dipeptide differ with the dosing protocol but not with gastric acidity or in patients with acute Dengue fever. *J Nutr* 130, 177–182.

Krause, M.S. and P.I.H.J de Bittencourt. 2008. Type 1 diabetes: Can exercise impair the autoimmune event? The L-arginine/glutamine coupling hypothesis. *Cell Biochem Funct* 26, 406–433.

Krebs, H.A. 1935. Metabolism of amino-acids: The synthesis of glutamine from glutamic acid and ammonia, and the enzymic hydrolysis of glutamine in animal tissues. *Biochem J* 29, 1951–1969.

Labow, B.I., W.W. Souba, and S.F. Abcouwer. 2001. Mechanisms governing the expression of the enzymes of glutamine metabolism–glutaminase and glutamine synthetase. *J Nutr* 131, 2467S–2474S; discussion 2486S–2487S.

Lamb, G.D. and H. Westerblad. 2011. Acute effects of reactive oxygen and nitrogen species on the contractile function of skeletal muscle. *J Physiol* 589, 2119–2127.

Lightfoot, A., A. McArdle, and R.D. Griffiths. 2009. Muscle in defense. *Crit Care Med* 37, S384–S390.

Manso Filho, H.C., K.H. McKeever, M.E. Gordon, H.E. Manso, W.S. Lagakos, G. Wu, and M. Watford. 2009. Developmental changes in the concentrations of glutamine and other amino acids in plasma and skeletal muscle of the Standardbred foal. *J Anim Sci* 87, 2528–2535.

Meister, A. 1983. Selective modification of glutathione metabolism. *Science* 220, 472–477.

Moley, K.H. and M.M. Mueckler. 2000. Glucose transport and apoptosis. *Apoptosis* 5, 99–105.

Mondello, S., D. Italiano, M.S. Giacobbe, P. Mondello, G. Trimarchi, C. Aloisi, P. Bramanti, and E. Spina. 2010. Glutamine-supplemented total parenteral nutrition improves immunological status in anorectic patients. *Nutrition* 26, 677–681.

Mora, J. 2012. *Glutamine: Metabolism, Enzymology, and Regulation.* Amsterdam, Netherlands: Elsevier Science.

Nässl, A-M., I. Rubio-Aliaga, H. Fenselau, M.K. Marth, G. Kottra, and H. Daniel. 2011. Amino acid absorption and homeostasis in mice lacking the intestinal peptide transporter PEPT1. *American Journal of Physiology—Gastrointestinal and Liver Physiology* 301, G128–G137.

Neu, J., V. Shenoy, and R. Chakrabarti. 1996. Glutamine nutrition and metabolism: Where do we go from here? *FASEB J* 10, 829–837.

Newsholme, F., R. Curi, T.C.P. Curi, C.J. Murphy, C. Garcia, and M.P. de Melo. 1999. Glutamine metabolism by lymphocytes, macrophages, and neutrophils: Its importance in health and disease. *J Nutr Biochem* 10, 316–324.

Newsholme, P. 2001. Why is L-glutamine metabolism important to cells of the immune system in health, postinjury, surgery or infection? *J Nutr* 131, 2515S–2522S; discussion 2523S–2514S.

Newsholme, P., F. Abdulkader, E. Rebelato, T. Romanatto, C.H. Pinheiro, K.F. Vitzel, E.P. Silva. et al. 2011a. Amino acids and diabetes: Implications for endocrine, metabolic and immune function. *Front Biosci* 16, 315–339.

Newsholme, P., L. Brennan, B. Rubi, and P. Maechler. 2005. New insights into amino acid metabolism, beta-cell function and diabetes. *Clin Sci (Lond)* 108, 185–194.

Newsholme, P., V. Cruzat, F. Arfuso, and K. Keane. 2014. Nutrient regulation of insulin secretion and action. *J Endocrinol* 221, R105–R120.

Newsholme, P., S. Gordon, and E.A. Newsholme. 1987. Rates of utilization and fates of glucose, glutamine, pyruvate, fatty acids and ketone bodies by mouse macrophages. *Biochem J* 242(3), 631–636.

Newsholme, P., M. Krause, E.A. Newsholme, S.J. Stear, L.M. Burke, and L.M. Castell. 2011b. BJSM reviews: A to Z of nutritional supplements: Dietary supplements, sports nutrition foods and ergogenic aids for health and performance—Part 18. *Br J Sports Med* 45, 230–232.

Newsholme, P., M.M. Lima, J. Procopio, T.C. Pithon-Curi, S.Q. Doi, R.B. Bazotte, and R. Curi. 2003a. Glutamine and glutamate as vital metabolites. *Braz J Med Biol Res* 36, 153–163.

Newsholme, P., J. Procopio, M.M. Lima, T.C. Pithon-Curi, and R. Curi. 2003b. Glutamine and glutamate— Their central role in cell metabolism and function. *Cell Biochem Funct* 21, 1–9.

Nicastro, H., C.R. da Luz, D.F. Chaves, L.R. Bechara, V.A. Voltarelli, M.M. Rogero, and A.K. Lancha, Jr. 2012. Does branched-chain amino acids supplementation modulate skeletal muscle remodeling through inflammation modulation? Possible mechanisms of action. *J Nutr Metab* 2012, 136937.

Nicklin, P., P. Bergman, B. Zhang, E. Triantafellow, H. Wang, B. Nyfeler, H. Yang et al. 2009. Bidirectional transport of amino acids regulates mTOR and autophagy. *Cell* 136, 521–534.

Oliveira-Yamashita, F., R.F. Garcia, A.M. Felisberto-Junior, R. Curi, and R.B. Bazotte. 2009. Evidence that L-glutamine is better than L-alanine as gluconeogenic substrate in perfused liver of weaned fasted rats submitted to short-term insulin-induced hypoglycaemia. *Cell Biochem Funct* 27, 30–34.

Petry, E.R., V.F. Cruzat, T.G. Heck, J.S. Leite, P.I. Homem de Bittencourt, Jr., and J. Tirapegui. 2014. Alanyl-glutamine and glutamine plus alanine supplements improve skeletal redox status in trained rats: Involvement of heat shock protein pathways. *Life Sci* 94, 130–136.

Rodas, P.C., O. Rooyackers, C. Hebert, A. Norberg, and J. Wernerman. 2012. Glutamine and glutathione at ICU admission in relation to outcome. *Clin Sci (Lond)* 122, 591–597.

Rogero, M.M., P. Borelli, R.A. Fock, M.C. Borges, M.A.R. Vinolo, R. Curi, K. Nakajima, A.R. Crisma, A.D. Ramos, and J. Tirapegui. 2010. Effects of glutamine on the nuclear factor-kappaB signaling pathway of murine peritoneal macrophages. *Amino Acids* 39, 435–441.

Rogero, M.M., P. Borelli, M.A. Vinolo, R.A. Fock, I.S.D. Pires, and J. Tirapegui. 2008. Dietary glutamine supplementation affects macrophage function, hematopoiesis and nutritional status in early weaned mice. *Clin Nutr* 27, 386–397.

Rogero, M.M., M.C. Borges, R.A. Fock, A.D. Ramos, I.S. Pires, M.A. Vinolo, R. Curi, P. Borelli and J. Tirapegui. 2009. Glutamine *in vitro* supplementation decreases glucose utilization by the glycolytic pathway in Lps-activated peritoneal macrophages. *Ann Nutr Metab* 55, 455–455.

Roth, E. 2008. Nonnutritive effects of glutamine. *J Nutr* 138, 2025S–2031S.

Rowbottom, D.G., D. Keast, and A.R. Morton. 1996. The emerging role of glutamine as an indicator of exercise stress and overtraining. *Sports Med* 21, 80–97.

Rutten, E.P., M.P. Engelen, A.M. Schols, and N.E. Deutz. 2005. Skeletal muscle glutamate metabolism in health and disease: State of the art. *Curr Opin Clin Nutr Metab Care* 8, 41–51.

Santos, R.V., E.C. Caperuto, and L.F. Costa Rosa. 2007. Effects of acute exhaustive physical exercise upon glutamine metabolism of lymphocytes from trained rats. *Life Sci* 80, 573–578.

Sartorelli, V. and M. Fulco. 2004. Molecular and cellular determinants of skeletal muscle atrophy and hypertrophy. *Sci STKE* 2004, re11.

Shimomura, Y., T. Honda, M. Shiraki, T. Murakami, J. Sato, H. Kobayashi, K. Mawatari, M. Obayashi and R.A. Harris. 2006. Branched-chain amino acid catabolism in exercise and liver disease. *J Nutr* 136, 250S–253S.

Shimomura, Y., T. Murakami, N. Nakai, M. Nagasaki, and R.A. Harris. 2004. Exercise promotes BCAA catabolism: Effects of BCAA supplementation on skeletal muscle during exercise. *J Nutr* 134, 1583S–1587S.

Singleton, K.D. and P.E. Wischmeyer. 2007. Glutamine's protection against sepsis and lung injury is dependent on heat shock protein 70 expression. *Am J Physiol Regul Integr Comp Physiol* 292, R1839–R1845.

Spittler, A., T. Sautner, A. Gornikiewicz, N. Manhart, R. Oehler, M. Bergmann, R. Fugger, and E. Roth. 2001. Postoperative glycyl-glutamine infusion reduces immunosuppression: Partial prevention of the surgery induced decrease in HLA-DR expression on monocytes. *Clin Nutr* 20, 37–42.

Valencia, E., A. Marin, and G. Hardy. 2001. Glutathione-nutritional and pharmacologic viewpoints: Part I. *Nutrition* 17, 428–429.

van de Poll, M.C.G., P.B. Soeters, N.E.P. Deutz, K.C.H. Fearon, and C.H.C. Dejong. 2004. Renal metabolism of amino acids: Its role in interorgan amino acid exchange. *Am J Clin Nutr* 79, 185–197.

Vina, J., R. Hems, and H.A. Krebs. 1978. Maintenance of glutathione content is isolated hepatocyctes. *Biochem J* 170, 627–630.

Wang, Y., Z.M. Jiang, M.T. Nolan, H. Jiang, H.R. Han, K. Yu, H.L. Li, B. Jie, and X.K. Liang. 2010. The impact of glutamine dipeptide-supplemented parenteral nutrition on outcomes of surgical patients: A meta-analysis of randomized clinical trials. *JPEN J Parenter Enteral Nutr* 34, 521–529.

Weitzel, L.R. and P.E. Wischmeyer. 2010. Glutamine in critical illness: The time has come, the time is now. *Crit Care Clin* 26, 515–525, ix–x.

Wernerman, J. 2008. Clinical use of glutamine supplementation. *J Nutr* 138, 2040S–2044S.

Wischmeyer, P.E. 2002. Glutamine and heat shock protein expression. *Nutrition* 18, 225–228.

Xue, H., D. Slavov, and P.E. Wischmeyer. 2012. Glutamine-mediated dual regulation of heat shock transcription factor-1 activation and expression. *J Biol Chem* 287, 40400–40413.

Yamauchi, K., T. Komatsu, A.D. Kulkarni, Y. Ohmori, H. Minami, Y. Ushiyama, M. Nakayama, and S. Yamamoto. 2002. Glutamine and arginine affect Caco-2 cell proliferation by promotion of nucleotide synthesis. *Nutrition* 18, 329–333.

Young, V.R. and A.M. Ajami. 2001. Glutamine: The emperor or his clothes? *J Nutr* 131, 2449S–2459S; discussion 2486S–2447S.

Zachara, N.E. and G.W. Hart. 2006. Cell signaling, the essential role of O-GlcNAc! *Biochim Biophys Acta* 1761, 599–617.

Zachara, N.E., N. O'Donnell, W.D. Cheung, J.J. Mercer, J.D. Marth, and G.W. Hart. 2004. Dynamic O-GlcNAc modification of nucleocytoplasmic proteins in response to stress. A survival response of mammalian cells. *J Biol Chem* 279, 30133–30142.

Ziegler, T.R., L.S. Young, K. Benfell, M. Scheltinga, K. Hortos, R. Bye, F.D. Morrow et al. 1992. Clinical and metabolic efficacy of glutamine-supplemented parenteral nutrition after bone marrow transplantation. A randomized, double-blind, controlled study. *Ann Intern Med* 116, 821–828.

Section II

New Data on the Biochemistry
of Glutamine

2 Intestinal Glutamine Synthetase Colocalizes with Goblet Cells and Decreases Enterocyte Proliferation

Theodorus B.M. Hakvoort, Youji He,
Irene van Herk, Jacqueline L.M. Vermeulen,
Jan M. Ruijter, and Wouter H. Lamers

CONTENTS

2.1 INTRODUCTION

Glutamine is, at a concentration of ~600 µmol/L, the most abundant amino acid in mammalian plasma (Tapiero et al. 2002). It is considered to be the principle metabolic fuel for rapidly dividing cells, including enterocytes (Windmueller 1982), as is underscored by the bowel dysfunction and necrosis that develops upon infusion of glutaminase (Baskerville et al. 1980). Even though the effects of glutaminase infusion, which reduced circulating glutamine to nondetectable levels (Hambleton et al. 1980), were more pronounced in the colon than in the small intestine, the few studies that were carried out on glutamine synthesis in the gut have focused on the small intestine. The only enzyme capable of glutamine synthesis is glutamine synthetase (GS; L-glutamate: ammonia ligase (ADP); EC 6.3.1.2). GS expression was undetectable in the small intestine of adult mice (Kuo et al. 1991). In adult rats, GS activity in the intestine was considered low relative to the distal stomach, but the colon expressed a ~10-fold higher activity than the small intestine (Arola et al. 1981; James et al. 1998b). Both GS protein and mRNA were reportedly present in all enterocytes (Kong et al. 2000) or mainly in the crypt regions (Roig et al. 1995). Fasting for 2 days reduced mucosal mass of the small intestine to ~70% but increased GS activity by 1.2–1.4-fold (Kong et al. 2000).

Some time ago, we showed in adult mice that the colon contained an 8–10-fold higher concentration of GS mRNA, protein, and activity than did the jejunum and that these numbers were ~2-fold higher in females than in males (van Straaten et al. 2006). We, therefore, deemed it of interest to investigate the role of GS in the intestine. To do so, we generated mice that were selectively deficient for GS in their intestines by crossing mice carrying a GS^{fl} allele (He et al. 2010b) with mice carrying a Vil-Cre allele (B6.SJL-Tg(Vil-cre)997Gum/J) (Madison et al. 2002). The flanking of the coding regions in the GS^{fl} allele does not alter GS functionality (He et al. 2010b). The effects of a specific deletion of the GS^{fl} alleles in astrocytes and myocytes were described earlier (He et al. 2010a,b). The Vil-Cre mice express the loxP sequence-specific Cre recombinase enzyme (Orban et al. 1992) in the enterocytes of the intestine (Madison et al. 2002). Villin is an actin-bundling protein in the apical brush border of absorptive tissues that is expressed in the intestinal epithelium from crypt to villus tip and from duodenum to the rectum from embryonic day 12.5 onward (Madison et al. 2002).

2.2 DISTRIBUTION OF GS IN THE INTESTINES

GS activity in the colon exceeds that seen in the small intestine ~10-fold (Figure 2.1a). Figure 2.2 shows that GS expression is confined to goblet cells and virtually absent from absorptive entero-cytes. Note that the anti-GS antibody did not stain the mucus itself. Although GS expression in small-intestinal villi and crypts was low, it was strongly expressed in Brunner's glands of the proximal duodenum (Figure 2.2). Figure 2.2 also shows that the expression of CPS, a marker for all enterocytes on the villus, is virtually absent from the deeper parts of the intestinal crypts, including Brunner's glands, and from the colon. The expression patterns of GS and CPS in the respective parts of the intestine are, therefore, mostly supplemental.

The number of goblet cells in the colon is much higher than in the small intestine. The selective expression of GS in goblet cells raised the question whether the high enzyme activity in the colon relative to the small intestine was due to the much higher number of goblet cells in the colon or to a difference in enzyme activity per goblet cell. We, therefore, quantified the Alcian blue-positive areas in the proximal third of the small intestine and in the colon as a fraction of the total area occupied by intestinal epithelium in the respective sections, using ImageJ software. Figure 2.1b shows that the mucus-containing area was ~8-fold bigger in the colon than in the small intestine. This difference does not differ significantly from the ratio of enzyme activity. We conclude that the goblet cells of both the small intestine and the colon contain a similar quantity of GS enzyme.

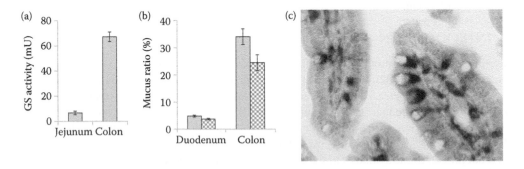

FIGURE 2.1 **(See color insert.)** (a) GS enzyme activity in jejunum and colon. GS activity was measured in tissue homogenates. Activity was determined spectrophotometrically with the γ-glutamyltransferase assay and expressed as nmoles/min mg total protein (mU) at 37°C. (b) Percentage of intestinal epithelial surface occupied by mucus in jejunum and colon of control (homogeneous gray) and GS-KO/I mice (cross-hatched). The "stained surface" of Alcian blue-stained sections was determined in four random pictures with ImageJ. (c) Ileal villus stained for the presence of GS in a wild-type mouse. The presence of GS was demonstrated with mouse monoclonal antibodies (clone GS-6, R&D Systems, UK). Antibody binding was visualized with the appropriate alkaline phosphatase-coupled secondary antisera. Specific staining is seen in the goblet cells only. Positive cells in the submucosa represent immune cells containing immunoglobulins that are recognized by the second antibody (see also Figures 2.3 and 2.4).

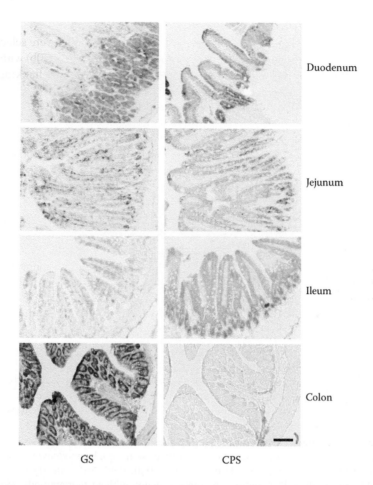

FIGURE 2.2   (See color insert.) Serial sections of the intestine in fed control mice were stained for the presence of GS or carbamoyl-phosphate synthetase (CPS). The presence of CPS was visualized with a rabbit antiserum (Charles et al. 1983) and an alkaline phosphatase-coupled secondary antiserum. Note the roughly reciprocal staining pattern of GS and CPS. The staining intensity of GS is relatively low in the small intestine, except for Brunner's glands in the duodenum, whereas its staining in the colon is intense. CPS is present in the epithelium of the small intestine, except for Brunner's glands and the colon, where it is nearly absent. Magnification: 10× (bar: 0.1 mm).

2.3   EFFECT OF ENTEROCYTE-SPECIFIC DELETION OF GS ON THE INTESTINE

Constitutive GS-deficient mice die in the blastocyst phase of development (He et al. 2007). Crossing Vil-Cre mice (Madison et al. 2002) with ROSA26R-LacZ reporter mice (Soriano 1999) demonstrated that Cre was expressed in all the epithelial cells of the duodenum, jejunum, ileum, and colon but not in the nonepithelial intestinal cells (not shown). On the basis of this experiment, we concluded that the Vil-Cre mouse was an efficient deleter strain. Expression was already complete at postnatal day 10. Crossing Vil-Cre with GS$^{fl/fl}$ or GS$^{fl/LacZ}$ mice yielded apparently healthy, enterocyte-specific GS-deficient mice (GS-KO/I). Enterocyte-specific deletion of GS expression was complete, even in the colon (cf. Figures 2.3 and 2.4).

The duodenum, jejunum, ileum, and colon of fasted and nonfasted male and female GS-KO/I and control mice were stained for the expression of GS, CPS (a marker for small intestinal epithelium), BrdU (a marker for the proliferative capacity), and activated caspase-2 (a marker for apoptosis). The number of Alcian blue-positive and GS-positive goblet cells increases progressively

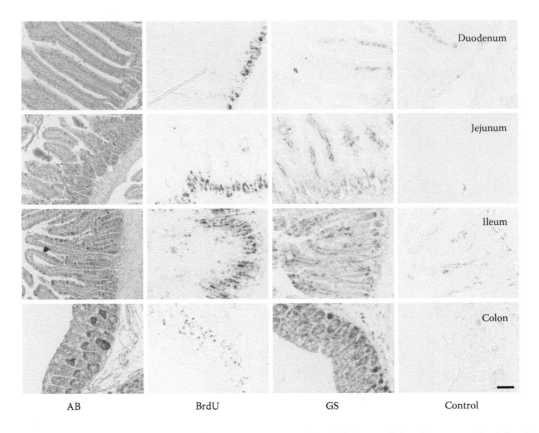

AB   BrdU   GS   Control

FIGURE 2.3 **(See color insert.)** Serial sections of the intestine of fed control females were stained for the presence of mucus (Alcian Blue with nuclear fast red counter staining), bromodeoxyuridine (BrdU), or GS; 32.5 μmol (10 mg) BrdU per 10 g body weight dissolved in 50 μL 0.9% NaCl was injected intraperitoneally 150 and 30 min before sacrifice. The control represents a section without first antibody. Magnification: 10× (bar: 0.1 mm).

between the duodenum and the colon (columns 1 and 3 in Figures 2.3 and 2.4), a higher degree of incorporation of BrdU in the small intestine than in the colon (column 2), and a varying degree of background staining with the secondary antibody (column 4). The background staining, which was also seen in sections stained for the presence of GS in GS-KO/I mice (Figure 2.4), stained the lamina propria and not the enterocytes and was only seen in sections incubated with anti-mouse IgG antiserum. We, therefore, hypothesize that the staining cells are immune cells that contain antibodies.

2.3.1 Effect of Enterocyte-Specific Deletion of GS on Portal-Vein Amino Acid Concentrations

Compared to fed mice, fasting only slightly decreased portal-vein concentrations of all amino acids (−8%) in control mice (Figure 2.5). As expected, glutamine and alanine behaved differently. The concentration of glutamine in the fasted condition was ~175% of that in the fed condition (P = 0.03), whereas in the case of alanine it was only ~80% (P = 0.009). The increase in glutamine concentration was similar to the decrease in alanine concentration. GS-KO/I mice differed from control mice in that fasting decreased the portal-vein concentrations of all amino acids to ~78%. The difference in the response of amino acids to fasting significant ($P_{lines} = 0.014$; Figure 2.5). The portal-vein

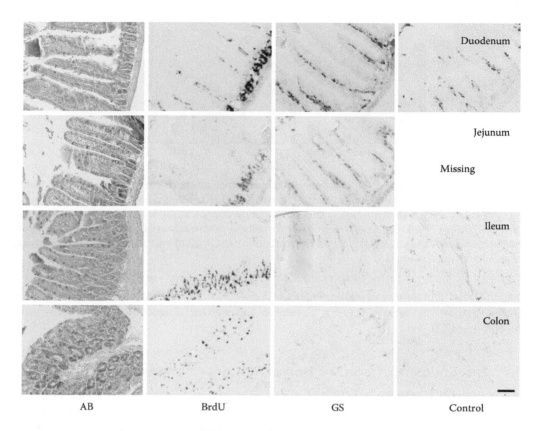

FIGURE 2.4 **(See color insert.)** Serial sections of the intestine of fed GS-KO/I females were stained for the presence of mucus, BrdU, or GS. Note that the stain in the duodenum and jejunum after incubation with the GS antibody is present in the stem of the villus and not in the epithelium. This staining pattern is also seen in the section incubated with the secondary antiserum only. The jejunal control section ("missing") was lost in the course of the immunohistochemical procedure. Bar: 0.1 mm.

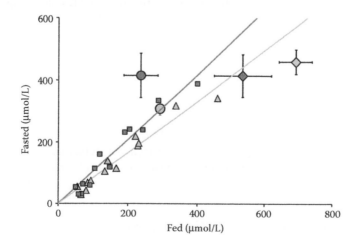

FIGURE 2.5 **(See color insert.)** Correlation between fed and 24-h-fasted portal-vein amino acid concentrations in control and GS/KO/I mice. Amino acid concentrations in deproteinized plasma samples were determined by HPLC (van Eijk et al. 1993). Control mice are represented by red symbols (regression line in red as well) and GS-KO/I mice by blue symbols (regression line: blue). Circles represent glutamine and diamonds alanine. Please note that amino acids, except for glutamine and alanine, are not identified by name.

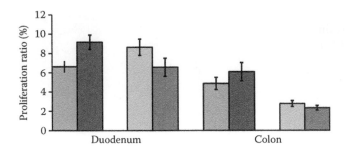

FIGURE 2.6   (See color insert.) BrdU incorporation into epithelial cells of the duodenum or colon. Control (red columns) or GS-KO/I (blue columns) mice were either fed (light columns) or 24-h-fasted (dark columns) when they were treated with BrdU. BrdU incorporation in the colon was ~70% of that in the duodenum and sensitive to fasting (~2-fold decrease), irrespective of whether the animal was or was not GS-deficient in the intestinal epithelium. The effect of fasting was most prominent in GS-KO/I mice and may also have decreased incorporation in the duodenum.

concentration of glutamine was similar in fed and GS-KO/I mice, whereas that of alanine declined to ~65%, that is, the balance between glutamine and alanine concentrations remained similar (260–300 μmol/L).

2.3.2   Effect of Enterocyte-Specific Deletion of GS on the Number of Goblet Cells

Figure 2.1b shows that the fraction of Alcian blue-positive areas in both the proximal third of the small intestine and the colon as a fraction of the total area occupied by intestinal epithelium in that section decreased to 77% in the duodenum (P = 0.028) and to 72% in the colon (P = 0.004) of GS-KO/I mice.

2.3.3   Effect of Enterocyte-Specific Deletion of GS on Enterocyte Proliferation

BrdU incorporation was much higher in the small intestine than in the colon (Figures 2.3 and 2.4). Figure 2.6 shows that the proliferating cells occupied ~1.5-fold larger relative volume of duodenal epithelium than of colonic epithelium (P < 0.001), irrespective of the genotype. Fasting had no significant effect on BrdU incorporation in the duodenum (P = 0.63), but in colon fasting decreased the proliferation of enterocytes to ~60% of fed mice in controls and to ~35% in GS-KO/I mice (both: P < 0.001).

2.4   DISCUSSION

The main findings of our study were that GS expression per goblet cell is similar in the small intestine and the colon and that fasting reduced intestinal cell proliferation in GS-deficient mice only.

2.4.1   Restriction of GS Expression to Goblet Cells

The finding that GS protein was only found in goblet cells and that the density of goblet cells determined the distribution of GS in the intestines was unexpected in view of earlier immune and *in situ* hybridization stainings (Roig et al. 1995; Kong et al. 2000). Our estimate of the number of goblet cells in the intestine concurs with earlier reports (Sharma and Schumacher 1995). Since the ratio of GS activity in the duodenum and colon was similar to that of goblet cells, the GS content per goblet cell was similar at both locations. In fish intestine, GS (Mommsen et al. 2003) and goblet cells (Hur et al. 2013) are also predominantly expressed in the distal part of the intestines, suggesting an evolutionarily conserved, and hence probably an important, function of GS in these cells. Goblet cells are known for their production and secretion of mucus and also secrete cysteine-rich peptides such as intestinal trefoil factor (TFF3), which play a key role in intestinal defense and repair (Kim and Ho 2010). Glutaminase activity far exceeds GS activity in the intestines (James et al. 1998a,b; McCauley et al. 1999; Kong et al. 2000), which explains why the (small) intestine is known as a glutamine-consuming organ (Windmueller 1982; Quan et al. 1998; Haisch et al. 2000; van de Poll et al. 2007). The restricted presence of GS in goblet cells also rules out enterocyte glutamine synthesis (Reeds and Burrin 2001). Instead, the presence of GS in goblet cells suggests a local function of the enzyme. Most likely, this function is the provision of glutamine as substrate for L-glutamine: D-fructose-6-phosphate amidotransferase (GFAT) to produce glucosamine-6-phosphate. Glucosamine-6-phosphate, in turn, is metabolized to uridine 5′-diphospho-N-acetyl-D-glucosamine (UDP-GlcNAc), which controls the biosynthesis of amino sugar-containing macromolecules, such as mucins (Milewski 2002). In agreement, the activity of GFAT is lower in the small intestine than in the colon (Winslet et al. 1994).

2.4.2 EFFECT OF FASTING AND GS DEFICIENCY ON ENTEROCYTE PROLIFERATION

Fasting decreased proliferation of the enterocytes, in particular in the colon, and was more prominent in GS-KO/I than in control mice. *In vitro*, ambient glutamine concentration has to be ~1 mmol/L for maximal growth of rat IEC-6 intestinal cells (DeMarco et al. 1999), which is similar to the mucosal concentration of glutamine (~1 and ~2 mmol/L in the small and large intestine of rats, respectively; Arola et al. 1981). We previously showed that fasting increased intestinal cell turnover (Sokolovic et al. 2007), but the effects after 24 h of fasting were still small.

2.4.3 EFFECT OF FASTING AND GS DEFICIENCY ON PORTAL AMINO ACID CONCENTRATIONS

Feeding caused the concentration of amino acids in the portal vein to increase ~8% relative to the corresponding amino acids in 24 h-fasted control mice, whereas the concentration of glutamine declined to ~55% and that of alanine increased ~30%. We did not measure arterial amino acid concentrations in these mice, but in an earlier experiment (He et al. 2010a) the arterial concentrations of corresponding amino acids were ~25% higher in fed than fasted control mice, whereas the "glutamine effect" was not seen. Fasting apparently reduces the intestinal consumption of amino acids (~1.4-fold) and especially that of glutamine (~2.5-fold) in a pronounced manner. There are few direct comparisons between amino acid consumption in fed and fasted intestines, but Windmueller and Spaeth's experiments also showed an ~2-fold higher glutamine and glucose consumption in fed than in post-absorptive rat jejunum, which was only partly compensated for by an increased ketone body metabolism in fasting jejunum (Windmueller and Spaeth 1978, 1980). In GS-KO/I mice, in contrast, the concentrations of all amino acids in the portal vein were ~20% lower in the fasted state than in the fed state, suggesting that, in the absence of food, the intestine did extract more arterial amino acids. The only difference between both sets of mice was their GS deficiency in the goblet cells and perhaps the associated decrease in their number, which was observed in 70%–75% of controls. It is tempting to speculate that the decline in the number of goblet cells accounts for the disappearance of the "glutamine effect" and the increased amino acid extraction is due to the loss of their capacity to synthesize glutamine. In other words, the goblet cells appear to be the main consumers of glutamine in the intestine.

REFERENCES

Arola, L., A. Palou, X. Remesar, and M. Alemany. 1981. Glutamine synthetase activity in the organs of fed and 24-hours fasted rats. *Horm Metab Res* 13 (4):199–202.

Baskerville, A., P. Hambleton, and J. E. Benbough. 1980. Pathological features of glutaminase toxicity. *Br J Exp Pathol* 61 (2):132–8.

Charles, R., A. De Graaf, W. H. Lamers, and A. F. Moorman. 1983. Control of the changes in rat-liver carbamoyl-phosphate synthase (ammonia) protein levels during ontogenesis: Evidence for a perinatal change in immunoreactivity of the enzyme. *Mech Ageing Dev* 22 (3–4):193–203.

DeMarco, V., K. Dyess, D. Strauss, C. M. West, and J. Neu. 1999. Inhibition of glutamine synthetase decreases proliferation of cultured rat intestinal epithelial cells. *J Nutr* 129 (1):57–62.

Haisch, M., N. K. Fukagawa, and D. E. Matthews. 2000. Oxidation of glutamine by the splanchnic bed in humans. *Am J Physiol Endocrinol Metab* 278 (4):E593–602.

Hambleton, P., J. E. Benbough, A. Baskerville, and P. W. Harris-Smith. 1980. Clinical biochemical aspects of glutaminase toxicity in rabbits and Rhesus monkeys. *Br J Exp Pathol* 61 (2):208–16.

He, Y., T. B. Hakvoort, S. E. Kohler et al. 2010a. Glutamine synthetase in muscle is required for glutamine production during fasting and extrahepatic ammonia detoxification. *J Biol Chem* 285 (13):9516–24.

He, Y., T. B. Hakvoort, J. L. Vermeulen et al. 2010b. Glutamine synthetase deficiency in murine astrocytes results in neonatal death. *Glia* 58 (6):741–54.

He, Y., T. B. Hakvoort, J. L. Vermeulen, W. H. Lamers, and M. A. Van Roon. 2007. Glutamine synthetase is essential in early mouse embryogenesis. *Dev Dyn* 236 (7):1865–75.

Hur, S. W., C. H. Lee, S. H. Lee et al. 2013. Characterization of cholecystokinin-producing cells and mucus-secreting goblet cells in the blacktip grouper, *Epinephelus fasciatus*. *Tissue Cell* 45 (2):153–7.

James, L. A., P. G. Lunn, and M. Elia. 1998a. Glutamine metabolism in the gastrointestinal tract of the rat assess by the relative activities of glutaminase (EC 3.5.1.2) and glutamine synthetase (EC 6.3.1.2). *Br J Nutr* 79 (4):365–72.

James, L. A., P. G. Lunn, S. Middleton, and M. Elia. 1998b. Distribution of glutaminase and glutamine synthetase activities in the human gastrointestinal tract. *Clin Sci (Lond)* 94 (3):313–9.

Kim, Y. S., and S. B. Ho. 2010. Intestinal goblet cells and mucins in health and disease: Recent insights and progress. *Curr Gastroenterol Rep* 12 (5):319–30.

Kong, S. E., J. C. Hall, D. Cooper, and R. D. McCauley. 2000. Starvation alters the activity and mRNA level of glutaminase and glutamine synthetase in the rat intestine. *J Nutr Biochem* 11 (7–8):393–400.

Kuo, F. C., W. L. Hwu, D. Valle, and J. E. Darnell, Jr. 1991. Colocalization in pericentral hepatocytes in adult mice and similarity in developmental expression pattern of ornithine aminotransferase and glutamine synthetase mRNA. *Proc Natl Acad Sci USA* 88 (21):9468–72.

Madison, B. B., L. Dunbar, X. T. Qiao, K. Braunstein, E. Braunstein, and D. L. Gumucio. 2002. Cis elements of the villin gene control expression in restricted domains of the vertical (crypt) and horizontal (duodenum, cecum) axes of the intestine. *J Biol Chem* 277 (36):33275–83.

McCauley, R., S. E. Kong, K. Heel, and J. C. Hall. 1999. The role of glutaminase in the small intestine. *Int J Biochem Cell Biol* 31 (3–4):405–13.

Milewski, S. 2002. Glucosamine-6-phosphate synthase–the multi-facets enzyme. *Biochim Biophys Acta* 1597 (2):173–92.

Mommsen, T. P., E. R. Busby, K. R. von Schalburg, J. C. Evans, H. L. Osachoff, and M. E. Elliott. 2003. Glutamine synthetase in tilapia gastrointestinal tract: Zonation, cDNA and induction by cortisol. *J Comp Physiol B* 173 (5):419–27.

Orban, P. C., D. Chui, and J. D. Marth. 1992. Tissue- and site-specific DNA recombination in transgenic mice. *Proc Natl Acad Sci USA* 89 (15):6861–5.

Quan, J., M. D. Fitch, and S. E. Fleming. 1998. Rate at which glutamine enters TCA cycle influences carbon atom fate in intestinal epithelial cells. *Am J Physiol* 275 (6 Pt 1):G1299–308.

Reeds, P. J. and D. G. Burrin. 2001. Glutamine and the bowel. *J Nutr* 131 (9 Suppl):2505S–8S; discussion 2523S–4S.

Roig, J. C., V. B. Shenoy, R. Chakrabarti, J. Y. Lau, and J. Neu. 1995. Localization of rat small intestine glutamine synthetase using immunofluorescence and *in situ* hybridization. *JPEN J Parenter Enteral Nutr* 19 (3):179–81.

Sharma, R. and U. Schumacher. 1995. Morphometric analysis of intestinal mucins under different dietary conditions and gut flora in rats. *Dig Dis Sci* 40 (12):2532–9.

Sokolovic, M., D. Wehkamp, A. Sokolovic et al. 2007. Fasting induces a biphasic adaptive metabolic response in murine small intestine. *BMC Genomics* 8:361.

Soriano, P. 1999. Generalized lacZ expression with the ROSA26 Cre reporter strain. *Nat Genet* 21 (1):70–1.

Tapiero, H., G. Mathe, P. Couvreur, and K. D. Tew. 2002. II. Glutamine and glutamate. *Biomed Pharmacother* 56 (9):446–57.

van de Poll, M. C., G. C. Ligthart-Melis, P. G. Boelens, N. E. Deutz, P. A. van Leeuwen, and C. H. Dejong. 2007. Intestinal and hepatic metabolism of glutamine and citrulline in humans. *J Physiol* 581 (Pt 2):819–27.

van Eijk HM, Rooyakkers DR, Deutz NE. 1993. Rapid routine determination of amino acids in plasma by high-performance liquid chromatography with a 2–3 microns Spherisorb ODS II column. *J Chromatogr* 620:143–8.

van Straaten, H. W., Y. He, M. M. van Duist et al. 2006. Cellular concentrations of glutamine synthetase in murine organs. *Biochem Cell Biol* 84 (2):215–31.

Windmueller, H. G. 1982. Glutamine utilization by the small intestine. *Adv Enzymol Relat Areas Mol Biol* 53:201–37.

Windmueller, H. G. and A. E. Spaeth. 1978. Identification of ketone bodies and glutamine as the major respiratory fuels *in vivo* for postabsorptive rat small intestine. *J Biol Chem* 253 (1):69–76.

Windmueller, H. G. and A. E. Spaeth. 1980. Respiratory fuels and nitrogen metabolism *in vivo* in small intestine of fed rats. Quantitative importance of glutamine, glutamate, and aspartate. *J Biol Chem* 255 (1):107–12.

Winslet, M. C., V. Poxon, A. Allan, and M. R. Keighley. 1994. Mucosal glucosamine synthetase activity in inflammatory bowel disease. *Dig Dis Sci* 39 (3):540–4.

3 Glutaminase Isoforms and Glutamine Metabolism

Norman P. Curthoys

CONTENTS

3.1 INTRODUCTION

Glutamine is the most abundant free amino acid in the human body. With an arterial plasma concentration of 0.5–0.8 mM, the circulating pool of glutamine constitutes 20%–25% of the plasma amino acids. In addition, this pool turns over with a rate (350 µmol/kg h) similar to the turnover of plasma glucose (Gerich et al. 2000). The rapid turnover of plasma glutamine reflects the fact that it functions as the primary nontoxic carrier for the interorgan transport of nitrogen. Glutamine is also among the most abundant free intracellular amino acids, particularly in muscle tissue where cytosolic concentrations range from 10 to 30 mM (Rennie et al. 1996). This pool serves as a glutamine reserve that is released to the plasma in response to stress or during hypercatabolic states. To emphasize the importance of glutamine metabolism, this chapter will provide a brief overview of the interorgan metabolism of glutamine followed by a more detailed discussion of the biosynthesis, kinetic and biophysical properties, and the regulation of the various glutaminase isoforms. It concludes with a discussion of the role of glutaminase in the tissue-specific metabolism of glutamine and attempts to provide some insight for future research.

3.2 INTERORGAN METABOLISM OF GLUTAMINE

Glutamine also has a broad range of metabolic functions. Through amidotransferase reactions, the amide nitrogen of glutamine serves as the precursor for *de novo* synthesis of purines, pyrimidines, amino sugars, and asparagine in humans. In other organisms, glutamine also contributes to the synthesis of histidine and tryptophan. Glutamine also functions as the primary metabolic fuel for many rapidly dividing cells, including intestinal epithelial cells (Wu 1998), lymphocytes

(Newsholme 2001), and various cancer cells (Hensley et al. 2013). Within the brain, glutamine participates in an intercellular cycle (Albrecht et al. 2007) that generates and removes the primary excitatory and inhibitory neurotransmitters of the central nervous system. In liver, glutamine is an important precursor for ureagenesis and gluconeogenesis (Watford et al. 2002). In contrast, during metabolic acidosis, the renal catabolism of glutamine supports ammoniagenesis and glucose synthesis (Curthoys 2012).

Most of the ingested glutamine is rapidly catabolized within the epithelial cells of the small intestine (Wu 1998). The exogenous glutamine that is absorbed intact is catabolized primarily in the liver. Therefore, the abundant pool of glutamine within the body is maintained largely through *de novo* synthesis, which is catalyzed by glutamine synthetase (EC 6.3.1.2, L-glutamine:ammonia ligase [ATP]). This enzyme catalyzes the ATP-dependent addition of an ammonium ion to glutamate to form glutamine (Equation 3.1).

$$\text{L-Glutamate}^- + \text{NH}_4^+ + \text{ATP} \rightarrow \text{L-Glutamine} + \text{ADP} + \text{P}_i \tag{3.1}$$

By contrast, the catabolism of glutamine is initiated primarily by a mitochondrial glutaminase (EC 3.5.1.2, L-glutamine amidohydrolase) that catalyzes the hydrolytic cleavage of glutamine to form glutamate and an ammonium ion (Equation 3.2).

$$\text{L-Glutamine} + \text{H}_2\text{O} \rightarrow \text{L-Glutamate}^- + \text{NH}_4^+ \tag{3.2}$$

In mammals, glutamine synthetase is a cytosolic enzyme that is expressed in most cells. However, it is most abundant in muscle, lung, and adipose tissues (Taylor and Curthoys 2004). These tissues contain low levels of glutaminase and as a result constitute the major sites of net synthesis and release of glutamine to the blood. In tissues that contain high levels of both enzymes, glutamine synthetase and glutaminase are expressed in different cells. For example, glutamine synthetase is highly expressed in glial cells or astrocytes within the brain (Albrecht et al. 2010). In contrast, the brain mitochondrial glutaminase is expressed primarily in neurons and to a lesser extent in glial cells. The rapid uptake of glutamate by the glial cells and its conversion to glutamine ensure that the extracellular concentration of glutamate is maintained in the μM range, which allows secreted glutamate to function as an effective neurotransmitter while preventing excitatory neurotoxicity. In the liver, glutaminase is expressed primarily within the periportal hepatocytes (Watford and Smith 1990), while glutamine synthetase is expressed only in a small layer of perivenous hepatocytes (Gebhardt 1990). Similarly in rat kidney, glutamine synthetase is expressed predominantly in the straight portion or distal segment of the proximal tubule (Burch et al. 1978), a cell type that contains very low levels of the mitochondrial glutaminase (Curthoys and Lowry 1973). The different cellular and subcellular localizations of the two enzymes contribute to their physiological functions and may reduce the futile cycling that would result from co-localization.

3.3 PROPERTIES OF GLUTAMINASE

3.3.1 *GLS1* AND *GLS2* GENES

The human *GLS1* gene, which spans 82 kb on chromosome 2, contains 19 exons and uses alternative splicing and different polyadenylation sites to form multiple mRNAs that encode two isoforms of glutaminase (Porter et al. 2002). The kidney-type glutaminase (KGA) mRNA is the primary glutaminase transcript expressed in kidney, brain, and intestine (Shapiro et al. 1991). The KGA mRNA is derived from exons 1–14 and 16–19 and is terminated at alternative polyadenylation signals to produce mRNAs that encode a 74-kDa precursor containing 669 amino acids (Figure 3.1). The first 16 amino acids of the KGA sequence form an amphipathic α-helix that functions as a mitochondrial

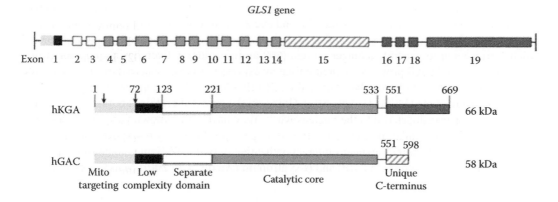

FIGURE 3.1 Structure of the human *GLS1* gene and the encoded proteins. The gene contains 19 exons that produce an initial transcript, which is alternatively spliced to encode two isoforms of glutaminase. The hKGA protein is derived from exons 1–14 and 16–19, while the hGAC protein is derived from exons 1–15. The two proteins share 550 amino acids in common but differ in their C-terminal sequences. The arrows indicate sights of cleavage by the mitochondrial processing protease.

targeting sequence (Shapiro et al. 1991). Following translocation into mitochondria, the matrix processing protease initially removes the mitochondrial targeting sequence and subsequently generates the mature 66-kDa subunit through a second cleavage after amino acid residue 72 (Srinivasan et al. 1995). A variant of the original KGA cDNA, termed GAC, was initially cloned from a human carcinoma cDNA library (Elgadi et al. 1999). The GAC mRNA is derived from exons 1 to 15 and contains a unique C-terminal coding sequence and 3′-untranslated region. The shorter GAC precursor protein contains 598 amino acids. It is also translocated into the mitochondria and similarly processed to produce a 58-kDa subunit. The N-terminus of the mature KGA and GAC proteins contain an unstructured region of low amino acid complexity. The central core region, which contains the catalytic domain, is highly conserved from bacteria to humans (Brown et al. 2008).

The human *GLS2* gene contains 18 exons (Porter et al. 2002) that span 18 kb on chromosome 12 (Aledo et al. 2000). It uses alternative promoters to transcribe two distinct mRNAs (Martin-Rufian et al. 2012), the liver-type glutaminase (LGA) and GAB (Figure 3.2). The LGA mRNA is transcribed from exons 2 to 18 to from a single 2.7-kb mRNA, which encodes a protein containing 565 amino acids that is expressed in periportal hepatocytes of the postnatal liver, pancreas, and brain (Aledo et al. 2000). The lengths of exons 3–17 of the human *GLS2* gene are identical to the lengths

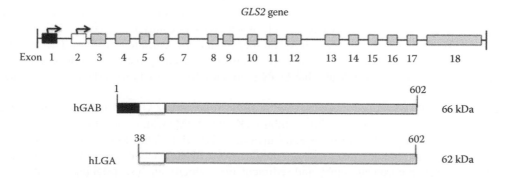

FIGURE 3.2 Structure of the human *GLS2* gene and the encoded proteins. The gene contains 18 exons with separate promoters in exons 1 and 2. Transcription of the hGAB mRNA is initiated at the promoter in exon 1, while the hLGA mRNA is transcribed from the promoter in exon 2. As a result, the hGAB protein contains 37 additional amino acids at the N-terminus. The arrows indicate the separate promoters.

of the corresponding exons in the *GLS1* gene (Porter et al. 2002). The nucleotide sequences derived from the conserved exons have a 69% identity and encode amino sequences that have 77% identity. Transcription from a separate promoter in exon 1 of the *GLS2* gene generates the GAB mRNA, which is translated to generate a longer protein (602 amino acids) in liver, brain, and some cancer cells. The LGA and GAB proteins are predominately expressed in liver, where they are translocated into the mitochondria. In brain, the LGA and GAB mRNAs constitute only about 5% of the total glutaminase transcripts (Marquez et al. 2013). However, the encoded proteins are primarily retained in the cytosol or translocated into the nucleus where they have an unknown function (Olalla et al. 2002). The different cellular distribution of the *GLS2* gene products may result from the fact that in brain their unique C-terminal segments interact with either of two PDZ-domain containing proteins, Glutaminase-interacting protein (GIP) and α-syntrophin (Aledo et al. 2001; Marquez et al. 2013).

3.3.2 KINETICS AND INHIBITORS OF GLUTAMINASE

A unique catalytic property of both the KGA and GAC isoforms is their potent activation by phosphate and other polyvalent anions (Curthoys et al. 1976). Phosphate activation correlates with the association of inactive dimers to form active tetramers (Godfrey et al. 1977; Morehouse and Curthoys 1981) and larger oligomers (Ferreira et al. 2013). In addition, the K_M for glutamine decreases from 36 to 4 mM in the presence of increasing phosphate concentration (Shapiro et al. 1982). Glutamate is a competitive inhibitor with respect to glutamine at both high and low phosphate concentrations. However, the K_I for glutamate is increased from 5 to 52 mM with increasing concentrations of phosphate. These data indicate that glutamate and glutamine bind to the same active site, but the conformation and specificity of the site are determined by the phosphate concentration and possibly the state of oligomerization.

In the postnatal liver, LGA is located in the mitochondrial matrix in loose association with the inner membrane (Kovacevic and McGivan 1983), similar to KGA (Curthoys and Weiss 1974; Kalra and Brosnan 1974). When contained in intact mitochondria, LGA exhibits a hyperbolic saturation profile for glutamine with a K_M of 6 mM, but is only slightly activated by phosphate (Kovacevic and McGivan 1983). However, purified LGA exhibits sigmoidal kinetics and a much higher $K_{0.5}$ for glutamine. In contrast to KGA, the activity of LGA is not inhibited by glutamate, but is strongly activated by ammonia, one of its products (McGivan and Bradford 1983).

Purified rat renal KGA is inactivated by the covalent and stoichiometric binding of L-2-amino-4-oxo-5-chloropentanoic acid (Shapiro, Clark, and Curthoys 1978) or 6-diazo-5-L-norleucine (DON) (Shapiro, Clark, and Curthoys 1979; Clark, Shapiro, and Curthoys 1982) (Figure 3.3a). The interaction of KGA with chloroketone is blocked by glutamate, but not glutamine, and increasing concentrations of phosphate that activate KGA decrease the rate of inactivation. Thus, this inhibitor preferentially binds to the dimeric form of KGA, which has a higher affinity for glutamate. By contrast, inactivation by DON occurs only when KGA is catalytically active. KGA activity and DON inhibition exhibit similar phosphate-dependent concentration profiles. The ability of glutamate to protect against DON inactivation is also decreased by increasing concentrations of phosphate. Thus, these data indicate that DON preferentially interacts with the active tetrameric form of KGA.

By contrast, BPTES, bis-2[5-phenylacetamido-1,2,4-thiadiazol-2-yl]ethylsulfide (Figure 3.3b), is a very specific and potent uncompetitive inhibitor (K_i of 0.2 μM) with respect to glutamine of both KGA and GAC but not LGA (Hartwick and Curthoys 2011). BPTES blocks the allosteric activation caused by phosphate binding and promotes the formation of an inactive complex (Robinson et al. 2007). Gel filtration chromatography and sedimentation velocity analysis established that BPTES prevents the formation of large phosphate-induced oligomers and instead promotes the formation of a single oligomeric species with distinct physical properties. Sedimentation equilibrium studies established that the oligomer produced by binding of BPTES is a stable tetramer. Therefore, BPTES is a potent and specific inhibitor of KGA and GAC that binds to a site other than the active site and

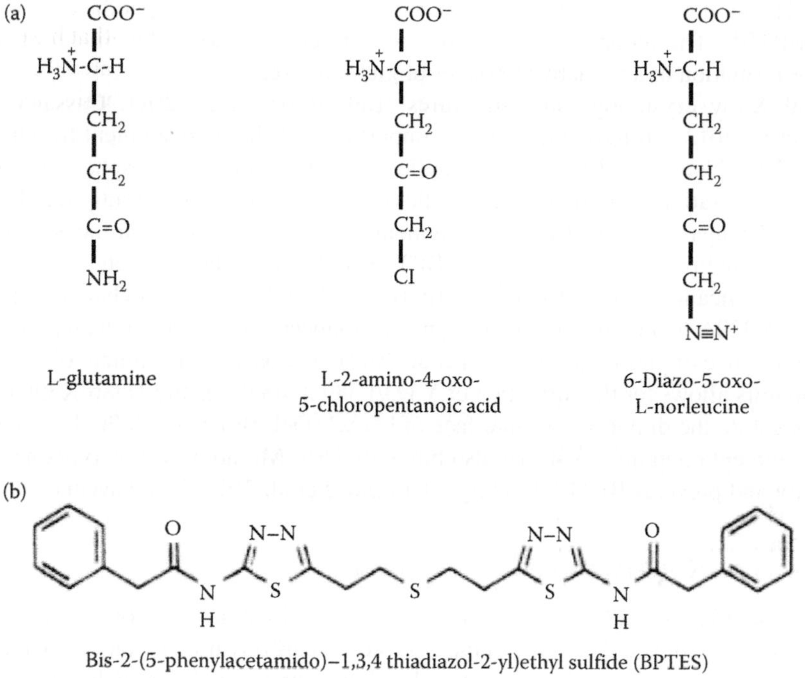

(a)

| L-glutamine | L-2-amino-4-oxo-5-chloropentanoic acid | 6-Diazo-5-oxo-L-norleucine |

COO⁻ structures:

$$COO^-$$
$$H_3\overset{+}{N}-C-H$$
$$CH_2$$
$$CH_2$$
$$C=O$$
$$NH_2$$

L-glutamine

$$COO^-$$
$$H_3\overset{+}{N}-C-H$$
$$CH_2$$
$$C=O$$
$$CH_2$$
$$Cl$$

L-2-amino-4-oxo-5-chloropentanoic acid

$$COO^-$$
$$H_3\overset{+}{N}-C-H$$
$$CH_2$$
$$CH_2$$
$$C=O$$
$$CH_2$$
$$N\equiv N^+$$

6-Diazo-5-oxo-L-norleucine

(b)

Bis-2-(5-phenylacetamido)–1,3,4 thiadiazol-2-yl)ethyl sulfide (BPTES)

FIGURE 3.3 Structure of various glutaminase inhibitors. Panel A. L-2-amino-4-oxo-5-chloropentanoic acid (chloroketone) and 6-diazo-5-oxo-L-norleucine (DON) are affinity-labeling agents that have a structure similar to the substrate, L-glutamine. Panel B. Bis-2-[(5-phenylacetamido)-1,3,4 thiadiazol-2-yl]ethyl sulfide (BPTES) is a potent allosteric inhibitor, which is specific for the KGA and GAC isoforms of glutaminase.

prevents a conformational change required for glutaminase activity. BPTES was the lead compound for the development of CB-893, which is currently being tested as an oral cancer chemotherapeutic agent that inhibits glutaminolysis (Parlati et al. 2013; Gross et al. 2014).

3.3.3 X-RAY STRUCTURE OF GLUTAMINASE

The Structural Genomics Consortium expressed the segment of human KGA (hKGA$_{221-533}$) corresponding to the catalytic domain in *E. coli*, purified and crystallized it in the presence of glutamate, and solved the 3-dimensional structure by X-ray crystallography (PDB:3CZD). This region forms a compact globular structure that is composed of two domains. One domain is entirely α-helical and the other contains both α-helices and β-sheets. The two domains form a pocket, which contains the active site serine residue. The co-crystallized glutamate molecule is tightly bound within this grove and is appropriately positioned adjacent to the active site serine residue.

More recently, the structure of hGAC$_{71-598}$ bound to BPTES was determined (DeLaBarre et al. 2011). The hGAC forms a highly symmetrical tetramer containing two molecules of BPTES that are positioned at the dimer–dimer interfaces (PDB:3UO9). The N-terminal regions of low complexity (residues 71–135) and the unique C-terminal segment (residues 547–598) were not evident in the X-ray crystallographic structure, suggesting that they are highly flexible or disordered. Residues 137–224 form small helical domains that are positioned on the sides of the tetramer opposite from the dimer–dimer interfaces. The function of this domain is unknown. The catalytic core of hGAC (residues 224–546) forms the highly conserved structure that is characteristic of all crystallized forms of glutaminase (Brown et al. 2008; DeLaBarre et al. 2011; Cassago et al. 2012; Thangavelu et al. 2012). Each BPTES interacts in a highly symmetrical fashion with residues in the loop sequences (residues 309–334) and α-helix-13 (residues 386–399) that forms the interface between two dimers. The loop sequence is normally unstructured, but it adopts a specific conformation upon binding of BPTES. The reported structure provides a detailed molecular model of how BPTES promotes the formation of an inactive tetramer of glutaminase.

Additional X-ray crystallographic structures (DeLaBarre et al. 2011; Cassago et al. 2012; Thangavelu et al. 2012) strongly implicate the importance of the loop segment (residues 309–334) and α-helix-13 (residues 386–399) in the catalytic mechanism and the phosphate-dependent oligomerization and activation of glutaminase. The flexible loop segment apparently regulates access to the active site (Thangavelu et al. 2012). This segment contains three of the amino acids (L321, F322, and L323) that form binding interactions with BPTES. Individual alanine mutations of each of these amino acids significantly reduce catalytic activity and BPTES binding (Thangavelu et al. 2012). By contrast, a K320A mutation in the loop segment enhances oligomerization and greatly activates hGAC in the absence of phosphate (Ferreira et al. 2013). Antiparallel alignment of the α-helices-13 from two subunits allows for the formation of Y393/F389 π-stacking and D386/K396 ionic interactions that constitute the dimer–dimer interface of hGAC (DeLaBarre et al. 2011; Thangavelu et al. 2012). This segment contains Y394 that also binds BPTES. Mutation of this tyrosine also reduces hGAC activity and prevents BPTES binding (DeLaBarre et al. 2011; Thangavelu et al. 2012).

3.3.4 Effects of N-Acetylation of Glutaminase

Acute regulation of KGA and GAC activity may be achieved by N-acetylation of specific lysine residues. Recent studies indicate that many of the enzymes of carbohydrate metabolism, the TCA cycle, β-oxidation, and amino acid oxidation are regulated by lysine acetylation (Choudhary et al. 2009; Zhao et al. 2010). Previous mass spectrometric screens identified K311 (Choudhary et al. 2009), K320 (Weinert et al. 2013), K328 (Wisniewski et al. 2010), and K396 (Still et al. 2013) as sites of lysine acetylation in hKGA and hGAC. All of these sites occur within the loop sequence or the α-helix-13 that binds BPTES. Mutations of residues within these segments have pronounced effects on oligomerization and activation of glutaminase. For example, K396 forms a salt bridge with D386 in the complementary α-helix that contributes to the dimer–dimer association (DeLaBarre et al. 2011). Thus, acetylation of this lysine residue would prevent this interaction and reduce formation of active tetramers. Recent mass spectrometric analysis demonstrated that acetylation of this residue in mouse LGA is significantly decreased upon re-feeding after an overnight fast (Still et al. 2013). Thus, N-acetylation of specific residues in glutaminase may regulate its activity.

When expressed in *E. coli*, the full-length recombinant rat KGA forms inclusion bodies (Shapiro et al. 1991). The N-terminal segment, containing the mitochondrial targeting signal and the region of low complexity, is encoded by exon 1. A construct that lacks this sequence (rKGA$_{\Delta 1}$) is readily expressed in *E. coli* as a soluble and fully active protein (Kenny et al. 2003). This form of purified recombinant rKGA was used to perform the initial characterization of the effects of BPTES inhibition (Robinson et al. 2007). More recently, the hKGA$_{\Delta 1}$, hGAC$_{\Delta 1}$, and hGA$_{124-551}$ segments were cloned into pET-15b and expressed with an N-terminal His$_6$-tag. The latter construct lacks the unique C-terminal sequences from either isoform. Kinetic experiments established that all three purified proteins exhibit a normal phosphate activation profile and a K_M for glutamine that is similar to the native enzyme (Hartwick and Curthoys 2011). Therefore, neither C-terminal domain is essential for catalysis.

To test the potential role of lysine acetylation, K to A mutations were introduced in the hGAC$_{\Delta 1}$ plasmid and the phosphate activation profiles of the four mutated proteins were compared to the wild-type enzyme (McDonald et al. 2015). Three of the mutations (K311A, K328A, and K396A) require significantly greater concentrations of phosphate to produce half maximal activation and exhibit increased Hill Coefficients. The fourth mutation (K320A) is highly active in the absence of phosphate and is only slightly activated by increasing concentrations of phosphate. When compared at physiological concentrations of mitochondrial phosphate, the mutations produce either a pronounced activation or significant inhibition of glutaminase activity. In addition, the K311A,

K328A, and K396A mutations exhibit increased sensitivity to BPTES, whereas the K320A mutant is resistant to BPTES inhibition. These data strongly suggest that lysine acetylation may constitute a potential mechanism to acutely regulate glutaminase activity and may alter the efficacy of this class of inhibitors.

3.4 TISSUE SPECIFIC FUNCTION OF GLUTAMINE METABOLISM

3.4.1 INTESTINE

Intestinal epithelial cells are generated in the crypt region, undergo differentiation as they migrate up the villus, and are eventually sloughed into the lumen. The continuous turnover of these cells requires significant synthesis of proteins, lipids, and nucleic acids. Dietary and plasma glutamine are quantitatively the most important precursor of both the carbon and the nitrogen used to support the *de novo* synthesis of these macromolecules. In addition, glutamine is the most important metabolic fuel for the epithelial cells of the small intestine (Reeds and Burrin 2001).

In the fed state, both dietary and arterial glutamine are rapidly extracted and catabolized by the epithelial cells of the small intestine (Windmueller and Spaeth 1980). The catabolism of glutamine, along with dietary glutamate and aspartate, accounts for nearly 80% of the CO_2 produced by these cells. By contrast, dietary and arterial glucose account for less than 10% of the total CO_2 production. The catabolism of glutamine requires its transport into mitochondria where it is deamidated by KGA. About 75% of the resulting ammonia is released to the venous blood as ammonium ions. A large portion of the remaining ammonia is used as a substrate for the mitochondrial carbamoyl phosphate synthetase and ultimately is incorporated into the ureido-nitrogen of citrulline. Some of the glutamate produced from glutamine or extracted from the lumen is consumed in the net production of ornithine, citrulline, and proline. However, most of the amino-nitrogen of glutamate is transaminated to pyruvate or glutamate semialdehyde to form alanine or ornithine, respectively. The combined release of ammonium ions, alanine, ornithine, citrulline, and proline account for 97% of the nitrogen derived from the catabolized glutamine. The α-ketoglutarate, generated in the transamination reactions, is partially oxidized in the TCA cycle to produce CO_2, lactate, and pyruvate.

In the post-absorptive state, the small intestine continues to extract and catabolize significant amounts of arterial glutamine through the same pathways (Windmueller and Spaeth 1978). The catabolism of this single amino acid now generates approximately one-third of the total CO_2 produced by the epithelial cells. This catabolism continues to generate ammonium ions and alanine, but lesser amounts of ornithine, citrulline, and proline. The bulk of the CO_2 production (50%) is now derived from the catabolism of ketone bodies, while glucose and lactate are still extracted and catabolized at slow rates to produce less than 10% of the total CO_2. A significant portion of the citrulline generated from the catabolism of glutamine is subsequently extracted by the kidney and converted to arginine (Windmueller and Spaeth 1981; Reeds and Burrin 2001). Thus, glutamine is an important metabolic fuel for the small intestine and an important precursor for the synthesis of various nonessential amino acids.

3.4.2 LIVER

The liver plays a major role in glutamine homeostasis (Watford et al. 2002). The expression of high levels of LGA and glutamine synthetase allows the liver to both catabolize and synthesize glutamine. In the fed state, the two processes occur at similar rates and there is little net extraction or release of glutamine across the liver. However, the combined reactions contribute significantly to the ability of the liver to detoxify the ammonium ions that are derived from the portal venous blood and generated by the hepatic catabolism of amino acids.

The portal venous blood contains a high concentration of ammonium ions that are derived from bacterial metabolism in the colon and the catabolism of glutamine in the small intestine. This blood passes through the liver where it accounts for 70%–80% of the hepatic blood supply. The removal of ammonium ions is facilitated by the differential expression of various enzymes within discrete zones of the hepatic acinar (Haussinger et al. 1992). LGA and the enzymes of urea synthesis are most abundant in periportal hepatocytes that are located near the portal venule (Watford et al. 2002). The levels of these enzymes decrease in the hepatocytes that are progressively encountered as the blood diffuses through the liver. By contrast, glutamine synthetase is localized solely in perivenous hepatocytes, the final layer of 1–3 cells that surround the hepatic venule (Gebhardt 1990). As a result of this zonal distribution, the bulk of ammonium ions, derived from the portal blood and from the hepatic catabolism of glutamine and other amino acids, are used to synthesize urea. This pathway has a high capacity, but low affinity for ammonium ions. Most of the remaining ammonium ions are used as a substrate for glutamine synthetase, an enzyme that has a higher affinity for ammonium ions. The sequential synthesis of urea and glutamine creates a highly efficient system to ensure that systemic levels of ammonium ions are maintained at nontoxic levels (Haussinger 1998).

A unique property of LGA is its activation by ammonium ions (Haussinger 1998; Watford et al. 2002). This property may provide a mechanism by which intestinal catabolism of glutamine activates hepatic utilization. Alternatively, ammonium ions may function as a feed-forward activator of LGA to ensure sufficient synthesis of mitochondrial glutamate and N-acetylglutamate (Brosnan and Brosnan 2002). The latter compound is an essential activator of urea synthesis. Thus, this pathway may constitute a regulatory loop that maintains an appropriate balance between the rate of ammonium ion production and urea cycle activity.

Hepatic utilization and synthesis of glutamine are significantly affected by changes in acid–base balance (Haussinger 1997). This adaptation occurs without significant changes in the levels of LGA or glutamine synthetase, but may due to the reciprocal pH activation profiles of the two enzymes (Watford 1991). A slight decrease in intracellular pH causes a decrease in LGA activity but activates the glutamine synthetase (Haussinger et al. 1992; Haussinger 1997). Therefore, the onset of metabolic acidosis results in a sparing of glutamine and a corresponding decrease in urea synthesis. As a result, the liver becomes a net producer of glutamine, which supports the increased renal extraction of glutamine. In the kidney, the catabolism of glutamine generates 2 moles of NH_4^+ and HCO_3^- ions that are differentially partitioned into the urine and the plasma, respectively (Curthoys 2012). Thus, total nitrogen excretion remains constant. However, the combined processes result in a net production of HCO_3^- ions that partially compensate the metabolic acidosis.

3.4.3 Brain

In the brain, KGA participates in the intercellular glutamate–glutamine cycle that generates and removes the excitatory neurotransmitter, glutamate (Masson et al. 2006). The cycle effectively ensures that extracellular glutamate is maintained at a very low μM concentration within the brain. Glutamate is normally removed from the extracellular fluid through its efficient uptake by glial cells. These cells contain a high level of glutamine synthetase, which rapidly converts glutamate to glutamine, which is then transported into the extracellular fluid where it is maintained at a high concentration (0.2–1 mM). Glutamine is also transported across the plasma membrane and into the mitochondria of specific neurons that express a high level of KGA, which regenerates glutamate. The resulting glutamate is then stored in secretory vesicles and is released by exocytosis in response to a neuronal impulse. The released glutamate binds to specific receptors on the adjacent neuron where it initiates an electrical impulse. The stimulation is made transient due to the rapid removal of glutamate by the glial cells and its recycling to glutamine.

An increase in extracellular glutamate causes excitotoxicity and contributes to neuronal cell death resulting from stroke, trauma, and chronic neurodegenerative diseases (Rothman and Olney 1986; Choi and Rothman 1990; Meldrum 1994; Muir and Lees 1995). The release of glutaminase from damaged neurons in cell culture results in the formation of extracellular glutamate and initiates a progression of excitotoxicity (Newcomb et al. 1997). Additional studies demonstrated that following brain injury, high levels of released glutaminase activity may contribute to the expanding zone of neuronal damage that evolves for 24–48 h after a stroke (Newcomb et al. 1998). Thus, gradual release of glutaminase from disrupted neurons is a potential contributor to the *in vivo* development of glutamate excitotoxicity. Subsequent studies indicated that release of glutaminase from HIV-infected macrophages (Zhao et al. 2004) and microglia (Huang et al. 2011) may also contribute to HIV-associated dementia. The observed effects were prevented by BPTES inhibition or siRNA knockdown of GA (Erdmann et al. 2007, 2009; Huang et al. 2011). Based on these observations, it was proposed that a non-membrane permeable inhibitor of the released glutaminase would be an effective treatment to reduce the morbidity associated with a stroke or HIV-associated dementia. More recent studies have also demonstrated that BPTES selectively inhibits the growth of glioblastoma cells that express the R134 mutation in isocitrate dehydrogenase (Seltzer et al. 2010). This mutation is frequently found in gliomas and acute myelogenous leukemia (Dang et al. 2009; Ward et al. 2010). The effect of BPTES was reproduced by selective siRNA knockdown of glutaminase and was reversed by providing an exogenous source of α-ketoglutarate.

3.4.4 KIDNEY

Previous micropuncture studies (Sajo et al. 1981) and assays using microdissected nephron segments (Good and Burg 1984) established that the preponderance of renal glutamine catabolism in normal or acidotic rats occurs within the proximal convoluted tubule. Most of the ammonium ions, which enter the lumen of the proximal tubule, are subsequently reabsorbed within the medullary thick ascending limb to produce an elevated concentration of ammonium ions within the renal medulla (Karim et al. 2002; Karim et al. 2006). This gradient provides the driving force for the final transport of ammonium ions into the urine, which occurs via the specific ammonia transporters, Rhbg and Rhcg, which are located in the basolateral and apical membranes of the distal tubule and collecting duct (Weiner and Verlander 2014). However, during normal acid–base balance, KGA activity is greatest in the medullary thick ascending limb, the distal convoluted tubule, and the inner medullary collecting duct (Curthoys and Lowry 1973; Wright and Knepper 1990a,b). By contrast, during chronic acidosis, a pronounced increase in KGA expression occurs only in the early segments of the proximal tubule.

During normal acid–base balance, the kidneys extract and metabolize very little of the plasma glutamine. For example, the measured rat renal arterial-venous difference is less than 3% of the arterial concentration of glutamine (Squires et al. 1976), and only 7% of the plasma glutamine is extracted by the human kidneys after an overnight fast (Meyer et al. 2002). Therefore, renal uptake is significantly less than the 20% of plasma glutamine that is filtered by the glomeruli. Nearly all of the filtered glutamine is reabsorbed within the proximal convoluted tubule and transported across the basolateral membrane (Silbernagl 1980). Utilization of the small fraction of extracted plasma glutamine requires its transport into the mitochondrial matrix where glutamine is deamidated by KGA. A mitochondrial glutamine transporter was partially purified from rat kidney and shown by reconstitution in lipid vesicles to be specific for glutamine and asparagine (Indiveri et al. 1998). Neither the amino acid sequence nor the gene that encodes this transporter has been identified. However, the KGA activity, measured in crude extracts, is much greater than that required to accomplish the normal catabolism of glutamine. Therefore, in order to accomplish the effective reabsorption of glutamine either the activity of the mitochondrial glutamine transporter or KGA must be largely inhibited or inactivated *in vivo* during normal acid–base balance.

Acute onset of a metabolic acidosis produces rapid changes in the interorgan metabolism of glutamine (Tamarappoo et al. 1990) that support a rapid and pronounced increase in renal catabolism of glutamine. The arterial plasma glutamine concentration is rapidly increased twofold (Hughey et al. 1980) due primarily to an increased release of glutamine from muscle tissue (Schrock et al. 1980). Renal extraction of glutamine is evident within 1 h and by 3 h net extraction by the kidneys reaches 35% of the plasma glutamine (Hughey et al. 1980), a level that significantly exceeds the 20% filtered by the glomeruli. Thus, the direction of basolateral glutamine transport must be reversed in order for the proximal convoluted tubule to extract glutamine from both the glomerular filtrate and the venous blood. During the first 4 h following onset of acidosis, the net excretion of ammonium ions is increased sixfold (Sleeper et al. 1978). To accomplish this adaptation, the transport of glutamine into the mitochondria (Sastrasinh and Sastrasinh 1990) and/or KGA activity must be acutely activated. Additional responses include a prompt acidification of the urine that results from translocation (Yang et al. 2000) and acute activation (Horie et al. 1990) of NHE3, the apical Na^+/H^+ exchanger. NHE3 can also transport NH_4^+ ions in place of H^+. Thus, the increased NHE3 activity also facilitates the rapid removal of cellular ammonium ions (Tannen and Ross 1979) and ensures that the bulk of the ammonium ions generated from the amide and amine nitrogens of glutamine are excreted in the urine. Finally, during acute acidosis, the cellular concentrations of glutamate and α-ketoglutarate are significantly decreased within the rat renal cortex (Lowry and Ross 1980). The two compounds are products of the KGA and glutamate dehydrogenase (GDH) reactions, respectively. Therefore, the acute increase in renal ammoniagenesis results from an increased availability of glutamine and the rapid activation of key transport processes and KGA and GDH activities. All of these adaptations precede the increased expression of the enzymes of renal ammoniagenesis (Hwang and Curthoys 1991; Wright et al. 1992; Schoolwerth et al. 1994). Thus, the cells of the renal proximal convoluted tubule must sense acute changes in extracellular or intracellular pH and/or HCO_3^- concentration and activate a signaling pathway that enhances flux through the existing GA, GDH, and TCA cycle enzymes.

During chronic acidosis, acute decreases in cellular glutamate and α-ketoglutarate are partially reversed and the arterial plasma concentration of glutamine is decreased to 70% of normal (Squires et al. 1976; Lowry and Ross 1980). However, more than a third of the plasma glutamine is still extracted in a single pass through the kidneys. Increased expression of genes that encode key transporters and enzymes of glutamine metabolism now contribute to the sustained increase in renal catabolism of glutamine. The most rapid adaptation is the pronounced increase (sixfold) in phosphoenolpyruvate carboxykinase (PEPCK) that also occurs only in the proximal convoluted tubule, but requires 8–24 h to achieve (Schoolwerth et al. 1994). The basolateral SNAT3 (SLC38A3), a high-affinity glutamine transporter, is also increased with similar kinetics in the early segments of the proximal tubule (Moret et al. 2007). The latter adaptation may contribute to the basolateral uptake of glutamine during chronic acidosis. More gradual increases in levels of mitochondrial KGA (Curthoys and Lowry 1973; Wright and Knepper 1990a,b) and GDH (Wright and Knepper 1990a,b) also occur within the proximal convoluted tubule but require 4–7 days to accomplish. Glutamine uptake in mitochondria from normal rats is mediated through two glutamine antiporters, whereas a highly active glutamine uniporter is evident only in mitochondria prepared from chronic acidotic rats (Atlante et al. 1994). Acute activation and subsequent increase in expression of NHE3 (Preisig and Alpern 1988; Ambuhl et al. 1996; Wu et al. 1996) acidifies the fluid in the tubular lumen and contributes to the active transport of ammonium ions (Tannen and Ross 1979). As a result, increased renal ammoniagenesis continues to provide an expendable cation that facilitates excretion of strong acids while conserving sodium and potassium ions. The filtered HCO_3^- load is decreased in metabolic acidosis, but the percent recovered in the proximal tubule is increased. In rats (Pagliara and Goodman 1970; Roobol and Alleyne 1974) and humans (Gerich et al. 2001), the α-ketoglutarate generated from renal catabolism of glutamine is primarily converted to glucose. This process requires PEPCK activity to divert oxaloactetate, derived from intermediates of the TCA cycle, into the pathway of gluconeogenesis. The combined pathways of ammoniagenesis and gluconeogenesis result in a net production of 2 NH_4^+ and 2 HCO_3^- ions per glutamine. Activation of NBCe1A (Preisig and Alpern 1988), the basolateral $Na^+/3 HCO_3^-$ co-transporter, facilitates the translocation of reabsorbed and *de novo*-synthesized HCO_3^- ions into the renal venous blood. Thus, the combined adaptations also create a net renal release of HCO_3^- ions that partially restores acid–base balance.

Acute recovery from metabolic acidosis results in an abrupt decrease in renal ammoniagenesis that is accompanied by rapid ($t_{1/2} = 5$ h) and coordinate decreases in PEPCK and KGA mRNAs (Hwang and Curthoys 1991; Hwang et al. 1991). However, it requires 4–7 days for the induced level of KGA protein to return to normal. This observation provides further evidence that the *in vivo* activities of the mitochondrial glutamine transporter and/or KGA are rapidly inactivated when normal acid–base balance is restored. This acute regulation may result from rapid changes in N-acetylation of specific lysine residues in KGA.

3.4.5 CANCER CELLS

Most cancer cells take up large amounts of glucose that are consumed primarily by aerobic glycolysis to form lactate (Warburg et al. 1927). To maintain mitochondrial function, transformed cells also exhibit an increased catabolism of glutamine to lactate (DeBerardinis et al. 2008). This pathway, termed glutaminolysis, generates ATP, NADPH, and the precursors necessary to support the synthesis of the nucleotides and lipids that are required for cell division. As a result, many transformed cells require glutamine as an essential nutrient. To support this addiction to glutamine, transformed cells frequently exhibit an increased expression of a mitochondrial glutaminase (DeBerardinis et al. 2007; Erickson and Cerione 2010). Early studies used Ehrlich ascites tumor cells to demonstrate the role of KGA in maintaining a transformed phenotype (Segura et al. 2001). The tumor cells, which were stably transfected with a plasmid that encoded a KGA antisense RNA, lost their transformed phenotype and failed to produce tumors when injected into mice. Interest in glutaminase as a potential cancer chemotherapeutic target was kindled further by two recent studies. The initial study demonstrated that increased expression of the c-Myc oncogene in human P-493 B lymphoma cells resulted in increased expression of KGA (Gao et al. 2009). Further experiments demonstrated that c-Myc expression suppressed the synthesis of two microRNAs, miR-23a/b, that inhibit KGA expression. The authors also demonstrated that siRNA knockdown of KGA significantly decreased the rates of proliferation of P493 B cells and human PC3 prostate cancer cells, two transformed cell lines that exhibit oncogenic levels of c-Myc. In the second study (Wang et al. 2010), compound 968 was identified as a potent inhibitor of the cellular transformation that was produced by expression of an oncogenic Dbl, a mutated form of a Rho-family guanine nucleotide exchange factor. Subsequent pull-down and mass spectrometric analysis identified GAC as the target of 968. Additional studies established that siRNA knockdown of GAC mimicked the effects of 968. Both treatments inhibited the ability of three constitutively activated Rac or Rho GTPases to stimulate growth in low serum or in soft agar. GAC knockdown also inhibited proliferation of transformed NIH3T3 fibroblasts and of breast cancer cells. As a result, mitochondrial glutaminase has become an important target for development of an effective cancer chemotherapeutic drug.

3.5 CONCLUSIONS AND PROSPECTIVE

Glutamine is the central metabolite in nitrogen metabolism. It serves as the most abundant nontoxic carrier of ammonium ions, which is used for hepatic urea synthesis and renal ammoniagenesis. The α-amino and amide nitrogens of glutamine also serve as precursors for the biosynthesis of most other nitrogen-containing compounds. In addition, the oxidation of glutamine generates the bulk of the ATP and the precursors for lipid synthesis in rapidly growing cells. Many of the biosynthetic reactions, which utilize glutamine, are catalyzed by an amidotransferase. However, the bulk of glutamine metabolism is initiated by a mitochondrial glutaminase that is encoded by the *GLS1* or *GLS2* gene. The mechanisms, which regulated increased expression of KGA in the kidney during acidosis or various glutaminase isoforms in cancer cells, have been partially characterized. However, much less is known regarding the acute regulation of glutaminase activity. Maximal *in vitro* activation of KGA and GAC requires very high nonphysiological concentrations of phosphate. It is unknown if some other polyvalent anion functions as the physiological activator. Alternatively, lysine acetylation may acutely regulate glutaminase activity. Interestingly, the $K_{320}A$ mutation enhances oligomerization and greatly activates hGAC in the absence of phosphate. Thus, this mutation may lock the enzyme in a conformation that mimics the phosphate-activated form of glutaminase. All of the previously reported structures of KGA and GAC are thought to model the inactive form of the enzyme. Therefore, it would be interesting to crystallize and solve the structure of the $K_{320}A$ mutant. This mutant is also resistant to BPTES inhibition, which was the lead compound for the development of CB-839, a potential cancer chemotherapeutic agent. Thus, it will also be important to determine if acetylation of specific lysine residues affects the sensitivity of GAC to this class of inhibitors.

REFERENCES

Albrecht, J., M. Sidoryk-Wegrzynowicz, M. Zielinska et al. 2010. Roles of glutamine in neurotransmission. *Neuron Glia Biol* 6 (4):263–276.

Albrecht, J., U. Sonnewald, H. S. Waagepetersen et al. 2007. Glutamine in the central nervous system: Function and dysfunction. *Front Biosci* 12:332–343.

Aledo, J. C., P. M. Gomez-Fabre, L. Olalla et al. 2000. Identification of two human glutaminase loci and tissue-specific expression of the two related genes. *Mamm Genome* 11 (12):1107–1110.

Aledo, J. C., A. Rosado, L. Olalla et al. 2001. Overexpression, purification, and characterization of glutaminase-interacting protein, a PDZ-domain protein from human brain. *Protein Expr Purif* 23 (3):411–418.

Ambuhl, P. M., M. Amemiya, M. Danczkay et al. 1996. Chronic metabolic acidosis increases NHE3 protein abundance in rat kidney. *Am J Physiol* 271 (4 Pt 2):F917–F925.

Atlante, A., S. Passarella, G. M. Minervini et al. 1994. Glutamine transport in normal and acidotic rat kidney mitochondria. *Arch Biochem Biophys* 315 (2):369–381.

Brosnan, J. T. and M. E. Brosnan. 2002. Hepatic glutaminase—A special role in urea synthesis? *Nutrition* 18 (6):455–457.

Brown, G., A. Singer, M. Proudfoot et al. 2008. Functional and structural characterization of four glutaminases from *Escherichia coli* and Bacillus subtilis. *Biochemistry* 47 (21):5724–5735.

Burch, H. B., S. Choi, W. Z. McCarthy et al. 1978. The location of glutamine synthetase within the rat and rabbit nephron. *Biochem Biophys Res Commun* 82 (2):498–505.

Cassago, A., A. P. Ferreira, I. M. Ferreira et al. 2012. Mitochondrial localization and structure-based phosphate activation mechanism of Glutaminase C with implications for cancer metabolism. *Proc Natl Acad Sci USA* 109 (4):1092–1097.

Choi, D. W. and S. M. Rothman. 1990. The role of glutamate neurotoxicity in hypoxic-ischemic neuronal death. *Ann Rev Neurosci* 13 (1):171–182.

Choudhary, C., C. Kumar, F. Gnad et al. 2009. Lysine acetylation targets protein complexes and co-regulates major cellular functions. *Science* 325:834–840.

Clark, V. M., R. A. Shapiro, and N. P. Curthoys. 1982. Comparison of the hydrolysis and the covalent binding of 6-diazo-5-oxo-L-[6-14C]norleucine by rat renal phosphate-dependent glutaminase. *Arch Biochem Biophys* 213 (1):232–239.

Curthoys, N. P. 2012. Renal ammonium ion production and excretion. In *The Kidney: Physiology and Pathophysiology*, 5th ed. (R. J. Alpern, O. W. Moe, and M. Caplan, Eds.), Elsevier, San Diego, 1993–2018.

Curthoys, N. P., T. Kuhlenschmidt, and S. S. Godfrey. 1976. Regulation of renal ammoniagenesis. Purification of phosphate-dependent glutaminase from rat kidney. *Arch Biochem Biophys* 174:82–89.

Curthoys, N. P. and O. H. Lowry. 1973. The distribution of glutaminase isoenzymes in the various structures of the nephron in normal, acidotic, and alkalotic rat kidney. *J Biol Chem* 248 (1):162–168.

Curthoys, N. P. and R. F. Weiss. 1974. Regulation of renal ammoniagenesis. Subcellular localization of rat kidney glutaminase isoenzymes. *J Biol Chem* 249 (10):3261–3266.

Dang, L., D. W. White, S. Gross et al. 2009. Cancer-associated IDH1 mutations produce 2-hydroxyglutarate. *Nature* 462 (7274):739–744.

DeBerardinis, R. J., J. J. Lum, G. Hatzivassiliou et al. 2008. The biology of cancer: Metabolic reprogramming fuels cell growth and proliferation. *Cell Metab* 7 (1):11–20.

DeBerardinis, R. J., A. Mancuso, E. Daikhin et al. 2007. Beyond aerobic glycolysis: Transformed cells can engage in glutamine metabolism that exceeds the requirement for protein and nucleotide synthesis. *Proc Natl Acad Sci USA* 104 (49):19345–19350.

DeLaBarre, B., S. Gross, C. Fang et al. 2011. Full-length human glutaminase in complex with an allosteric inhibitor. *Biochemistry* 50 (50):10764–10770.

Elgadi, K. M., R. A. Meguid, M. Qian et al. 1999. Cloning and analysis of unique human glutaminase isoforms generated by tissue-specific alternative splicing. *Physiol Genomics* 1 (2):51–62.

Erdmann, N., C. Tian, Y. Huang et al. 2009. *In vitro* glutaminase regulation and mechanisms of glutamate generation in HIV-1-infected macrophage. *J Neurochem* 109 (2):551–561.

Erdmann, N., J. Zhao, A. L. Lopez et al. 2007. Glutamate production by HIV-1 infected human macrophage is blocked by the inhibition of glutaminase. *J Neurochem* 102 (2):539–549.

Erickson, J. W. and R. A. Cerione. 2010. Glutaminase: A hot spot for regulation of cancer cell metabolism? *Oncotarget* 1 (8):734–740.

Ferreira, A. P., A. Cassago, A. Goncalves Kde et al. 2013. Active glutaminase C self-assembles into a supra-tetrameric oligomer that can be disrupted by an allosteric inhibitor. *J Biol Chem* 288 (39):28009–28020.

Gao, P., I. Tchernyshyov, T. C. Chang et al. 2009. c-Myc suppression of miR-23a/b enhances mitochondrial glutaminase expression and glutamine metabolism. *Nature* 458 (7239):762–765.

Gebhardt, R. 1990. Heterogeneous intrahepatic distribution of glutamine synthetase. *Acta Histochem Suppl* 40:23–28.

Gerich, J. E., C. Meyer, and M. W. Stumvoll. 2000. Hormonal control of renal and systemic glutamine metabolism. *J Nutr* 130 (4S Suppl):995S–1001S.

Gerich, J. E., C. Meyer, H. J. Woerle et al. 2001. Renal gluconeogenesis: Its importance in human glucose homeostasis. *Diabetes Care* 24 (2):382–391.

Godfrey, S. S., T. Kuhlenschmidt, and N. P. Curthoys. 1977. Correlation between activation and dimer formation of rat renal phosphate-dependent glutaminase. *J Biol Chem* 252:1927–1931.

Good, D. W. and M. B. Burg. 1984. Ammonia production by individual segments of the rat nephron. *J Clin Invest* 73 (3):602–610.

Gross, M. I., S. D. Demo, J. B. Dennison et al. 2014. Antitumor activity of the glutaminase inhibitor CB-839 in triple-negative breast cancer. *Mol Cancer Ther* 13 (4):890–901.

Hartwick, E. W. and N. P. Curthoys. 2011. BPTES inhibition of hGA(124-551), a truncated form of human kidney-type glutaminase. *J Enzyme Inhib MedChem* 27 (6):861–867.

Haussinger, D. 1997. Liver regulation of acid–base balance. *Miner Electrolyte Metab* 23 (3–6):249–452.

Haussinger, D. 1998. Hepatic glutamine transport and metabolism. *Adv Enzymol Relat Areas Mol Biol* 72:43–86.

Haussinger, D., W. H. Lamers, and A. F. Moorman. 1992. Hepatocyte heterogeneity in the metabolism of amino acids and ammonia. *Enzyme* 46 (1–3):72–93.

Hensley, C. T., A. T. Wasti, and R. J. DeBerardinis. 2013. Glutamine and cancer: Cell biology, physiology, and clinical opportunities. *J Clin Invest* 123 (9):3678–3684.

Horie, S., O. Moe, A. Tejedor et al. 1990. Preincubation in acid medium increases Na/H antiporter activity in cultured renal proximal tubule cells. *Proc Natl Acad Sci USA* 87 (12):4742–4745.

Huang, Z., L. Zhao, B. Jia et al. 2011. Glutaminase dysregulation in HIV-1-infected human microglia mediates neurotoxicity: Relevant to HIV-1 associated neurocognitive disorders. *J Neurosci* 31:15195–15204.

Hughey, R. P., B. B. Rankin, and N. P. Curthoys. 1980. Acute acidosis and renal arteriovenous differences of glutamine in normal and adrenalectomized rats. *Am J Physiol* 238 (3):F199–F204.

Hwang, J. J. and N. P. Curthoys. 1991. Effect of acute alterations in acid–base balance on rat renal glutaminase and phosphoenolpyruvate carboxykinase gene expression. *J Biol Chem* 266 (15):9392–9396.

Hwang, J. J., S. Perera, R. A. Shapiro et al. 1991. Mechanism of altered renal glutaminase gene expression in response to chronic acidosis. *Biochemistry* 30 (30):7522–7526.

Indiveri, C., G. Abruzzo, I. Stipani et al. 1998. Identification and purification of the reconstitutively active glutamine carrier from rat kidney mitochondria. *Biochem J* 333 (Pt 2):285–290.

Kalra, J. and J. T. Brosnan. 1974. The subcellular localization of glutaminase isoenzymes in rat kidney cortex. *J Biol Chem* 249 (10):3255–3260.

Karim, Z., A. Attmane-Elakeb, and M. Bichara. 2002. Renal handling of NH_4^+ in relation to the control of acid–base balance by the kidney. *J Nephrol* 15 (Suppl 5):S128–S134.

Karim, Z., M. Szutkowska, C. Vernimmen et al. 2006. Recent concepts concerning the renal handling of NH_3/NH_4^+. *J Nephrol* 19 (Suppl 9):S27–S32.

Kenny, J., Y. Bao, B. Hamm et al. 2003. Bacterial expression, purification, and characterization of rat kidney-type mitochondrial glutaminase. *Protein Expr Purif* 31 (1):140–148.

Kovacevic, Z. and J. D. McGivan. 1983. Mitochondrial metabolism of glutamine and glutamate and its physiological significance. *Physiol Rev* 63 (2):547–605.

Lowry, M. and B. D. Ross. 1980. Activation of oxoglutarate dehydrogenase in the kidney in response to acute acidosis. *Biochem J* 190 (3):771–780.

Marquez, J., C. Cardona, J. A. Campos-Sandoval et al. 2013. Mammalian glutaminase isozymes in brain. *Metab Brain Dis* 28 (2):133–137.

Martin-Rufian, M., M. Tosina, J. A. Campos-Sandoval et al. 2012. Mammalian glutaminase Gls2 gene encodes two functional alternative transcripts by a surrogate promoter usage mechanism. *PLoS One* 7 (6):e38380.

Masson, J., M. Darmon, A. Conjard et al. 2006. Mice lacking brain/kidney phosphate-activated glutaminase have impaired glutamatergic synaptic transmission, altered breathing, disorganized goal-directed behavior and die shortly after birth. *J Neurosci* 26 (17):4660–4671.

McDonald, C. J., E. Acheff, R. Kennedy et al. 2015. Effect of lysine to alanine mutations on the phosphate activation and BPTES inhibition of glutaminase. *Neurochem Internat* 88:10–14.

McGivan, J. D. and N. M. Bradford. 1983. Characteristics of the activation of glutaminase by ammonia in sonicated rat liver mitochondria. *Biochim Biophys Acta* 759 (3):296–302.

Meldrum, B. S. 1994. The role of glutamante in epilepsy and other CNS disorders. *Neurology* 44 (Suppl 8):S14–S23.

Meyer, C., M. Stumvoll, J. Dostou et al. 2002. Renal substrate exchange and gluconeogenesis in normal postabsorptive humans. *Am J Physiol Endocrinol Metab* 282 (2):E428–E434.

Morehouse, R. F. and N. P. Curthoys. 1981. Properties of rat renal phosphate-dependent glutaminase coupled to sepharose. Evidence that dimerization is essential for activation. *Biochem J* 193:709–716.

Moret, C., M. H. Dave, N. Schulz et al. 2007. Regulation of renal amino acid transporters during metabolic acidosis. *Am J Physiol Renal Physiol* 292 (2):F555–F566.

Muir, K. W. and K. R. Lees. 1995. Clinical experience with excitatory amino acid antagonist drugs. *Stroke* 26:503–513.

Newcomb, R., A. R. Pierce, T. Kano et al. 1998. Characterization of mitochondrial glutaminase and amino acids at prolonged times after experimental focal cerebral ischemia. *Brain Res* 813 (1):103–111.

Newcomb, R., X. Sun, L. Taylor et al. 1997. Increased production of extracellular glutamate by the mitochondrial glutaminase following neuronal death. *J Biol Chem* 272 (17):11276–11282.

Newsholme, P. 2001. Why is L-glutamine metabolism important to cells of the immune system in health, postinjury, surgery or infection? *J Nutr* 131 (9 Suppl):S2515–S2522.

Olalla, L., A. Gutierrez, J. A. Campos et al. 2002. Nuclear localization of L-type glutaminase in mammalian brain. *J Biol Chem* 277 (41):38939–38944.

Pagliara, A. S. and A. D. Goodman. 1970. Relation of renal cortical gluconeogenesis, glutamate content, and production of ammonia. *J Clin Invest* 49 (11):1967–1974.

Parlati, F., S. Bromley-Dulfano, S. Demo et al. 2013. Antitumor activity of the glutaminase inhibitor CB-839 in hematological malignances. *Blood* 122:4226.

Porter, L. D., H. Ibrahim, L. Taylor et al. 2002. Complexity and species variation of the kidney-type glutaminase gene. *Physiol Genomics* 9 (3):157–166.

Preisig, P. A. and R. J. Alpern. 1988. Chronic metabolic acidosis causes an adaptation in the apical membrane Na/H antiporter and basolateral membrane Na(HCO$_3$)$_3$ symporter in the rat proximal convoluted tubule. *J Clin Invest* 82 (4):1445–1453.

Reeds, P. J. and D. G. Burrin. 2001. Glutamine and the bowel. *J Nutr* 131 (9 Suppl):S2505–S2508.

Rennie, M. J., A. Ahmed, S. E. Khogali et al. 1996. Glutamine metabolism and transport in skeletal muscle and heart and their clinical relevance. *J Nutr* 126 (4 Suppl):S1142–S1149.

Robinson, M. M., S. J. McBryant, T. Tsukamoto et al. 2007. Novel mechanism of inhibition of rat kidney-type glutaminase by bis-2-(5-phenylacetamido-1,2,4-thiadiazol-2-yl)ethyl sulfide (BPTES). *Biochem J* 406 (3):407–414.

Roobol, A. and G. A. Alleyne. 1974. Control of renal cortex ammoniagenesis and its relationship to renal cortex gluconeogenesis. *Biochim Biophys Acta* 362 (1):83–91.

Rothman, S. M. and J. W. Olney. 1986. Glutamate and the pathopysiology of hypoxic-ischemic brain damage. *Ann Neurol* 2:105–111.

Sajo, I. M., M. B. Goldstein, H. Sonnenberg et al. 1981. Sites of ammonia addition to tubular fluid in rats with chronic metabolic acidosis. *Kidney Int* 20 (3):353–358.

Sastrasinh, M. and S. Sastrasinh. 1990. Effect of acute pH change on mitochondrial glutamine transport. *Am J Physiol* 259 (6 Pt 2):F863–F866.

Schoolwerth, A. C., P. A. deBoer, A. F. Moorman et al. 1994. Changes in mRNAs for enzymes of gluta-mine metabolism in kidney and liver during ammonium chloride acidosis. *Am J Physiol* 267 (3 Pt 2):F400–406.

Schrock, H., C. J. Cha, and L. Goldstein. 1980. Glutamine release from hindlimb and uptake by kidney in the acutely acidotic rat. *Biochem J* 188 (2):557–560.

Segura, J. A., M. A. Ruiz-Bellido, M. Arenas et al. 2001. Ehrlich ascites tumor cells expressing anti-sense glu-taminase mRNA lose their capacity to evade the mouse immune system. *Int J Cancer* 91 (3):379–384.

Seltzer, M. J., B. D. Bennett, A. D. Joshi et al. 2010. Inhibition of glutaminase preferentially slows growth of glioma cells with mutant IDH1. *Cancer Res* 70 (22):8981–8987.

Shapiro, R. A., V. M. Clark, and N. P. Curthoys. 1978. Covalent interaction of L-2-amino-4-oxo-5-chloropentanoic acid with rat renal phosphate-dependent glutaminase. Evidence for a specific glutamate binding site and of subunit heterogeneity. *J Biol Chem* 253 (19):7086–7090.

Shapiro, R. A., V. M. Clark, and N. P. Curthoys. 1979. Inactivation of rat renal phosphate-dependent gluta-minase with 6-diazo-5-oxo-L-norleucine. Evidence for interaction at the glutamine binding site. *J Biol Chem* 254 (8):2835–2838.

Shapiro, R. A., L. Farrell, M. Srinivasan et al. 1991. Isolation, characterization, and *in vitro* expression of a cDNA that encodes the kidney isoenzyme of the mitochondrial glutaminase. *J Biol Chem* 266 (28):18792–18796.

Shapiro, R. A., R. F. Morehouse, and N. P. Curthoys. 1982. Inhibition by glutamate of phosphate-dependent glutaminase of rat kidney. *Biochem J* 207 (3):561–566.

Silbernagl, S. 1980. Tubular reabsorption of L-glutamine studied by free-flow micropuncture and microperfu-sion of rat kidney. *Int J Biochem* 12 (1–2):9–16.

Sleeper, R. S., L. L. Vertuno, F. Strauss et al. 1978. Effects of acid challenge on *in vivo* and *in vitro* rat renal ammoniagenesis. *Life Sci* 22 (18):1561–1571.

Squires, E. J., D. E. Hall, and J. T. Brosnan. 1976. Arteriovenous differences for amino acids and lactate across kidneys of normal and acidotic rats. *Biochem J* 160 (1):125–128.

Srinivasan, M., F. Kalousek, and N. P. Curthoys. 1995. *In vitro* characterization of the mitochondrial processing and the potential function of the 68-kDa subunit of renal glutaminase. *J Biol Chem* 270 (3):1185–1190.

Still, A. J., B. J. Floyd, A. S. Hebert et al. 2013. Quantification of mitochondrial acetylation dynamics high-lights prominent sites of metabolic regulation. *J Biol Chem* 288 (36):26209–26219.

Tamarappoo, B. K., S. Joshi, and T. C. Welbourne. 1990. Interorgan glutamine flow regulation in metabolic acidosis. *Miner Electrolyte Metab* 16 (5):322–330.

Tannen, R. L. and B. D. Ross. 1979. Ammoniagenesis by the isolated perfused rat kidney: The critical role of urinary acidification. *Clin Sci (Lond)* 56 (4):353–364.

Taylor, L. and N. P. Curthoys. 2004. Glutamine metabolism: Role in acid–base balance. *Biochem Molec Biol Ed* 32:291–304.

Thangavelu, K., C. Q. Pan, T. Karlberg et al. 2012. Structural basis for the allosteric inhibitory mechanism of human kidney-type glutaminase (KGA) and its regulation by Raf-Mek-Erk signaling in cancer cell metabolism. *Proc Natl Acad Sci USA* 109 (20):7705–7710.

Wang, J. B., J. W. Erickson, R. Fuji et al. 2010. Targeting mitochondrial glutaminase activity inhibits onco-genic transformation. *Cancer Cell* 18 (3):207–219.

Warburg, O., F. Wind, and E. Negelein. 1927. The metabolism of tumors in the body. *J Gen Physiol* 8 (6):519–530.

Ward, P. S., J. Patel, D. R. Wise et al. 2010. The common feature of leukemia-associated IDH1 and IDH2 mutations is a neomorphic enzyme activity converting alpha-ketoglutarate to 2-hydroxyglutarate. *Cancer Cell* 17 (3):225–234.

Watford, M. 1991. Regulation of expression of the genes for glutaminase and glutamine synthetase in the acidotic rat. *Contrib Nephrol* 92:211–217.

Watford, M., V. Chellaraj, A. Ismat et al. 2002. Hepatic glutamine metabolism. *Nutrition* 18 (4):301–303.

Watford, M. and E. M. Smith. 1990. Distribution of hepatic glutaminase activity and mRNA in perivenous and periportal rat hepatocytes. *Biochem J* 267 (1):265–267.

Weiner, I. D. and J. W. Verlander. 2014. Ammonia transport in the kidney by Rhesus glycoproteins. *Am J Physiol Renal Physiol* 306 (10):F1107–F1120.

Weinert, B. T., C. Scholz, S. A. Wagner et al. 2013. Lysine succinylation is a frequently occurring modifica-tion in prokaryotes and eukaryotes and extensively overlaps with acetylation. *Cell Rep* 4 (4):842–851.

Windmueller, H. G. and A. E. Spaeth. 1978. Identification of ketone bodies and glutamine as the major respira-tory fuels *in vivo* for postabsorptive rat small intestine. *J Biol Chem* 253 (1):69–76.

Windmueller, H. G. and A. E. Spaeth. 1980. Respiratory fuels and nitrogen metabolism *in vivo* in small intestine of fed rats. Quantitative importance of glutamine, glutamate, and aspartate. *J Biol Chem* 255 (1):107–112.

Windmueller, H. G. and A. E. Spaeth. 1981. Source and fate of circulating citrulline. *Am J Physiol* 241 (6):E473–E480.

Wisniewski, J. R., N. Nagaraj, A. Zougman et al. 2010. Brain phosphoproteome obtained by a FASP-based method reveals plasma membrane protein topology. *J Proteome Res* 9 (6):3280–3289.

Wright, P. A. and M. A. Knepper. 1990a. Glutamate dehydrogenase activities in microdissected rat nephron segments: Effects of acid–base loading. *Am J Physiol* 259 (1 Pt 2):F53–F59.

Wright, P. A. and M. A. Knepper. 1990b. Phosphate-dependent glutaminase activity in rat renal cortical and medullary tubule segments. *Am J Physiol* 259 (6 Pt 2):F961–F970.

Wright, P. A., R. K. Packer, A. Garcia-Perez et al. 1992. Time course of renal glutamate dehydrogenase induction during NH4Cl loading in rats. *Am J Physiol* 262 (6 Pt 2):F999–F1006.

Wu, G. 1998. Intestinal mucosal amino acid catabolism. *J Nutr* 128 (8):1249–1252.

Wu, M. S., D. Biemesderfer, G. Giebisch et al. 1996. Role of NHE3 in mediating renal brush border Na$^+$-H$^+$ exchange. Adaptation to metabolic acidosis. *J Biol Chem* 271 (51):32749–32752.

Yang, X., M. Amemiya, Y. Peng et al. 2000. Acid incubation causes exocytic insertion of NHE3 in OKP cells. *Am J Physiol Cell Physiol* 279 (2):C410–419.

Zhao, J., A. L. Lopez, D. Erichsen et al. 2004. Mitochondrial glutaminase enhances extracellular glutamate production in HIV-1-infected macrophages: Linkage to HIV-1 associated dementia. *J Neurochem* 88 (1):169–180.

Zhao, S., W. Xu, W. Jiang et al. 2010. Regulation of cellular metabolism by protein lysine acetylation. *Science* 327 (5968):1000–1004.

Section III

Molecular and Cellular Aspects
of Glutamine Metabolism

4 Importance of Glutamine to Insulin Secretion, Insulin Action, and Glycemic Control

Gaewyn Ellison, Cyril Mamotte, Vinicius Fernandes Cruzat, and Philip Newsholme

CONTENTS

4.1 INTRODUCTION

Glutamine affects not only insulin secretion, but also insulin action, including reducing insulin resistance and improving glycemic control in certain physiological conditions. In this chapter we outline the action of insulin, identify metabolic states associated with positive effects of glutamine supplementation, summarize findings from studies of the effects of glutamine supplementation on insulin action and glycemic control and discuss possible mechanisms by which glutamine affects insulin secretion and action.

4.2 INSULIN ACTION

Insulin is essential for life, having both stimulatory and inhibitory functions that are exquisitely primed to maintain metabolic homeostasis. Insulin receptors are present on almost all mammalian tissues, though differential receptor and signaling expression profile makes tissues such as skeletal muscle, adipose, and hepatic tissue far more sensitive to its effects (Kahn and White 1988). Insulin has multiple effects on protein, fat, and particularly glucose metabolism. Glutamine has some effects on protein and fat metabolism that are broadly parallel to those of insulin. For example, glutamine can reduce protein catabolism in critical illness (Matthews and Battezzati 1993) and decrease serum free fatty acids (Cui et al. 2014). Hence glutamine has influences on protein, fat, and carbohydrate metabolism, but the focus here will be specifically on the effect of glutamine on insulin action relating to carbohydrate metabolism and glycemic control.

4.3 METABOLIC STATES ASSOCIATED WITH POSITIVE EFFECTS OF GLUTAMINE SUPPLEMENTATION

In certain states associated with insulin resistance, an apparent increased tissue requirement for glutamine occurs, often resulting in low levels of plasma glutamine (Borel et al. 1998). These include Type 2 Diabetes Mellitus (T2DM) (Samocha-Bonet et al. 2011), severe exercise (Iwashita et al. 2005), and catabolic settings such as seen in burns (Peng et al. 2006), trauma (Bakalar et al. 2006; Dechelotte et al. 2006), surgery (Wilmore 2001; Dechelotte et al. 2006; Awad and Lobo 2012; Cui et al. 2014), sepsis and fasting, including perioperative fasting (Awad and Lobo 2012). A normal dietary intake of <10 g plus the endogenous production of 40–70 g per 24 h (Tjader et al. 2007) would thus appear to be insufficient for the increased demand in spite of increased release of glutamine from skeletal muscle and accelerated synthesis (Lacey and Wilmore 1990) under these conditions. A summary of metabolic changes associated with the catabolic state can be found in Figure 4.1. Biological requirements for glutamine clearly differ between homeostatic and catabolic bioenergetic states. Thus it is possible that glutamine supplementation may have different effects on insulin action and glycemic control in these different states.

To counteract glutamine depletion in catabolic states, supplementation studies have been undertaken in varying contexts. While two clinical studies found glutamine supplementation may have a negative effect on glycemic control (Duska et al. 2008; Breitman et al. 2011), many others found patient outcomes (e.g., rate of infection, length of time on ventilator or in ICU, and nitrogen balance) improved with glutamine intake (Iwashita et al. 2005; Dechelotte et al. 2006; Bakalar et al. 2006; Grau et al. 2011; Hissa et al. 2011; Samocha-Bonet et al. 2011; Dock-Nascimento et al. 2012; Bashandy et al. 2013). This was often ascribed to its effect on insulin action, where observed improvements in glycemic control (Dechelotte et al. 2006; Grau et al. 2011; Hissa et al. 2011; Samocha-Bonet et al. 2011) were attributed to an attenuation of insulin resistance (Bakalar et al. 2006; Bashandy et al. 2013; Cui et al. 2014). A summary of these studies follows, including studies on healthy subjects and trauma patients, diabetics and animal models. It is important to note that variations in several factors may influence results and the interpretation of the effect of glutamine on insulin action. These include (a) differences in delivery, including oral, parenteral, and enteral delivery; (b) differences in administration, including glutamine given in isolation, in an amino-acid cocktail, in combination with either free alanine or as the alanyl–glutamine dipeptide, or with lipids or other substances such as growth hormone; and (c) differing metabolic states of recipients, ranging from healthy, through T2DM to severely catabolic such as in major trauma. These variations can, for example, affect activation of gut hormones, confound or compliment results, or otherwise affect physiologic response (Table 4.1).

4.4 GLUTAMINE SUPPLEMENTATION STUDIES

In a study of healthy young males, Iwashita et al. observed that increases in energy expenditure, and both carbohydrate and fat oxidation after glutamine supplementation with a meal may be related to the effect of glutamine on insulin action and glucose disposal (Borel et al. 1998; Iwashita et al. 2006). Awad et al. (2011) also observed blunted postprandial glucose and insulin responses in healthy subjects and hypothesized that glutamine may reduce insulin resistance. This hypothesis

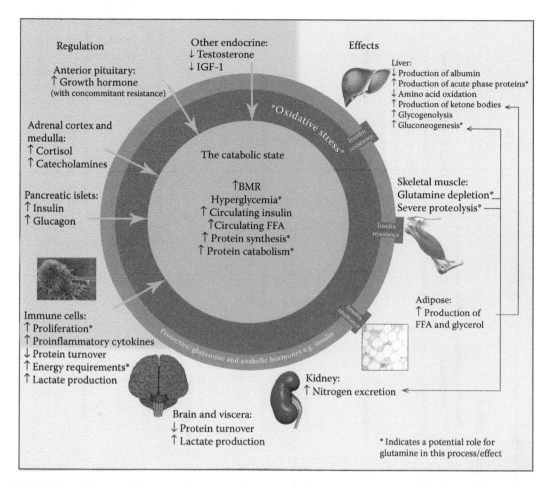

FIGURE 4.1 The catabolic state. Factors regulating catabolic metabolism include hormones and immunological responses. Net metabolic changes occurring after physiological disturbance such as trauma or sepsis, when catabolic and anabolic influences become unbalanced in favor of catabolism, are summarized here. Regulatory and specific organ effects (indicated around the perimeter), particularly in insulin-sensitive tissue, contribute to the net metabolic response (center) and glutamine is important in potentiating several of these effects.

has been supported in clinical situations. For example, in heart surgery patients the use of a preoperative nutriceutic dose of glutamine diminished postoperative stress hyperglycemia (Hissa et al. 2011).

Samocha-Bonet et al. (2011) found T2DM subjects benefited from the reduction of postprandial hyperglycemia mediated by glutamine, and indeed it has been proposed as a potential therapeutic agent for diabetics (Greenfield et al. 2009). In contrast, Chang et al. (2013) found that glutamine given to healthy and T2DM men by intraduodenal infusion did not lower glycemia after glucose, despite stimulating insulin and incretin hormones. Higher glucagon levels (discussed later) were proposed to affect glycemia in this study.

Rat studies confirm the generally observed glucose-lowering effect of glutamine (Opara et al. 1996). Studies in obese or induced Type 1 or 2 diabetic rat or mouse models have found that glutamine (a) decreased plasma glucose and increased circulating insulin (Badole et al. 2013), (b) increased circulating levels of the active form of the incretin hormone glucagon-like peptide 1 (GLP-1) (Badole et al. 2013), and (c) improved glycemic control (Opara et al. 1996; Badole et al.

TABLE 4.1
Studies of the Effect of Glutamine on Insulin Action and Glycemic Control

Reference	Subjects	Glutamine dose and Control/s	Effect on Insulin Sensitivity	Effect on Glycemic Control	Other Effects of Glutamine
Iwashita et al. (2006)	10 Healthy males	1.05 kcal/kg glutamine administered orally or isocaloric amino acid mix containing alanine:glycerine:serine (2:1:0.5) with a mixed meal	Not measured	Not measured	Glutamine increased post-meal energy expenditure by increasing carbohydrate and fat oxidation in early and late post-meal phase, respectively
Awad et al. (2011)	10 Healthy males	15 g glutamine administered orally or isocaloric-isovolumetric (50 g carbohydrate OR 36 g carbohydrate + 7 g lipid) drink	Not measured	Improved	Blunted postprandial insulin and glucose responses
Hissa et al. (2011)	22 Patients with coronary artery occlusion	250 mL L-alanyl-glutamine dipeptide 20% + saline administered parenterally or saline	Not measured	Improved significantly	
Samocha-Bonet et al. (2011)	15 T2DM patients	30 or 15 g L-glutamine or L-glutamine + sitagliptin in water orally or water	Not measured	Improved postprandially	Increased postprandial insulin response (possibly affecting clearance rather than secretion). Increased GLP-1 concentrations and possibly slowed gastric emptying
Greenfield et al. (2009)	24 subjects: 8 lean healthy, 8 each obese nondiabetic, and obese with Type 2 diabetes/impaired glucose tolerance	30 g glutamine administered orally or water or glucose	Not measured	Not measured	Increased circulating GLP-1 and GIP concentrations Significantly increased circulating plasma insulin concentrations Stimulated glucagon secretion
Chang et al. (2013)	20 subjects: 10 healthy and 10 with T2DM	7.5 g or 15 g glutamine administered by intraduodenal infusion or saline	Not measured	No effect	Stimulated incretin hormone (GLP-1, GIP, glucagon, and insulin secretion Increased pyloric motility

(Continued)

TABLE 4.1 (*Continued*)
Studies of the Effect of Glutamine on Insulin Action and Glycemic Control

Reference	Subjects	Glutamine dose and Control/s	Effect on Insulin Sensitivity	Effect on Glycemic Control	Other Effects of Glutamine
Opara et al. (1996)	40 C57BL/6J mice: 10 per diet	2.87% L-glutamine with a high-fat diet or high fat, low-sucrose diet Low fat or low sucrose, high fat with 3.5% L-alanine	Not measured	Prevented or attenuated hyperglycemia	Prevented or reduced body weight and attenuated hyperinsulinemia
Badole et al. (2013)	36 Streptozotocin-induced diabetic rats	250, 500, or 1000 mg/kg/day L-glutamine or distilled water for 8 weeks	Not measured	Significant reduction in plasma glucose and glycosylated hemoglobin	500 and 1000 mg/kg doses reduced food intake and body weight compared to diabetic controls, significantly decreased plasma cholesterol, triglycerides, VLDL, and LDL; increased HDL, active GLP-1, plasma and pancreatic insulin levels, and endogenous liver antioxidants compared to diabetic control. Sitagliptin 5 mg/kg/day had a similar effect
Tsai, Liu et al. (2012)	28 Type II diabetic rats	Glutamine as 25% of total amino acid nitrogen replacing casein or casein in a common semi-purified diet for 8 weeks	Not measured	No change	No difference in food intake or body weights compared to diabetic controls Higher total plasma antioxidant capacity Decreased oxidative stress-related gene expression
Tsai et al. (2011)	27 Type 1 diabetic mice	Glutamine as 25% of total amino acid nitrogen or casein in a common semi-purified diet for 6 weeks	Not measured	No change	Leukocyte adhesion may be reduced; Reduced neutrophil infiltration in the liver Reduced nitrotyrosine (marker for oxidative damage to proteins) in organs Increased GSH:GSSG ratio
Borel et al. (1998)	5 dogs	0.72 mM/kg/hr glutamine administered by intravenous infusion or saline	Enhanced responsiveness suggested by results	Hyperinsulinemic-euglycemic clamp used	Whole-body glucose production was increased Enhanced insulin-mediated glucose utilization 3-fold compared to changes in glucose production

(Continued)

TABLE 4.1 (Continued)
Studies of the Effect of Glutamine on Insulin Action and Glycemic Control

Reference	Subjects	Glutamine dose and Control/s	Effect on Insulin Sensitivity	Effect on Glycemic Control	Other Effects of Glutamine
Iwashita et al. (2005)	6 dogs during, before, and after exercise (hyperinsulinemic, euglycemic clamp conditions)	12 μM/kg/min L-glutamine administered by intravenous infusion or saline	Not measured	Hyperinsulinemic-euglycemic clamp used	Increased net hepatic glucose output by 7-fold during exercise
Cui et al. (2013)	60 patients with colorectal cancer	0.5 g/kg of 3.4% alanyl-L-glutamine diluted in 8.5% mixed amino acid vehicle, saline OR vehicle administered by intravenous infusion	Significantly improved in the glutamine group ($p < 0.05$) measured by HOMA-IR and QUICKI	Postoperatively increased blood glucose attenuated by glutamine	Serum TNF-α and free fatty acid concentrations reduced
Bashandy et al. (2013)	40 patients with cancer	0.4 g/kg L-alanyl-L-glutamine dipeptide or saline administered by intravenous infusion	Significantly improved in the glutamine group ($p < 0.05$) measured by HOMA-IR	Postoperatively increased blood glucose attenuated by glutamine	Plasma reduced glutathione levels higher in the glutamine group
Dock-Nashimento et al. (2012)	48 patients submitted for elective laparoscopic cholecystectomy	Average 0.77 g/kg (range, 0.61–0.97 g/kg) glutamine with maltodextrine and water administered orally or water only, water with maltodextrine or fasting	Significantly improved in the glutamine and other intervention groups compared to fasting ($p < 0.05$) measured by HOMA-IR	Not measured	Improved antioxidant defenses (serum glutathione) Reduced proinflammatory cytokines (IL-6, C-reactive protein) No difference in serum triglycerides or VLDL cholesterol Nitrogen balance less negative
Cunha Filho et al. (2011)	30 children submitted to palatoplasty	0.5 g/kg L-alanyl-L-glutamine dipeptide or saline	Not measured	Improved	Attenuated inflammatory response (C-reactive protein, but not IL-6)

(Continued)

TABLE 4.1 (Continued)
Studies of the Effect of Glutamine on Insulin Action and Glycemic Control

Reference	Subjects	Glutamine dose and Control/s	Effect on Insulin Sensitivity	Effect on Glycemic Control	Other Effects of Glutamine
Bakalar et al. (2006)	40 multiple trauma patients	0.4 g/kg/day L-analyl-glutamine (parenteral) + 1.1 g/kg/day mixed amino acids (parenteral or enteral) or balanced amino acid solution (1.5 g/ kg/day parenteral or enteral)	Prevented insulin resistance as seen in control group	Lower glycemia in glutamine group	Higher oxidation of carbohydrates rather than lipids Lower C-peptide plasma concentration on Day 8 indicating reduced insulin expression compared to controls Improved insulin-mediated glucose disposal
Dechelotte et al. (2006)	114 ICU patients admitted for: multiple trauma (38) complicated surgery (65), or pancreatitis (11)	0.5 g/kg L-alanyl-L-glutamine dipeptide/day with total parenteral nutrition or isocaloric, isonitrogenous L-alanine + L-proline with total parenteral nutrition	Not measured	Less frequent hyperglycemic events amongst glutamine patients	Lower infection rate and incidence of pneumonia (both p < 0.05) Fewer patients required insulin
Grau et al. (2011)	127 ICU patients requiring parenteral nutrition for 5–9 days	0.5 g/kg L-alanyl-L-glutamine dipeptide/day with total parenteral nutrition or isonitrogenous, isocaloric total parenteral nutrition	Not measured	Improved	A 54% reduction in the amount of insulin required for the same levels of glycemia Less pneumonia per days of mechanical ventilation (p = 0.02) Less urinary tract infections per days of urinary catheter (p = 0.04)
Duska et al. (2008)	30 multiple-trauma patients	0.3 g/kg L-alanyl-L-glutamine dipeptide/day with total parenteral nutrition or isonitrogenous, isocaloric total parenteral nutrition	Worsened in the growth hormone + glutamine group, improved in both glutamine and control groups	Not measured	Nitrogen economy was improved with growth hormone plus glutamine

2013) as well as potentially improving insulin sensitivity due to a reduction of oxidative stress (Tsai et al. 2011; Tsai, Liu et al. 2012; Tsai, Yeh et al. 2012; Badole et al. 2013).

Likewise, in canine models, glutamine was shown to enhance insulin-mediated glucose utilization but blunt insulin action on inhibition of glucose production both at rest as well as during and post-exercise (Iwashita et al. 2005). Insulin secretion is usually low post-exercise, but the glutamine effects persisted even upon application of a hyperinsulinemic-euglycemic clamp (Iwashita et al. 2006).

Several randomized controlled trials have shown that glutamine delivered by the oral or parenteral route can improve insulin resistance and glycemic control in surgical (Cunha Filho et al. 2011; Hissa et al. 2011; Dock-Nascimento et al. 2012; Bashandy et al. 2013; Cui et al. 2014) and trauma patients (Bakalar et al. 2006; Dechelotte et al. 2006; Grau et al. 2011). A recent review of glutamine supplementation trials in intensive care patients supports the view that it benefits patients by reducing length of hospital stay and rate of infectious complications (Coeffier and Dechelotte 2005).

In contrast, a pilot study of multiple trauma patients in intensive care given growth hormone plus alanyl-glutamine (AG) or AG supplements alone did not clearly show an attenuation of insulin resistance (inferred from glucose disposal rate) or incidence of hyperglycemia after enteral and parenteral nutrition in the AG group. Differences in timing of measurements and AG administration, dose, weight, and age of subjects were noted as possible reasons for this apparent reduced effect (Duska et al. 2008). Interestingly, this study used AG in combination with growth hormone for ethical reasons due to a previous report of increased mortality among patients receiving growth hormone treatment, with hyperglycemia and sepsis being more frequently reported in the growth hormone group. It was anticipated that glutamine would counter these adverse effects.

4.5   TISSUE SPECIFICITY AND IMPROVEMENT IN INSULIN RESISTANCE

While most studies cited above found that glutamine or AG supplementation attenuated insulin resistance, it is not yet clear whether this effect applies to all insulin-sensitive tissues since studies by Prada et al. (2007) found glutamine induced an improvement in insulin resistance in liver, muscle, and overall, but increased insulin resistance in adipose tissue. These tissue-specific effects could help explain the reduction in weight potentiated by glutamine (Opara et al. 1996), since insulin resistance in adipose tissue results in both reduced inhibition of non-esterified fatty acid (NEFA) release from adipocytes and reduced activation of adipose tissue lipoprotein lipase which is required for the hydrolysis of chylomicron and VLDL triglyceride to fatty acids (Frayn 2001).

In summary, the majority of studies have found glutamine given either in isolation or in combination with other amino acids to be beneficial to glycemic control and/or insulin sensitivity, but there are some exceptions. Differences in metabolic state may be more important in determining the efficacy of supplementation than variations in administration and delivery, though comparisons can be difficult due to inconsistencies in parameters measured in different studies.

4.6   MECHANISM OF ACTION

The mechanisms by which glutamine improves glycemic control and insulin sensitivity are not fully understood and continue to be explored. Promising lines of investigation currently include effects mediated via stimulation of the incretin hormone GLP-1 and decreased insulin resistance through influences on oxidative stress and inflammation. Some additional potential mechanisms are also briefly presented.

4.6.1   GLP-1

Glucagon-like peptide-1 (GLP-1) is an incretin hormone that is potently stimulated by glutamine (Reimann et al. 2004; Tolhurst et al. 2011) and, like other incretins, is secreted from the gut

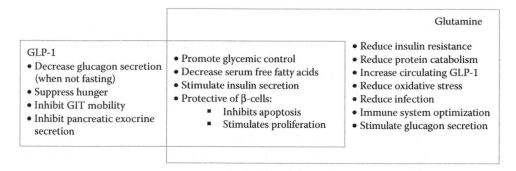

FIGURE 4.2 Effects common to GLP-1 and glutamine. Some commonality occurs between the effects of glutamine and glucagon-like peptide-1 (GLP-1), as summarized here.

in response to nutrients. GLP-1 is known to stimulate glucose-dependent insulin release (Holst 2007; Greenfield et al. 2009; Mansour et al. 2013); reduce levels of blood glucose, non-esterified fatty acids, and triglycerides (Greenfield et al. 2009); slow gastric emptying (Holst 2007); suppress hunger (Kim and Egan 2008; Mansour et al. 2013); and inhibit glucagon secretion (Holst 2007; Kim and Egan 2008), all actions that can help to improve glycemic control. Several of these effects have also been attributed to glutamine (see Figure 4.2). Other studies also outline the protective and proliferative effect of GLP-1 on pancreatic β-cells, which can lead to upregulation of glucokinase and glucose transporter 2 expression, both key elements of insulin secretion and insulin gene transcription.

GLP-1 levels are thought to be comparatively diminished postprandially among obese and insulin-resistant patients (Mansour et al. 2013), and, while this finding is still under debate (Samocha-Bonet et al. 2011), studies in humans have prompted the suggestion that GLP-1 can potentially promote glycemic control in T2DM patients (Greenfield et al. 2009). The possibility of using glutamine specifically as a GLP-1 secretagogue for T2DM therapy has been suggested (Tolhurst et al. 2011). In addition, two drugs based on GLP-1, exenatide (a synthetic incretin[*]) and sitagliptin (an inhibitor of the GLP-1 degrading enzyme DPP4[†]), have recently become available for use in the treatment of T2DM (Kim and Egan 2008).

Glutamine is thought to stimulate GLP-1 secretion by binding to the GLP-1 receptor, as seen in docking studies in glutamine-supplemented rats. It may also be involved in GLP-1 activation, as increased concentrations of the GLP-1 (7-36) amide, the active form of colonic GLP-1, were found after glutamine administration in the same rat study (Badole et al. 2013). In a randomized controlled crossover study of T2DM patients, glutamine (30 g) or glutamine (15 g) plus sitagliptin, which inhibits GLP-1 catabolism, were found to reduce postprandial glycemia relative to control. Glutamine was also found to increase both total and active GLP-1 concentrations, suggesting its glucose-lowering effect, at least in part, was linked to increased GLP-1 action (Samocha-Bonet et al. 2011). Another study in healthy subjects, however, failed to see increased GLP-1 after glutamine ingestion, although glucose and insulin responses were similarly blunted (Awad et al. 2011). The authors did not include an explanation for this result but alluded to a possible difference in the role of glutamine in elective surgery as opposed to critical illness, implying that its GLP-1 stimulating action may be more important in times of increased glutamine demand.

Gastric emptying time is an important factor determining postprandial blood glucose levels (Mansour et al. 2013). Slowed gastric emptying is a well-documented effect of GLP-1 (Holst 2007)

---

[*] Exenatide is a synthetic form of an incretin mimetic discovered in the saliva of a Gila monster lizard that became available for clinical use in T2DM in 2005. It has 53% homology to GLP-1 and binds with greater affinity than GLP-1 to GLP-1 receptors. It is not degraded by DPP4 due to having no recognition site for this enzyme, thus it's biological effect remains for up to 8 h after subcutaneous injection (Kim 2008).

[†] DPP4 degrades GLP-1 very quickly, resulting in a half-life of approximately 2 min.

and is thought to be the main cause of reduced postprandial glycemia in the glutamine and glutamine + sitagliptin study mentioned above. However, an effect of glutamine on gastric emptying time has not yet clearly been demonstrated. In a study measuring antral and duodenal pressure waves it was found that glutamine had a stimulatory effect on pyloric motility, while the effect of GLP-1 on gastric motility is typically inhibitory. Diminished glycemia after glutamine plus glucose was not observed in this study (Chang et al. 2013). In addition, a study of healthy subjects showed, scintigraphically, no difference in gastric emptying time after glutamine- or lipid-supplemented isocaloric-isovolumetric carbohydrate drinks (Awad et al. 2011).

Given that glutamine can stimulate GLP-1 release and increase its circulation, resulting in reduced postprandial glycemia in T2DM patients and stimulation of insulin secretion, this line of enquiry holds merit in the quest to understand glutamine's effect on glycemic control.

4.6.2 INSULIN RESISTANCE

The molecular mechanisms that contribute to the development of insulin resistance are not well understood, but factors such as oxidative stress, inflammation, and gluco- and lipo-toxicity are considered to play a central role (Turner et al. 2014). There are clear links between these: When reactive oxygen species (ROS), which are byproducts of normal mitochondrial metabolism, exceed antioxidant capacity, the resulting oxidative stress can damage macromolecules and stimulate an immune response, including the production of proinflammatory cytokines. As outlined below, glutamine has been shown to exert a beneficial influence on many of these different aspects, including effects on oxidative stress, for example, by increasing generation of glutathione, a critically important antioxidant, and by reducing inflammation, for example, by a balancing effect on cellular and humoral immunity.

4.6.3 INFLUENCES ON OXIDATIVE STRESS AND ASSOCIATED PROCESSES

Glutamine, with cysteine and glycine, can be metabolized to glutathione, a critical cellular antioxidant (Newsholme et al. 2003) with the capacity to scavenge reactive oxygen species (ROS) and reactive nitrogen species (RNS) produced during metabolic processes, thus protecting cells from oxidative damage (Petry et al. 2014). The ratio of reduced glutathione (GSH) to oxidized glutathione (GSSH) regulates the redox potential of the cell (Bashandy et al. 2013) and plasma glutathione levels give an indication of tissue redox potential. Under catabolic conditions, this ratio is shifted due to high demand for antioxidant activity. A randomized controlled study found that patients undergoing abdominal surgery for neoplasms who were given a preoperative glutamine infusion had significantly higher levels of plasma glutathione and lower insulin resistance (Bashandy et al. 2013). Similarly, higher serum GSH concentrations were seen after glutamine in a randomized controlled clinical study of elective cholecystectomy patients (Dock-Nascimento et al. 2012).

These human studies are supported by animal studies. GSH levels in the skeletal muscle of rats conditioned to high-intensity exercise doubled after 21 days of glutamine supplementation by gavage, compared to non-supplemented animals. This effectively increased the GSH:GSSH ratio (by 40%), leading to a more balanced redox status in muscle tissue (Petry et al. 2014). In endotoxemic mice, a reduction in redox potential >2.7-fold in erythrocytes and muscle tissue was returned to normal by a combination of glutamine and alanine, either in free form or as a dipeptide (Cruzat, Bittencourt et al. 2014). In an *in vitro* study, lipopolysaccharide-stimulated primary alveolar type II epithelial cells from rat lung showed a significant decrease in GSH concentration, but this was reversed by ≥2 mM glutamine. Inhibition of GSH synthesis blocked the protective effect of glutamine entirely, indicating that the mechanism of action is via GSH synthesis (Zhang et al. 2008).

There are also some less direct influences on processes linked to oxidative stress. The cytoprotective heat shock proteins are a well-described family (Lindquist and Craig 1988) expressed under physiologically stressful conditions such as hypoxia, oxidative stress, and inflammation. They are considered to be potent anti-inflammatory agents (Krause and de Bittencourt 2008). Upregulation of the 70 kDa member, HSP70, has been associated with glutamine supplementation in a variety of contexts (Wischmeyer 2007) including rat pancreatic islet transplantation (Jang et al. 2008); rat or mouse muscle during exhaustive exercise (Petry et al. 2014) or endotoxemia (Cruzat, Pantaleao et al. 2014), respectively; and in the serum of surgical intensive care unit patients (Ziegler et al. 2005). HSP70 expression correlated with an attenuation of ischemic damage, improved redox status, and fewer days spent on ventilation and/or in ICU. In addition, glutamine improved survival in wild-type mice after experimental sepsis but not in mice that had a gene deletion for HSP70 (Singleton and Wischmeyer 2007; Wischmeyer 2007).

Glutamine influences HSP70 regulation via the hexosamine biosynthetic pathway (HBP), in which glutamine is a key substrate (Figure 4.3) (Hamiel et al. 2009). However, increased flux

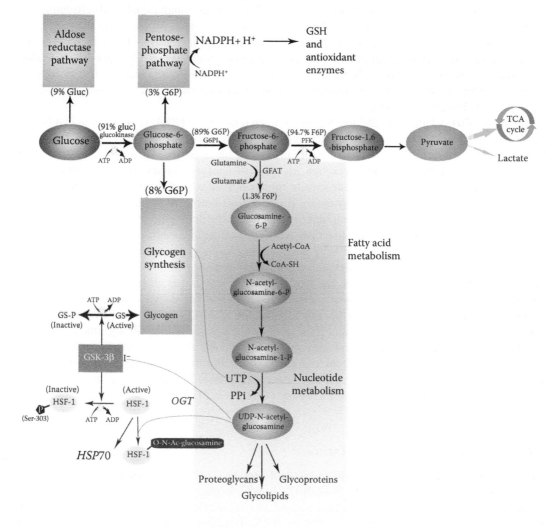

FIGURE 4.3 The hexosamine biosynthetic pathway and the role of glutamine in HSP70 synthesis. Glutamine can upregulate glucose flux through the hexosamine biosynthetic pathway (HBP) and thereby stimulate heat shock protein (HSP) 70 production. Basal flux balance in β-cells is indicated in parentheses, which show the proportional amount of metabolite consumed in the various metabolic pathways. GSH: glutathione; GFAT: glutamine:fructose-6-phosphate aminotransferase; TCA: tricarboxylic acid cycle; GSK-3β: glycogen synthase kinase-3β; HSF-1: heat shock factor-1; OGT: O-linked N-acetylglucosaminyl transferase; PPi: inorganic phosphate. (Adapted from Newsholme, P. et al. 2013.)

through the HBP also occurs in hyperglycemia due to mitochondrial superoxide overproduction (Du et al. 2000; Buse 2006). In primary adipose cells (Marshall et al. 1991; Hawkins et al. 1997) and rat muscle (Hawkins et al. 1997), insulin resistance is thought to be closely linked to increased flux through the HBP due to high glucose or free fatty acid stimulation, although not all studies support this (Choi et al. 2001). Thus, it appears that enhanced HBP flux can be beneficial but overenhanced flux may be detrimental to insulin action. The fact that glutamine is a key substrate in this pathway (Prada et al. 2007; Hamiel et al. 2009) is a clue to a complex relationship between glutamine, insulin resistance, and the products and effects of the HBP.

Another member of the heat shock protein family (HSP-32) found to be activated by glutamine is the inducible form of hemeoxygenase (HO-1) (Uehara et al. 2005). Experiments in an *in vitro* model of ischemia/reperfusion injury using human proximal renal tubular epithelial cells found that glutamine rescued cells from apoptosis due to upregulation of HO-1, probably via the p38MAPK signal transduction pathway (Shi et al. 2009). The same study demonstrated that HO-1 provided protection by three downstream effects: (a) increased carbon monoxide (CO), a potent antioxidant and product of the metabolism of heme (from hemoglobin) to biliverdin, a reaction that HO-1 catalyzes; (b) reduced iNOS activation (proinflammatory, discussed later); and (c) increased Bcl-2 (an anti-apoptotic molecule) activity.

Inducible nitric oxide synthase (iNOS), shown to be reduced by HO-1, is an enzyme involved in catalyzing nitric oxide (NO) synthesis from L-arginine during an immune response. Besides having a protective function in immunity (Radomski 1995), NO has a number of roles in insulin action, including insulin signaling, insulin secretion, and glucose uptake (Newsholme et al. 2010). In high concentrations, however, NO can destructively inhibit mitochondrial ATP synthesis and upregulate expression of proinflammatory genes in β-cells, contributing to β-cell stress and apoptosis (Wang et al. 2010). In combination with superoxide it forms the damaging free radical peroxynitrite (ONOO⁻). Glutamine has been found to reduce NF-κB signaling (Esposito et al. 2011) (which drives iNOS expression—see Figure 4.4) as well as circulating levels of iNOS and NO (Lu et al. 2009; Mondello et al. 2011) in zymosan-treated mice and in rat hepatocytes incubated in the presence of IL-1β. This led to reduced nitrosative and oxidative stress and enhanced insulin sensitivity in the mouse study, but these parameters were not measured in the rat hepatocyte study.

In summary, there is evidence of the redox balancing effects of glutamine being via glutathione, the heat shock proteins HSP70 and HO-1, and/or nitric oxide (either via arginine or directly). Oxidative status and inflammatory responses are closely linked, and there is evidence that both are affected by glutamine, as flow-on effects from each other and/or independently. Glutamine has also been shown to mediate aspects of the cellular immune response. These effects are important to the discussion of insulin action because of increasing evidence of their significant influence on insulin signaling and uptake.

4.6.4 GLUTAMINE AND INSULIN SECRETION

Under appropriate conditions, specific amino acids enhance insulin secretion from primary islet β-cells and β-cell lines (Newsholme et al. 2011). *In vivo*, L-glutamine and L-alanine are quantitatively the most abundant amino acids in the blood and extracellular fluids, closely followed by the branched chain amino acids (Newsholme et al. 2005). However, many amino acids do not evoke insulin-secretory responses *in vitro* when added at physiological concentrations but rather combinations of physiological concentrations of amino acids or high concentrations of individual amino acids are much more effective. *In vivo*, amino acids derived from dietary proteins or intestinal epithelial cells, in combination with glucose, stimulate insulin secretion, thereby leading to protein synthesis and amino acid transport in target tissues such as skeletal muscle (Cunningham et al. 2005; Newsholme et al. 2011, 2014).

While amino acids can potentially affect a number of aspects of β-cell function, a relatively small number of amino acids promote or synergistically enhance insulin release from pancreatic

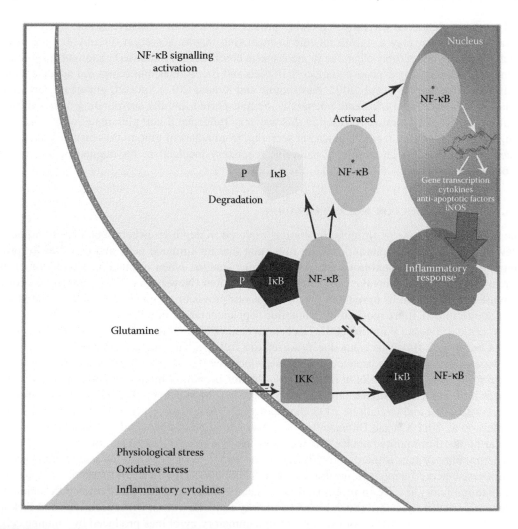

FIGURE 4.4   Effect of glutamine on NF-κB signal activation. Stressors activate inhibitor of kappa B kinase (IKK), prompting phosphorylation of inhibitor of kappa B (IκB), which allows nuclear factor-κB(NF-κB) translocation to the nucleus, where it promotes transcription of inducible nitric oxide synthase (iNOS), various cytokines, and anti-apoptotic factors. *Glutamine inhibits the phosphorylation of IκB.

β-cells. The mechanisms by which amino acids enhance insulin secretion are understood to primarily rely on: (i) direct depolarization of the plasma membrane (e.g., cationic amino acid, L-arginine); (ii) metabolism (e.g., glutamine, leucine); and (iii) co-transport with Na^+ and cell membrane depolarization (e.g., L-alanine). Notably, partial oxidation, for example, of L-alanine may also initially increase the cellular content of ATP impacting on K_{ATP} channel closure prompting membrane depolarization, Ca^{2+} influx, and insulin exocytosis (Newsholme et al. 2007, 2011).

Both rat islets and rat derived BRIN-BD11 β-cells consume glutamine at high rates, but notably while glutamine can potentiate glucose stimulated insulin secretion (GSIS) and interact with other nutrient secretagogues, it does not initiate an insulin-secretory response (Corless et al. 2006). In rat islets, glutamine is converted to γ-amino butyric acid (GABA) and aspartate and, in the presence of leucine, oxidative metabolism is increased due to activation of glutamate dehydrogenase and entry of glutamine carbon into the TCA cycle (Newgard et al. 2009; Newsholme, Gaudel, and Krause 2012). Production of glutamate from glutamine (Cruzat and Tirapegui 2009) may also contribute to β-cell antioxidant defense with entry into the γ-glutamyl cycle, thereby enhancing glutathione synthesis (Cunningham et al. 2005; Newsholme et al. 2014).

Therefore, glutamine derivatives possibly protect β-cells from oxidative insult. Interestingly, glutamate may also play a significant role in mediating insulin secretion directly, but the exact mechanisms are not entirely clear due to inconsistent observations. Increased glutamate levels have been detected following exposure to glucose in islets and β-cell lines, but others did not detect any significant changes (Hoy et al. 2002; Newsholme and Krause 2012). Indeed, glutamate can accumulate within insulin vesicles and, potentially, be transported into the surrounding matrix during insulin exocytosis. Glutamate released in this way may influence β-cell glutamate receptor activation. In addition, it may regulate glucagon secretion from adjacent glutamate-sensitive pancreatic α-cells and is possibly an additional paracrine regulatory mechanism for maintenance of blood carbohydrate levels.

4.6.5 IMMUNE FUNCTION AND INFLAMMATION

The effect of glutamine on immune function is explored in depth elsewhere, but a brief outline is relevant here. Given that glutamine is an important fuel for immune cells and essential for proliferation, it could be tempting to assume that during trauma, when immune cell proliferation is increased and glutamine uptake can increase up to 5–8-fold (Newsholme 1996; Peng et al. 2006), immune activity would be upregulated with exogenous provision of glutamine. Indeed, complications due to infection are reduced by glutamine supplementation in clinical studies after surgery and in critical illness (Wilmore 2001; Dechelotte et al. 2006; Grau et al. 2011; Bollhalder et al. 2013; Chen et al. 2014). This is not due, however, to a full-spectrum increase in number of immune cells together with cytokine production increase, which could lead to increased oxidative stress and insulin resistance. Instead, glutamine is responsible for immune function optimization, involving changes in immune cell populations (Esposito et al. 2011; Mondello et al. 2011), reduced cytokine secretion (Coeffier and Dechelotte 2005; Singleton et al. 2005; Prada et al. 2007; Wischmeyer 2007; Mondello et al. 2011; Cruzat, Bittencourt et al. 2014), and improved pro- and anti-inflammatory and cellular/humoral immunity balance (Chang, Yang, and Shaio 1999; Yeh et al. 2005).

The immune system is increasingly being considered a major player in the pathophysiology of insulin resistance. Macrophage infiltration, proinflammatory cytokines, and specific components of innate immunity feature in recent studies as factors in the complex link between the immune system and insulin resistance (Su et al. 2009; Olefsky and Glass 2010; Fernandez-Real and Pickup 2012; Kammoun et al. 2014). For example, proinflammatory cytokines produced by immune cells interfere with both insulin signaling and sensitivity (Cai et al. 2005; Su et al. 2009) (see Figure 4.5). Several studies have found that glutamine-mediated immuno-modulation is paralleled by improved insulin action and glycemic control as reviewed by Wischmeyer (2007).

4.6.6 GLUTAMINE IMPACT ON GLYCEMIA OR INSULIN RESISTANCE AND INFLAMMATION

In a notable exception glutamine was associated with significantly poorer insulin sensitivity, higher fasting serum insulin concentrations, and upregulated inflammatory markers (C-reactive protein and IL-6) in a study on obese subjects. It is possible that glutamine may have quite different results in more severe metabolic derangements, such as the morbidly obese subjects of this study (BMI 43.3 ± 4.1 kg/m^2) (Breitman et al. 2011). In addition, a mixed amino acid supplement (glutamine, arginine, and leucine) was used in the study, and poorer recovery of insulin sensitivity could be due to a known effect of leucine to reduce glucose uptake. Several studies have shown varying results within a group of inflammatory markers. For example, a study of children undergoing cleft palate surgery found no significant difference in IL-6 levels between the glutamine and control groups, but attenuation of post-surgical trauma indicated by reduced C-reactive protein expression and absence of significant changes in postoperative glucose levels in glutamine-supplemented patients showed an overall attenuated inflammatory response and improved glycemic control (Cunha Filho et al. 2011).

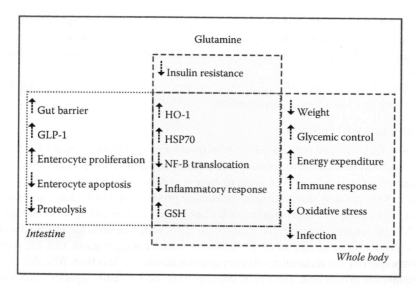

FIGURE 4.5   Role of glutamine in insulin sensitivity. Mechanisms potentially involved in the beneficial effects of glutamine on insulin sensitivity and glycemic control. (Adapted from Coeffier, M. and P. Dechelotte. 2005. *Nutr Rev* 63 (2):65–9.)

Thus, glutamine mostly has an optimizing effect on immune function, reducing inflammation and, via reduced oxidative stress, cellular damage and signaling interference, enhancing insulin action and improving glycemic control.

4.6.7   Additional Mechanisms

In addition to these main avenues of investigation, other observations about the possible metabolic effects of glutamine include glucagon stimulation, effects on mitochondrial function, and glutamine/glutamate cycling, as briefly summarized below.

4.6.7.1   Stimulation of Gluconeogenesis

Glutamine can be used as a substrate for gluconeogenesis and thus has the potential to increase blood glucose. For example, in a canine study, net hepatic glucose output was found to increase 7-fold during exercise in the glutamine group compared to a 4-fold increase in the control group. This was supported by a significantly increased net hepatic uptake of gluconeogenic amino acids (particularly, but not exclusively, glutamine) in the glutamine group (Iwashita et al. 2005). Glutamine's gluconeogenic potential is particularly important in the small intestine. While this organ has not traditionally been considered a site of gluconeogenesis, under insulinopenic conditions such as fasting or diabetes (type-1 or advanced type-2), gene expression studies have confirmed that phosphoenol pyruvate carboxykinase, which is required for incorporation of glutamine carbons into glucose via the TCA cycle, is strongly induced in this site. In fact, glucose released by the small intestine was found to account for a significant amount (13%) of total glucose production in diabetic rats (Mithieux 2001). In addition, much of the glutamine taken up by the small intestine during fasting is converted, via alanine transaminase activity, to alanine and subsequently used as a substrate for hepatic gluconeogenesis (Mithieux 2001).

4.6.7.2   Stimulation of Glucagon Secretion

Glutamine stimulates pancreatic release of glucagon in healthy (lean and obese) and diabetic subjects (Greenfield et al. 2009). This is in spite of the well-known inhibitory effect of the coincidently stimulated GLP-1 secretion. Though this is likely to affect glycemic status, the mechanism and specific impact of glucagon secretion on insulin action and glycemic control in the context of glutamine stimulation are yet to be explored but are clearly not sufficient to diminish the overall antiglycemic effects of glutamine.

In spite of its gluconeogenic and glucagon-stimulating potential, glutamine generally increases insulin sensitivity and has a hypoglycemic effect.

4.6.7.3 Mitochondrial Function

Due to the close link between mitochondrial ROS production and insulin resistance, mitochondrial dysfunction has been considered as a contributing factor in the insulin-resistant state (Turner et al. 2014). Glutamine oxidation is also thought to have a profound effect on mitochondrial function (Mates et al. 2009), possibly due to excess superoxide production, but to date no clear conclusion can be drawn. For example, a bioenergetics study has found an association between high-dose (500 and 5000 μM) glutamine treatment and suboptimal mitochondrial function (Krajcova et al. 2015). These supra-physiologic concentrations of glutamine (albeit concentrations that are routinely used in cell culture experiments) reduced respiratory chain efficiency to less than 70% due to uncoupling and inner-membrane proton leak, but had no effect on respiratory chain capacity, anaerobic glycolysis rate, or non-mitochondrial oxygen consumption.

In a similar study, insulin acutely reduced mitochondrial inner membrane proton leak, enhancing respiratory chain efficiency after 20 min of treatment (Nisr and Affourtit 2014). A comparison of these real-time studies on glutamine- or insulin-treated skeletal muscle cells show opposite effects on mitochondrial coupling efficiency, dependent on glutamine dose. A sub-physiological glutamine concentration (but consistent with moderate clinical hypoglutaminemia) of 300 μM did not adversely affect respiratory chain efficiency. It was suggested that increased energy expenditure as seen by Iwashita et al. (2006) in healthy volunteers after glutamine supplementation may be a result of futile cycles and heat generation. However, it was deemed more likely evidence of an uncontrolled leak explained by mitochondrial toxicity due to intracellular breakdown of glutamine to glutamate and ammonia (Krajcova et al. 2015). To date, no bioenergetics studies have been undertaken to elucidate the effect of simultaneous treatment with both insulin and glutamine, which would more closely reflect the *in vivo* situation.

Mitochondrial glutamine oxidation may be important in β-cell adaptation to insulin resistance. In islets from insulin-resistant (but not diabetic) mice, Fex et al. (2007) observed a 2-fold increase in mitochondrial area in conjunction with an improvement in oxidation of fuels such as glutamine requiring mitochondrial metabolism, which they proposed may indicate compensation for observed impaired glucose oxidation due to increased lipid flux.

4.6.7.4 Glutamine/Glutamate Cycling

An interesting recent study used liquid chromatography/mass spectrometry to profile plasma metabolites from subjects enrolled in the Framingham Heart Study and the Malmo Diet and Cancer Study to link metabolic pathways with cardiometabolic risk factors (Cheng et al. 2012). They found that metabolic risk factors, including high plasma insulin levels and insulin resistance, were strongly associated with high circulating glutamate compared to glutamine. This was also a risk factor for future diabetes.

This is the first time an association has been reported between the glutamine/glutamate ratio and multiple metabolic risk factors in humans. The researchers then conducted diet intervention studies to test the effect of glutamine on glucose tolerance. Less extreme glycemic fluctuations and plasma glucose levels were recorded for the glutamine-supplemented mice compared to the glutamate-supplemented or control mice. From these results, it appears that low glutamine concentrations, particularly in relation to glutamate and other precursor amino acids, may be a contributing factor in the development of metabolic diseases. In addition, it has been suggested that liver transaminases, responsible for converting precursor amino acids to glutamine and back again and currently considered biomarkers for liver damage, may be involved in the pathophysiology of insulin resistance and other aspects of metabolic syndrome (Sookoian and Pirola 2012).

4.7 SUMMARY AND CONCLUSION

It is clear that there is a high level of complexity in the processes involved in glutamine utilization and its effects on insulin action and glycemic control. Overall, and in spite of its gluconeogenic function, glutamine improves glycemic control and increases insulin sensitivity by various mechanisms, including reduced oxidative stress and inflammation, which can interfere with insulin signaling.

REFERENCES

Awad, S., P. E. Blackshaw, J. W. Wright et al. 2011. A randomized crossover study of the effects of glutamine and lipid on the gastric emptying time of a preoperative carbohydrate drink. *Clin Nutr* 30 (2):165–71.

Awad, S. and D. N. Lobo. 2012. Metabolic conditioning to attenuate the adverse effects of perioperative fasting and improve patient outcomes. *Curr Opin Clin Nutr Metab Care* 15 (2):194–200.

Badole, S. L., P. P. Bagul, S. P. Mahamuni et al. 2013. Oral L-glutamine increases active GLP-1 (7–36) amide secretion and improves glycemic control in stretpozotocin-nicotinamide induced diabetic rats. *Chem Biol Interact* 203 (2):530–41.

Bakalar, B., F. Duska, J. Pachl et al. 2006. Parenterally administered dipeptide alanyl-glutamine prevents worsening of insulin sensitivity in multiple-trauma patients. *Crit Care Med* 34 (2):381–6.

Bashandy, G., N. Boules, and F. Taha. 2013. Effects of a single preoperative dose of N(2)-L-alanyl-L-glutamine on insulin resistance and plasma glutathione levels in the early postoperative period. *Eg J Anaesth* 29:319–24.

Bollhalder, L., A. M. Pfeil, Y. Tomonaga et al. 2013. A systematic literature review and meta-analysis of randomized clinical trials of parenteral glutamine supplementation. *Clin Nutr* 32 (2):213–23.

Borel, M. J., P. E. Williams, K. Jabbour et al. 1998. Parenteral glutamine infusion alters insulin-mediated glucose metabolism. *JPEN J Parenter Enteral Nutr* 22 (5):280–5.

Breitman, I., N. Saraf, M. Kakade et al. 2011. The effects of an amino acid supplement on glucose homeostasis, inflammatory markers, and incretins after laparoscopic gastric bypass. *J Am Col Surg* 212 (4):617–25; discussion 625–7.

Buse, M. G. 2006. Hexosamines, insulin resistance, and the complications of diabetes: Current status. *Am J Physiol Endocrinol Metab* 290 (1):E1–E8.

Cai, D., M. Yuan, D. F. Frantz et al. 2005. Local and systemic insulin resistance resulting from hepatic activation of IKK-beta and NF-kappaB. *Nat Med* 11 (2):183–90.

Chang, J., T. Wu, J. R. Greenfield et al. 2013. Effects of intraduodenal glutamine on incretin hormone and insulin release, the glycemic response to an intraduodenal glucose infusion, and antropyloroduodenal motility in health and type 2 diabetes. *Diabetes Care* 36 (8):2262–5.

Chang, W. K., K. D. Yang, and M. F. Shaio. 1999. Effect of glutamine on Th1 and Th2 cytokine responses of human peripheral blood mononuclear cells. *Clin Immunol* 93 (3):294–301.

Chen, Q. H., Y. Yang, H. L. He et al. 2014. The effect of glutamine therapy on outcomes in critically ill patients: A meta-analysis of randomized controlled trials. *Critical Care* 18 (1):R8.

Cheng, S., E. P. Rhee, M. G. Larson et al. 2012. Metabolite profiling identifies pathways associated with metabolic risk in humans. *Circulation* 125 (18):2222–31.

Choi, C. S., F. N. Lee, and J. H. Youn. 2001. Free fatty acids induce peripheral insulin resistance without increasing muscle hexosamine pathway product levels in rats. *Diabetes* 50 (2):418–24.

Coeffier, M. and P. Dechelotte. 2005. The role of glutamine in intensive care unit patients: Mechanisms of action and clinical outcome. *Nutr Rev* 63 (2):65–9.

Corless, M., A. Kiely, N. H. McClenaghan et al. 2006. Glutamine regulates expression of key transcription factor, signal transduction, metabolic gene, and protein expression in a clonal pancreatic beta-cell line. *J Endocrinol* 190 (3):719–27.

Cruzat, V. F., A. Bittencourt, S. P. Scomazzon et al. 2014. Oral free and dipeptide forms of glutamine supplementation attenuate oxidative stress and inflammation induced by endotoxemia. *Nutrition* 30 (5):602–11.

Cruzat, V. F., L. C. Pantaleao, J. Donato, Jr. et al. 2014. Oral supplementations with free and dipeptide forms of L-glutamine in endotoxemic mice: Effects on muscle glutamine-glutathione axis and heat shock proteins. *J Nutr Biochem* 25 (3):345–52.

Cruzat, V. F. and J. Tirapegui. 2009. Effects of oral supplementation with glutamine and alanyl-glutamine on glutamine, glutamate, and glutathione status in trained rats and subjected to long-duration exercise. *Nutrition* 25 (4):428–35.

Cui, Y., L. Hu, Y. J. Liu et al. 2014. Intravenous alanyl-L-glutamine balances glucose-insulin homeostasis and facilitates recovery in patients undergoing colonic resection: A randomised controlled trial. *Eur J Anaesthesiol* 31 (4):212–8.

Cunha Filho, J. F., Goncalves, II, S. B. Guimaraes et al. 2011. L-alanyl-glutamine pretreatment attenuates acute inflammatory response in children submitted to palatoplasty. *Acta Cirurgica Brasileira/Sociedade Brasileira para Desenvolvimento Pesquisa em Cirurgia* 26 (Suppl 1):72–6.

Cunningham, G. A., N. H. McClenaghan, P. R. Flatt et al. 2005. L-Alanine induces changes in metabolic and signal transduction gene expression in a clonal rat pancreatic beta-cell line and protects from pro-inflammatory cytokine-induced apoptosis. *Clin Sci (Lond)* 109 (5):447–55.

Dechelotte, P., M. Hasselmann, L. Cynober et al. 2006. L-alanyl-L-glutamine dipeptide-supplemented total parenteral nutrition reduces infectious complications and glucose intolerance in critically ill patients: The French controlled, randomized, double-blind, multicenter study. *Crit Care Med* 34 (3):598–604.

Dock-Nascimento, D. B., J. E. de Aguilar-Nascimento, M. S. Magalhaes Faria et al. 2012. Evaluation of the effects of a preoperative 2-hour fast with maltodextrine and glutamine on insulin resistance, acute-phase response, nitrogen balance, and serum glutathione after laparoscopic cholecystectomy: A controlled randomized trial. *JPEN Journal of Parenteral and Enteral Nutrition* 36 (1):43–52.

Du, X. L., D. Edelstein, L. Rossetti et al. 2000. Hyperglycemia-induced mitochondrial superoxide overproduction activates the hexosamine pathway and induces plasminogen activator inhibitor-1 expression by increasing Sp1 glycosylation. *Proc Natl Acad Sci USA* 97 (22):12222–6.

Duska, F., M. Fric, P. Waldauf et al. 2008. Frequent intravenous pulses of growth hormone together with glutamine supplementation in prolonged critical illness after multiple trauma: Effects on nitrogen balance, insulin resistance, and substrate oxidation. *Cri Care Med* 36 (6):1707–13.

Esposito, E., S. Mondello, R. Di Paola et al. 2011. Glutamine contributes to ameliorate inflammation after renal ischemia/reperfusion injury in rats. *Naunyn Schmiedebergs Arch Pharmacol* 383 (5):493–508.

Fernandez-Real, J. M. and J. C. Pickup. 2012. Innate immunity, insulin resistance and type 2 diabetes. *Diabetologia* 55 (2):273–8.

Fex, M., M. D. Nitert, N. Wierup et al. 2007. Enhanced mitochondrial metabolism may account for the adaptation to insulin resistance in islets from C57BL/6J mice fed a high-fat diet. *Diabetologia* 50 (1):74–83.

Frayn, K. N. 2001. Adipose tissue and the insulin resistance syndrome. *Proc Nutr Soc* 60 (3):375–80.

Grau, T., A. Bonet, E. Minambres et al. 2011. The effect of L-alanyl-L-glutamine dipeptide supplemented total parenteral nutrition on infectious morbidity and insulin sensitivity in critically ill patients. *Crit Care Med* 39 (6):1263–8.

Greenfield, J. R., I. S. Farooqi, J. M. Keogh et al. 2009. Oral glutamine increases circulating glucagon-like peptide 1, glucagon, and insulin concentrations in lean, obese, and type 2 diabetic subjects. *Am J Clin Nutr* 89 (1):106–13.

Hamiel, C. R., S. Pinto, A. Hau et al. 2009. Glutamine enhances heat shock protein 70 expression via increased hexosamine biosynthetic pathway activity. *Am J Physiol Cell Physiol* 297 (6):C1509–19.

Hawkins, M., N. Barzilai, R. Liu et al. 1997. Role of the glucosamine pathway in fat-induced insulin resistance. *J Clin Invest* 99 (9):2173–82.

Hissa, M. N., R. C. Vasconcelos, S. B. Guimaraes et al. 2011. Preoperative glutamine infusion improves glycemia in heart surgery patients. *Acta Cirurgica Brasileira/Sociedade Brasileira para Desenvolvimento Pesquisa em Cirurgia* 26 (Suppl 1):77–81.

Holst, J. J. 2007. The physiology of glucagon-like peptide 1. *Physiol Rev* 87 (4):1409–39.

Hoy, M., P. Maechler, A. M. Efanov et al. 2002. Increase in cellular glutamate levels stimulates exocytosis in pancreatic beta-cells. *FEBS Lett* 531 (2):199–203.

Iwashita, S., C. Mikus, S. Baier et al. 2006. Glutamine supplementation increases postprandial energy expenditure and fat oxidation in humans. *JPEN J Parenter Enteral Nutr* 30 (2):76–80.

Iwashita, S., P. Williams, K. Jabbour et al. 2005. Impact of glutamine supplementation on glucose homeostasis during and after exercise. *J Appl Physiol* 99 (5):1858–65.

Jang, H. J., J. H. Kwak, E. Y. Cho et al. 2008. Glutamine induces heat-shock protein-70 and glutathione expression and attenuates ischemic damage in rat islets. *Transplant Proc* 40 (8):2581–4.

Kahn, C. R. and M. F. White. 1988. The insulin receptor and the molecular mechanism of insulin action. *J Clin Invest* 82 (4):1151–6.

Kammoun, H. L., M. J. Kraakman, and M. A. Febbraio. 2014. Adipose tissue inflammation in glucose metabolism. *Rev Endocr Metab Disord* 15 (1):31–44.

Kim, W. and J. M. Egan. 2008. The role of incretins in glucose homeostasis and diabetes treatment. *Pharmacol Rev* 60 (4):470–512.

Krajcova, A., J. Ziak, K. Jiroutkova, J. Patkova, M. Elkalaf, V. Dzupa, J. Trnka, and F. Duska. 2015. Normalizing glutamine concentration causes mitochondrial uncoupling in an *in vitro* model of human skeletal muscle. *JPEN J Parenter Enteral Nutr* 39:180–189.

Krause, M. S. and P. I. H. Jr. de Bittencourt. 2008. Type 1 diabetes: Can exercise impair the autoimmune event? The L-arginine/glutamine coupling hypothesis. *Cell Biochem Funct* 26 (4):406–33.

Lacey, J. M. and D. W. Wilmore. 1990. Is glutamine a conditionally essential amino acid? *Nutr Rev* 48 (8):297–309.

Lindquist, S. and E. A. Craig. 1988. The heat-shock proteins. *Annu Rev Genet* 22:631–77.

Lu, J., X. Y. Wang, and W. H. Tang. 2009. Glutamine attenuates nitric oxide synthase expression and mitochondria membrane potential decrease in interleukin-1beta-activated rat hepatocytes. *Eur J Nutr* 48 (6):333–9.

Mansour, A., S. Hosseini, B. Larijani et al. 2013. Nutrients related to GLP1 secretory responses. *Nutrition* 29 (6):813–20.

Marshall, S., V. Bacote, and R. R. Traxinger. 1991. Discovery of a metabolic pathway mediating glucose-induced desensitization of the glucose transport system. Role of hexosamine biosynthesis in the induction of insulin resistance. *J Biol Chem* 266 (8):4706–12.

Mates, J. M., J. A. Segura, J. A. Campos-Sandoval et al. 2009. Glutamine homeostasis and mitochondrial dynamics. *Int J Biochem Cell Biol* 41 (10):2051–61.

Matthews, D. E. and A. Battezzati. 1993. Regulation of protein metabolism during stress. *Curr Opin Gen Surg* 72–7.

Mithieux, G. 2001. New data and concepts on glutamine and glucose metabolism in the gut. *Curr Opin Clin Nutr Metab Care* 4 (4):267–71.

Mondello, S., M. Galuppo, E. Mazzon et al. 2011. Glutamine treatment attenuates the development of organ injury induced by zymosan administration in mice. *Eur J Pharmacol* 658 (1):28–40.

Newgard, C. B., J. An, J. R. Bain et al. 2009. A branched-chain amino acid-related metabolic signature that differentiates obese and lean humans and contributes to insulin resistance. *Cell Metab* 9 (4):311–26.

Newsholme, E. A. 1996. The possible role of glutamine in some cells of the immune system and the possible consequence for the whole animal. *Experientia* 52 (5):455–9.

Newsholme, P., F. Abdulkader, E. Rebelato et al. 2011. Amino acids and diabetes: Implications for endocrine, metabolic and immune function. *Front Biosci* 16:315–39.

Newsholme, P., K. Bender, A. Kiely et al. 2007. Amino acid metabolism, insulin secretion and diabetes. *Biochem Soc Trans* 35 (Pt 5):1180–6.

Newsholme, P., L. Brennan, B. Rubi, and P. Maechler. 2005. New insights into amino acid metabolism, beta-cell function and diabetes. *Clin Sci (Lond)* 108 (3):185–94.

Newsholme, P., V. Cruzat, F. Arfuso et al. 2014. Nutrient regulation of insulin secretion and action. *J Endocrinol* 221 (3):R105–20.

Newsholme, P., C. Gaudel, and M. Krause. 2012. Mitochondria and diabetes. An intriguing pathogenetic role. *Adv Exp Med Biol* 942:235–47.

Newsholme, P., P. I. Homem De Bittencourt, C. O' Hagan et al. 2010. Exercise and possible molecular mechanisms of protection from vascular disease and diabetes: The central role of ROS and nitric oxide. *Clin Sci* 118 (5):341–9.

Newsholme, P. and M. Krause. 2012. Nutritional regulation of insulin secretion: Implications for diabetes. *Clin Biochem Rev* 33 (2):35–47.

Newsholme, P., K. Keane, P. I. Homem (Jr) de Bittencourt et al. 2013. The impact of inflammation on pancreatic β-cell metabolism, function and failure in T1DM and T2DM: Commonalities and differences. In *Type 1 Diabetes*, edited by A. P. Escher and Alice Li. Available online at http://library.umac.mo/ebooks/b28356184.pdf.

Newsholme, P., J. Procopio, M. M. Lima et al. 2003. Glutamine and glutamate—Their central role in cell metabolism and function. *Cell Biochem Funct* 21 (1):1–9.

Nisr, R. B. and C. Affourtit. 2014. Insulin acutely improves mitochondrial function of rat and human skeletal muscle by increasing coupling efficiency of oxidative phosphorylation. *Biochimica et Biophysica Acta* 1837 (2):270–6.

Olefsky, J. M. and C. K. Glass. 2010. Macrophages, inflammation, and insulin resistance. *Annu Rev Physiol* 72:219–46.

Opara, E. C., A. Petro, A. Tevrizian et al. 1996. L-glutamine supplementation of a high fat diet reduces body weight and attenuates hyperglycemia and hyperinsulinemia in C57BL/6J mice. *J Nutr* 126 (1):273–9.

Peng, X., H. Yan, Z. You et al. 2006. Glutamine granule-supplemented enteral nutrition maintains immunological function in severely burned patients. *Burns* 32 (5):589–93.

Petry, E. R., V. F. Cruzat, T. G. Heck et al. 2014. Alanyl-glutamine and glutamine plus alanine supplements improve skeletal redox status in trained rats: Involvement of heat shock protein pathways. *Life Sci* 94 (2):130–6.

Prada, P. O., S. M. Hirabara, C. T. de Souza et al. 2007. L-glutamine supplementation induces insulin resistance in adipose tissue and improves insulin signalling in liver and muscle of rats with diet-induced obesity. *Diabetologia* 50 (9):1949–59.

Radomski, M. W. 1995. Nitric oxide: Biological mediator, modulator and effector. *Ann Med* 27 (3):321–9.

Reimann, F., L. Williams, G. da Silva Xavier et al. 2004. Glutamine potently stimulates glucagon-like peptide-1 secretion from GLUTag cells. *Diabetologia* 47 (9):1592–601.

Samocha-Bonet, D., O. Wong, E. L. Synnott et al. 2011. Glutamine reduces postprandial glycemia and augments the glucagon-like peptide-1 response in type 2 diabetes patients. *J Nutr* 141 (7):1233–8.

Shi, Q., Y. N. Feng, J. Fang et al. 2009. Pretreatment with glutamine attenuates anoxia/reoxygenation injury of human proximal renal tubular epithelial cells via induction of heme oxygenase-1. *Pharmacology* 84 (1):1–8.

Singleton, K. D., V. E. Beckey, and P. E. Wischmeyer. 2005. Glutamine prevents activation of NF-kappaB and stress kinase pathways, attenuates inflammatory cytokine release, and prevents acute respiratory distress syndrome (ARDS) following sepsis. *Shock* 24 (6):583–9.

Singleton, K. D. and P. E. Wischmeyer. 2007. Glutamine's protection against sepsis and lung injury is dependent on heat shock protein 70 expression. *Am J Physiol Regul Integr Comp Physiol* 292 (5):R1839–45.

Sookoian, S. and C. J. Pirola. 2012. Alanine and aspartate aminotransferase and glutamine-cycling pathway: Their roles in pathogenesis of metabolic syndrome. *World J Gastroenterol* 18 (29):3775–81.

Su, D., G. M. Coudriet, D. Hyun Kim et al. 2009. FoxO1 links insulin resistance to proinflammatory cytokine IL-1beta production in macrophages. *Diabetes* 58 (11):2624–33.

Tjader, I., A. Berg, and J. Wernerman. 2007. Exogenous glutamine—Compensating a shortage? *Crit Care Med* 35 (9 Suppl):S553–6.

Tolhurst, G., Y. Zheng, H. E. Parker et al. 2011. Glutamine triggers and potentiates glucagon-like peptide-1 secretion by raising cytosolic Ca2+ and cAMP. *Endocrinology* 152 (2):405–13.

Tsai, P. H., J. J. Liu, W. C. Chiu et al. 2011. Effects of dietary glutamine on adhesion molecule expression and oxidative stress in mice with streptozotocin-induced type 1 diabetes. *Clin Nutr* 30 (1):124–9.

Tsai, P. H., J. J. Liu, C. L. Yeh et al. 2012. Effects of glutamine supplementation on oxidative stress-related gene expression and antioxidant properties in rats with streptozotocin-induced type 2 diabetes. *Br J Nutr* 107 (8):1112–8.

Tsai, P. H., C. L. Yeh, J. J. Liu et al. 2012. Effects of dietary glutamine on inflammatory mediator gene expressions in rats with streptozotocin-induced diabetes. *Nutrition* 28 (3):288–93.

Turner, N., G. J. Cooney, E. W. Kraegen et al. 2014. Fatty acid metabolism, energy expenditure and insulin resistance in muscle. *J Endocrinol* 220 (2):T61–79.

Uehara, K., T. Takahashi, H. Fujii et al. 2005. The lower intestinal tract-specific induction of heme oxygenase-1 by glutamine protects against endotoxemic intestinal injury. *Crit Care Med* 33 (2):381–90.

Wang, C., Y. Guan, and J. Yang. 2010. Cytokines in the progression of pancreatic beta-cell dysfunction. *Int J Endocrinol* 2010:515136.

Wilmore, D. W. 2001. The effect of glutamine supplementation in patients following elective surgery and accidental injury. *J Nutr* 131 (9 Suppl):2543S–9S; discussion 2550S-1S.

Wischmeyer, P. E. 2007. Glutamine: Mode of action in critical illness. *Critical Care Medicine* 35 (9 Suppl):S541–4.

Yeh, C. L., C. S. Hsu, S. L. Yeh et al. 2005. Dietary glutamine supplementation modulates Th1/Th2 cytokine and interleukin-6 expressions in septic mice. *Cytokine* 31 (5):329–34.

Zhang, F., X. Wang, W. Wang et al. 2008. Glutamine reduces TNF-alpha by enhancing glutathione synthesis in lipopolysaccharide-stimulated alveolar epithelial cells of rats. *Inflammation* 31 (5):344–50.

Ziegler, T. R., L. G. Ogden, K. D. Singleton et al. 2005. Parenteral glutamine increases serum heat shock protein 70 in critically ill patients. *Intensive Care Med* 31 (8):1079–86.

5 Glutamine and Autophagy

Rolf Gebhardt

CONTENTS

5.1 INTRODUCTION: BACKGROUND AND DRIVING FORCES

It is known for decades that glutamine can act as a signal providing valuable information about the nitrogen status and other important aspects associated with amino acid and energy metabolism to cells, organs, and even the entire organism. Although several different mechanisms for sensing glutamine concentration and various physiological targets have been elucidated (for review see Curi et al. 2005; Häussinger and Schliess 2007; Roth 2008; Rhoads and Wu 2009; Ghavami et al. 2014), we are far from comprehensively understanding the rich spectrum of different functions involved. One process that has come into special focus in recent years is autophagy. First experimental evidence for an outstanding role of glutamine in the regulation of autophagy dates back to the early 1980s, when high glutamine concentrations were found to inhibit mass protein degradation in the liver (Seglen et al. 1980; Mortimore and Pösö 1984). Since then, however, it became obvious that the influence of glutamine on autophagy is much more complex and can range from inhibition to activation and indirect modulation depending on the cell type or tissue under consideration.

Autophagy is a highly conserved homeostatic mechanism for the degradation and recycling of bulk cytoplasm, long-lived proteins, and cell organelles (Mizushima and Komatsu 2011). It is triggered and modulated by a plethora of different stimuli such as nutrient deprivation and other stress signals. The amino acid-responsive form is called macroautophagy from its morphological characteristics (for review and other forms of autophagy see Ghavami et al. 2014). The process of autophagosome formation proceeds via initiation, elongation, and maturation steps leading to autophagic vesicles that, together with the cargo to be degraded, finally fuse with lysosomes to form the autophagolysosomes (Figure 5.1). The entire process of macroautophagy (hereafter simply called autophagy), in particular the initial steps, are controlled by a large variety of autophagy related genes (ATGs) that are involved in the sequential formation of multimeric complexes.

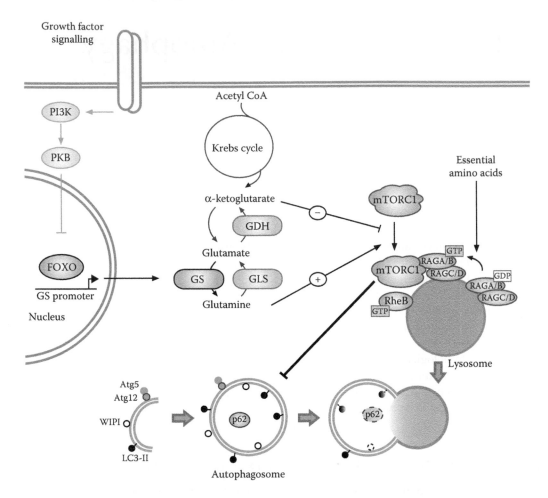

FIGURE 5.1 Schematic illustration of the interplay between glutamine metabolism, mTOR activation, and autophagy. (Taken from van der Vos, K.E. and Coffer, P.J. 2012. *Autophagy*, 8: 1862–1864.)

Although the details of the pre-autosomal complex formation and of its subsequent transformation are not fully established, there is convincing evidence that PI3 kinases class III and, particularly, the mTOR kinase complex 1 (mTORC1) play a dominant role in the control of these processes and, thus, in the regulation of autophagy (Ghavami et al. 2014; Noguchi et al. 2014). In this chapter, the central role of glutamine in this regulatory network is addressed.

5.2 THE PUZZLING SPECTRUM OF GLUTAMINE EFFECTS ON AUTOPHAGY

Ten years ago, glutamine was considered as a potent inhibitor of autophagy sharing its influence with several other plasma amino acids such as leucine and tyrosine, which collectively were called regulatory amino acids (Kadowaki and Kanazawa 2003). This view was based mainly on studies in liver or isolated hepatocytes and was in line with the observation that autophagic proteolysis is a major source of amino acids in starvation (Mortimore and Kadowaki 2001). Although the effect of amino acids on autophagy was discovered long ago (Buse and Reid 1975; Fulks et al. 1975; Seglen et al. 1980; Mortimore and Pösö 1984), the mechanisms remained largely obscure, particularly in the case of glutamine. The past decade, however, has seen a tremendous increase in the number of investigations of these questions paralleled by the discovery that the effects of glutamine on autophagy were quite variable in different types of cells and tissues and could result not only in

TABLE 5.1

Different Effects of Glutamine on Autophagy

	Primary Mechanism	Secondary Mechanism	References
		Activation	
5.2.1	FoxO-induced GS activation	Glutamine inhibition of mTORC1	Van der Vos et al. (2012)
5.2.2	Glutaminolysis → NH$_3$	Activation of autophagy (not defined)	Eng and Abraham (2010)
			Eng et al. (2010)
	NH$_3$ production	mTOR-dependent and AMPK-dependent	Harder et al. (2014)
5.2.3	Glutaminolysis → NH$_3$ (in tumor)	Diffusion of NH$_3$	Ko et al. (2011)
		Activation of autophagy by NH$_3$ in stroma	Albanese et al. (2011)
5.2.4	Hexosamine pathway activation or N-Acetyl-glucosamine	Unclear	Denzel et al. (2014)
		Inhibition	
5.2.5	Bidirectional transport of amino acids	Leucine activation of mTOR	Nicklin et al. (2009)
5.2.6	Glutaminolysis → α-ketoglutarate	Activation of mTORC1	Durán et al. (2012)

inhibition but also in activation of autophagy. Concomitantly, these studies provided deep insight into a surprising complex regulatory mechanism that underlies the context-dependent variation of glutamine action. For the sake of clarity, the major findings are classified in Table 5.1 and discussed in detail in the following sections.

5.2.1 THE FoxO-MEDIATED GLUTAMINE SYNTHETASE-DEPENDENT ACTIVATION PATHWAY

Forkhead box O (FoxO) transcription factors can influence a wide range of biological processes in many cell types, including stress resistance, nutrient deprivation, cell cycle progression, and apoptosis (Calnan and Brunet 2008; Dansen and Burgering 2008). They are inactivated trough phosphorylation by the PI3K-AKT1 axis in response to insulin, insulin-like growth factors (IGFs), and other growth factors. In their active, non-phosphorylated form FoxO3 and FoxO4 transcription factors enhance the expression of specific genes, including certain ATGs such as LC3 and Bnip3 in skeletal muscle (Mammucari et al. 2008) and the enzyme glutamine synthetase in liver (Gebhardt and Hovhannisyan 2010, van der Vos et al. 2012). Elevated enzyme levels of glutamine synthetase led to a selective increase in intracellular glutamine at the expense of glutamate and eventually of α-ketoglutarate (see Figure 5.1). As convincingly shown by van der Vos et al. (2012), high intracellular glutamine abrogates the lysosomal localization of mTORC1 and leads to the activation of autophagy. Of particular interest is that L-methionine sulphoximine, a specific inhibitor of glutamine synthetase, abrogates autophagosome formation in this system indicating that glutamine synthesis in an essential step. This mechanism seems to be evolutionarily conserved as it could be demonstrated in *C. elegans* as well as in several mammalian cell types (van der Vos et al. 2012). A link between FoxO transcription factors and autophagy was also reported in cardiomyocytes (Sengupta et al. 2009) and neurons (Xu et al. 2011).

5.2.2 THE GLUTAMINOLYSIS/AMMONIA-DEPENDENT ACTIVATION PATHWAY

The first step in glutaminolysis is catalyzed by glutaminase (GLS) resulting in deamination to glutamate and ammonia. The increased rate of glutaminolysis in tumor cells has been recognized for a long time. One particular role is replenishment of the tricarboxylic acid (TCA) cycle, which is critical for the production of biosynthetic precursor molecules. When studying the reasons for the sustained increase in autophagic flux in cultured cancer cells, Eng and colleagues discovered a link between glutaminolysis and the production of a diffusible stimulator of autophagy that turned out to be ammonia at low millimolar concentrations (2–4 mM) (Eng et al. 2010). Although the molecular mechanism by which ammonia activates autophagy is not yet fully established, there is evidence against the exclusive dependence on mTORC1. This was confirmed by Harder and colleagues using MCF7 cancer cells (Harder et al. 2014). In a noteworthy phosphoproteomic study comparing the effects of ammonia and rapamycin, these authors could partially exclude the participation of mTORC1 and of MAPK3 from the cellular response to ammonia. Instead, they provided evidence for an upregulation of 5' AMP-activated protein kinase (AMPK) and the unfolded protein response (UPR) as possible links between ammonia and autophagy (Harder et al. 2014).

Besides various tumor cells, T lymphocytes may represent a normal cell type that undergoes explosive rounds of rapid proliferation using the glutaminolysis pathway for fuelling cell growth and survival (Eng and Abraham 2010).

5.2.3 THE TRANSCELLULAR AMMONIA-DEPENDENT ACTIVATION PATHWAY

This pathway resembles that described in Section 5.2.2. Now, however, the cell producing ammonia (e.g., the tumor cell) is no longer considered the (exclusive) target of ammonia. Instead, it is assumed that ammonia is extruded from the producing cell and diffuses into a different cell (type) in the vicinity (e.g., a tumor cell in a different location or a tumor-associated fibroblast) (Ko et al. 2011). In the receiving cell (e.g., the fibroblast), ammonia subsequently induces autophagy according to the mechanism described before (Section 5.2.2).

5.2.4 THE HEXOSAMINE-DEPENDENT ACTIVATION PATHWAY

Induction of autophagy has been associated with increased life span because it provides a quality-control mechanism that contributes to the turnover of aggregation-prone proteins and organelle homeostasis (Menzies et al. 2011). Focusing on *C. elegans*, a model organism frequently used is studies on lifespan extensions, Denzel and colleagues demonstrated that hexosamine pathway activation or N-acetylglucosamine supplementation induces distinct protein quality-control mechanisms, including autophagy, which result in extended life span (Denzel et al. 2014). Increased autophagy was shown by condensation of the light chain 3 (LC3) homolog LGG-1 I puncta as well as by an increase in the lipidated form of LGG-1. Apparently, autophagy was increased by N-acetylglucosamine in a posttranscriptional manner. Generally, transcriptional events could virtually be excluded from participating in this type of mechanism (Denzel et al. 2014).

Since glutamine is the primary nitrogen donor in the synthesis of hexosamines, there is an obvious glutamine dependence of this activating mechanism of autophagy. In an earlier report a similar influence was described for glucosamine (Carames et al. 2013). In that study activation of autophagy was induced via inhibition of the Akt/Forkhead box O(FoxO)/mechanistic target of rapamycin (mTOR) pathway. Moreover, D-glucosamine supplementation was found to extend the life span of nematodes and of aging mice (Weimer et al. 2014).

5.2.5 THE BIDIRECTIONAL AMINO ACID TRANSPORT-DEPENDENT INHIBITION PATHWAY

This pathway was originally described in HeLa cells and MCF7 cells. When these cells are preloaded with glutamine (up to 1 mM), which is taken up via the SLC1A5 transporter (Fuchs and Bode 2005), they respond to the subsequent extracellular exposure to essential amino acids (EAA) by an activation of mTORC1 (Nicklin et al. 2009). The role of glutamine in this mechanism is to drive the uptake of EAA such as leucine via exchange by the antiporter SLC7A5-SLC3A2. As a result, sufficiently high intracellular concentrations of leucine are reached. How leucine activates mTORC1 and whether the Rag GTPases play a role in this process remains unanswered in this study. Alternate mechanisms such as leucine-dependent activation of GDH (see below) were also not tested.

The strength of this investigation, however, is the broad and convincing evidence that the effect of glutamine and leucine is dependent on the presence and functional activity of the two amino acid transport systems, SLC1A5 and SLC7A-SLC3A2 (Nicklin et al. 2009). Thus, this mechanism may be of importance in cell populations simultaneously expressing both transport systems. Prominent examples may be found among epithelial cell types particularly in kidney and intestine (Bode 2001), but generalization is difficult, because of the large cellular variation in the expression of transporter subtypes.

Another important point is that rising the extracellular concentration of glutamine in combination with EAA leads to sustained activation of mTORC1 as indicted by the phosphorylation and activation of ribosomal protein S6 kinase 1 (S6K1) in cultured cells (Nicklin et al. 2009). This observation reveals that it is the extracellular glutamine that matters in this type of mechanism, not the intracellular one (which has a low steady-state). This was emphasized also in a recent hypothesis about the possible role of this mechanism in the periportal zone of the liver (Gebhardt and Coffer 2013).

5.2.6 THE GLUTAMINOLYSIS-DEPENDENT INHIBITION PATHWAY

Glutaminolysis to glutamate and further to α-ketoglutarate proceeds via GLS reaction followed by either transaminase or glutamate dehydrogenase (GDH) reactions that preserve the α-amino nitrogen or liberate it as ammonia, respectively. The latter pathway is moderately stimulated by leucine in most mammalian cells that possess only one gene for GDH (Smith and Stanley 2008). Whereas in humans a similar gene (GDH1) is widely expressed as a type of housekeeping gene, a second gene (GDH2) is expressed only in certain cells and tissues (e.g., neurons, testicular cells, and pancreatic β-cells) (Spanaki and Plaitakis 2012). This is important because leucine is a much stronger allosteric activator of GDH2 than of GDH1 (Kanavouras et al. 2007; Smith and Stanley 2008). Thus, human cells expressing GDH2 are expected to produce much more α-ketoglutarate from glutamate (or glutamine) in the presence of leucine than do other cells.

Recently, Duran and colleagues reported that the end-product of glutaminolysis, α-ketoglutarate, is a specific activator of mTORC1 by enhancing its translocation to the surface of lysosomes (Durán et al. 2012). Specifically, α-ketoglutarate was found to directly activate mTORC1 via activation of prolyl hydroxylases (Durán et al. 2012), a family of α-ketoglutarate-dependent dioxygenases (Boulahbel et al. 2009). These findings provide an interesting explanation on how α-ketoglutarate might transduce the inhibitory effect of glutaminolysis on autophagy.

5.3 GENERAL MECHANISTIC CONSIDERATIONS

5.3.1 THE GLUTAMINE/α-KETOGLUTARATE RATIO

Because of the different scenarios by which glutamine metabolism can affect autophagy (Table 5.1), it is intriguing to find out whether they can be grouped into a general mechanistic scheme. In Figure 5.2 the major chemical reactions of glutamine metabolism are depicted. They include transport possibilities across the plasma membrane, GLS, and glutamine synthetase reactions, and conversion of glutamate to α-ketoglutarate via GDH that results in additional ammonia or via transaminases that lead to an additional amino acid molecule. Apparently, not all reactions are active in the same manner at the same time and in the same cells. More likely, different cells preferentially express different transporters and/or certain subsets of reactions as exemplified in Table 5.2 and, thus, show different metabolic fluxes and ratios between intracellular levels of glutamine and α-ketoglutarate. In particular, the balance between the intracellular concentrations of

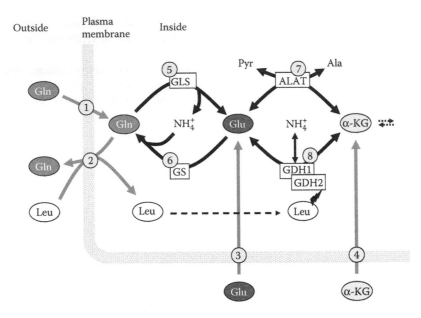

FIGURE 5.2 Scheme of major transport and enzyme reactions of cellular glutamine metabolism, Gln: glutamine, Glu: glutamate, α-KG: α-ketoglutarate, Leu: leucine, 1 to 4: transport reactions defined in Table 5.2, 5/GLS: glutaminase, 6/GS: glutamine synthetase, 7/ALAT: alanine amino transferase, 8/GDH: glutamate dehydrogenase.

glutamine, on one hand, and α-ketoglutarate, on the other, seems to be a potent regulatory parameter determining mTORC1 activity and, consequently, autophagy (van der Vos and Coffer 2012). For instance, intracellular glutamine is high in cells expressing glutamine synthetase (e.g., pericentral hepatocytes; astrocytes). Here, levels of glutamate, α-ketoglutarate, and ammonia, which are all substrates of glutamine synthesis, are low at the same time, resulting in an especially high glutamine/α-ketoglutarate ratio.

TABLE 5.2
Examples of Cellular Diversity in Glutamine Uptake and Metabolism

Reaction Sequence[a]	Transport Details	Cell Type/Organ	Function
1, 2, 5, (7) 8	1 = SNAT3 (Slc38a3) (2 Na⁺ in, 1 H⁺ out)	Hepatocyte (periportal)	Glutaminolysis
	2 = LAT1/CD98 (Slc7a5/Slc3a2)		
4, (7) 8, 3, 6,1	4 = OAT	Hepatocyte (pericentral)	Glutamine synthesis
	3 = GLT1		
	1 = SNAT3 (Slc38a3) (2 Na⁺ in, 1 H⁺ out)		
1, 5, 7 (8)	1 = SNAT3 (Slc38a3)	Skeletal muscle	Glutaminolysis
3, 6, 1	3 = SNAT1 (Slc38a1)	Astrocyte	Glutamine release
	1 = SNAT3 (Slc38a1)		
1, 5, 8	1 = SNAT1 (Slc38a1)	Many tumor cells	Glutamine accumulation/
	or		Glutaminolysis
	1 = ASCT2 (Slc1a5)		
(a) 1, 2	1 = ASCT2 (Slc1a5) (apical)	Enterocyte	(a) Transcellular transport
(b) 1, 5, 8	2 = LAT1/CD98 (Slc7a5/Slc3a2)	and	(b) (partial) Glutaminolysis
	(basolateral)	kidney	

[a] Numbers refer to transporter and enzyme reactions specified in Figure 5.2.

In contrast, cells with high activities of GLS (e.g., periportal hepatocytes, tumor cells) may show an especially low glutamine/α-ketoglutarate ratio. In this case, further aspects have to be taken into account. First, as pointed out by Shanware et al. (2011), availability of glucose may considerably influence the source and amount of α-ketoglutarate in the TCA cycle, thus, additionally influencing this ratio. Second, the concentration of NH_4^+, which is a byproduct of both GLS and GDH reactions, may counteract the inhibitory influence of α-ketoglutarate on autophagy. Whether ammonia is retained within the cell as NH_4^+ or escapes from the cell as NH_3 depends on the intracellular pH. Therefore, pH may be an additional regulatory factor under conditions of a low glutamine/α-ketoglutarate ratio.

5.3.2 REGULATION OF AUTOPHAGY BY MORPHOGENS

In recent years, accumulating evidence points to an important role of morphogen signaling pathways such as Wnt/β-catenin signaling (Gebhardt and Coffer 2013) and hedgehog signaling (Jimenez-Sanchez et al. 2012; Gagné-Sansfaçon et al. 2014) in the regulation of autophagy. Since morphogens are well known as indispensable regulators not only in embryogenesis, organogenesis, and tissue regeneration (Wartlick et al. 2009, Ingham et al. 2011) but also in carcinogenesis (Brechbiel et al. 2014, Kahn 2014), it seems plausible that they also seek control over cellular processes as powerful as autophagy in the context of these developmental phenomena. Surprisingly, within the past decade it was realized that morphogens are also powerful regulators of metabolism, particularly in mature cells and tissues (Matz-Soja et al. 2013, Gebhardt and Matz-Soja 2014, Teperino 2014). To date, only few experimental studies have explored this promising field, the majority of which have been carried out in liver. In these studies, it was shown that the zonal expression of glutamine synthetase and of GLS is reciprocally regulated by wnt/β-catenin signaling in the pericentral and periportal zone of liver parenchyma, respectively (Gebhardt and Hovhannisyan 2010). Thus, important enzymes of glutamine synthesis and glutaminolysis are under the control of morphogens (Gebhardt and Matz-Soja 2014). In the context of the considerations made in the previous section one may wonder whether other enzymes and transport systems such as SLC7A5 and GDH are also under the control of these morphogens. These and other questions have prompted us to advance a hypothesis that assembles most of the isolated findings of glutamine metabolism into an overarching concept that is specifically tailored to explain the conditions of liver tissue (Gebhardt and Coffer 2013). It culminates in the conjecture that autophagy may be controlled in a zonal fashion by different mechanisms, a concept that may be valid also for many other tissues. Briefly, autophagy is controlled by the bidirectional amino acid transport pathway in the periportal zone and by the FoxO-mediated glutamine synthesis pathway in the pericentral zone (Gebhardt and Coffer 2013). However, it needs to be emphasized that glutamine metabolism may only be one of many different targets of morphogen signaling and that other mechanisms controlling autophagy may be targeted as well.

Likewise, the interplay of morphogens and autophagy may not be a one-way road. Indeed, there is evidence that autophagy may feed-back on morphogen signaling. For instance, autophagy was found to regulate Wnt signaling by promoting disheveled degradation (Gao et al. 2010). Taken together, these findings imply that autophagy is not only subject to regulation by morphogens but also may contribute to shaping graded morphogen action, an as yet unsolved problem at least in liver (Gebhardt and Hovhannisyan 2010).

5.4 IMPLICATIONS

The implications of the complex effects of glutamine on autophagy are manifold and documented by a vast amount of literature. Since it is beyond the scope of this chapter to present a comprehensive overview, we focus on three major aspects and cite only a selection of reviews or outstanding research papers.

5.4.1 PHYSIOLOGICAL AND PATHOPHYSIOLOGICAL EFFECTS

When dealing with glutamine regulation of autophagy two major aspects come into focus: nutrient sensing and homeostasis. Although glutamine is a nonessential amino acid, its availability is of considerable importance for the proper function (including energy supply) of many cells. In its absence (glutamine deprivation) compensating mechanisms have to be switched on at the cellular or the tissue level, to maintain nutrient homeostasis. One such mechanism is autophagy, which may allow recycling of excess or unwanted cellular material to ensure the supply of suitable substrates including glutamine. Several recent publications have highlighted these interactions in different cell types and tissues such as connective tissue, brain, liver, and heart (Lin et al. 2012; Dunlop and Tee 2014; Fader et al. 2015; Kesidou et al. 2013). Interestingly, there is an additional amino acid–sensing mechanism inside the lysosomes that is relayed via the vacuolar H^+-ATPase (v-ATPase) to the Ragulator complex at the outside (Zoncu et al. 2011). The Ragulator complex includes the Rag GTPases, RagA and RagB, that switch to the active GTP-bound state when amino acids are plentiful (Sancak et al. 2010). The v-ATPase is also involved in energy sensing (Dunlop and Tee 2014). Such mechanisms may impact on more than just amino acid metabolism. For instance, Ezaki et al. (2011) have shown that liver autophagy contributes to the maintenance of blood glucose in an amino acid- and insulin-dependent manner. Furthermore, these processes may enhance the fitness of the cells and extend life span (Menzies et al. 2011, Rubinsztein et al. 2011, Lapierre et al. 2012). With respect to cellular fitness, it is highly interesting that autophagy and exosome formation appear as coordinated mechanisms to alleviate stress particularly in diseased conditions (reviewed in Baixauli et al. 2014).

Concerning lipid metabolism the specific role of autophagy in the digestion of lipid droplets was appreciated by coining the term "lipophagy" (reviewed in Singh and Cuervo 2012). Although lipophagy plays a natural role in adipose tissue (Christian et al. 2013) it may become considerably important in other tissues such as liver under conditions of pathological lipid accumulation (Gebhardt and Coffer 2013). Important links between the regulation of autophagy and liver complications associated with obesity and nonalcoholic fatty liver disease (NAFLD) have been reported, reports provide only an incoherent and controversial picture (Kwanten et al. 2014; Lavallard and Gual 2014). If disease progresses, fibrotic alterations are common. Autophagy seems to play an important role in this development as reviewed by Mallat et al. (2014). More important, their review illustrates the wide spectrum of how autophagy in different cell types, such as hepatocytes and hepatic stellate cells, contributes to this process. Apart from NAFLD, autophagy seems to play a role in various other liver diseases (Cursio et al. 2015), but addressing these aspects in detail would go beyond the scope of this review.

5.4.2 GLUTAMINE, AUTOPHAGY, AND AGING

It has already been discussed above that autophagy plays an important role in aging. In general, all cellular mechanisms involved in the removal of deteriorated proteins from cells contribute to longevity (Vilchez et al. 2014; Madeo et al. 2015; Martinez-Lopez et al. 2015; Schloesser et al. 2015) particularly in organs with low cell turnover such as the heart (Linton et al. 2015) or the brain (Perluigi et al. 2015). Mitophagy, the autophagic removal of damaged mitochondria, has received special attention with respect to life extension (Biala et al. 2015). As pointed out above, normal autophagy as well as mitophagy is under the control of mTOR activity, and, thus, it is no surprise that inhibition of mTORC1 activity by various drugs is expected to prolong life span (Kroemer 2015). The same should hold for glutamine according to the mechanisms described in Sections 5.2.1 and 5.3.1, but direct experimental evidence for a life-extending role of glutamine is still lacking. Intriguingly, however, overexpression of FOXO1 in skeletal muscle increased glutamine synthetase protein but did not alter longevity in mice (Chiba et al. 2009). In this context, it is interesting to note that in humans serum glutamine level increases with age in healthy females while it remained unchanged in males (Kouchiwa et al. 2012). In human skeletal muscle, however, age negatively correlated with the cytosolic concentration ratio of glutamine to total branched chain amino acids (Stuerenburg et al. 2006), indicating that relative loss of muscle glutamine contributes to sarcopenia. It is not clear whether glutamine supplementation can reverse these phenomena. Experiments in adult and very old female rats revealed an increased glutamine requirement during aging (Mignon et al. 2007) that may be associated with the stimulation of glutamine synthetase activity in muscle tissue in rats with advanced age (Mezzarobba et al. 2003; Pinel et al. 2006). In contrast, in some rats with very advanced age (29–32 months) lower values of glutamine synthetase activity were determined (Pinel et al. 2006). These variable results call for additional studies on the influence of endogenous glutamine and glutamine supplementation on life expectancy.

5.4.3 Effects on Cancer Cells

The role of autophagy in tumorigenesis, tumor progression, and cancer therapeutics is indifferent and highly context dependent. It can promote tumor cell survival as well as death, and, thus, tumor therapeutics influencing autophagy can be either pro-survival or pro-death for tumor cells (reviewed in Lui and Ryan 2012; Lorin et al. 2013; Lozy and Karantza 2012). Generally, macroautophagy can be tumor-suppressive by removing aberrant proteins and organelles or it can aid cancer cells to overcome metabolic stress and cytotoxicity of chemotherapeutic agents.

Herein we focus on glutamine effects in tumor cells. The vast majority of tumor cells is prone to glutaminolysis for a number of reasons, including (a) support of cell growth and proliferation by providing carbon and nitrogen for energy production and biosynthetic reactions (e.g., nucleotide and lipid synthesis) and (b) support of cell survival under stressful conditions, for example, scarcity of glucose and enhanced production of reactive oxygen species (ROS). These reactions are under the complex control by oncogens. This is exemplified by Ras-driven signals in pancreatic tumor cells such as B-Raf signaling and the PI3 K/AKT axis which interfere directly with the various possibilities for regulating glutamine metabolism and its effect on autophagy outlined above (Shanware et al. 2011; White 2013; Blum and Kloog 2014). Simultaneously, they can also affect autophagy directly through transcriptional effects (Kubisch et al. 2013).

Another important aspect is the cooperation between cancer cells and stromal cells in their environment (reviewed in Martinez-Outschoorn et al. 2011; Icard et al. 2014). In this respect, the production of ammonia via GLS and/or GDH in tumor cells may be of particular interest as NH_3 may diffuse out of the tumor cells and stimulate autophagy in neighboring stroma cells, a concept that has been advanced by Ko et al. (2011). In these cells, autophagy may serve as means to supply the tumor with substrates for continuous growth and expansion (Martinez-Outschoorn et al. 2014).

5.5 CONCLUSION AND PERSPECTIVES

The findings reviewed convincingly demonstrate that glutamine is a potent regulator of autophagy, the effect of which, however, is strongly dependent on cell type and physiological context. Obviously, there is an emerging concept based on cellular glutamine metabolism that can explain many aspects of its regulatory spectrum. It will be a challenge for future research to elaborate this concept in more detail and to combine it with the regulation through additional signals, nutritional and hormonal, that can interfere at different levels. Another challenge may be to investigate the various molecular events through which glutamine may exert its effects on autophagy and, eventually, on aging. Given the conflicting effects of autophagy, particularly in cancer cells, only a deeper understanding of the molecular mechanisms may allow us to identify appropriate and selective targets for therapeutic intervention.

REFERENCES

Albanese, C., Machado, F.S. and Tanowitz, H.B. 2011. Glutamine and the tumour microenvironment: Understanding the mechanisms that fuel cancer progression. *Cancer Biol Ther* 12, 1098–1100.

Baixauli, F., Lopez-Otin, C. and Mittelbrunn, M. 2014. Exosomes and autophagy: Coordinated mechanisms for the maintenance of cellular fitness. *Front Immunol* 5, 403.

Biala, A.K., Dhingra, R. and Kirshenbaum, L.A. 2015. Mitochondrial dynamics: Orchestrating the journey to advanced age. *J Mol Cell Cardiol* 83, 37–43.

Blum, R. and Kloog, Y. 2014. Metabolism addiction in pancreatic cancer. *Cell Death Dis* 5, e1065.

Bode, B.P. 2001. Recent molecular advances in mammalian glutamine transport. *J Nutr* 131, 2475S–2485S; discussion 2486S–2487S.

Boulahbel, H., Duran, R.V. and Gottlieb, E. 2009. Prolyl hydroxylases as regulators of cell metabolism. *Biochem Soc Trans* 37, 291–294.

Brechbiel, J., Miller-Moslin, K. and Adjei, A.A. 2014. Crosstalk between hedgehog and other signalling pathways as a basis for combination therapies in cancer. *Cancer Treat Rev* 40, 750–759.

Buse, M.G. and Reid, S.S. 1975. Leucine. A possible regulator of protein turnover in muscle. *J Clin Invest* 56, 1250–1261.

Calnan, D.R. and Brunet, A. 2008. The FoxO code. *Oncogene* 27, 2276–2288.

Carames, B., Kiosses, W.B., Akasaki, Y. et al. 2013. Glucosamine activates autophagy *in vitro* and *in vivo*. *Arthritis Rheum* 65, 1843–1852.

Chiba, T., Kamei, Y., Shimizu, T. et al. 2009. Overexpression of FOXO1 in skeletal muscle does not alter longevity in mice. *Mech Ageing Dev* 130, 420–428.

Christian, P., Sacco, J. and Adeli, K. 2013. Autophagy: Emerging roles in lipid homeostasis and metabolic control. *Biochimica et biophysica acta* 1831, 819–824.

Curi, R., Lagranha, C.J., Doi, S.Q. et al. 2005. Molecular mechanisms of glutamine action. *J Cell Physiol* 204, 392–401.

Cursio, R., Colesetti, P., Codogno, P. et al. 2015. The role of autophagy in liver diseases: Mechanisms and potential therapeutic targets. *BioMed Res Int* ID 480508.

Dansen, T.B. and Burgering, B.M.T. 2008. Unravelling the tumour-suppressive functions of FOXO proteins. *Trends Cell Biol* 18, 421–429.

Denzel, M.S., Storm, N.J., Gutschmidt, A. et al. 2014. Hexosamine pathway metabolites enhance protein quality control and prolong life. *Cell* 156, 1167–1178.

Dunlop, E.A. and Tee, A.R. 2014. mTOR and autophagy: A dynamic relationship governed by nutrients and energy. *Semin Cell Dev Biol* 36, 121–129.

Durán, R.V., Oppliger, W., Robitaille, A.M. et al. 2012. Glutaminolysis activates Rag-mTORC1 signalling. *Molecular Cell* 47, 349–358.

Eng, C.H. and Abraham, R.T. 2010. Glutaminolysis yields a metabolic by-product that stimulates autophagy. *Autophagy* 6, 968–970.

Eng, C.H., Yu, K., Lucas, J. et al. 2010. Ammonia derived from glutaminolysis is a diffusible regulator of autophagy. *Science Signalling* 3, ra31.

Ezaki, J., Matsumoto, N., Takeda-Ezaki, M. et al. 2011. Liver autophagy contributes to the maintenance of blood glucose and amino acid levels. *Autophagy* 7, 727–736.

Fader, C.M., Aguilera, M.O. and Colombo, M.I. 2015. Autophagy response: Manipulating the mTOR-controlled machinery by amino acids and pathogens. *Amino Acids* 47, 2101–2112.

Fuchs, B.C. and Bode, B.P. 2005. Amino acid transporters ASCT2 and LAT1 in cancer: Partners in crime? *Semin Cancer Biol* 15, 254–266.

Fulks, R.M., Li, J.B. and Goldberg, A.L. 1975. Effects of insulin, glucose, and amino acids on protein turnover in rat diaphragm. *J Biol Chem* 250, 290–298.

Gagné-Sansfaçon, J., Allaire, J.M., Jones, C. et al. 2014. Loss of Sonic hedgehog leads to alterations in intestinal secretory cell maturation and autophagy. *PloS One* 9, e98751.

Gao, C., Cao, W., Bao, L. et al. 2010. Autophagy negatively regulates Wnt signalling by promoting Disheveled degradation. *Nat Cell Biol* 12, 781–790.

Gebhardt, R. and Coffer, P.J. 2013. Hepatic autophagy is differentially regulated in periportal and pericentral zones—A general mechanism relevant for other tissues? *CCS* 11, 21.

Gebhardt, R. and Hovhannisyan, A. 2010. Organ patterning in the adult stage: The role of Wnt/beta-catenin signalling in liver zonation and beyond. *Developmental Dynamics: An Official Publication of the American Association of Anatomists* 239, 45–55.

Gebhardt, R. and Matz-Soja, M. 2014. Liver zonation: Novel aspects of its regulation and its impact on homeo-stasis. *World J Gastroenterol* 20, 8491–8504.

Ghavami, S., Shojaei, S., Yeganeh, B. et al. 2014. Autophagy and apoptosis dysfunction in neurodegenerative disorders. *Prog Neurobiol* 112, 24–49.

Harder, L.M., Bunkenborg, J. and Andersen, J.S. 2014. Inducing autophagy: A comparative phosphoproteomic study of the cellular response to ammonia and rapamycin. *Autophagy* 10, 339–355.

Häussinger, D. and Schliess, F. 2007. Glutamine metabolism and signalling in the liver. *Front Biosci* 12, 371–391.

Icard, P., Kafara, P., Steyaert, J.-M. et al. 2014. The metabolic cooperation between cells in solid cancer tumours. *Biochim Biophys Acta* 1846, 216–225.

Ingham, P.W., Nakano, Y. and Seger, C. 2011. Mechanisms and functions of Hedgehog signalling across the metazoa. *Nature Reviews. Genetics* 12, 393–406.

Jimenez-Sanchez, M., Menzies, F.M., Chang, Y.-Y. et al. 2012. The Hedgehog signalling pathway regulates autophagy. *Nat Commun* 3, 1200.

Kadowaki, M. and Kanazawa, T. 2003. Amino acids as regulators of proteolysis. *J Nutr* 133, 2052S–2056S.

Kahn, M. 2014. Can we safely target the WNT pathway? *Nat Rev Drug Discov* 13, 513–532.

Kanavouras, K., Mastorodemos, V., Borompokas, N. et al. 2007. Properties and molecular evolution of human GLUD2 (neural and testicular tissue-specific) glutamate dehydrogenase. *J Neurosci Res* 85, 3398–3406.

Kesidou, E., Lagoudaki, R., Touloumi, O. et al. 2013. Autophagy and neurodegenerative disorders. *Neural Regen Res* 8, 2275–2283.

Ko, Y.-H., Lin, Z., Flomenberg, N. et al. 2011. Glutamine fuels a vicious cycle of autophagy in the tumour stroma and oxidative mitochondrial metabolism in epithelial cancer cells: Implications for preventing chemotherapy resistance. *Cancer Biol Ther* 12, 1085–1097.

Kouchiwa, T., Wada, K., Uchiyama, M. et al. 2012. Age-related changes in serum amino acid concentrations in healthy individuals. *Clin Chem Lab Med* 50, 861–870.

Kroemer, G. 2015. Autophagy is a druggable process that is deregulated in aging and human disease. *J Clin Invest* 125, 1–4.

Kubisch, J., Turei, D., Foldvari-Nagy, L. et al. 2013. Complex regulation of autophagy in cancer—Integrated approaches to discover the networks that hold a double-edged sword. *Semin Cancer Biol* 23, 252–261.

Kwanten, W.J., Martinet, W., Michielsen, P.P. et al. 2014. Role of autophagy in the pathophysiology of nonal-coholic fatty liver disease: A controversial issue. *World J Gastroenterol* 20, 7325–7338.

Lapierre, L.R., Meléndez, A. and Hansen, M. 2012. Autophagy links lipid metabolism to longevity in *C. elegans*. *Autophagy* 8, 144–146.

Lavallard, V.J. and Gual, P. 2014. Autophagy and non-alcoholic fatty liver disease. *Biomed Res Int* 2014, 120179.

Lin, T.-C., Chen, Y.-R., Kensicki, E. et al. 2012. Autophagy: Resetting glutamine-dependent metabolism and oxygen consumption. *Autophagy* 8, 1477–1493.

Linton, P.J., Gurney, M., Sengstock, D. et al. 2015. This old heart: Cardiac aging and autophagy. *J Moll Cell Med* 83, 44–54.

Liu, E.Y. and Ryan, K.M. 2012. Autophagy and cancer—Issues we need to digest. *J Cell Sci* 125, 2349–2358.

Lorin, S., Hamai, A., Mehrpour, M. et al. 2013. Autophagy regulation and its role in cancer. *Semin Cancer Biol* 23, 361–379.

Lozy, F. and Karantza, V. 2012. Autophagy and cancer cell metabolism. *Semin Cell Dev Biol* 23, 395–401.

Madeo, F., Zimmermann, A., Maluri, M.C. et al. 2015. Essential role for autophagy in life span extension. *J Clin Invest* 125, 85–93.

Mallat, A., Lodder, J., Teixeira-Clerc, F. et al. 2014. Autophagy: A multifaceted partner in liver fibrosis. *Biomed Res Int* 2014, 869390.

Mammucari, C., Schiaffino, S. and Sandri, M. 2008. Downstream of Akt: FoxO3 and mTOR in the regulation of autophagy in skeletal muscle. *Autophagy* 4, 524–526.

Marc Rhoads, J. and Wu, G. 2009. Glutamine, arginine, and leucine signalling in the intestine. *Amino Acids* 37, 111–122.

Martinez-Lopez, N., Athonvarangkul, D. and Singh, R. 2015. Autophagy and aging. *Adv Exp Med Biol* 847, 73–87.

Martinez-Outschoorn, U.E., Lisanti, M.P. and Sotgia, F. 2011. Stromal-epithelial metabolic coupling in can-cer: Integrating autophagy and metabolism in the tumour microenvironment. *Int J Biochem Cell Biol* 43, 1045–1051.

Martinez-Outschoorn, U., Sotgia, F., and Lisanti, M.P. 2014. Tumor microenvironment and metabolic synergy in breast cancers: Critical importance of mitochondrial fuels and function. Semin Oncol 41 (2), 195–216.

Matz-Soja, M., Hovhannisyan, A. and Gebhardt, R. 2013. Hedgehog signalling pathway in adult liver: A major new player in hepatocyte metabolism and zonation? Med Hypotheses 80, 589–594.

Menzies, F.M., Moreau, K. and Rubinsztein, D.C. 2011. Protein misfolding disorders and macroautophagy. Cur Op Cell Biol 23, 190–197.

Mezzarobba, V., Torrent, A., Leydier, I. et al. 2003. The role of adrenal hormones in the response of glutamine synthetase to fasting in adult and old rats. Clin Nutr 22, 569–575.

Mignon, M., Lévêque, L., Bonnel, E. et al. 2007. Does glutamine supplementation decrease the response of muscle glutamine synthetase to fasting in muscle in adult and very old rats? J Parenter Enteral Nutr 31, 26–31.

Mizushima, N. and Komatsu, M. 2011. Autophagy: Renovation of cells and tissues. Cell 147, 728–741.

Mortimore, G. and Kadowaki, M. 2001. Regulation of protein metabolism in liver. In: The Endocrine Pancreas and Regulation of Metabolism (Jefferson, L.S. and Goodman H.M., eds.). In: Handbook of Physiology (Geiger, S.R., ed.) pp. 553–557. Bethesda, MD: American Physiological Society.

Mortimore, G.E. and Pösö, A.R. 1984. Lysosomal pathways in hepatic protein degradation: Regulatory role of amino acids. Fed Proc 43, 1289–1294.

Nicklin, P., Bergman, P., Zhang, B. et al. 2009. Bidirectional transport of amino acids regulates mTOR and autophagy. Cell 136, 521–534.

Noguchi, M., Hirata, N. and Suizu, F. 2014. The links between AKT and two intracellular proteolytic cascades: Ubiquitination and autophagy. Biochim Biophys Acta 1846, 342–352.

Perluigi, M., Di Domenico, F. and Butterfield, D.A. 2015. mTOR signaling in aging and neurodegeneration: At the crossroad between metabolism dysfunction and impairment of autophagy. Neurobiol Dis (e-pub ahead of print), doi: 10.1016/j.bbadis.2015.08.002.

Pinel, C., Coxam, V., Mignon, M. et al. 2006. Alterations in glutamine synthetase activity in rat skeletal muscle are associated with advanced age. Nutrition 22, 778–785.

Roth, E. 2008. Nonnutritive effects of glutamine. J Nutr 138, 2025S–2031S.

Rubinsztein, D.C., Marino, G. and Kroemer, G. 2011. Autophagy and aging. Cell 146, 682–695.

Sancak, Y., Bar-Peled, L., Zoncu, R. et al. 2010. Ragulator-Rag complex targets mTORC1 to the lysosomal surface and is necessary for its activation by amino acids. Cell 141, 290–303.

Schloesser, A., Campbell, G., Glüer, C.C. et al. 2015. Restriction on an energy-dense diet improves markers of metabolic health and cellular aging in mice through decreasing hepatic mTOR activity. Rejuvenation Res 18, 30–39.

Seglen, P.O., Gordon, P.B. and Poli, A. 1980. Amino acid inhibition of the autophagic/lysosomal pathway of protein degradation in isolated rat hepatocytes. Biochim Biophys Acta 630, 103–118.

Sengupta, A., Molkentin, J.D. and Yutzey, K.E. 2009. FoxO transcription factors promote autophagy in cardiomyocytes. J Biol Chem 284, 28319–28331.

Shanware, N.P., Mullen, A.R., DeBerardinis, R.J. et al. 2011. Glutamine: Pleiotropic roles in tumour growth and stress resistance. J Mol Med (Berlin, Germany) 89, 229–236.

Singh, R. and Cuervo, A.M. 2012. Lipophagy: Connecting autophagy and lipid metabolism. Int J Cell Biol 2012, 282041.

Smith, T.J. and Stanley, C.A. 2008. Untangling the glutamate dehydrogenase allosteric nightmare. Trends Biochem Sci 33, 557–564.

Spanaki, C. and Plaitakis, A. 2012. The role of glutamate dehydrogenase in mammalian ammonia metabolism. Neurotox Res 21, 117–127.

Stuerenburg, H.J., Stangneth, B. and Schoser, B.G. 2006. Age related profiles of free amino acids in human skeletal muscle. Neuro Endocrinol Lett 27, 133–136.

Teperino, R., Aberger, F., Esterbauer, H. et al. 2014. Canonical and non-canonical Hedgehog signalling and the control of metabolism. Sem Develop Biol 33, 81–92.

van der Vos, K.E. and Coffer, P.J. 2012. Glutamine metabolism links growth factor signalling to the regulation of autophagy. Autophagy 8, 1862–1864.

van der Vos, K.E., Eliasson, P., Proikas-Cezanne, T. et al. 2012. Modulation of glutamine metabolism by the PI(3)K-PKB-FOXO network regulates autophagy. Nat Cell Biol 14, 829–837.

Vilchez, D., Saez, I. and Dillin, A. 2014. The role of protein clearance mechanisms in organismal ageing and age-related diseases. Nat Cummun 5, 6659.

Wartlick, O., Kicheva, A. and González-Gaitán, M. 2009. Morphogen gradient formation. Cold Spring Harb Perspect Biol 1, a001255.

Weimer, S., Priebs, J., Kuhlow, D. et al. 2014. D-Glucosamine supplementation extends life span of nematodes and of ageing mice. *Nat Commun* 5, 3563.

White, E. 2013. Exploiting the bad eating habits of Ras-driven cancers. *Genes Dev* 27, 2065–2071.

Xu, P., Das, M., Reilly, J. et al. 2011. JNK regulates FoxO-dependent autophagy in neurons. *Genes Dev* 25, 310–322.

Zoncu, R., Bar-Peled, L., Efeyan, A. et al. 2011. mTORC1 senses lysosomal amino acids through an inside-out mechanism that requires the vacuolar H(+)-ATPase. *Science* 334, 678–683.

6 Regulation of Hepatic Glutamine and Ammonia Metabolism by Morphogens

Madlen Matz-Soja, Jan Böttger, and Rolf Gebhardt

CONTENTS

6.1 INTRODUCTION: BACKGROUND AND DRIVING FORCES

Blood glutamine levels are important for ensuring the proper development of mammalian organisms because glutamine acts as a potent precursor for biosynthetic processes/reactions and is a metabolic signal. In many pathological conditions, blood glutamine levels may vary with considerable consequences, particularly for immune response and regeneration in cases of decrease.

The liver plays a central role in maintaining proper blood glutamine concentrations. In principle, this organ can either supply or take up glutamine via net production or net consumption. Recently, it has been revealed that morphogenic signals are master regulators of liver glutamine and ammonia metabolism. Morphogens can strongly modulate the balance between biosynthetic and catabolic pathways of glutamine metabolism by differentially influencing the expression of the appropriate transporters and enzymes in different zones of the liver lobules. These findings raise two important questions: (a) Does impairment or stimulation of morphogen signaling in the liver contribute to the alterations of blood glutamine levels in specific diseases? (b) Can morphogenic signaling provide novel therapeutic targets for improving blood glutamine levels in diseased states? In this chapter, we review basic findings concerning the regulation of liver glutamine metabolism by morphogens and attempt to answer the questions raised in the context of current knowledge.

6.2 SYSTEMIC GLUTAMINE LEVELS AND THE LIVER

Glutamine is the most abundant free amino acid in the blood of mammals, including in humans. It is required for many biosynthetic reactions, for example, pyrimidine and purine bases, amino sugars and asparagine, but it may also be used as a fuel for cellular energy production in the form

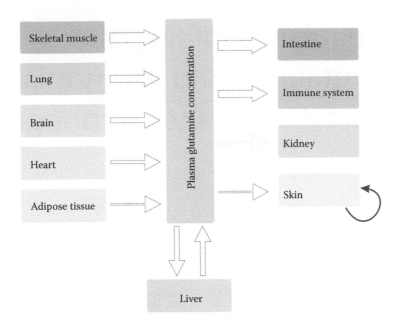

FIGURE 6.1 Glutamine exchange between different organs and the blood in the post-absorptive state. The arrows indicate the estimated amount and direction of glutamine delivery and uptake.

of adenosine triphosphate (ATP). With respect to glutamine metabolism, the different tissues can be subdivided into glutamine-producing and glutamine-consuming tissues (Figure 6.1).

Skeletal muscle, lungs, brain, adipose tissue, and heart (listed in decreasing order of their contribution) are glutamine-producing organs, while the intestine, immune cells, and kidney are glutamine-consuming organs. The skin, although equipped with high glutamine synthetase (GS) activity in keratinocytes, is neutral or even slightly consuming because it uses all of the formed glutamine for the synthesis of glutamine-rich proteins necessary for crosslinking via transglutaminase reactions during keratinization (Danielyan et al. 2009). Thus, in this regard, the liver is considered one of the few organs that is capable of both glutamine production and consumption. Under normal physiological conditions, the contribution of the liver to plasma glutamine levels is neutral because glutamine uptake/breakdown and biosynthesis/secretion are nearly balanced. However, this contribution can easily be shifted to one of the other states under specific physiological and pathological conditions (Watford 2000). For example, in acidosis, hepatic bicarbonate consumption is decreased, thereby limiting bicarbonate-consuming urea synthesis, which in turn results in an increased production of glutamine by the liver to avoid hyperammonemia (Häussinger 1998). Another example is consuming a protein-rich diet, which causes an upregulation of ureogenesis associated with increased net glutamine consumption by the liver, despite a simultaneous increase in glutamine-synthesizing capacity (Lal and Agarwal 1975; Boon et al. 1999).

6.3 EFFECT OF ZONATION ON HEPATIC GLUTAMINE METABOLISM

The features described above, and particularly the remarkable flexibility of the liver with respect to glutamine metabolism, are highly connected to the metabolic zonation of the liver parenchyma. Figure 6.2 schematically shows the zonation of glutamine metabolism and that of other amino acids of the glutamate family.

Glutaminase catalyzes the breakdown of glutamine to glutamate and is expressed in periportal hepatocytes (Moorman et al. 1994), while the opposite reaction, catalyzed by GS, is restricted to a small rim of hepatocytes surrounding the central vein of each lobule (Gebhardt and Mecke 1983).

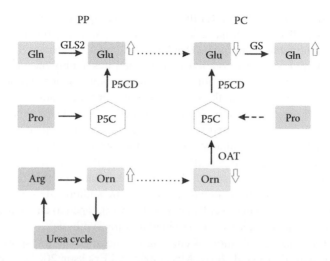

FIGURE 6.2 Schematic depiction of the zonal distribution of metabolic pathways among members of the glutamate family of amino acids in the healthy liver lobule. PP, periportal zone; PC, pericentral zone. Normal arrows indicate single or sequential reactions, dashed arrows indicate possible reactions, and dotted arrows indicate intrahepatic transport to downstream hepatocytes. Increased and decreased concentrations of amino acids are marked by up- and down-oriented filled arrows, respectively. (Substrates: Gln, glutamine; Glu, glutamate; Pro, proline; Orn, ornithine; Arg, arginine; P5C, 1-pyrroline-5-carboxylic acid; enzymes: GLS2, glutaminase 2; GS, glutamine synthetase; P5CD, P5C dehydrogenase [aldehyde dehydrogenase 4 family, member A1]; OAT, ornithine aminotransferase.)

Thus, the liver shows extensive glutamine cycling that is of utmost importance for body nitrogen balance and, simultaneously, also contributes to acid–base balance in the blood (Häussinger 1998). However, liver heterogeneity cannot be understood in the simple terms of "periportal" and "pericentral" localizations but shows a much more facetted pattern, which in the case of glutamine and ammonia metabolism and the relationship with other metabolic pathways (e.g., carbohydrate metabolism) is just emerging and presents with unexpected details (Brosnan and Brosnan 2009; Vasilj et al. 2012; Gebhardt and Matz-Soja 2014).

Briefly, glutamine is synthesized from and broken down to glutamate via GS and glutaminase reactions (Figure 6.2). Because glutamine synthesis is an endergonic reaction driven by the hydrolysis of adenosine triphosphate (ATP), the coexistence of these reactions in one and the same cell facilitates a futile cycle, resulting in the unwanted waste of energy. Thus, it is reasonable to separate these reactions not only within the cell into different organelles but also to separate the different cells along the porto-central axis of the liver lobules. Indeed, glutaminase is mitochondrial and is expressed in hepatocytes located in the periportal area of the lobule (Moorman et al. 1994), whereas GS is cytoplasmic and expressed exclusively in a few hepatocytes (usually less than 7%), which surround the central vein (Gebhardt et al. 1988, 1989). This sophisticated separation serves several physiological purposes.

First, the liberation of ammonia from glutamine in the mitochondrial matrix fuels ureogenesis by increasing the ammonia concentration for low-affinity enzyme carbamoyl phosphate synthase I, which catalyzes the initial step of ureogenesis and is also mitochondrial. However, this supporting function is not absolutely necessary because ureogenesis is highly active in hepatocytes located further downstream (i.e., in the midzonal area) even without prior glutaminolysis (Comar et al. 2010). Furthermore, the glutamate resulting from the glutaminase reaction can be further disseminated by periportal glutamate dehydrogenase, resulting in additional ammonium ions and alpha-oxoglutarate that can be used in the citric acid cycle.

Second, the localization of GS in the pericentral zone (Figure 6.2) ensures reformation of normal high glutamine concentrations in peripheral blood because the newly synthesized glutamine is rapidly exported from the cytoplasm via the system N transporter (SN1/SNAT3) in the plasma membrane (Bode 2001). Because GS has a low affinity for ammonia, this reaction also serves to detoxify the low concentrations of ammonia that have escaped ureogenesis. However, restriction of the expression of glutamine synthesis to a few cells (sometimes to only one cell layer at the border of the central veins) requires the cooperation of several enzymatic steps to render ammonia detoxification as efficient as possible. Indeed, the specific transporter for ammonia, RhBG, the glutamate transporter Glu1, and the enzyme ornithine aminotransferase (OAT) share the restricted localization of GS (Gebhardt et al. 2007). In contrast, pyrrolin-5-carboxylate dehydrogenase (P5CD) is not zonated and is involved in forming glutamate from proline throughout the parenchyma (Figure 6.2). Nevertheless, it can transform ornithine to glutamate only in the pericentral zone due to the strict and limited expression of OAT to this zone. Furthermore, glutamate dehydrogenase in the pericentral area may form glutamate from alpha-oxoglutarate by additionally removing stoichiometric amounts of ammonia. Thus, pericentral cells are optimally equipped to channel glutamate (or various precursors of it) to ammonia detoxification via glutamine synthesis.

Consistent with the zonal localization of enzymatic reactions, the transport of glutamine and glutamate is also zonated (Baird et al. 2004; Mackenzie and Erickson 2004). System N amino acid transporters exhibit shallow gradients with periportal (SNAT5) and pericentral (SNAT3) preference (Baird et al. 2004). Although both transporters are able to regulate bidirectional glutamine fluxes, the SNAT5 transporter may have a particular importance for the modulation of net hepatic glutamine flux (Baird et al. 2004).

6.4　REGULATION OF HEPATIC GLUTAMINE METABOLISM

6.4.1　Metabolic Regulation

Hepatic glutamine metabolism is affected by various types of signals. Metabolic cues, including ammonia levels, glutamate and alpha-oxoglutarate concentrations, pH, and several amino acids, act on the level of transporters and enzymes by modulating the activity of these proteins (Meister 1985; Baird et al. 2004; Brosnan and Brosnan 2009). Such signals are involved in short-term regulation, which respond directly to intracellular conditions.

Hormone levels, particularly members of the hypothalamo-pituitary axis, such as growth hormone and glucocorticoids, influence the expression of specific enzymes, such as GS (Gebhardt et al. 1994; Abcouwer et al. 1995; Lie-Venema et al. 1998), and are involved in adapting liver glutamine metabolism to nutritional changes and other environmental cues, including circadian rhythm (Gebhardt and Matz-Soja 2014). Cell swelling due to changes in osmolarity or cellular levels of specific osmolytes considerably influence hepatic glutamine metabolism (Häussinger and Schliess 2007). In this respect, glutamine itself is an important cellular osmolyte. Recently, morphogens, particularly Wnt factors, were identified as master regulators of liver zonation that specifically contribute to the zonated expression of GS (Benhamouche et al. 2006; Gebhardt et al. 2007).

6.4.2　The Role of Wnt/Beta-Catenin Signaling in Controlling Glutamine Synthesis

The zonation of glutamine metabolism is differentially regulated. The periportal localization of glutaminase is dynamic and is directly dependent on the metabolic need that the pericentral localization GS is static, that is, cannot be easily changed by daily nutritional variations and other acute signals (Gebhardt et al. 1994). Consistent with this finding, various hormones simply controlled the magnitude of expression rather than its zonal distribution in the parenchyma (Gebhardt et al. 1994; Gebhardt et al. 2007). However, the enigma regarding which factors are responsible for the zonated expression of GS was revealed in 2002 when several groups simultaneously discovered that the Wnt signaling pathway is a major player in this regulation (for a review, see

Gebhardt et al. 2007). Wnt morphogens are most active during development and govern embryogenesis and organogenesis via a beta-catenin-dependent (canonical) and several beta-catenin-independent (non-canonical) pathways (van Amerongen et al. 2012). Liver zonation is one of the first examples that Wnt signaling is active in the adult stage and is involved in metabolic regulation. In this case, only canonical signaling via beta-catenin appears to be involved and is active across the porto-central axis by a shallow increasing gradient from the portal tract toward the central vein (for review, see Gebhardt and Hovhannisyan 2010). This was shown using transgenic mice in which beta-catenin was hepatocellularly knocked out. These mice do not express any GS as well as some other enzymes (e.g., some cytochrome P450s), which are also regulated by Wnt/beta-catenin signaling (Sekine et al. 2006; Tan et al. 2006). Conversely, hepatocyte-specific knockouts of the tumor suppressor gene, adenomatous polyposis coli (APC), which is a component of the destruction complex for beta-catenin, results in an activation of Wnt/beta-catenin signaling (Benhamouche et al. 2006). In such livers, GS is strongly upregulated and may spread from the pericentral to the periportal zone, while periportal functions, such as ureogenesis, are downregulated and limit their expression zone to a small periportal area (Benhamouche et al. 2006). Similar changes (although less pronounced) are found in the so-called APCloxPNeo mice (generated by Shibata et al. 1997) in the homozygous state (APChomo mice) compared to WT mice as depicted in Figure 6.3 for GS and CPS1 as well as the zonation markers, E-cadherin (periportal) and Cyp2E1 (pericentral). These images demonstrate how the pericentral GS-positive area expands toward the portal triad if Wnt/beta-catenin signaling is activated, while the carbamoyl phosphate synthase 1–positive area shrinks in APChomo mice.

What is the molecular mechanism by which the zonal expression of enzymes is controlled? Usually, the expression of Wnt-responsive genes is activated by the binding of beta-catenin to the T-cell/lymphoid enhancer (TCF/LEF) transcription factor, which subsequently binds to TCF-binding sites in the respective genes (van Amerongen et al. 2012). However, it must be emphasized that GS is not a direct TCF-target gene (Gebhardt et al. 2007). Many interactions of beta-catenin with other transcription factors, such as forkhead box O3 (FoxO3), exist that contribute in a combinatorial manner to the expression of this enzyme (for review, see Gebhardt and Hovhannisyan 2010). Moreover, such mechanisms integrate the effect of other factors, such as hormones, and form the basis for the dominant role of beta-catenin as a master regulator of zonation.

6.5 METABOLIC CONSEQUENCES OF ZONATION AND REGULATION OF HEPATIC GLUTAMINE METABOLISM

In a normal mouse liver, glutamine consumption and production are almost balanced as indicated by only slightly lower blood concentrations leaving the organ compared to the blood concentrations entering the organ *in vivo* (Schliess et al. 2014). In the same study, it was shown that glutamate net consumption is much higher than that of glutamine in the normal liver *in vivo*. Because it is complicated to study the effect of zonation on metabolism *in vivo*, the contribution of hepatocytes from the periportal or pericentral zone was examined in cell culture. When the metabolic rates were determined in the culture medium, the differences between periportal and pericentral hepatocytes were determined as shown for glutamate consumption and urea synthesis in Figure 6.4b.

However, in the case of glutamine, metabolic fluxes are underestimated because the culture medium contains a high concentration of glutamine (2 mM), and cultured cells generally show a much higher consumption of glutamine as hepatocytes *in situ*. Thus, pericentral production of glutamine is reflected only by a lower net consumption compared with periportal hepatocytes (Figure 6.4b). Consistent with the *in vivo* findings, arginine is consumed and converted into ornithine via arginase 1 particularly in the periportal zone (Figure 6.4b). Only part of the ornithine produced is converted by the strongly pericentral OAT into glutamate-γ-semialdehyde and further into pyrroline-5-carboxylate. Thus, ornithine delivers extra glutamate via the pyrroline-5-carboxylate

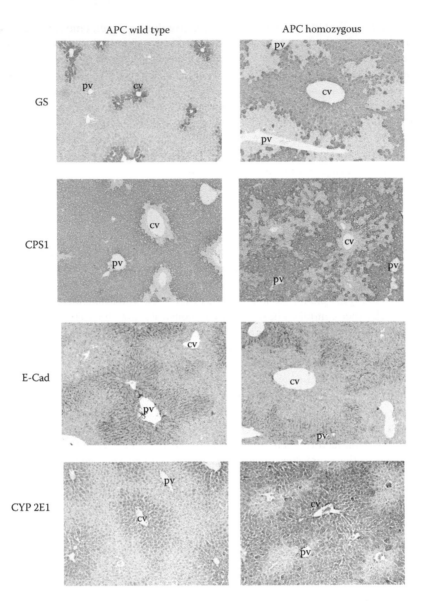

FIGURE 6.3 Influence of the moderate upregulation of Wnt/beta-catenin signaling in transgenic APC mice on liver zonation. Immunohistochemistry was performed on liver sections obtained from APC wild-type mice (controls) and homozygous APCloxPNeo mice for glutamine synthetase (GS), carbamoyl-phosphate synthase 1 (CPS1), E-cadherin, and CYP2E1. GS and CPS1 show the typical pericentral and periportal localization in APC wild-type mice, as the markers CYP2E1 and E-cadherin, respectively. After upregulation of Wnt/ beta-catenin signaling in APC homozygous mice markers of pericentral metabolism increased toward the periportal zone and markers of periportal metabolism decreased. Sections were stained with peroxidase and counterstained with hematoxylin. Magnification: ×100, pv, portal vein; cv, central vein.

dehydrogenase (P5CD) reaction for glutamine synthesis (Gebhardt et al. 2007). *In vivo*, this can occur only after the intrahepatic transfer of periportally secreted ornithine to the pericentral zone (Figure 6.2). Because the majority of ornithine is not metabolized, a normal liver may be an ornithine-producing organ. Proline is also converted to pyrroline-5-carboxylate, a reaction that is preferentially performed in the periportal area but may also occur in the pericentral zone, though with less activity (Figure 6.2). Thus, proline is consumed by the normal liver.

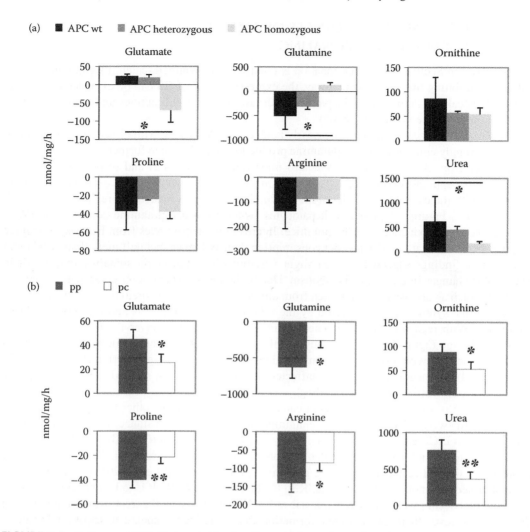

FIGURE 6.4 Influence of Wnt/beta-catenin signaling activity and zonation on metabolomic profile of cultured hepatocytes. Extracellular metabolite flux rates of hepatocytes after 2 h of cultivation. (a) Hepatocytes were isolated from APCloxPNeo mice of different genotypes and (b) from periportal (pp) and pericentral (pc) regions of liver parenchyma. Positive values represent production rates; negative values represent uptake rates. Values are means ± SD (n(wild type) = 3, n(heterozygous) = 2, n(homozygous) = 5, n(pp) = 3, n(pc) = 4). Statistical evaluation was performed using the Mann–Whitney U Test for APC hepatocytes and the unpaired t-test for pp/pc hepatocytes; $*p < 0.05$, $**p < 0.01$.

One possibility to confirm these findings and interpretations *in vivo* is to examine damage of the pericentral zone by exposing the animals to CCl4, which results in the loss of glutamine synthetic activity (Gebhardt et al. 1988). In such mice, the liver converts to a glutamine-consuming tissue (Schliess et al. 2014). In contrast, net consumption of glutamate decreases to a nearly balanced state after CCl4-induced liver damage (unpublished observation). This finding indicates that net glutamate uptake is needed to ensure proper synthesis of glutamine under normal conditions. Similarly, arginine converted into urea and ornithine by periportally localized arginase 1 (Figure 6.2) shows a high net consumption in normal mouse liver, which is maintained in CCl4-treated mice. Thus far, the effect of CCl4 damage in the liver on the metabolism of ornithine and proline *in vivo* remains to be established. However, given that OAT activity is minimal and P5CD activity is reduced under these conditions, it is most likely that production of ornithine increases and the consumption of proline is slightly reduced.

6.6 FUNCTIONAL CONSEQUENCES OF ALTERED WNT/BETA-CATENIN SIGNALING

As discussed in Section 6.4.2, liver zonation is controlled by Wnt/beta-catenin signaling. By activating or inhibiting this signaling pathway, the expression zone of GS can be extended or limited. Generally speaking, activation of the pathway increases pericentral functions and reduces periportal functions and vice versa (Figure 6.5).

Uptake and release of glutamine are nearly balanced in WT livers, while livers from APChomo mice are strongly committed to net glutamine production. This has been further studied in cultured hepatocytes from APChomo and APChetero mice (see Section 6.4.2) and respective WT mice. These *in vitro* approaches adequately reflect the metabolic consequences of activated beta-catenin signaling with the exception that glutamine production is underestimated as previously discussed. As depicted in Figure 6.4a, cultured hepatocytes switch from net glutamine consumption (WT) to net glutamine production (APChomo) mice. Interestingly, hepatocytes from heterozygous mice range in between, that is, show less net consumption than WT mice, but still more than APChomo mice. These findings suggest that even slight variations in beta-catenin signaling may result in remarkable changes in glutamine metabolism. Due to the inverse changes observed with periportal functions, such as ureogenesis, the switch from ammonia excretion (via urea) to ammonia retention (via glutamine synthesis), best reflected by the ratio of these pathways, is an even more sensitive parameter. With regard to the other reactions involved in the interconversion of glutaminogenic amino acids (see Figure 6.2), it is obvious that the reduction of ureogenesis in APChomo hepatocytes is associated with less arginine consumption and less ornithine production (Figure 6.4a). In contrast, proline consumption remains unaffected because P5CD is not zonated and does not appear to be a target of Wnt/beta-catenin signaling.

Modulation of the activity of Wnt/beta-catenin signaling by means other than genetic manipulation may likewise affect intrahepatic glutamine metabolism. For instance, the pathway can be activated with LiCl, an inhibitor of glycogen synthase kinase 3 beta (GSK3β), which phosphorylates beta-catenin and marks it for proteolytic breakdown (see Gebhardt et al. 2007). Exposure of hepatocytes to LiCl results in enhanced glutamine production (Bartl et al. 2015). Similar results were obtained for another inhibitor of GSK3β (Gebhardt et al. 2010). It is to be expected that such a mechanism occurs with any therapeutic use of LiCl, for instance, in the treatment of bipolar brain disorders. However, there is no current information about whether therapeutic doses of LiCl result in

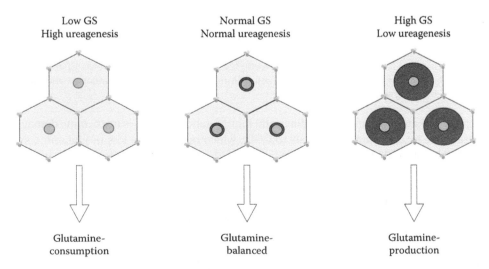

FIGURE 6.5 Illustration of the relationship between the lobular expression pattern of glutamine synthetase or ureogenesis and the resulting glutamine consumption or production of the liver.

a significant increase in circulating glutamine levels under all conditions and whether this increase might contribute to the therapeutic success.

6.7   PATHOLOGICAL AND BENEFICIAL ROLE OF GLUTAMINE

In specific pathological conditions, glutamine supply is limited because of either increasing demand or lower circulating concentrations due to improper *de novo* synthesis. Well-known examples are most types of cancer (independent of affected organs), specific heart diseases, and inflammation (Watford et al. 2002). Thus, glutamine is sometimes classified as a conditionally essential amino acid (Watford 2008), and supplementation of glutamine may be beneficial, particularly in heart disease (Shahzad et al. 2011). However, a number of diseases, such as liver cirrhosis, acute liver failure, or chronic kidney disease are accompanied by increasing plasma levels of glutamine (Ytrebo et al. 2006; Fadel et al. 2014). In these cases, glutamine is produced in excess amounts by skeletal muscle compensating for the drying up of other sources.

However, glutamine supplementation is highly controversial (Soeters and Grecu 2012). On one hand, glutamine supplementation did not increase glutamine stores in different tissues and plasma (Boza et al. 2000); on the other, preconditioning glutamine protects against ischemia/reperfusion-induced liver injury (Xu et al. 2014). It seems that a general answer is not possible and that each case should be carefully studied and discussed independently. This endeavor should include a detailed investigation of the specific role of the liver because this has not been comprehensively performed in the past. In particular, it should be taken into account that moderate liver damage by many environmental toxins and carcinogens has been shown to severely reduce the number of GS-positive cells in the liver without acutely affecting major liver functions and behavior (Umemura et al. 1998; Williams et al. 1998). Unfortunately, it is not known whether circulating glutamine levels are altered (most probably decreased) under these conditions.

An alternative to glutamine supplementation would be the enhancement of the glutamine-synthesizing capacity of the liver to increase the availability of glutamine in the body. Such an approach has not been considered because it is almost impossible to increase GS activity in the liver by dietary regimens or hormonal treatment (Gebhardt et al. 1994, 2007). Considering the specific role of morphogen signaling in determining the zonal distribution of hepatic glutamine metabolisms, this situation has changed. Moderate activation of the Wnt/beta-catenin signaling by small molecular activators (e.g., LiCl) may increase endogenous glutamine levels in a transient and regulated manner. However, activation of Wnt/beta-catenin signaling may be a double-edged sword due to its role in tumor formation (Niehrs and Acebron 2012). However, a wide therapeutic range of adverse reactions may manifest because a considerable increase in the GS-positive region can be achieved by repeated starvation (Ueberham et al. 2004) without any harmful effects on the mice.

6.8   CONCLUSIONS AND PERSPECTIVES

The findings reviewed herein clearly demonstrate that liver zonation is a dominant determinant of whether the liver is a glutamine-consuming or glutamine-producing organ. Zonation is determined by morphogenic signaling, which is relatively stable in adulthood and does not vary in response to nutritional changes in a similar temporal manner as do hormones involved in nutritional adaptation. However, liver diseases may result in a broad spectrum of changes in morphogenic signaling, ranging from small, almost undetectable, changes to moderate and even dramatic alterations of signaling activity. However, consequences of such changes to the liver's glutamine metabolism have not yet received adequate attention, although they may have a considerable effect on immune function, regeneration, and other important features. Another point of concern is the potential therapeutic use of this interdependence. A full understanding of how morphogenic signaling controls liver zonation may reveal new therapeutic targets and open new avenues for the design of new drugs for modulating morphogenic signaling in an adequate manner, thereby avoiding adverse reactions.

REFERENCES

Abcouwer, S.F., Bode, B.P., Souba, W.W. 1995. Glucocorticoids regulate rat glutamine synthetase expression in a tissue-specific manner. *J. Surg. Res.* 59(1):59–65.

Baird, F.E., Beattie, K.J., Hyde, A.R. et al. 2004. Bidirectional substrate fluxes through the system N (SNAT5) glutamine transporter may determine net glutamine flux in rat liver. *J. Physiol.* 559(Pt 2):367–381.

Bartl, M., Pfaff, M., Ghallab, A. et al. 2015. Optimality in the zonation of ammonia detoxification in rodent liver. *Arch. Toxicol.* 89(11):2069–2078.

Benhamouche, S., Decaens, T., Godard, C. et al. 2006. APC tumor suppressor gene is the "zonation-keeper" of mouse liver. *Dev. Cell* 10(6):759–770.

Bode, B.P. 2001. Recent molecular advances in mammalian glutamine transport. *J. Nutr.* 131(9 Suppl):2475S–2485S; discussion 2486S–2487S.

Boon, L., Geerts, W.J., Jonker, A. et al. 1999. High protein diet induces pericentral glutamate dehydrogenase and ornithine aminotransferase to provide sufficient glutamate for pericentral detoxification of ammonia in rat liver lobules. *Histochem. Cell Biol.* 111(6):445–452.

Boza, J.J., Moennoz, D., Jarret, A.R. et al. 2000. Neither glutamine nor arginine supplementation of diets increase glutamine body stores in healthy growing rats. *Clin. Nutr.* 19(5):319–325.

Brosnan, M.E., Brosnan, J.T. 2009. Hepatic glutamate metabolism: A tale of 2 hepatocytes. *Am. J Clin. Nutr.* 90(3):857S.

Comar, J.F., Suzuki-Kemmelmeier, F., Constantin, J. et al. 2010. Hepatic zonation of carbon and nitrogen fluxes derived from glutamine and ammonia transformations. *J. Biomed. Sci.* 17(1):1.

Danielyan, L., Zellmer, S., Sickinger, S. et al. 2009. Correction: Keratinocytes as depository of ammonium-inducible glutamine synthetase: Age- and anatomy-dependent distribution in human and rat skin. *PLoS ONE* 4(3):e4416.

Fadel, F.I., Elshamaa, M.F., Essam, R.G. et al. 2014. Some amino acids levels: Glutamine, glutamate, and homocysteine, in plasma of children with chronic kidney disease. *Int. J. Biomed. Sci.* 10(1):36–42.

Gebhardt, R., Baldysiak-Figiel, A., Krügel, V. et al. 2007. Hepatocellular expression of glutamine synthetase: An indicator of morphogen actions as master regulators of zonation in adult liver. *Prog. Histochem. Cytochem.* 41(4):201–266.

Gebhardt, R., Ebert, A., Bauer, G. 1988. Heterogeneous expression of glutamine synthetase mRNA in rat liver parenchyma revealed by *in situ* hybridization and Northern blot analysis of RNA from periportal and perivenous hepatocytes. *FEBS Lett.* 241(1–2):89–93.

Gebhardt, R., Gaunitz, F., Mecke, D. 1994. Heterogeneous (positional) expression of hepatic glutamine synthetase: Features, regulation and implications for hepatocarcinogenesis. *Adv. Enzyme Regul.* 34:27–56.

Gebhardt, R., Hovhannisyan, A. 2010. Organ patterning in the adult stage: The role of Wnt/beta-catenin signaling in liver zonation and beyond. *Dev. Dyn.* 239(1):45–55.

Gebhardt, R., Lerche, K.S., Götschel, F. et al. 2010. 4-Aminoethylamino-emodin—A novel potent inhibitor of GSK-3β- acts as an insulin-sensitizer avoiding downstream effects of activated β-catenin. *J. Cell. Mol. Med.* 14(6a):1276–1293.

Gebhardt, R., Matz-Soja, M. 2014. Liver zonation: Novel aspects of its regulation and its impact on homeostasis. *World J. Gastroenterol.* 20(26):8491–8504.

Gebhardt, R., Mecke, D. 1983. Glutamate uptake by cultured rat hepatocytes is mediated by hormonally inducible, sodium-dependent transport systems. *FEBS Lett.* 161(2):275–278.

Gebhardt, R., Schmid, H., Fitzke, H. 1989. Immunohistochemical localization of glutamine synthetase in human liver. *Experientia* 45(2):137–139.

Häussinger, D. 1998. Hepatic glutamine transport and metabolism. *Adv. Enzymol. Relat. Areas Mol. Biol.* 72:43–86.

Häussinger, D., Schliess, F. 2007. Glutamine metabolism and signaling in the liver. *Front. Biosci.* 12:371–391.

Lal, A., Agarwal, K.N. 1975. Influence of carbohydrate-free protein-rich diet on free alpha-amino nitrogen changes in plasma, erythrocytes and leucocytes. *Nutr. Metab.* 18(3):152–156.

Lie-Venema, H., Hakvoort, T.B., van Hemert, F.J. et al. 1998. Regulation of the spatiotemporal pattern of expression of the glutamine synthetase gene. *Prog. Nucleic Acid Res. Mol. Biol.* 61:243–308.

Mackenzie, B., Erickson, M.D. 2004. Sodium-coupled neutral amino acid (System N/A) transporters of the SLC38 gene family. *Pflugers Arch.* 447(5):784–795.

Meister, A. 1985. Glutamate synthase from *Escherichia coli*, *Klebsiella aerogenes*, and *Saccharomyces cerevisiae*. *Methods Enzymol.* 113:327–337.

Moorman, A.F., Boer, P.A. de, Watford, M. et al. 1994. Hepatic glutaminase mRNA is confined to part of the urea cycle domain in the adult rodent liver lobule. *FEBS Lett.* 356(1):76–80.

Niehrs, C., Acebron, S.P. 2012. Mitotic and mitogenic Wnt signalling. *EMBO J.* 31(12):2705–2713.

Schliess, F., Hoehme, S., Henkel, S.G. et al. 2014. Integrated metabolic spatial-temporal model for the prediction of ammonia detoxification during liver damage and regeneration. *Hepatology* 60(6):2040–2051.

Sekine, S., Lan, B.Y., Bedolli, M. et al. 2006. Liver-specific loss of beta-catenin blocks glutamine synthesis pathway activity and cytochrome p450 expression in mice. *Hepatology* 43(4):817–825.

Shahzad, K., Chokshi, A., Schulze, P.C. 2011. Supplementation of glutamine and omega-3 polyunsaturated fatty acids as a novel therapeutic intervention targeting metabolic dysfunction and exercise intolerance in patients with heart failure. *Curr. Clin. Pharmacol.* 6(4):288–294.

Shibata, H., Toyama, K., Shioya, H. et al. 1997. Rapid colorectal adenoma formation initiated by conditional targeting of the Apc gene. *Science* 278(5335):120–123.

Soeters, P., Grecu, I. 2012. Have we enough glutamine and how does it work? A clinician's view. *Ann. Nutr. Metab.* 60(1):17–26.

Tan, X., Behari, J., Cieply, B. et al. 2006. Conditional deletion of beta-catenin reveals its role in liver growth and regeneration. *Gastroenterology* 131(5):1561–1572.

Ueberham, E., Arendt, E., Starke, M. et al. 2004. Reduction and expansion of the glutamine synthetase expressing zone in livers from tetracycline controlled TGF-beta1 transgenic mice and multiple starved mice. *J. Hepatol.* 41(1):75–81.

Umemura, T., Takada, K., Schulz, C. et al. 1998. Cell proliferation in the livers of male mice and rats exposed to the carcinogen P-dichlorobenzene: Evidence for thresholds. *Drug Chem. Toxicol.* 21(1):57–66.

van Amerongen, R., Bowman, A.N., Nusse, R. 2012. Developmental stage and time dictate the fate of Wnt/beta-catenin-responsive stem cells in the mammary gland. *Cell Stem Cell* 11(3):387–400.

Vasilj, A., Gentzel, M., Ueberham, E. et al. 2012. Tissue proteomics by one-dimensional gel electrophoresis combined with label-free protein quantification. *J. Proteome Res.* 11(7):3680–3689.

Watford, M. 2000. Glutamine and glutamate metabolism across the liver sinusoid. *J. Nutr.* 130(4S Suppl):983S–987S.

Watford, M. 2008. Glutamine metabolism and function in relation to proline synthesis and the safety of glutamine and proline supplementation. *J. Nutr.* 138(10):2003S–2007S.

Watford, M., Chellaraj, V., Ismat, A. et al. 2002. Hepatic glutamine metabolism. *Nutrition* 18(4):301–303.

Williams, G.M., Iatropoulos, M.J., Wang, C.X. et al. 1998. Nonlinearities in 2-acetylaminofluorene exposure responses for genotoxic and epigenetic effects leading to initiation of carcinogenesis in rat liver. *Toxicol. Sci.* 45(2):152–161.

Xu, F., Dai, C., Peng, S. et al. 2014. Preconditioning with glutamine protects against ischemia/reperfusion-induced hepatic injury in rats with obstructive jaundice. *Pharmacology* 93(3–4):155–165.

Ytrebo, L.M., Sen, S., Rose, C. et al. 2006. Interorgan ammonia, glutamate, and glutamine trafficking in pigs with acute liver failure. *Am. J. Physiol. Gastrointest Liver Physiol.* 291(3):G373–G381.

Section IV

Glutamine, the Brain and Neurological Diseases

7 Brain Glutamine
Roles in Norm and Pathology

Jan Albrecht, Monika Szeliga, and Magdalena Zielińska

CONTENTS

7.1 GENERAL COMMENTS: SCOPE OF THE CHAPTER

In the brain, glutamine (Gln) participates in numerous metabolic processes that are common to all the mammalian tissues. These ubiquitous roles of Gln and also its contributions to processes that are specific to tissues other than brain will not be dealt with here. The scope of this chapter is confined to the distinct roles of Gln in neurotransmission, a function specific to the nervous system, and to abnormalities of Gln metabolism critical for the pathogenesis of selected central nervous system diseases. We commence with a brief description of the distribution of Gln in the brain tissues and subcellular fractions (Section 2.1). Next, we discuss—in a natural history mode—the evidence that Gln serves as a precursor of the excitatory neurotransmitter glutamate (Glu) and the inhibitory neurotransmitter, gamma-aminobutyric acid (GABA; Section 2.2). We focus on the so-called glutamine/glutamate cycle (GGC), the mechanistic basis of the interplay between nerve cells (neurons) and their supporting cells, astrocytes in generating neurotransmitter pools of Glu and GABA. Within this section, we also characterize the brain-specific aspects of glutamine transport, underscoring the distinct properties of glutamine carriers located in astrocytic and neuronal plasma membranes that couple Gln transport to GGC activity. Furthermore, we briefly discuss Gln transport to mitochondria, a process critical for the pathogenesis of hyperammonemic encephalopathies. Discussing the role of Gln in brain pathology (Section 3), we dwell on a strictly pre-selected group of diseases, considering only those where the prominent roles of altered Gln status in their pathogenesis appears beyond doubt. In addition to the aforementioned hyperammonemic encephalopathies, we focus on hepatic encephalopathy (Section 3.1), an issue also dealt with in Chapter 8, where the reader will find some complementary data and views. In what follows, we discuss the peculiarities of epilepsy (Section 3.2) and brain tumors (Section 3.3). The chapter concludes with an attempt to draw perspectives for therapies that would be based on correcting the Gln tissue imbalance in the discussed pathological conditions (Section 4).

7.2 GLUTAMINE IN THE HEALTHY BRAIN

7.2.1 BRAIN GLUTAMINE CONTENT AND DISTRIBUTION

Glutamine is relatively evenly distributed between different brain structures or regions. Its concentrations in the rat brain range from ca 5 nmoles/mg in the hippocampus to ca 7 nmoles/mg in the cerebellum (Jacobson et al. 1985) and in the rabbit brain from ca 4 nmoles/mg in the frontal cortex to ca 8 nmoles/mg in the hippocampus (Nitsh et al. 1983). While the tissue contents of Gln are equal or even slightly lower than of other common amino acids like Glu or taurine (Tossman et al. 1987), its contents in the extracellular fluid (Gln_{ECF}) are remarkably high, exceeding by at least an order of magnitude the extracellular contents of the other amino acids, falling in the range of 0.2–0.5 mM (Hamberger and Nyström 1985; Kanamori and Ross 2004). Also as opposed to other amino acids, Gln_{ECF} is very close to its blood concentration (Xu et al. 1998). The relatively flat brain tissue/extracelluar fluid (ECF)/blood Gln facilitates its movements between different compartments, which is of advantage for its role in coordinating the astrocytic and neuronal aspects of the GGC and thus the synthesis of the neurotransmitters Glu and GABA (see the following).

7.2.2 GLUTAMINE AS A PRECURSOR OF NEUROTRANSMITTERS GLU AND GABA: A ROUTE FROM SIMPLE PRECURSOR/PRODUCT DEMONSTRATIONS TO THE VISUALIZATION OF THE ASTROCYTIC-NEURONAL INTERPLAY IN THE GLN/GLU/GABA CYCLE (GGC)

Sound evidence that Gln may serve as a direct precursor of Glu and GABA has been already obtained in the late 1970s/early 1980s. Depolarization of slices of different brain regions preloaded with radiolabeled Gln evoked the release of radiolabeled Glu (Reubi et al. 1978; Hamberger et al. 1979a,b) and/or GABA (Reubi et al. 1978; Tapia and Gonzalez 1978). Glu release turned out to be partly calcium dependent, a feature mimicking the working brain *in situ* (Hamberger et al. 1979a). The seminal observation that inhibition of the Gln-degrading enzyme, phosphate-activated glutaminase (GA), reduced the synaptosomal pool of Glu and Asp and decreased the depolarization dependent release of Glu opened the venue for later more sophisticated studies of the coupling of Gln metabolism to glutamatergic neurotransmission (Bradford et al. 1989). The precursor role of Gln for releasable Glu has also been demonstrated in cultures of cerebellar granule cells (CGC), a model of glutamatergic neurons (Gallo et al. 1982). These *in vitro* findings have found support in *in vivo* experiments in which radiolabeled Gln was directly administered to the brain: This resulted in the labeling of cellular and extracellular Glu and GABA (Gauchy et al. 1980; Thanki et al. 1983; Ward et al. 1983).

The advent of the nuclear magnetic resonance (NMR) technique facilitated more direct demonstration that Gln is indeed feeding the releasable pools of Glu and GABA. Successful studies toward this end were performed using ^{13}C- or ^{15}N-labeled Gln not only in the *in vivo* setting (Patel et al. 2001; Kanamori and Ross 2004; Wang et al. 2007) but also in pertinent *in vitro* preparations: cultured CGC (Waagepetersen et al. 2005), GABA-ergic neurons (Waagepetersen et al. 2001), or brain tissue slices and prisms (Rae et al. 2003).

The discovery that glutamine synthetase (GS, EC 6.3.1.2), the enzyme synthesizing Gln from Glu and ammonia is located predominantly, if not exclusively, in astrocytes (Martinez-Hernandez et al. 1977), crystallized the concept of Gln metabolism being compartmented between astrocytes and neurons. In the first study directly demonstrating the astrocytic leg of the GGC, incubation of cultured primary astrocytes with ^{14}C-labelled Glu resulted in the production of [14]C Gln and its export to the extracellular space (Waniewski and Martin 1986). The concept of the GGC cycle was successfully advanced in multiple studies in which the fate of ^{13}C or ^{15}N-labelled Gln and other precursors was followed in astrocytic neuronal co-cultures (reviewed in Bak et al. 2006; Albrecht et al. 2007) and has led to the elucidation of metabolic reactions constituting the GGC. The essential steps of the cycle, representing the key mechanism of generation of Glu and GABA from Gln, are illustrated in Figure 7.1.

Briefly, a major proportion of Gln that is synthesized in astrocytes and not metabolized in there is exported to neurons, where it is degraded back to Glu and ammonia by phosphate-activated glutaminase (GA, EC 3.5.1.2). A portion of so formed Glu feeds the neurotransmitter pool of Glu; one other portion is converted to GABA by glutamic acid decarboxylase (GAD, EC 4.1.1.15). Glu released in the neurotransmission process from neurons is taken up to astrocytes to initiate a new round of the GGC. The released GABA is taken up both by neurons and astrocytes and further metabolized by GABA aminotransferase (GABA-T, EC 2.6.1.19) that transaminates pyruvate to alanine, a process taking place outside the GGC. The cycle is partly open: Gln not used in Glu or GABA synthesis leaves the brain via the cell membranes of endothelial cells forming the blood–brain barrier. Mechanism of Gln transport across the different points of entry/exit located in the brain are described below.

As described in different chapters of this book, Gln transport across the cell membranes of mammalian tissues is mediated by multiple proteinaceous carriers belonging to the four major systems: the sodium-independent system L, and the sodium-dependent systems ASC, A, and N (reviewed by Palacín et al. 1998). The functioning of the GGC cycle is specifically fine-tuned via the involvement of non-overlapping Gln-transporting moieties located in astrocytes in neurons. By now it is well established that Gln efflux from astrocytes is promoted by system N transporters, SN1 (SNAT3) (Chaudhry et al. 2001) and SN2 (SNAT5) (Cubelos et al. 2005), which are primarily located in

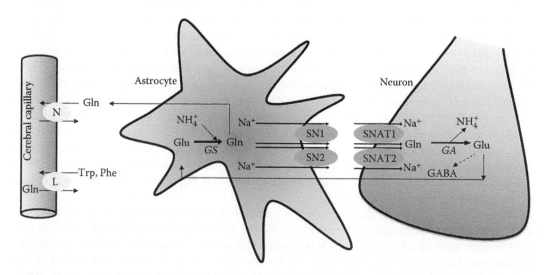

FIGURE 7.1 The glutamine–glutamate cycle in the brain. The scheme shows how glutamine is synthesized, shuttled between the different compartments of the CNS, and degraded and/or transferred out of the CNS, and illustrates contribution of the major amino acid transport systems or individual carriers to the Gln fluxes. Newly synthesized Gln exits astrocytes using N system carriers, SN1 (SNAT3) and SN2 (SNAT5), and is taken up by neurons by A system carriers SNAT1 and SNAT2. A portion of Gln is transported from brain to blood by system N carriers. Gln also leaves the brain in exchange of large neutral amino acids, which is mediated by a sodium-independent system L. Abbreviations: GABA, gamma-amino butyric acid; Glu, glutamate; Gln, glutamine; GS, glutamine synthetase; GA, phosphate-activated glutaminase; Phe, phenylalanine; Trp, tryptophan. (Scheme based on Albrecht, J. et al. 2007. *Front Biosci.* 12: 332–343, modified.)

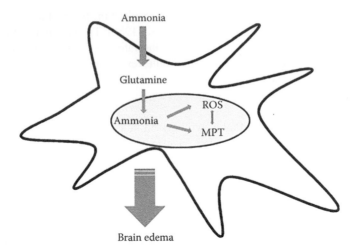

FIGURE 7.2 The "Trojan horse" hypothesis of glutamine toxicity in hepatic encephalopathy. Glutamine (the "Trojan Horse") derived from ammonia in astrocytic cytoplasm is transferred to mitochondria, where it is reconverted to ammonia ("unloads the troops"). The "troops" ("Ammonia") devastate mitochondria, which leads to mitochondrial permeability transition (MPT) associated with accumulation of reactive oxygen species (ROS) and astrocytic swelling. In this way "the troops" become guilty of brain edema associated with HE. (After Albrecht, J. and M.D. Norenberg. 2006. *Hepatology* 44 (4):788–794.)

astrocytic processes enwrapping the glutamatergic terminals (Figure 7.1). The preferably outward mode of action of N transporters, their Gln/Na^+ cotransport/H^+ antiport mechanism and electroneutrality, render them particularly well suited for carrying out the efflux in the way of fulfilling the needs of the adjacent neurons. In turn, neuronal Gln uptake is catalyzed by system A transporters, SNAT1 and SNAT2 (Figure 7.2), which (i) are exclusively located in neurons, (ii) work in the unidirectional, inward mode, and (iii) cotransport Gln with Na^+ ions (reviewed by Chaudhry et al. 2002). The fact that system A–mediated Gln uptake is specifically inhibited by methyl-aminobutyric acid (MeAiB) has been elegantly used to provide electrophysiological evidence for the precursor role of Gln. MeAiB suppressed spontaneous glutamatergic transmission in neurons of organotypic hippocampal cultures or hippocampal slices, and this effect was reversed upon enrichment of the bathing medium with Gln (Bacci et al. 2002). In a similar experimental setting, MeAiB served as a tool to demonstrate the role of Gln in stimulation of the inhibitory GABA-ergic transmission in the pyramidal cells of the hippocampus (Liang et al. 2006; Fricke et al. 2007). Most recently, a vicious circle of events encompassing seizure-related changes in Gln distribution have been demonstrated; in rats with kainic-acid-induced TLE, seizure-induced decrease of GLN_{ECF} reflected its increased uptake into neurons (Kanamori and Ross, 2013).

Gln turnover within GGC also involves Gln uptake to brain mitochondria, which is predominantly saturable and stereospecific (Roberg et al. 1999). Two features of mitochondrial Gln uptake are in concert with its role in GGC: (i) It is inhibited by a series of different amino acids, including histidine (His) and leucine, which also inhibit GA (Albrecht et al. 2000); (ii) the pool of Gln transported by the His-sensitive carrier is preferentially metabolized to Glu (Ziemińska et al. 2004).

7.3 GLUTAMINE IN BRAIN PATHOLOGIES

7.3.1 HYPERAMMONEMIA/HEPATIC ENCEPHALOPATHY

7.3.1.1 General Characteristics

Hepatic encephalopathy (HE) is the most common representative of so-called hyperammonemic encephalopathies, diseases whose pathomechanism reflects neurotoxic effects of blood-derived

TABLE 7.1

Grades (Clinical Stages) of Hepatic Encephalopathy

Stage	Mental State
I	Mild confusion, euphoria, or depression; decreased attention; slowing of ability to perform mental tasks; untidiness; slurred speech; irritability; reversal of sleep rhythm
II	Drowsiness, lethargy, gross deficits in ability to perform mental tasks, obvious personality changes, inappropriate behavior, intermittent disorientation (especially for time), lack of sphincter control
III	Somnolence, loss of ability to perform mental tasks, persistent disorientation with respect to time and/or place, amnesia, occasional fits of rage, speech present but incoherent, pronounced confusion
IV	Coma, with (IVA) or without (IVB) response to painful stimuli

Source: Modified from Albrecht, J. and E.A. Jones. 1999. *J Neurol. Sci.* 170 (2):138–146.

ammonia. Since the impact of HE is not much publicized and intuitively underestimated, different aspects of HE will be presented here in some detail.

HE is a complex neuropsychiatric disorder that results from impaired liver function, that is, impaired clearance from blood of toxins that eventually enter the brain (Albrecht and Jones 1999). Ammonia is by far not the only pathogen in HE; recent studies underscore the role of neuroinflammation in its pathogenesis (Su et al. 2015). However, since the direct substrate of Gln synthesis and pronounced derangements of Gln metabolism in HE are almost exclusively related to ammonia only the hyperammonemia (HA)-related aspects of HE will be subject of consideration in this section.

Diagnosis of the increasing severity of the HE patients' condition is subject to grading of the major neuropsychiatric and behavioral symptoms: Detailed description of the HE symptoms characteristic of the subsequent grades of HE are illustrated in Table 7.1.

There is a consensus that development of HE symptoms is mainly associated with ammonia-induced imbalance between the inhibitory GABA-ergic and the excitatory Glu-ergic neurotransmission in disfavor of the former.

Impaired ammonia detoxification by the liver is associated with liver cirrhosis, which is a serious epidemiological, social, and economic burden. In EU countries, as many as 1,000,000 people are affected with liver cirrhosis, of which most show symptoms of HE, with average survival time of about 15 years. Average yearly treatment cost of one patient (lactulose, one hospitalization) is about 9000€ (estimate from Neff et al. 2006). The death rate of liver cirrhosis in EU countries (per 100,000) for male population amounts to about 25, which is only slightly belowthe rate for diabetes (23) (Eurostat, online data code: hlth_cd_asdr, 2012). In addition to patients with overt HE, who show gross mental deficits, about 50%–60% of cirrhotic are affected by subclinical hepatic encephalopathy (US statistics, discussed in Leevy and Phillips 2007), characterized by mild cognitive, attention, and motor skill deficits that escape detection during routine clinical tests. Subclinical encephalopathy (SHE) subjects suffer decreased quality of life and impaired working efficiency and pose increased risks of motor vehicle accidents.

Ammonia affects mainly astrocytes making impaired astrocyte–neuron interactions a key player in neurotransmission imbalance. Moreover, astrocytic swelling is the primary cause of cerebral edema, increased intracranial pressure, and herniation, the immediate causes of death in acute HE. In what follows, we focus on the role of glutamine in the development of ammonia-evoked derangement of the pertinent astrocytic functions.

7.3.1.2 Mediation of Ammonia Neurotoxicity by Glutamine

For many decades, the dominating view has been that the key HE symptoms are due to direct neurotoxic action of ammonia on central nervous system (CNS) cells, while Gln has been considered as a benign ammonia detoxification product. Indeed, increase of blood ammonia level, along

TABLE 7.2

Effects of L-Methionine-DL-Sulfoximine (MSO, Glutamine Synthase Inhibitor) on the Major HE Parameters in Hyperammonemic (HA) Rats

	Control	HA	HA + MSO
Ammonia (blood) (µM)	29 ± 3	601 ± 38	908 ± 196
GS (brain) (IU/g)	38.8 ± 0.8	39.9 ± 0.3	14.1 ± 0.2
Gln (brain) (mmol/kg)	5.6 ± 0.4	18.8 ± 0.4	2.6 ± 0.4
Glu (brain) (mmol/kg)	10.1 ± 1.0	6.6 ± 0.4	9.5 ± 0.6
Specific gravity (brain)	1.0452	1.0424	1.0446
Water content (brain) (%)	0.783	0.804	0.784

Source: Data from Takahashi, H. et al. 1991. *Am. J Physiol.* 261 (3 Pt 2):H825–H829.

with electroencephalogram (EEG) abnormalities and impairment of psychometric score, constitute a basic triad for parametric evaluation of HE grade (Conn and Bircher 1994). The concept that excess glutamine accumulating under increased ammonia load to the brain mediates ammonia neurotoxicity was derived from observations made in the early 1990s with the use of a relatively specific inhibitor of GS, L-methionine-DL-sulfoximine (MSO). Administration of MSO to experimental animals with HE or HA evoked by systemic administration of ammonium acetate evoked by systemic administration of ammonium ions ameliorated pathophysiological manifestations of ammonia neurotoxicity (Takahashi et al. 1991; Hawkins et al. 1993, see Tables 7.2 and 7.3). Most significantly, the recovery to normal values included a return to control value of the specific gravity and relative water content of the brain (Table 7.2).

Subsequent experimental studies *in vitro* and *in vivo* with the use of MSO confirmed the role of Gln in causing astrocytic swelling and cerebral edema. The effects of MSO included abrogation of ammonia-induced swelling of cortical astrocytes in culture (Norenberg and Bender 1994); attenuation of swelling of perivascular astrocytes and pericytes (Willard-Mack et al. 1996; Tanigami et al. 2005) and reduction of potassium accumulation in the intracellular space in the cerebral cortex of rats with HA (Sugimoto et al. 1997); and attenuation of the increase of cerebral blood flow and intracranial pressure in the cerebral cortex of rats with chronic HE and subsequently challenged with extra ammonia load (Master et al. 1999). Excessive glutamine accumulation in the brain has been proven to be the HE-inducing factor in humans. Advancement of the NMR technique led in 1990 to the first demonstration of increased Gln content in the brain of a symptomatic HE patient

TABLE 7.3

Effects of L-Methionine-DL-Sulfoximine (MSO, Glutamine Synthase Inhibitor) on the Major HE Parameters in Portacaval Shunted (PCS) Rats

	Control	PCS	PCS + MSO
Ammonia (blood) (nmol/L)	97 ± 8	227 ± 15	265 ± 27
Ammonia (brain) (nmol/g)	146 ± 6	384 ± 22	424 ± 46
Gln (brain) (nmol/g)	5580 ± 360	8780 ± 570	5180 ± 540
Tryptophan (brain) (nmol/g)	17 ± 1	45 ± 3	25 ± 2
Glucose consumption (brain) (nmol/min/g)	861 ± 53	614 ± 39	733 ± 87
BBB transport of tryptophan (µL/min/g)	18 ± 2	31 ± 5	15 ± 3

Source: Data from Hawkins, R.A. et al. 1993. *J Neurochem.* 60 (3):1000–1006.

(Kreis et al. 1990). A few years later a well-documented study has appeared demonstrating good correlation between the cerebral Gln content and the HE grade (Laubenberger et al. 1997). A bedside brain microdialysis study revealed that in patients with acute HE awaiting liver transplantation due to cirrhosis, blood ammonia correlated with cerebral (microdialysate) Gln, which in turn correlated with the intracranial pressure value (Tofteng et al. 2006).

Initial interpretation of the edema-inducing effect of Gln was that it acted as an osmolyte that by increasing osmotic pressure in astrocytes promoted their swelling. However, relative contribution of accumulating Gln to the osmotic pressure produced by the sum of different contributing osmolytes (lactate, alanine) appeared insufficient to account for this effect (discussed in Albrecht 2003). On top of that, in chronic HE, increase of brain Gln is accompanied by loss of different osmolytes at low molecular weight, including myo-inositol, taurine, and betaine (Cordoba et al. 1996). Ever since, strong evidence has accumulated that Gln impairs mitochondrial function and that it occurs as a consequence of excessive accumulation in mitochondria:

- Ammonia stimulated Gln uptake in isolated non-synaptic mitochondria (Dolińska et al. 1996).
- Gln induced permeability transition and swelling of mitochondria when added to mitochondrial preparation (Ziemińska et al. 2000) or cultured astrocytes (Pichili et al. 2007): In either case, this effect was blocked by the mitochondrial Gln uptake inhibitor, His.
- In cultured astrocytes, MSO suppressed ammonia-induced formation of reactive oxygen species (ROS) (Murthy et al. 2001).
- Gln dose-dependently increased ROS synthesis in astrocytes (Jayakumar et al. 2004).
- Cyclosporine A (CsA) suppressed ROS induction by Gln in astrocytes (Jayakumar et al. 2004) and swelling of mitochondria in a non-synaptic mitochondrial preparation (Ziemińska et al. 2000).

The effects of Gln required Gln degradation: Gln accumulation in ammonia-treated astrocytes preceded for some hours peak astrocytic swelling (Jayakumar et al. 2006), and swelling of ammonia-treated astrocytes was prevented by a GA inhibitor (DON) (Jayakumar et al. 2006). Histidine, which, as mentioned before, preferentially blocks transport to mitochondria of the Gln pool accessible to deamidation (Ziemińska et al. 2004), cooperated with MSO in reducing ammonia-induced swelling of astrocytes. These observations led to formulation of the "Trojan Horse" hypothesis of action of Gln. Accordingly, Gln carries and unloads excess ammonia in mitochondria, thus behaving in a "Trojan horse" style, and the Gln-derived ammonia triggers mitochondrial impairment and the ensuing chain of deleterious reactions leading to astrocytic swelling and brain edema. This hypothesis, as formulated by Albrecht and Norenberg (2006), is illustrated by a diagram (Figure 7.2).

More recently, the Trojan horse hypothesis found support in both *in vitro* and *in vivo* experiments. HE was found to lower the expression of the Gln transporter SN1 that mediates Gln efflux from astrocytes; the effect paralleled induction of cerebral cortical edema (Zielińska et al. 2014), and His added i.p. to rats with HE-abolished brain edema and symptoms of oxidative stress in these rats (Rama Rao et al. 2010; for a recent review, see Rama Rao et al. 2014).

7.3.1.3 Glutamine as a Modulator of the Cyclic Guanosine Monophosphate (cGMP)/Nitric Oxide (NO) Pathway in Hyperammonemic Brain: Role of the Glutamine/Arginine Exchange Carrier, y+LAT2

Alterations in NO and cGMP levels play varied and independent roles in the pathomechanism of HE. In acute HE, activation of NO synthesis, is usually but not necessarily associated with the activation of N-methyl-D-aspartate (NMDA) receptors, contributes to oxidative nitrosative stress and cGMP serves as marker of this activation (Hermenegildo et al. 2000; Hilgier et al. 2005). However, chronic HE is associated with decreased activity of this pathway and cGMP deficit, which is held responsible for cognitive and memory impairments (Erceg et al. 2005). The authors' laboratory has shown that pharmacological manipulations increasing extracellular Gln in the brain to the level found in acute HE patients decrease NO and cGMP production both in healthy and ammonia-exposed brain, by limiting the transport to the cells of the NO precursor, arginine (Arg) (Hilgier et al. 2009). Accordingly, preincubation with Gln stimulates Arg efflux from the rat brain slices pre-incubated with Gln, a situation reflecting that occurring in the early stages of HE, when newly synthesized Gln accumulates in the extracellular space (Zielińska et al. 2011). More recently studies were able to prove the involvement the hybrid y+LAT2 transporter in this process serves to exchange Arg for Gln, and for which Gln and Arg compete (Zielińska et al. 2012). Ammonia was shown to specifically activate y+LAT2 in astrocytes and subsequently Arg uptake, by a mechanism encompassing increased expression of the transporter at the messenger RNA (mRNA) and protein level (Zielińska et al. 2012). Upregulation of y(+) LAT2 transporter was found to be coupled with increased inducible nitric oxide synthase (iNOS) expression, leading to increased nitric oxide (NO) synthesis and protein nitration, a deleterious consequence of oxidative/nitrosative stress (Zielińska et al. 2015). These variable effects of y+LAT2 activation on the direction of Arg fluxes may partly explain the stage-dependent variations of NO synthesis and cGMP accumulation in the astrocytes.

In summary, the available evidence suggests that during HE, ammonia-derived Gln (i) deranges synthesis of amino acid neurotransmitters Glu and GABA, contributing to excitation/inhibition imbalance; (ii) increases osmotic pressure of cytoplasm; (iii) impairs mitochondrial function subsequent to liberation of ammonia; (iv) modulates the NO/cGMP pathway by interfering with Arg transport across the cell membrane. As such, the evidence justifies description of Gln in HE as a "multifacet intruder." Though hyperosmosis and mitochondrial impairment primarily and directly affect astrocytes, their dysfunction bears upon neural transmission. On the other hand, it is not yet entirely clear whether Gln interference with Arg transport and with the NO/cGMP pathway involves astrocytes only or also neurons and the physiologic implications (beneficial vs. detrimental) of this interference remain to delineated.

7.3.2 Epilepsy

Epilepsy is a neurological disorder characterized by sudden and temporary discharges of neurons (epileptic seizures). Depending on the number of neurons involved, epilepsy is defined as partial, focal, or general epilepsy. Temporal lobe epilepsy (TLE) is the most common form, whereby mesial temporal lobe epilepsy (MTLE) with hippocampal sclerosis has so far been subjected to the most thorough mechanistic analysis (ILAE Commission Report 2004). Epilepsy is a severe socio-economic burden: 50 million individuals worldwide have a confirmed diagnosis of this disease. Reported regional prevalence (per 1000) varies from 2.7 (Rochester, MN) to 17.6 (Chile), while incidence (per 100,000) ranges from 26 (Norway) to 111 (Chile; based on Banerjee et al. 2009).

Epileptic discharges are due to the imbalance between the excitatory glutamatergic and the inhibitory GABA-ergic transmission in favor of the former. In MTLE patients who in EEG present the onset of epileptogenic activity, an excessive accumulation of Glu and concomitant reduction of GABA is recorded in the extracellular space (microdialysates) of the brain (During and Spencer 1993). The fact that this condition was accompanied by decreased extracellular Gln/Glu (Cavus et al. 2005) directly implicated deranged Gln metabolism in the pathogenesis of epilepsy. Indeed, increased glutamatergic activity in MTLE was found to be well correlated with GGC dysfunction, including impairment of enzymes involved in this cycle. A lower rate of Glu–Gln cycling was found in hippocampi of MTLE patients, as revealed by ^{13}C NMR spectroscopy (Petroff et al. 2002), and appeared to be related to a decrease of GS expression and activity, specifically confined to the epilepsy-affected regions of the hippocampus (CA1 but not subiculum; Eid et al. 2004). Opposite to GS, GA immunostaining was found increased in surviving neurons of all regions of epilepsy-affected brain, and co-localized with Glu immunostaining in pre- and post-synaptic mitochondria (Eid et al. 2007). A recent study using *in situ* hybridization technique on histologic sections of hippocampi preformed on a large population of patients demonstrated dysregulation of GS and GA expression at the mRNA level (Eid et al. 2013). In rats in which epilepsy was modeled by pentylentetrazole (PTZ) treatment, decreased GS activity was associated with, and mechanistically related to, increased nitration of tyrosine residues (Bidmon et al. 2008). Collectively, increased GA and decreased GS activity remain the most likely cause of excessive Glu accumulation and, successively, increased Glu-ergic tone. However, the involvement of GS may not be the rule in all the brain regions affected by epilepsy; no changes in this enzyme activity were detected in brain tissue of frontal cortical epilepsy patients (Steffens et al. 2005). Most recently, a vicious circle of events encompassing seizure-related changes in Gln distribution in the epilepsy-vulnerable brain region has been demonstrated; in rats with kainic-acid-induced TLE, seizure-induced decrease of GLN_{ECF} reflected its increased uptake into neurons, promoting increased Glu production and thus seizures (Kanamori and Ross 2013).

Impaired Gln metabolism may also be a cause of GABA-ergic hypofunction associated with epilepsy. In a rat model of juvenile model of TLE, an early excessive accumulation of Gln in the brain is accompanied by a profound decrease of GABA content as revealed by magnetic resonance spectroscopy (MRS) analysis; at the morphological level the decrease of GABA was coincident with GABA-ergic neuronal loss (van der Hel et al. 2013). In mouse hippocampus, experimentally induced reactive astrocytosis that mimics epilepsy-associated tissue sclerosis resulted in profound inhibition of Gln synthesis that was associated with the depression of inhibitory GABA-ergic currents and coupled with hyper-excitation. These changes in hippocampal currents could be reversed by Gln administration (Ortinski et al. 2010).

7.3.3 GLUTAMINE AND THE PATHOGENESIS OF BRAIN TUMORS

The incidence of primary brain tumors is 4–11 per 100,000 population per year, and the annual mortality rates are 3–7 per 100,000 (Ohgaki et al. 2008). Although many risk factors such as genetic susceptibility, exposure to ionizing and non-ionizing radiation, neurocarcinogenes and metals, and virus infections have been postulated, the etiology of these neoplasms remains unclear. Gliomas of astrocytic, ependymal, or oligodendroglial origin account for more than 70% of brain tumors (Ohgaki 2009). In spite of progress in understanding biology of gliomas, they are still among the deadliest human tumors: median survival time of patients with the most aggressive glioblastoma (WHO IV) is less than one year (Weller et al. 2013).

Gln is a central metabolite in many neoplastic cells and tissues, including gliomas. It provides a major substrate for respiration and is a source of nitrogen for the production of nucleotides, proteins, and other molecules essential for cell growth (Cheng et al. 2011). Moreover, Gln is both necessary and sufficient for modulation of glioma cell volume and thereby facilitates cell migration (Ernest and Sontheimer 2007).

High demands for Gln can be met by upregulated Gln uptake. Transporter ASCT2, belonging to the ASC system, is abundantly expressed in glioma cell lines (Dolińska et al. 2003) and tissues (Sidoryk et al. 2004). Consistently, Gln uptake in glioma cells is predominantly mediated by ASCT2 (Dolińska et al. 2003).

Gln, as was mentioned before, is metabolized to Glu and ammonia by phosphate-activated GA. In mammals, there are two genes coding for GA isoforms: The *Gls* gene encodes kidney-type GLS isoforms—kidney-type glutaminase (KGA) and glutaminase C (GAC), whereas the *Gls2* gene encodes liver-type GLS2 isoforms—GAB and LGA (Aledo et al. 2000). Deregulated expression and activity of GA isoforms is a characteristic feature of different tumors and neoplastic cell lines (Szeliga and Obara-Michlewska 2009). In human developed high-grade gliomas, the GLS isoforms are highly expressed, whereas transcripts arising from the GLS2 are hardly detectable (Szeliga et al. 2005).

Elevated glutaminolysis results in the intense production of Glu, which also plays an important role in malignant phenotype of glioma. Significant quantities of Glu released by glioma into the extracellular space exert peritumoral excitotoxicity and thus promote tumor expansion (Sontheimer 2008).

Release of Glu occurs via the system Xc cystine/glutamate antiporter, whose catalytic subunit xCT is upregulated in glioma tissues (Ye et al. 1999; Sontheimer 2008). Moreover, failure to express functional Glu transporters, EAAT1 and EAAT2, leads to significant decrease in Glu uptake (Ye et al. 1999). This lack of Glu reuptake mechanisms in glioblastomas results in accumulation of this neurotoxic amino acid in the vicinity of tumor, which in turn causes neuron death. Moreover, Glu released by gliomas contributes to peritumoral seizures and tumor-associated epilepsy (Watkins and Sontheimer 2012).

7.4 CONCLUDING COMMENTS: CAN MODULATION OF GLUTAMINE CONTENT OFFER TREATMENT MODALITIES FOR GLUTAMINE RELATED BRAIN DISORDERS?

Each of the above-discussed pathological conditions of the brain is associated with impairments of well-defined steps of GGC, with straightforward consequences for their pathogenesis. In HE, excess ammonia entry to the brain leads to Gln accumulation, which is one of the causative factors in cerebral edema and increased intracranial pressure. In epilepsy, inactivation of Gln synthesis plus its excessive degradation favor increased glutamatergic tone and epileptic discharges. In cerebral tumors, excessive Gln metabolism provides energy for proliferation and renders Glu as an agent fostering penetration of the surrounding tissues and invasion. In theory, thus, relevant pharmacological manipulations with GGC may in the future become useful treatment modalities in either of the pathological conditions. In particular, treatments with inhibitors of GS or GA might relieve symptoms of HE and epilepsy, respectively. However, the available inhibitors of these enzymes cannot be used because of severe side effects. The GS inhibitor MSO is a convulsing agent frequently used to model epileptic discharges in animals (Bidmon et al. 2008) by a mechanism related to increased glycogen synthesis (Cloix and Hevor 2009). The fact that primates are much less sensitive to the convulsive activity of MSO than rodents has raised hopes for using this compound as treatment modality in human HE (Cooper 2013). However, preclinical data supporting the notion are still preliminary. The common GA inhibitor DON interferes, among other processes, with the γ-glutamyl transpeptidase activity and amino acid transport at the blood–brain barrier (Cloix and Hevor 2009 and references therein). Attempts at designing nontoxic, side effect-free modulators of GS and GA appear warranted. By recent accounts, some light at the end of the tunnel has emerged with the discovery of a potent uncompetitive GA inhibitor bis-2-(5-phenylacetamido-1,2,4-thiadiazol-2-yl) ethyl sulfide (BPTES; Robinson et al. 2007), and its less toxic analogues (Shukla et al. 2012). With regard to brain tumors, targeted inhibition of the prevalent kidney-type glutaminase, GLS, appears to be a plausible task for future trials. Of note in this context, the liver-type glutaminase isoform, GLS2, which is normally underexpressed or absent in highly malignant gliomas, curbs their growth upon being transfected (Szeliga et al. 2009). Most recently, combination of inhibition of GLS1 and overexpression of GLS2 turned out effective in limiting the growth of glioma cells *in vitro* (Martín-Rufián et al. 2014; Szeliga et al. 2014). Clearly, further development efficient methods of targeted delivery of the modalities to the tumor tissue appear to be a prerequisite of therapeutic success.

REFERENCES

Albrecht, J. 2003. Glucose-derived osmolytes and energy impairment in brain edema accompanying liver failure: The role of glutamine reevaluated. *Gastroenterology* 125 (3):976–978.

Albrecht, J., M. Dolińska, W. Hilgier et al. 2000. Modulation of glutamine uptake and phosphate-activated glutaminase activity in rat brain mitochondria by amino acids and their synthetic analogues. *Neurochem. Int.* 36 (4–5):341–347.

Albrecht, J. and E.A. Jones. 1999. Hepatic encephalopathy: Molecular mechanisms underlying the clinical syndrome. *J Neurol. Sci.* 170 (2):138–146.

Albrecht, J. and M.D. Norenberg. 2006. Glutamine: A Trojan horse in ammonia neurotoxicity. *Hepatology* 44 (4):788–794.

Albrecht, J., U. Sonnewald, H.S. Waagepetersen et al. 2007. Glutamine in the central nervous system: Function and dysfunction. *Front Biosci.* 12:332–343.

Aledo, J.C., P.M. Gómez-Fabre, L. Olalla et al. 2000. Identification of two human glutaminase loci and tissue-specific expression of the two related genes. *Mamm. Genome* 11 (12):1107–1110.

Bacci, A., G. Sancini, C. Verderio et al. 2002. Block of glutamate-glutamine cycle between astrocytes and neurons inhibits epileptiform activity in hippocampus. *J Neurophysiol.* 88 (5):2302–2310.

Bak, L.K., A. Schousboe, and H.S. Waagepetersen. 2006. The glutamate/GABA-glutamine cycle: Aspects of transport, neurotransmitter homeostasis and ammonia transfer. *J Neurochem.* 98 (3):641–653.

Banerjee, P.N., D. Filippi, and W.A. Hauser. 2009. The descriptive epidemiology of epilepsy—A review. *Epilepsy Res.* 85 (1):31–45.

Bidmon, H.J., B. Görg, N. Palomero-Gallagher et al. 2008. Glutamine synthetase becomes nitrated and its activity is reduced during repetitive seizure activity in the pentylentetrazole model of epilepsy. *Epilepsia* 49 (10):1733–1748.

Bradford, H.F., H.K. Ward, and P. Foley. 1989. Glutaminase inhibition and the release of neurotransmitter glutamate from synaptosomes. *Brain Res.* 476 (1):29–34.

Cavus, I., W.S. Kasoff, M.P. Cassaday et al. 2005. Extracellular metabolites in the cortex and hippocampus of epileptic patients. *Ann Neurol.* 57 (2):226–235.

Chaudhry, F.A., D. Krizaj, P. Larsson et al. 2001. Coupled and uncoupled proton movement by amino acid transport system. *N. EMBO Journal* 20 (24):7041–7051.

Chaudhry, F.A., R.J. Reimer, and R.H. Edwards. 2002. The glutamine commute: Take the N line and transfer to the A. *J Cell Biol.* 157 (3):349–355.

Cheng, T., J. Sudderth, C. Yang et al. 2011. Pyruvate carboxylase is required for glutamine-independent growth of tumor cells. *Proc. Natl. Acad. Sci. USA* 108 (21):8674–8679.

Cloix, J.F. and T. Hevor. 2009. Epilepsy, regulation of brain energy metabolism and neurotransmission. *Curr. Med. Chem.* 16 (7):841–853.

Conn, H.O. and J. Bircher. 1994. *Hepatic Encephalopathies: Syndromes and Therapies*. Bloomington: Medi-Ed Press, 1–13.

Cooper, A.J. 2013. Possible treatment of end-stage hyperammonemic encephalopathy by inhibition of glutamine synthetase. *Metabol. Brain Dis.* 28 (2):119–125.

Cordoba, J., J. Gottstein, and A.T. Blei. 1996. Glutamine, myo-inositol, and organic brain osmolytes after portocaval anastomosis in the rat: Implications for ammonia-induced brain edema. *Hepatology* 24 (4):919–923.

Cubelos, B., I.M. Gonzalez-Gonzalez, C. Gimenez et al. 2005. Amino acid transporter SNAT5 localizes to glial cells in the rat brain. *Glia* 49 (2):230–244.

Dolińska, M., A. Dybel, B. Zabłocka et al. 2003. Glutamine transport in C6 glioma cells shows ASCT2 system characteristics. *Neurochem. Int.* 43 (4–5):501–507.

Dolińska, M., W. Hilgier, and J. Albrecht. 1996. Ammonia stimulates glutamine uptake to the cerebral non-synaptic mitochondria of the rat. *Neurosci. Lett.* 213 (1):45–48.

During, M.J. and D.D. Spencer. 1993. Extracellular hippocampal glutamate and spontaneous seizure in the conscious human brain. *Lancet* 341 (8861):1607–1610.

Eid, T., J. Hammer, E. Rundén-Pran et al. 2007. Increased expression of phosphate-activated glutaminase in hippocampal neurons in human mesial temporal lobe epilepsy. *Acta Neuropathologica* 113 (2):137–152.

Eid, T., T.S. Lee, Y. Wang et al. 2013. Gene expression of glutamate metabolizing enzymes in the hippocampal formation in human temporal lobe epilepsy. *Epilepsia* 54(2):228–238.

Eid, T., M.J. Thomas, D.D. Spencer et al. 2004. Loss of glutamine synthetase in the human epileptogenic hippocampus: Possible mechanism for raised extracellular glutamate in mesial temporal lobe epilepsy. *Lancet* 363(9402):28–37.

Erceg, S., P. Monfort, M. Hernández-Viadel et al. 2005. Oral administration of sildenafil restores learning ability in rats with hyperammonemia and with portacaval shunts. *Hepatology* 41(2):299–306.

Ernest, N.J. and H. Sontheimer. 2007. Extracellular glutamine is a critical modulator for regulatory volume increase in human glioma cells. *Brain Res.* 4:231–238.

Fricke, M.N., D.M. Jones-Davis, and G.C. Mathews. 2007. Glutamine uptake by System A transporters maintains neurotransmitter GABA synthesis and inhibitory synaptic transmission. *J. Neurochem.* 102 (6):1895–1904.

Gallo, V., M.T. Ciotti, A. Coletti et al. 1982. Selective release of glutamate from cerebellar granule cells differentiating in culture. *Proc. Natl. Acad. Sci. USA* 79 (24):7919–7923.

Gauchy, C., M.L. Kemel, J. Glowinski et al. 1980. *In vivo* release of endogenously synthesized [3H]GABA from the cat substantia nigra and the pallido-entopeduncular nuclei. *Brain Res.* 193 (1):129–141.

Hamberger, A.C., G.H. Chiang, E.S. Nylen et al. 1979a. Glutamate as a CNS transmitter. I. Evaluation of glucose and glutamine as precursors for the synthesis of preferentially released glutamate. *Brain Res.* 168 (3):513–530.

Hamberger, A.C., G.H. Chiang, E. Sandoval et al. 1979b. Glutamate as a CNS transmitter. II. Regulation of synthesis in the releasable pool. *Brain Res.* 168 (3):531–541.

Hamberger, A. and B. Nyström. 1984. Extra- and intracellular amino acids in the hippocampus during development of hepatic encephalopathy. *Neurochem. Res.* 9 (9):1181–1192.

Hauser, W.A. and L.T. Kurland. 1975. The epidemiology of epilepsy in Rochester, Minnesota, 1935 through 1967. *Epilepsia* 16 (1):1–66.

Hawkins, R.A., J. Jessy, A.M. Mans et al. 1993. Effect of reducing brain glutamine synthesis on metabolic symptoms of hepatic encephalopathy. *J Neurochem.* 60 (3):1000–1006.

Hermenegildo, C., P. Monfort, and V. Felipo. 2000. Activation of N-methyl-D-aspartate receptors in rat brain *in vivo* following acute ammonia intoxication: Characterization by *in vivo* brain microdialysis. *Hepatology* 31 (3):709–715.

Hilgier, W., I. Freśko, E. Klemenska et al. 2009. Glutamine inhibits ammonia-induced accumulation of cGMP in rat striatum limiting arginine supply for NO synthesis. *Neurobiol. Dis.* 35 (1):75–81.

Hilgier, W., S.S. Oja, P. Saransaari et al. 2005. Taurine prevents ammonia-induced accumulation of cyclic GMP in rat striatum by interaction with GABA$_A$ and glycine receptors. *Brain Res.* 1043 (1–2):242–246.

Hilgier, W., M. Puka, and J. Albrecht. 1992. Characteristics of large neutral amino acid-induced release of preloaded L-glutamine from rat cerebral capillaries *in vitro*: Effects of ammonia, hepatic encephalopathy, and gamma-glutamyl transpeptidase inhibitors. *J Neurosci. Res.* 32 (2):221–226.

Jacobson, I., M. Sandberg, and A. Hamberger. 1985. Mass transfer in brain dialysis devices—A new method for the estimation of extracellular amino acids concentration. *J Neurosci. Meth.* 15 (3):263–268.

Jayakumar, A.R., K.V. Rama Rao, A. Schousboe et al. 2004. Glutamine-induced free radical production in cultured astrocytes. *Glia* 46 (3):296–301.

Jayakumar, A.R., K.V. Rao, Ch.R. Murthy et al. 2006. Glutamine in the mechanism of ammonia-induced astrocyte swelling. *Neurochem. Int.* 48 (6–7):623–628.

Kanamori, K. and B.D. Ross. 2004. Quantitative determination of extracellular glutamine concentration in rat brain, and its elevation *in vivo* by system A transport inhibitor, alpha-(methylamino)isobutyrate. *J Neurochem.* 90 (1):203–210.

Kanamori, K. and B.D. Ross. 2013. Electrographic seizures are significantly reduced by *in vivo* inhibition of neuronal uptake of extracellular glutamine in rat hippocampus. *Epilepsy Res.* 107 (1–2):20–36.

Kreis, R., N. Farrow, and B.D. Ross. 1990. Diagnosis of hepatic encephalopathy by proton magnetic resonance spectroscopy. *Lancet* 336 (8715):635–636.

Laubenberger, J., D. Häussinger, S. Bayer et al. 1997. Proton magnetic resonance spectroscopy of the brain in symptomatic and asymptomatic patients with liver cirrhosis. *Gastroenterology* 112 (5):1610–1616.

Leevy, C.B. and J.A. Phillips. 2007. Hospitalizations during the use of rifaximin versus lactulose for the treatment of hepatic encephalopathy. *Dig. Dis. Sci.* 52 (3):737–741.

Liang, S.L., G.C. Carlson, and D.A. Coulter. 2006. Dynamic regulation of synaptic GABA release by the glutamate-glutamine cycle in hippocampal area CA1. *J Neurosci.* 26 (33):8537–8548.

Martinez-Hernandez, A., K.P. Bell, and M.D. Norenberg. 1977. Glutamine synthetase: Glial localization in brain. *Science* 195 (4284):1356–1358.

Martín-Rufián, M., R. Nascimento-Gomes, A. Higuero et al. 2014. Both GLS silencing and GLS2 overexpression synergize with oxidative stress against proliferation of glioma cells. *J Mol. Med.* 92 (3):277–290.

Master, S., J. Gottstein, and A. Blei. 1999. Cerebral blood flow and the development of ammonia-induced brain edema in rats after portacaval anastomosis. *Hepatology* 30:876–880.

Murthy, C.R., K.V. Rama Rao, G. Bai et al. 2001. Ammonia-induced production of free radicals in primary cultures of rat astrocytes. *J Neurosci. Res.* 66 (2):282–288.

Neff, G.W., N. Kemmer, V.C. Zacharias et al. 2006. Analysis of hospitalizations comparing rifaximin versus lactulose in the management of hepatic encephalopathy. *Transplant Proc.* 38 (10):3552–3555.

Nitsch, C., B. Schmude, and P. Haug. 1983. Alterations in the content of amino acid neurotransmitters before the onset and during the course of methoxypyridoxine-induced seizures in individual rabbit brain regions. *J Neurochem.* 40 (6):1571–1580.

Norenberg, M.D. and A.S. Bender. 1994. Astrocyte swelling in liver failure: Role of glutamine and benzodiazepines. *Acta Neurochirurgica Suppl (Wien)* 60:24–27.

Ohgaki, H. 2009. Epidemiology of brain tumors. *Methods Mol. Biol.* 472:323–342.

Ortinski, P.I., J. Dong, A. Mungenast et al. 2010. Selective induction of astrocytic gliosis generates deficits in neuronal inhibition. *Nat. Neurosci.* 13 (5):584–591.

Palacín, M., R. Estévez, J. Bertran et al. 1998. Molecular biology of mammalian plasma membrane amino acid transporters. *Physiol. Rev.* 78 (4):969–1054.

Patel, A.B., D.L. Rothman, G.W. Cline et al. 2001. Glutamine is the major precursor for GABA synthesis in rat neocortex *in vivo* following acute GABA-transaminase inhibition. *Brain Res.* 919 (2):207–220.

Petroff, O.A., L.D. Errante, D.L. Rothman et al. 2002. Glutamate-glutamine cycling in the epileptic human hippocampus. *Epilepsia* 43 (7):703–710.

Pichili, V.B., K.V. Rao, A.R. Jayakumar et al. 2007. Inhibition of glutamine transport into mitochondria protects astrocytes from ammonia toxicity. *Glia* 55 (8):801–809.

Rae, C., N. Hare, W.A. Bubb et al. 2003. Inhibition of glutamine transport depletes glutamate and GABA neurotransmitter pools: Further evidence for metabolic compartmentation. *J Neurochem.* 85 (2):503–514.

Rama Rao, K.V. and M.D. Norenberg. 2014. Glutamine in the pathogenesis of hepatic encephalopathy: The Trojan horse hypothesis revisited. *Neurochem. Res.* 39 (3):593–598.

Rama Rao, K.V., P.V. Reddy, X. Tong et al. 2010. Brain edema in acute liver failure: Inhibition by L-histidine. *Am. J Pathol.* 176:1400–1408.

Reubi, J.C., C. Van Der Berg, and M. Cuénod. 1978. Glutamine as precursor for the GABA and glutamate transmitter pools. *Neurosci. Lett.* 10 (1–2):171–174.

Roberg, B., I.A. Torgner, and E. Kvamme. 1999. Glutamine transport in rat brain synaptic and non-synaptic mitochondria. *Neurochem. Res.* 24(7):383–390.

Robinson, M.M., S.J. McBryant, T. Tsukamoto et al. 2007. Novel mechanism of inhibition of rat kidney-type glutaminase by bis-2-(5-phenylacetamido-1,2,4-thiadiazol-2-yl)ethyl sulfide (BPTES). *Biochem. J* 406 (3):407–414.

Shukla, K., D.V. Ferraris, A.G. Thomas et al. 2012. Design, synthesis, and pharmacological evaluation of bis-2-(5-phenylacetamido-1,2,4-thiadiazol-2-yl)ethyl sulfide 3 (BPTES) analogs as glutaminase inhibitors. *J Med. Chem.* 55 (23):10551–10563.

Sidoryk, M., E. Matyja, A. Dybel et al. 2004. Increased expression of a glutamine transporter SNAT3 is a marker of malignant gliomas. *Neuroreport* 15 (9):575–578.

Sontheimer, H. 2008. A role for glutamate in growth and invasion of primary brain tumors. *J. Neurochem.* 105 (2):287–295.

Steffens, M., H.J. Huppertz, J. Zentner et al. 2005. Unchanged glutamine synthetase activity and increased NMDA receptor density in epileptic human neocortex: Implications for the pathophysiology of epilepsy. *Neurochem. Int.* 47 (6):379–384.

Su, Y.Y., G.F. Yang, G.M. Lu et al. 2015. PET and MR imaging of neuroinflammation in hepatic encephalopathy. *Metab. Brain Dis.* 30(1):31–45.

Sugimoto, H., R.C. Koehler, D.A. Wilson et al. 1997. Methionine sulfoximine, a glutamine synthetase inhibitor, attenuates increased extracellular potassium activity during acute hyperammonemia. *J Cerebr. Blood Flow Metabol.* 17 (1):44–49.

Szeliga, M., M. Bogacińska-Karaś, A. Różycka et al. 2014. Silencing of GLS and overexpression of GLS2 genes cooperate in decreasing the proliferation and viability of glioblastoma cells. *Tumour Biol.* 35 (3):1855–1862.

Szeliga, M. and M. Obara-Michlewska. 2009. Glutamine in neoplastic cells: Focus on the expression and roles of glutaminases. *Neurochem. Int.* 55 (1–3):71–75.

Szeliga, M., M. Sidoryk, E. Matyja et al. 2005. Lack of expression of the liver-type glutaminase (LGA) mRNA in human malignant gliomas. *Neurosci. Lett.* 374 (3):171–173.

Takahashi, H., R.C. Koehler, S.W. Brusilow et al. 1991. Inhibition of brain glutamine accumulation prevents cerebral edema in hyperammonemic rats. *Am. J Physiol.* 261 (3 Pt 2):H825–H829.

Tanigami, H., A. Rebel, L.J. Martin et al. 2005. Effect of glutamine synthetase inhibition on astrocyte swelling and altered astroglial protein expression during hyperammonemia in rats. *Neurosci.* 131 (2):437–449.

Tapia, R. and R.M. Gonzalez. 1978. Glutamine and glutamate as precursors of the releasable pool of GABA in brain cortex slices. *Neurosci. Lett.* 10 (1–2):165–169.

Thanki, C.M., D. Sugden, A.J. Thomas et al. 1983. *In vivo* release from cerebral cortex of [14C]glutamate synthesized from [U-14C]glutamine. *J Neurochem.* 41 (3):611–617.

Tofteng, F., J. Hauerberg, B.A. Hansen et al. 2006. Persistent arterial hyperammonemia increases the concentration of glutamine and alanine in the brain and correlates with intracranial pressure in patients with fulminant hepatic failure. *J Cerebr. Blood Flow Metab.* 26 (1):21–27.

Tossman, J., A. Delin, L.S. Eriksson et al. 1987. Brain cortical amino acids measured by intracerebral dialysis in portacaval shunted rats. *Neurochem. Res.* 12 (3):265–269.

van der Hel, W.S., P. van Eijsden, I.W. Bos et al. 2013. *In vivo* MRS and histochemistry of status epilepticus-induced hippocampal pathology in a juvenile model of temporal lobe epilepsy. *NMR Biomed.* 26 (2):132–140.

Waagepetersen, H.S., H. Qu, U. Sonnewald et al. 2005. Role of glutamine and neuronal glutamate uptake in glutamate homeostasis and synthesis during vesicular release in cultured neurons. *Neurochem. Int.* 47 (1–2):92–102.

Waagepetersen, H.S., U. Sonnewald, G. Gegelashvili et al. 2001. Metabolic distinction between vesicular and cytosolic GABA in cultured GABAergic neurons using 13C magnetic resonance spectroscopy. *J Neurosci. Res.* 63 (4):347–355.

Wang, L., T.J. Maher, and R.J. Wurtman. 2007. Oral L-glutamine increases GABA levels in striatal tissue and extracellular fluid. *Fed. Am. Soc. Exp. Biol. J* 21 (4):1227–1232.

Waniewski, R.A. and D.L. Martin. 1986. Exogenous glutamate is metabolized to glutamine and exported by rat primary astrocyte cultures. *J Neurochem.* 47 (1):304–313.

Ward, H.K., C.M. Thanki, and H.F. Bradford. 1983. Glutamine and glucose as precursors of transmitter amino acids: Ex vivo studies. *J Neurochem.* 40 (3):855–860.

Watkins, S. and H. Sontheimer. 2012. Unique biology of gliomas: Challenges and opportunities. *Trends Neurosci.* 35 (9):546–556.

Weller, M., T. Cloughesy, J.R. Perry et al. 2013. Standards of care for treatment of recurrent glioblastoma— Are we there yet? *Neuro Oncol.* 15 (1):4–27.

Wieser, H.G. 2004. ILAE Commission Report: Mesial temporal lobe epilepsy with hippocampal sclerosis. *Epilepsia* 45 (6):695–714.

Willard-Mack, C.L., R.C. Koehler, T. Hirata et al. 1996. Inhibition of glutamine synthetase reduces ammonia-induced astrocyte swelling in rat. *Neurosci.* 71 (2):589–599.

Xu, G.Y., D.J. McAdoo, M.G. Hughes et al. 1998. Considerations in the determination by microdialysis of resting extracellular amino acid concentrations and release upon spinal cord injury. *Neurosci.* 86 (3):1011–1021.

Ye, Z.C., J.D. Rothstein, and H. Sontheimer. 1999. Compromised glutamate transport in human glioma cells: Reduction-mislocalization of sodium-dependent glutamate transporters and enhanced activity of cystine-glutamate exchange. *J Neurosci.* 19 (24):10767–10777.

Zielińska, M., K. Milewski, M. Skowrońska et al. 2015. Induction of iNOS expression in ammonia-exposed cultured astrocytes is coupled to increased arginine transport by upregulated y+ LAT2 transporter. *J Neurochem.* 35(6):1272–1278.

Zielińska, M., M. Popek, and J. Albrecht. 2014. Roles of changes in active glutamine transport in brain edema development during hepatic encephalopathy: An emerging concept. *Neurochem. Res.* 39 (3):599–604.

Zielińska, M., J. Ruszkiewicz, W. Hilgier et al. 2011. Hyperammonemia increases the expression and activity of the glutamine/arginine transporter y+ LAT2 in rat cerebral cortex: Implications for the nitric oxide/ cGMP pathway. *Neurochem. Int.* 58 (2):190–195.

Zielińska, M., M. Skowrońska, I. Fręśko et al. 2012. Upregulation of the heteromeric +LAT2 transporter contributes to ammonia-induced increase of arginine uptake in rat cerebral cortical astrocytes. *Neurochem. Int.* 61 (4):531–535.

Ziemińska, E., M. Dolińska, J.W. Lazarewicz et al. 2000. Induction of permeability transition and swelling of rat brain mitochondria by glutamine. *Neurotoxicology* 21 (3):295–300.

Ziemińska, E., W. Hilgier, H.S. Waagepetersen et al. 2004. Analysis of glutamine accumulation in rat brain mitochondria in the presence of a glutamine uptake inhibitor, histidine, reveals glutamine pools with a distinct access to deamidation. *Neurochem. Res.* 29 (11):2121–2123.

8 Brain Glutamine Accumulation in Liver Failure

Role in the Pathogenesis of Central Nervous System Complications

Roger F. Butterworth and Chantal Bemeur

CONTENTS

8.1 INTRODUCTION

Removal of excess ammonia in mammalian systems depends principally on its conversion to urea via the urea cycle, a metabolic pathway that is only expressed in the liver although other tissues, including the brain, may express some of its constituent enzymes.

Liver failure sufficient to cause central nervous system (CNS) dysfunction is referred to as hepatic encephalopathy (HE), which may result from acute or chronic liver failure with a wide range of etiology, including viral hepatitis, alcoholic liver injury, nonalcoholic steatohepatitis, ischemic liver damage, and a range of genetic abnormalities. HE is a common and debilitating neuropsychiatric complication of liver disease and is characterized by cognitive dysfunction starting with attention deficits, psychomotor slowing, and asterixis progressing to stupor and coma as well as disorders of motor coordination and sleep. Seizures may occur in acute liver failure (ALF).

Neuropathologic studies in material from patients with ALF reveal cytotoxic brain edema that, in extreme cases, may result in intracranial hypertension and death by brain herniation. Another feature is a characteristic alteration of astrocytes in chronic liver failure known as Alzheimer type 2 astrocytosis in which the nuclei of these cells are characterized by swelling, glycogen deposition, and margination of the normal chromatin pattern. Neuronal cell death has been reported in chronic liver failure (cirrhosis), the two most common presentations involving neuronal cell death being acquired hepatocerebral degeneration and "Parkinsonism in cirrhosis."

While the principal etiologic factor in the pathogenesis of HE appears to be increased levels of circulating and brain ammonia, glutamine (GLN) has also been implicated in the pathogenesis of HE. Blood and brain concentrations of GLN are increased in HE (Laubenberger et al. 1997, Lavoie et al. 1987a, Tofteng et al. 2006) consistent with the detoxification of ammonia via glutamine synthetase (GS), the only significant alternate pathway available in conditions in which hepatic urea synthesis is seriously impaired, as in liver failure.

8.2   GLUTAMINE: PHYSIOLOGICAL FUNCTIONS AND PATHOGENIC IMPLICATIONS

Glutamine, a nonessential amino acid, is found abundantly in the CNS where it participates in a variety of metabolic pathways. Its major role in the brain is that of precursor of the releasable pool of the excitatory neurotransmitter amino acid glutamate and the inhibitory amino acid, γ-amino butyric acid (GABA). During hepatocyte dysfunction, ammonia detoxification to GLN in brain and skeletal muscle is activated. In addition to ammonia detoxification, enhanced GLN synthesis may exert beneficial effects on the immune system and gut barrier. However, increased GLN production may stimulate branched-chain amino acids catabolism in skeletal muscle and adversely affect the CNS by inducing astrocyte swelling and altered neurotransmission.

8.3   BRAIN GLUTAMINE ACCUMULATION IN LIVER FAILURE

Brain GLN concentrations are significantly increased in liver failure; in general, the magnitude of the increase in GLN is significantly correlated with the severity of HE and, in the case of ALF, with the presence of brain edema and intracranial hypertension (Clemmesen et al. 1999). Proton-Nuclear Magnetic Resonance (NMR) studies in patients with decompensated liver cirrhosis reveal a significant correlation between brain GLN and severity of encephalopathy (Laubenberger et al. 1997) (Figure 8.1). Such findings have led to the suggestion that accumulation of the GLN molecule *per se* is somehow causally related to the neurological symptoms in liver failure independent of the etiology.

A series of mechanisms involving brain GLN accumulation have been proposed to explain its possible role in the pathogenesis of HE and such mechanisms include alterations in osmolarity resulting from the intracellular accumulation of GLN, GLN-induced increases of cerebral blood flow (hyperemia) (Cooper and Plum 1987), as well as mitochondrial dysfunction resulting in induction of the mitochondrial permeability transition, a calcium-dependent process that results in the collapse of the inner mitochondrial membrane and consequent production of free radicals and energy failure (Albrecht and Norenberg 2006, Bai et al. 2001).

However, although increases in brain GLN are consistently described in HE, direct evidence for a role of increased brain GLN synthesis rates *per se* remains rather less convincing.

8.4   BRAIN GLUTAMINE SYNTHESIS RATES IN LIVER FAILURE

Ammonia removal by the brain is an astrocytic responsibility since the enzyme responsible (GS) has a predominantly, and perhaps exclusively, astrocytic localization. The neuron has little, if any, measureable capacity for ammonia removal. It was shown that ammonia is incorporated almost exclusively into GLN via GS, rather than to glutamate via glutamate dehydrogenase and that, under normal physiological conditions, brain contains very little excess GS capacity over that required to maintain normal metabolic flux (Cooper and Plum 1987). Direct measurements of GS in autopsied brain tissue from patients who died in grade 4 HE actually showed a small but significant loss of GS enzyme activity (Lavoie et al. 1987b) and studies in an experimental animal model of minimal HE (MHE) resulting from end-to-side portacaval anastomosis in the rat likewise revealed losses of GS activity in several brain regions (Butterworth et al. 1988). One explanation that was proposed to explain this apparent limitation on GS activity in brain involves stimulation of post-synaptic glutamate (NMDA) receptors in the brain leading to the formation of nitric oxide that then goes on to inactivate GS in the neighboring astrocytes by protein tyrosine nitration (Schliess et al. 2002).

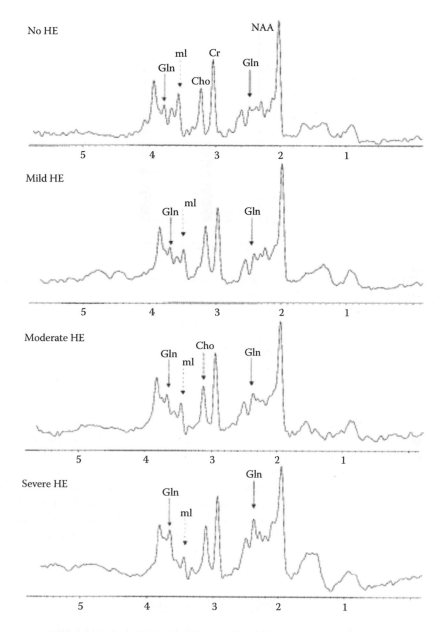

FIGURE 8.1 1H-NMR spectra from cirrhotic patients with varying severity of hepatic encephalopathy (HE). A: no HE, B: mild HE, C: moderate HE, D: HE. Note that increased intensities of glutamine (Gln) resonances with increasing severity of HE. mI: myoinositol, Cho: Choline, Cr: Creatine. (Modified from Laubenberger, J. et al. 1997. *Gastroenterology*. 112(5):1610–16, with permission.)

To directly assess GLN synthesis rates *per se* in ALF, the technique of 1H/13C NMR spectroscopy was utilized (Zwingmann and Butterworth 2005, Zwingmann et al. 2003). Using this technique, it was shown that, although *de novo* synthesis rates for GLN in brain were increased, neither the increased brain concentrations of GLN nor the magnitude of the increase in *de novo* GLN synthesis rates were significantly correlated with the severity of HE or with the occurrence of brain edema in these animals (Figure 8.2).

Moreover, mild hypothermia (sufficient to delay progression of HE and to prevent brain edema in ALF animals) had no significant effect on GLN synthesis rates in brain leaving open the possibility

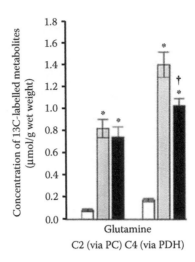

FIGURE 8.2 Increased *de novo* synthesis of brain glutamine from 13C-glucose is not correlated with the severity of encephalopathy in rats with ALF resulting from hepatic devascularization. C2 (PC) represents glutamine synthesis from 13C-glucose via pyruvate carboxylase; C4 (PDH) represents glutamine synthesis from 13C-glucose via the pyruvate dehydrogenase complex. Values represent mean +/− SEM. Values significantly different from sham-operated control values (sham) indicated by *$p < 0.01$. Significant differences between ALF precoma and ALF coma are indicated by †$p < 0.02$ by ANOVA. (White bars represent sham, grey bars represent precoma and black bars represent coma). (From Zwingmann, C. et al. 2003. *Hepatology.* 37(2):420–28, with permission.)

that the increase in brain GLN reported in HE may have resulted from alternative mechanisms such as the inhibition of GLN hydrolysis or GLN transamination. This issue has been reviewed (Zwingmann and Butterworth 2005).

Finally, inhibition of GS in an animal model of cirrhosis and HE (the bile-duct ligated rat) revealed that the brain and the kidney were important for metabolizing blood-borne ammonia (Fries et al. 2014). Furthermore, methionine sulfoximine (MSO), a GS inhibitor, has been shown to be neuroprotective in rodent models of hyperammonemia and ALF, confirming the pathogenetic role of GLN and suggesting that MSO may have clinical potential (Jeitner and Cooper 2014). However, applicability of such inhibitors in the prevention of HE has been limited by their potential adverse effects.

8.5　THE GLUTAMATE–GLUTAMINE CYCLE IN BRAIN

Ammonia removal as GLN in the astrocyte is an essential component of the so-called glutamate–glutamine cycle shown in simplified schematic form in Figure 8.3. The cycle involves the astrocyte and its adjoining neuron (in the interest of clarity, Figure 8.3 indicates the glutamatergic neuron only). Ammonia uptake into the astrocyte from the circulation is removed by GS (Section 8.3) and the GLN formed is then transported out of the cell by the neutral sodium-coupled amino acid transporters SNAT-1, SNAT-3, and SNAT-5, transporters that may directly influence both glutamatergic and GABAergic transmission in mammalian brain. SNAT-3 (previously SN-1) favors the release of GLN, rather than its uptake, from astrocytes (Chaudhry et al. 2001). SNAT-5, like SNAT-3, shares the Na^+/H^- coupling mechanism and is expressed in high concentrations by astrocyte cell bodies and their processes that surround glutamatergic, GABAergic, and glycinergic nerve terminals (Cubelos et al. 2005).

The GLN released from the perineuronal astrocyte may then be uptaken by the adjacent neuron where the action of GLNase results in the renewal of the transmitter pool of glutamate. Synaptic release of glutamate then occurs and any surplus glutamate is transported principally into the

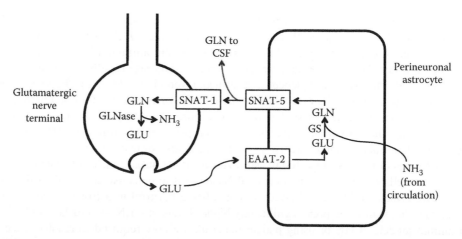

FIGURE 8.3 Schematic representation of the "Glutamate–Glutamine cycle" involving the perineuronal astrocyte and adjacent glutamatergic nerve terminal showing the role of the astrocytic glutamate (EAAT2) and glutamine (SNAT-5) transporters in relation to blood-borne ammonia removal by glutamine synthetase (GS) in the astrocyte and to transmitter glutamate (GLU) synthesis via glutaminase (GLNase) in the nerve terminal. CSF: cerebrospinal fluid; NH_3: ammonia; SNAT-1: neuronal glutamine transporter.

neighboring astrocyte by one of a series of high-affinity glutamate transporters including excitatory amino acid transporters EAAT-1 and EAAT-2 and the cycle continues. One turn of the cycle results in the removal of ammonia in the astrocyte but synthesis of ammonia in the neuron. It should be borne in mind, however, that the constituent enzymes and transporters of the cycle do not represent a concerted series of steps and represent possible metabolic conversions with no intended relationship to metabolic fluxes.

Ammonia-infused animals manifest suppression of brain GLN release to the extracellular fluid (Kanamori and Ross 2005) consistent with downregulation of one of the SNATs. ALF resulting from hepatic devascularization in the rat leads to significant downregulation of SNAT-5 (Desjardins et al. 2012) suggesting that restrictions of the transfer of GLN from the astrocyte (rather than increased GLN synthesis within the cell as had been previously presumed) could offer a cogent explanation for the increase in intracellular GLN leading to cytotoxic brain edema in ALF. Moreover, GLN trapping within the astrocyte has the potential to limit neuronal excitability by limiting the transfer of GLN from the astrocytic to the releasable neuronal pool and, in this way, result in encephalopathy in ALF. Further studies using techniques such as *in vivo* microdialysis are now required to assess these possibilities.

8.6 BRAIN GLUTAMINE METABOLISM IN LIVER FAILURE

8.6.1 GLUTAMINASE

The glutamate–glutamine cycle is predicated on the assumption that GLNase is localized exclusively in neurons and this was initially shown to be the case (Laake et al. 1995). However, the results of recent studies suggest that such a simplistic model may need to be adjusted. At least two GLNase isoforms are expressed in mammalian brain, namely the K-type and the L-type with different molecular structures and regulatory properties that are found to co-localize in cells throughout the brain. Moreover, L-type GLNase is localized to both neuronal mitochondria and nuclei (Márquez et al. 2009, 2012). Whether or not a fully functional GLNase is expressed in astrocytes remains a matter of debate. Immunohistochemical studies show that the K-type protein is expressed in rat brain astrocytes (Aoki et al. 1991). On the other hand, no GLNase signal was observed in astrocytes of rat cerebellum (Laake et al. 1999).

The notion of a possible astrocytic localization for one of the GLNase isoforms led to the "Trojan Horse" theory of HE. According to this theory, GLN synthesized in the astrocyte in liver failure serves as a "Trojan horse" and as an indirect carrier of nascent ammonia into the mitochondrion of the astrocyte where the action of the purported astrocytic GLNase rapidly regenerates ammonia with mitochondrial cytotoxic consequences (Albrecht and Norenberg 2006; this theory was recently revisited; Rama Rao and Norenberg 2014). This notion of GLNase-derived ammonia toxicity was based principally on the results of studies of the exposure of astrocytes in culture to GLN that led to cell swelling and activation of the mitochondrial permeability transition (Bai et al. 2001). The theory, while attracting some interest and debate, has also drawn criticism based on the relatively low activities of GLNase reported in astrocytes *in situ* (Laake et al. 1999). The likelihood of futile cycling in cells expressing both GS and GLNase needs to be considered as does the question of the selective effects of GLNase-derived ammonia being harmful to astrocytes but not neurons despite the fact that neurons express significantly higher levels of GLNase. Further studies, preferably in animal models of HE or using patient material, are now required to resolve these issues before full credence can be given to this theory and its possible role in the pathogenesis of HE.

8.6.2 GLUTAMINE TRANSAMINATION

An important but little-studied step in GLN metabolism involves GLN transamination resulting in the production of alpha-ketoglutaramate (AKGM) that may then be hydrolyzed to alpha-ketoglutarate and ammonia in a reaction catalyzed by omega-amidase, the so-called glutaminase-II pathway. This pathway is active in human brain (Cooper and Gross 1977) and studies in liver failure (Vergara et al. 1974) reveal significant increases of AKGM in circulation and in the brain. Moreover, in cirrhosis, the correlation between cerebrospinal fluid concentrations of AKGM and HE grade was found to be equal to that of ammonia or GLN (Vergara et al. 1974). It was recently proposed that serum concentrations of AKGM could afford an effective biomarker for hyperammonemic disorders (Cooper and Kuhara 2014, Halámková et al. 2012).

8.7 CONCLUSIONS

Liver failure leads to increased plasma and brain concentrations of ammonia and its detoxification product GLN. Increased brain GLN correlates well with HE grade in patients with cirrhosis. On the other hand, studies using 1H/13C NMR spectroscopy fail to show a significant correlation between increased GLN synthesis *per se* and either HE grade or brain edema in experimental ALF. This limitation on GLN synthesis capacity may be the consequence of tyrosine nitration of the GS protein. Skeletal muscle adapts metabolically to become the major organ responsible for ammonia removal in liver failure, an adaptation resulting from post-translational induction of the GS gene. This metabolic adaptation accounts for the importance of maintaining adequate dietary protein intake in patients with liver failure. However, it was recently reported that, in a rat model of cirrhosis, hyperammonemia was associated with inadequate compensation by muscle GS and increased gut GLNase activity (Jover-Cobos et al. 2014). These results suggest that GS and GLNase may serve as important future therapeutic targets.

Other GLN metabolic and regulatory pathways with the potential to impact on brain function in liver failure include GLN deamination by GLNase, and GLN transamination leading to the production of AKGM with possible neurotoxic properties. Recent findings of reduced expression of the GLN transporter SNAT-5 (responsible for GLN exit from the astrocyte) in an ALF model raises the possibility of "GLN trapping" within these cells, a mechanism that could contribute to cytotoxic brain edema and to the encephalopathy that results from an imbalance between excitatory and inhibitory neurotransmission. Additional studies are warranted to elucidate the mechanisms implicating GLN as a key player in the pathogenesis of CNS complications of liver failure. As the pathogenetic mechanisms are identified, insights for new therapeutic strategies will undoubtedly be uncovered.

REFERENCES

Albrecht, J. and Norenberg, M.D. 2006. Glutamine: A Trojan horse in ammonia neurotoxicity. *Hepatology.* 44(4):788–94.

Aoki, C., Kaneko, T., Starr, A. et al. 1991. Identification of mitochondrial and non-mitochondrial glutaminase within select neurons and glia of rat forebrain by electron microscopic immunocytochemistry. *J. Neurosci. Res.* 28(4):531–48.

Bai, G., Rao, K.V.R., Murthy, C.R. et al. 2001. Ammonia induces the mitochondrial permeability transition in primary cultures of rat astrocytes. *J. Neurosci. Res.* 66(5):981–91.

Butterworth, R.F., Girard, G., Giguère, J.F. 1988. Regional differences in the capacity for ammonia removal by brain following portocaval anastomosis. *J. Neurochem.* 51(2):486–90.

Chaudhry, F.A., Krizaj, D., Larsson, P. et al. 2001. Coupled and uncoupled proton movement by amino acid transport system N. *EMBO J.* 20(24):7041–51.

Clemmesen, J.O., Larsen, F.S., Kondrup, J. et al. 1999. Cerebral herniation in patients with acute liver failure is correlated with arterial ammonia concentration. *Hepatology.* 29(3):648–53.

Cooper, A.J., Gross, M. 1977. The glutamine transaminase-omega-amidase system in rat and human brain. *J. Neurochem.* 28(4):771–78.

Cooper, A.J. and Kuhara, T. 2014. α-Ketoglutaramate: An overlooked metabolite of glutamine and a biomarker for hepatic encephalopathy and inborn errors of the urea cycle. *Metab. Brain Dis.* 29(4):991–1006.

Cooper, A.J., Plum, F. 1987. Biochemistry and physiology of brain ammonia. *Physiol. Rev.* 67(2):440–519.

Cubelos, B., González-González, I.M., Giménez, C. et al. 2005. Amino acid transporter SNAT5 localizes to glial cells in the rat brain. *Glia.* 49(2):230–44.

Desjardins, P., Du, T., Jiang, W. et al. 2012. Pathogenesis of hepatic encephalopathy and brain edema in acute liver failure: Role of glutamine redefined. *Neurochem. Int.* 60(7):690–96.

Fries, A.W., Dadsetan, S., Keiding, S. et al. 2014. Effect of glutamine synthetase inhibition on brain and interorgan ammonia metabolism in bile duct ligated rats. *J. Cereb. Blood Flow Metab.* 34(3):460–66.

Halámková, L., Mailloux, S., Halámek, J. et al. 2012. Enzymatic analysis of α-ketoglutaramate–a biomarker for hyperammonemia. *Talanta.* 100:7–11.

Jeitner, T.M., Cooper, A.J.L. 2014. Inhibition of human glutamine synthetase by L-methionine-S,R-sulfoximine-relevance to the treatment of neurological diseases. *Metab Brain Dis.* 29(4):983–89.

Jover-Cobos, M., Noiret, L., Lee, K. et al. 2014. Ornithine phenylacetate targets alterations in the expression and activity of glutamine synthase and glutaminase to reduce ammonia levels in bile duct ligated rats. *J. Hepatol.* 60(3):545–53.

Kanamori, K., Ross, B.D. 2005. Suppression of glial glutamine release to the extracellular fluid studied in vivo by NMR and microdialysis in hyperammonemic rat brain. *J. Neurochem.* 94(1):74–85.

Laake, J.H., Slyngstad, T.A., Haug, F.M. et al. 1995. Glutamine from glial cells is essential for the maintenance of the nerve terminal pool of glutamate: Immunogold evidence from hippocampal slice cultures. *J. Neurochem.* 65(2):871–81.

Laake, J.H., Takumi, Y., Eidet, J. et al. 1999. Postembedding immunogold labelling reveals subcellular localization and pathway-specific enrichment of phosphate activated glutaminase in rat cerebellum. *Neurosci.* 88(4):1137–51.

Laubenberger, J., Häussinger, D., Bayer, S. et al. 1997. Proton magnetic resonance spectroscopy of the brain in symptomatic and asymptomatic patients with liver cirrhosis. *Gastroenterology.* 112(5):1610–16.

Lavoie, J., Giguère, J.F., Layrargues, G.P. et al. 1987a. Amino acid changes in autopsied brain tissue from cirrhotic patients with hepatic encephalopathy. *J. Neurochem.* 49(3):692–97.

Lavoie, J., Giguère, J.F., Layrargues, G.P. et al. 1987b. Activities of neuronal and astrocytic marker enzymes in autopsied brain tissue from patients with hepatic encephalopathy. *Metab. Brain Dis.* 2(4):283–90.

Márquez, J., Cardona, C., Campos-Sandoval, J.A. et al. 2012. Mammalian glutaminase isozymes in brain. *Metab. Brain Dis.* 28(2):133–37.

Márquez, J., Tosina, M., de la Rosa, V. et al. 2009. New insights into brain glutaminases: Beyond their role on glutamatergic transmission. *Neurochem. Int.* 55(1–3):64–70.

Rama Rao, K.V., Norenberg, M.D. 2014. Glutamine in the pathogenesis of hepatic encephalopathy: The Trojan Horse hypothesis revisited. *Neurochem. Res.* 39(3):593–8.

Schliess, F., Görg, B., Fischer, R. et al. 2002. Ammonia induces MK-801-sensitive nitration and phosphorylation of protein tyrosine residues in rat astrocytes. *FASEB J.* 16(7):739–41.

Tofteng, F., Hauerberg, J., Hansen, B.A. et al. 2006. Persistent arterial hyperammonemia increases the concentration of glutamine and alanine in the brain and correlates with intracranial pressure in patients with fulminant hepatic failure. *J. Cereb. Blood Flow Metab.* 26(1):21–27.

Vergara, F., Plum, F., Duffy, T.E. 1974. Alpha-ketoglutaramate: Increased concentrations in the cerebrospinal fluid of patients in hepatic coma. *Science*. 183(4120):81–83.

Zwingmann, C., Butterworth, R. 2005. An update on the role of brain glutamine synthesis and its relation to cell-specific energy metabolism in the hyperammonemic brain: Further studies using NMR spectroscopy. *Neurochem. Int.* 47(1–2):19–30.

Zwingmann, C., Chatauret, N., Leibfritz, D. et al. 2003. Selective increase of brain lactate synthesis in experimental acute liver failure: Results of a [H-C] nuclear magnetic resonance study. *Hepatology*. 37(2):420–28.

9 Glutamate/Glutamine Cycle
Evidence of Its Role in Parkinson's Disease Using In Vivo MRS Techniques

Carine Chassain, Guy Bielicki, Jean-Pierre Renou, and Franck Durif

CONTENTS

9.1 INTRODUCTION

Parkinson's disease (PD) is a common neurodegenerative disorder that affects the human population worldwide (Braak et al. 2003). It generally presents clinically in adults over the age of 60 years, and major symptoms include akinesia, rest tremor, bradykinesia, and postural instability (Beitz 2014). The disorder is characterized by progressive loss of dopaminergic neurons in the substantia nigra *pars compacta* (SNc) and a resulting decrease in dopamine in the dorsolateral and ventral striatum (Hornykiewicz 1998). The low level of dopamine in the striatum leads to dysfunction of corticobasal ganglio-thalamo cortical pathways in the brain and subsequently to clinical manifestations of PD. Currently, its diagnosis is based largely on assessment of these clinical symptoms. Unfortunately, this purely clinical diagnosis, combined with the similarities of PD symptoms with those of other movement disorders, results in frequent misdiagnosis (Meara 1999). PD can only be confirmed upon postmortem analysis through its pathological hallmark of Lewy bodies and Lewy neurites located in residual neurons or axons, respectively (Shults 2006).

To complicate matters, diagnosis is generally made at an advanced stage of neurodegeneration because motor symptoms occur after 60%–80% loss of dopaminergic neurons in the SNc (Goldstein et al. 2006). Thus, the introduction of new therapeutic strategies to prevent dopaminergic denervation and organize the PD management will depend on improved diagnosis, preferably at early, premotor stages when there is still a larger population of dopaminergic cells. Identifying sensitive, specific biomarkers for PD therefore becomes an exciting challenge.

Documented reports show that the loss of dopaminergic neurons in the SNc and the consecutive reduction in dopamine content within the striatum have effects on the biochemistry of these structures (Nagatsu and Sawada 2007; Obeso et al. 2010). Thus, there is evidence of inflammatory process (Nagatsu and Sawada 2007), cellular death by apoptosis (Nagatsu and Sawada 2007; Choi et al. 2008) in the SNc, and changes in neurotransmitter contents in the striatum (Kish et al. 1986; Tanaka et al. 1986; Soghomonian and Laprade 1997; Chassain et al. 2008, 2010; Emir et al. 2012). Changes in neurotransmission in the striatum induce dysregulation in corticobasal ganglio-thalamo cortical loops and can explain cardinal signs of PD, such as akinesia.

Continuing development of magnetic resonance spectroscopy (MRS) produced techniques for the measurement of cerebral neurotransmitters gamma-aminobutyric acid (GABA) and glutamate and of the energetic and neurotransmission fluxes associated with these compounds. Thus, the detection and quantification of brain metabolites selectively in brain structures involved in corticobasal ganglia-cortical pathways could improve the mechanistic understanding of the physiopathology of PD. In addition, this metabolite profile could be used as a tool for early diagnosis and for monitoring therapeutic responsiveness.

In this chapter, we describe some of the insights gained into the physiopathology of PD through the study of glutamate, glutamine, and GABA levels, and metabolic processes. The chapter is divided into two parts. The first section presents our current knowledge of biochemical changes in PD assessed by proton (^{1}H) MRS. ^{1}H MRS studies in animal models of PD have shown that the tissue levels of the neurotransmission-related metabolites glutamate, glutamine, and GABA are increased in the striatum (Chassain et al. 2008, 2010; Bagga et al. 2013; Coune et al. 2013) and that acute pharmacological treatment and acute, subchronic, and chronic deep brain stimulation of the subthalamic nucleus (STN) modify these levels (Melon et al. 2015; Chassain et al. 2016). In clinical studies, there is evidence to suggest that the metabolic profile of the striatum undergoes changes in PD (Mazuel et al. 2016).

In Section 2, we present the results of works examining the glutamate–glutamine cycle in PD. Early studies using carbon ^{13}C MRS found that levels of glutamate and glutamine labeled on C4 increased after [2-^{13}C] sodium acetate infusion in the brain of animal models of PD (Chassain et al. 2005). A more recent study reported altered energy metabolism in the striatum of the MPTP-intoxicated mouse, a murine model of PD (Bagga et al. 2013).

In the pathophysiology of PD, these results showed a significant role for glutamate metabolism, glutamate–glutamine cycle, and neuron–glia interactions, as expressed through glutamate and glutamine concentrations in the striatum.

9.2 BIOCHEMISTRY OF THE STRIATUM IN PD

9.2.1 GLUTAMATERGIC HYPERACTIVITY IN THE STRIATUM

The motor symptoms of PD are primarily attributed to dysfunction in the corticobasal ganglia-thalamo cortical loop circuits that results from degeneration of the dopaminergic neurons in SNc. Dopamine denervation-induced changes in glutamate and GABA neurotransmission systems are key components of the pathophysiology of PD. Alterations in the glutamatergic drive include increased glutamatergic transmission and maladaptive synaptic plasticity at the synapses formed by cortical afferents onto projection neurons of the striatum (Lindefors and Ungerstedt 1990; Calabresi et al. 1993; Centonze et al. 1999), the main basal ganglia input station, and pathological activation in bursts of STN (Hollerman et al. 1992; Bergman et al. 1994; Bevan et al. 2002). Dopamine denervation triggers opposite changes in the two populations of striatal projection neurons, decreased activity of the direct pathway neurons and increased activity of the indirect pathway neurons, which contribute, together with pathological activation of STN, to produce an overactivity of the BG output structures, the internal globus pallidus, and the substantia nigra pars reticulata (SNr) (Blandini et al. 2000; Obeso et al. 2008). The increased tonic activity of these structures enhances inhibition of thalamic neurons projecting to the sensorimotor cortex and then induces cortical hypoactivity (Figure 9.1).

According to this scheme, the striatum is a basal ganglia center that supports massive glutamatergic inputs arising from the brain cortex. Several experimental results have shown that corticostriatal glutamatergic transmission is increased in PD. Morphological study in human PD analyzing characteristics of the synapses formed by afferents in asymmetric contact with dendritic spines of neurons in the caudate nucleus of patients with PD evidenced synaptic plasticity (Anglade et al. 1996). In fact, the length of the postsynaptic densities and the number of perforated synapses are both significantly increased in PD patients (+24 and +88%, respectively). Furthermore, the size of these afferents and the surface area occupied by their mitochondria are also greater. This plasticity of corticostriatal synapses has been observed in the striatum of rats with a 6-hydroxydopamine-induced (6-OHDA) lesion of the SNc (Ingham et al. 1998; Meshul et al. 1999, 2000). More recently, a quantitative analysis of postsynaptic glutamatergic areas using 3D modeling shows that the length of these areas is increased in the non-human primate intoxicated with MPTP, model of PD. This is indicative of a remodeling of the glutamatergic synapses (Villalba et Smith 2011). Together, these results suggest hyperactivity of the glutamatergic synapses after dopamine depletion.

The hypothesis of a corticostriatal pathway hyperactivity after dopamine denervation is consistent with an increase in the basal extracellular level of striatal glutamate, as measured by *in vivo* microdialysis in 6-OHDA-lesioned rats (Lindefors et Ungerstedt 1990; Meshul et al. 1999; Jonkers et al. 2002).

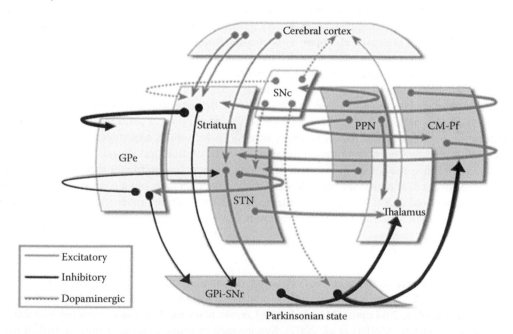

FIGURE 9.1 Functional organization of the basal ganglia in Parkinson's disease. Denervation of dopaminergic neurons in SNc (illustrated with gray-dotted arrows) induces hyperactivity of some basal ganglia-related nuclei such as the STN, GPi-SNr, CM-Pf, and PPN that are represented by a darker color. This results in hyperactivity of neurons in GPi/SNr and a decrease in thalamo-cortical glutamatergic activity. The diagram shows the presence of a number of transverse, modulatory loops. Black arrows indicate inhibitory projections and grey ones excitatory projections. The thickness of the arrows reflects changes in neuronal activity following dopaminergic denervation: The thinner arrows correspond to a decrease in activity, and the thick arrows indicate an increase. CM-Pf: centromedian-parafascicular thalamic nucleus, GPe: globus pallidus pars externa, GPi: globus pallidus pars interna, PPN: pedunculopontine nuclei, SNc: substantia nigra pars compacta, SNr: substantia nigra pars reticulate, STN: subthalamic nucleus, VL: ventral lateral nucleus. (Adapted from Obeso, J.A. and J.L. Lanciego. 2011. *Frontiers in Neuroanatomy*, 5:1–6.)

In association with this corticostriatal hyperactivity, ultrastructural data support synaptic changes in contacts between axio-spinous glutamatergic elements coming from the cortex and striatal astrocytes in MPTP-treated parkinsonian monkeys (Villalba et Smith 2011). The authors observed a significant expansion of the astrocytic coverage of striatal synapses in the parkinsonian state.

All these results show:

1. Lesions of dopamine nigrostriatal pathways increase corticostriatal glutamatergic transmission.
2. These changes are associated with compensatory modification of the astrocytic microenvironment in the striatum.

All the above factors could modify the biochemistry of the striatum.

9.2.2 *In vivo* MRS Measurements

The proton (^{1}H) nucleus is the most sensitive nucleus for NMR, both in terms of intrinsic NMR sensitivity (high gyromagnetic ratio) and high natural abundance (>99.9%). Since nearly all metabolites contain ^{1}H, *in vivo* ^{1}H MRS is a powerful technique to observe, identify, and quantify biologically important endogenous metabolites noninvasively *in vivo*.

However, the application of ^{1}H MRS *in vivo* is challenging for several reasons. First, owing to its high concentration, the water resonance is several orders of magnitude larger than the low-concentration metabolites, making metabolic detection difficult. Second, the chemical shift range of *in vivo* ^{1}H NMR spectra is narrow at 5 ppm. This creates strongly overlapping metabolite resonances making their detection and quantification difficult. Detection of glutamate metabolite at 2.34 ppm is hampered by spectral overlap with other metabolites: glutamine, N-acetyl aspartate (NAA), and GABA. At 3 T field strength, glutamate is detected by spectral editing that minimizes the contribution of other metabolites (Kicklers et al. 2007). However, the detection and quantification of metabolites in the brain requires high field strength (9.4 T) and very short echo time, as demonstrated by Peuffer et al. (1999). Third, NMR is a very insensitive technique, making the detection of low-concentration metabolites a compromise between time resolution and signal-to-noise ratio. This low sensitivity limits the detection to compounds with a concentration higher than about 0.5 mM.

With the advent of higher magnetic field strength scanners, an increasing sophistication of acquisition techniques and of water suppression methods, and also with improvement of spectral resolution, *in vivo* ^{1}H NMR spectra have many resonances from a wide range of metabolites.

Thus, after water suppression and with the use of a short echo time, the main resonances observed in a spectrum are from the following:

- The CH$_3$ groups of the combined N-acetyl resonances, mainly consisting of N-acetyl aspartate (NAA; 2.01 ppm) and with a smaller contribution from N-acetylaspartyl glutamate (NAAG; 2.04 ppm). Mainly located inside neurons, NAA is considered as a cell integrity marker (Moffett et al. 2007). Synthesized in mitochondria, it may be linked to neuronal energy metabolism (ATP synthesis) (Benarroch 2008).
- The N(CH$_3$)$_3$ groups of total choline (Cho; 3.22 ppm), which consist of phosphoryl choline and glycerophosphoryl-choline. These compounds are involved in membrane phospholipids, and variations in Cho levels reflect changes in cellular density.
- The CH$_3$ groups of total creatine (creatine and phosphocreatine, tCr; 3.03 ppm). Creatine is involved in cell energetic metabolism and thus it is used as a marker of energetic status (Andres et al. 2008).
- The myo-inositol (myo-Ins; 3.6 ppm) is observed only at short echo time. Mainly located in astrocytes and microglial cells, myo-Ins is considered to be a glial marker (Brand et al. 1993). It is thought to be involved in osmoregulation (Ross 1991).

- The glutamate and glutamine signals between 2 and 2.5 ppm. Glutamate is the main excitatory neurotransmitter; its degradation and recycling involve glutamine synthesis inside astrocytes.

These two metabolites traditionally constitute one pool owing to their striking structural similarity within the brain. As mentioned earlier, recent developments of the method have led to improved spectral resolution that allows the two molecules to be distinguished.

Some other metabolites in low concentrations in the brain, such as alanine, aspartate, γ-aminobutyric acid (GABA), glucose, glycine, scyllo-inositol, and taurine, can also be detected using short echo time and at high magnetic field.

In pathological situations such as in tumor tissues or cerebral ischemia, the lactate signal can be observed (Goergen et al. 2014). In addition, the metabolite resonances are typically superimposed on an intense baseline arising from macromolecules and lipids.

Carbon 13 (^{13}C) NMR spectroscopy is a useful tool in assessing metabolism in the intact brain. *In vivo* ^{13}C NMR spectroscopy of brain faces a number of problems that make its application more challenging. It is the appropriate method for monitoring the dynamics of metabolism in the Krebs cycle flux after the injection of substrates bearing labeled carbon atoms. Direct detection of ^{13}C label provides a wealth of highly specific information on metabolites and metabolic rates, such as the measurement of resolved carbon resonances of glutamate and glutamine in the brain. Despite yielding a well-resolved ^{13}C spectrum with good chemical shift dispersion, ^{13}C NMR spectroscopy is hampered by low sensitivity of the ^{13}C nucleus and the need for highly localized measurements in a functionally heterogeneous organ such as the brain. The protons bound to ^{13}C atoms can be detected by proton-observed, carbon-edited NMR spectroscopy. This pulse sequence (POCE) proposed as an alternative to direct ^{13}C NMR spectroscopy is therefore of great interest, as it would have the same sensitivity as a ^{1}H sequence. (Rothman et al. 1992; De Graaf et al. 2003). Thus, ^{13}C NMR spectroscopy, combined with the administration of ^{13}C-labeled substrates, allows for the detection of ^{13}C incorporation from ^{13}C-labeled precursors into various carbon positions of metabolites, such as tricarboxylic acid (TCA) cycle intermediates and the glutamate–glutamine cycle between the neuronal and glial compartments (de Graaf et al. 2011). In fact, the glial compartment uses glucose or acetate as substrates and contains GS. This allows the production of glutamine, which is transferred to the neuronal compartment and metabolized into glutamate and GABA (Figure 9.2). [2-^{13}C] sodium acetate is synthesized to [2-^{13}C] acetyl-CoA, which enters the glial TCA and is incorporated into C4 glutamate. The latter is quickly metabolized into C4 glutamine by the glial GS. Labeled C4 glutamine is recycled in the neuronal compartment, where labeled C4 glutamate and C2 GABA are produced. In subsequent TCA cycles, C2 and C3 glutamate are synthesized and then metabolized into C2 and C3 glutamine.

9.2.2.1 Applications in Animal Models of PD

^{1}H MRS has been used to detect cerebral metabolic changes in animal models of PD. The recent technical advances of NMR spectroscopy, including the availability of high magnetic fields and the development of reliable methods for absolute metabolite quantification and a better identification of metabolite signals, have yielded detailed *in vivo* information of pathophysiology of PD. However, studies performed in animal models of PD have yielded differing results, in part because they are extremely heterogeneous in terms of the animal model used (mouse or rat), the mode of neurotoxin injection (systemic or local), the site of injection, the toxin dose, and the time between injection and NMR acquisitions. The NMR spectroscopy techniques used to identify and to process the metabolite signals and the methods used to calculate the metabolite concentrations are also different. Technical NMR spectroscopy factors, including different echo and relaxation times, voxel sizes and locations, field strength, and POCE, could also account for the variations in results observed between studies.

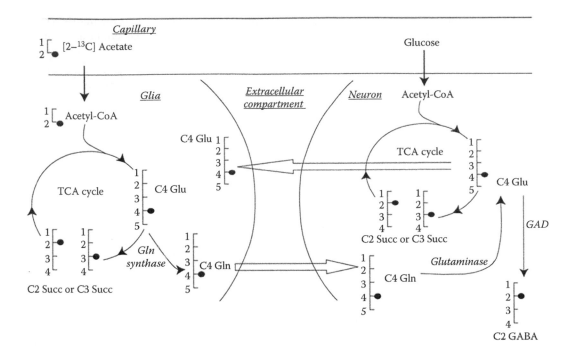

FIGURE 9.2 ¹³C labeling patterns of amino acids derived from [2-¹³C] sodium acetate in glial and neuronal compartments (from Chassain et al. 2005). Two metabolic compartments associated with the glial (left) or neuronal (right) compartment exist in the brain. [2-¹³C] sodium acetate is activated to [2-¹³C] acetyl-CoA, which enters the glial tricarboxylic acid (TCA) cycle and is incorporated into C4 glutamate. The latter is quickly metabolized into C4 glutamine by glial GS. Labeled glutamine is recycled in the neuronal compartment, where labeled C4 glutamate and C2 GABA are produced by glutaminase and GAD, respectively. Filled circles indicate the position of ¹³C-labeled carbon atoms. Abbreviations are as follows: C2 GABA: C2 gamma-aminobutyric acid; C4 Glu: C4 glutamate; C4 Gln: C4 glutamine; GAD: glutamic acid decarboxylase; Gln synthase: glutamine synthetase.

Thus, some studies reported higher intracellular glutamate, glutamine, and GABA levels in the striatum of the MPTP-intoxicated mouse, a mouse model of PD, than in the striatum of control mice (Chassain et al. 2008, 2010, 2013; Bagga et al. 2013) (Figure 9.3). High levels of glutamate and glutamine in the striatum support the hypothesis of overactive striatal glutamate transmission in response to dopamine denervation and the development of compensatory mechanisms to prevent excitotoxicity in the mouse model of PD. In addition, these adaptive processes are mainly synaptic because no change is observed in the cortex of MPTP-intoxicated mice relative to controls (Chassain et al. 2010). GABA levels in the striatum of MPTP-intoxicated mice provide further evidence that GABAergic neurons are hyperactive after lesions of the nigrostriatal dopaminergic pathway. This increase is in accordance with the well-documented increased activity of GABAergic striatopallidal neurons after experimental lesions of the dopaminergic nigrostriatal pathway (Calabresi et al. 1993; Carta et al. 2003). Interestingly, after acute L-dopa administration, the neurochemical profiles return to normal (Chassain et al. 2010, 2013). Furthermore, we show that dopaminergic denervation >59% is sufficient to induce these metabolic changes (Chassain et al. 2013) (Figure 9.4).

Other studies performed on different rat models of PD, the rat with a complete nigrostriatal lesion induced by 6-OHDA cerebral injection and a genetic model based on the nigral injection of an adeno-associated viral vector coding for human α-synuclein revealed no change (Kiclers et al. 2009) or significant decrease in glutamate levels and increase in GABA levels measured in the striatum (Coune et al. 2013).

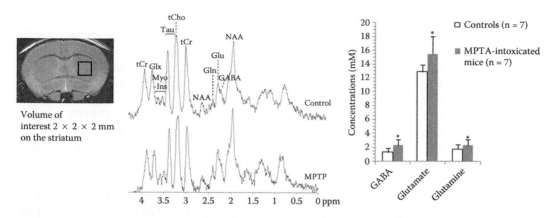

FIGURE 9.3 *In vivo* proton NMR spectra from the striatum of a control and an MPTP-intoxicated mouse at 9.4 T (Chassain et al. 2008) and absolute concentrations for GABA, glutamate, and glutamine. Spectra are acquired using a PRESS sequence for NMR localized spectroscopy in a voxel of 8 μL (2 × 2 × 2 mm) located on the striatum. Major acquisition parameters are TR = 4000 ms, TE = 8.8 ms, NS = 512. Free induction decay was 4096 points and Fourier transformed. Spectra are line broadened (5 Hz), and resonances are assigned as N-acetyl aspartate (NAA) at 2.008 ppm; GABA at 2.27 ppm, glutamate (Glu) at 2.34 ppm, glutamine (Gln) at 2.42 ppm; total creatine (tCr) at 3.022 ppm and 3.98 ppm, total choline (tCho) at 3.22 ppm; taurine (Tau) at 3.24–3.42 ppm; myo-inositol (Myo-Ins) at 3.48–3.52 ppm; and Glu + Gln complex (Glx) at 3.75 ppm. Absolute metabolite concentrations (mmol/L) defined by jMRUI software for spectra analyses are shown to the right of the figure. Data represent mean ± SD for seven animals in each group. Statistically significant differences are noted for comparison between metabolite concentrations of controls and MPTP-intoxicated mice using a Student's *t*-test. *$p < 0.05$.

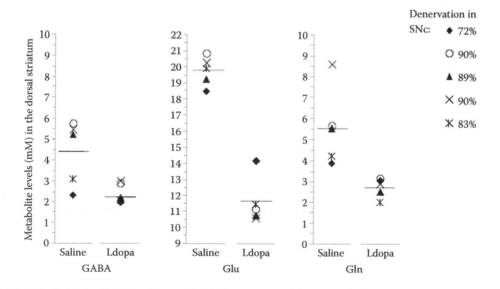

FIGURE 9.4 Individual data measured in the dorsal striatum in relation to dopaminergic (DA) denervation of the substantia nigra pars compacta (SNc). Plotted are the gamma-aminobutyric acid (GABA), glutamate (Glu), and glutamine (Gln) concentrations assessed by NMR spectroscopy in the dorsal striatum. Individual data points represent individual measurements for the MPTP-intoxicated mice, which were sacrificed for tyrosine hydroxylase (TH) immunohistochemical staining, after saline and levodopa administration (n = 5). The percentages of DA denervation in the SNc are indicated on the right. Horizontal bars are the mean value for each group of animals.

9.2.2.2 Clinical Applications in PD

Using ^{1}H MRS to measure changes in the striatum of PD patients could provide important information in terms of pathophysiology and would also allow as diagnosis of PD and an assessment of therapeutical response (see review of Ciurleo et al. 2014). Thus, changes in glutamate and GABA concentrations detected *in vivo* in basal ganglia of PD patients could be suggestive of dysfunction of neuronal excitatory and inhibitory activities that are involved in the control of movements. *In vivo* NMR spectroscopy meets many of the criteria of an ideal imaging biomarker. ^{1}H MRS has good test–retest reliability and, compared with other *in vivo* imaging techniques, such as positron emission tomography (PET) and single photon emission tomography (SPECT), is noninvasive and cheap, and it does not require contrast agents for the molecular imaging involving exposure to radioactive substances.

Again, previous studies provide conflicting results. Glutamate and glutamine levels in the putamen of PD patients were close to those measured in the putamen of healthy volunteers (Kicklers et al. 2007; Emir et al. 2012). Only one study at very high magnetic field showed a higher concentration of GABA in the striatum of PD patients compared to controls (Emir et al. 2012). Several factors might account for the discrepancies, including the measurement method, spectra analysis processes, absolute versus relative data, the number of PD patients enrolled, and their clinical heterogeneity. These studies included parkinsonian patients with or without dopaminergic treatment and those with large variation in disease duration. This clinical heterogeneity is almost certainly a key factor in explaining many of the differences observed. However, owing to the spectral overlap of the glutamate metabolite at 2.34 ppm with other metabolites, changes in glutamate levels could be masked by changes in the other direction of glutamine, NAA, and/or GABA. Studies on larger samples of homogeneous PD patients, MRS at high magnetic fields, standardized methods for the acquisition and processing of spectroscopic metabolite signals, and the use of absolute quantification of tissue metabolite concentrations are therefore required to definitively validate ^{1}H MRS for PD characterization. In regard with these points, a recent study performed on patients with a moderate PD at 3 T using a standard short-echo-time single-voxel MRS sequence showed metabolic changes in the putamen of parkinsonian patients compared to healthy volunteers (Mazuel et al. 2016). Determination of absolute concentrations by the LCModel software showed significantly lower putamen concentrations of tNAA, tCr, and myo-Ins in drug-OFF parkinsonian patients compared to healthy volunteers (Figure 9.5). Moreover, L-DOPA treatment restored tNAA and tCr levels while m-Ins levels remained unchanged. Interestingly, changes in tNAA and tCr could reflect mitochondrial energy impairment in the putamen of drug-OFF parkinsonian patients. These changes are reversed under dopaminergic treatment, which means tNAA and tCr could be used to assess responsiveness to treatment.

9.3 GLUTAMATE: GLUTAMINE CYCLING INVOLVED IN PD

High levels of glutamine concomitant with high levels of glutamate in the striatum after dopaminergic denervation in murine models of PD are suggestive of abnormalities in the glutamate–glutamine cycle.

9.3.1 GLUTAMATE: GLUTAMINE CYCLE

Our knowledge of the metabolism of glutamate in glutamine is long-standing, in particular owing to the use of radiotracers labeled with carbon 14. Then, the following studies suggest there are two pools of glutamate. The first corresponds to the glutamate stored in synaptic vesicles used for neurotransmission and which does not interact with the second pool of glutamate derived from the metabolism. This concept was challenged by an early work of ^{13}C carbon in human brain, in which authors describe synthesis of glutamate and glutamine after [1-^{13}C] glucose infusion (Gruetter et al. 1994). This study was the first to identify a rapid transfer of ^{13}C labeling of glutamate (principally

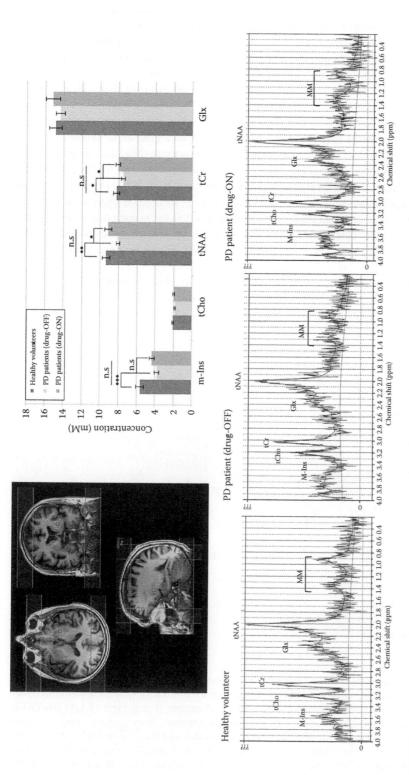

FIGURE 9.5 Three-plane T_1-weighted image from a healthy control showing a spectroscopic volume-of-interest located exactly on the left putamen. Volume-of-interest is boxed in white in axial (top left), coronal (top right), and sagittal (bottom) anatomical slices. Four outer-volume suppressions were located at the bone–brain interface. Individual spectra representative of mean spectral quality for healthy volunteers (LW = 0.067 ppm; S/N = 6), for PD patients in drug-OFF (LW = 0.076 ppm; S/N = 5), and for PD patients in drug-ON (LW = 0.067 ppm; S/N = 6). The resonances of selected metabolites were assigned as follows: NAA = 2.008 ppm, tCr (total creatine) = 3.02 ppm, tCho (total choline) = 3.2 ppm, m-Ins = 3.56 ppm, Glx (glutamate + glutamine) = 2.05–2.50 ppm, MM (macromolecules) = 0.9–1.3 ppm. For each condition, the *in vivo* spectrum (black spectrum) was estimated with LCModel output (red spectrum). The difference between spectra is plotted at the top and represents the residue. The thin signal under the experimental spectrum is the baseline spline estimate, determined with LCModel. Per our group findings, NAA, tCr, and m-Ins levels are lower in PD patients in drug-OFF condition than in the healthy volunteers group. In the PD patients in drug-ON condition, NAA and tCr levels are identical to each other than those measured in healthy volunteers. Metabolites that were significantly different between groups are flagged $*p < 0.05$, $**p < 0.01$ and $***p < 0.001$.

neuronal) to the glutamine (mainly astroglial) suggesting the existence of glutamate metabolism involving neuron–glia interactions. Furthermore, studies using [1-^{13}C] acetate, a precursor specifically metabolized inside the glial cells, reported a glutamine synthesis prior to the detection of the glutamate (Lebon et al. 2002; Deelchand et al. 2009). Together, these studies support the transfer of ^{13}C labeling from neurons to astrocytes and from astrocytes to neurons, which involves a metabolic cycle between glutamate and glutamine and neuron–astrocyte interaction.

Following its release in the synaptic cleft, glutamate is avidly taken up by astrocytes to start a process of recycling. Glutamate reuptake is efficiently performed by two glial glutamate transporters (EAAT1 or GLAST and EAAT2 or GLT-1) (Danbolt 2001) while the conversion of glutamate into glutamine is under the control of a specific astrocytic enzyme, glutamine synthetase (GS). Glutamate is then transported back to neurons via amino acid transporters (Mackenzie and Erickson 2004), transformed into glutamate by the phosphate-activated glutaminase and finally packed into vesicles by the vesicular glutamate transporters (VGLUT) (Fremeau et al. 2004) (Figure 9.6). Thus a "glutamate–glutamine cycle" between neurons and astrocytes is formed. It plays a vital part in preserving the low extracellular concentration of glutamate needed for proper receptor-mediated functions and in maintaining low concentrations of extracellular glutamate to prevent excitotoxicity and to replenish the glutamate vesicular pools (Schousboe 2003; Schousboe and Waagepetersen 2005).

A disturbance in this glutamate–glutamine equilibrium could play an important role in the pathogenesis of some brain diseases (Albrecht et al. 2016; Butterworth and Bemeur 2016). *In vivo* MRS has been used to demonstrate changes in the concentrations of glutamate and glutamine in

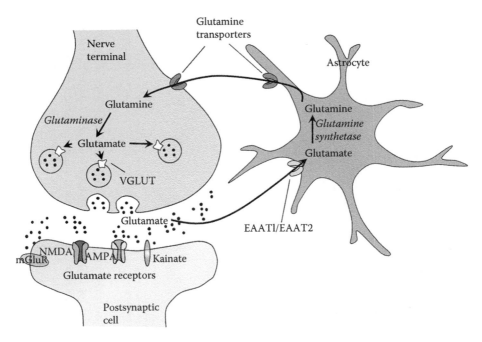

FIGURE 9.6 The glutamate–glutamine cycle. Glutamate is released in the synaptic cleft from glutamatergic neuronal vesicles via a calcium-dependant mechanism. To prevent excitotoxicity of high levels of extracellular glutamate, astrocytes avidly take up glutamate by specific glutamate transporters (EAAT1/EAAT2). Glutamate is then quickly converted into glutamine by glutamine synthetase. Some specific transmembrane transporters of glutamine allow the secretion of glutamine by astrocytes and then the reuptake of glutamine by neurons. This coupling of glutamine synthetase and glutamine traffic from glia to neurons allows glutamate to pass into the extracellular compartment in a non-neuroactive form (glutamine), thus avoiding toxicity. Neurons then hydrolyze glutamine into glutamate and ammoniac via the glutaminase and store the glutamate inside vesicles by using the vesicular glutamate transporters (VGLUT).

many neurological and psychiatric diseases (Ramadan et al. 2012), including also neurodegenerative disorders (Lin et al. 2003; Martin 2007).

9.3.2 GLUTAMATE–GLUTAMINE CYCLE IN PD

Changes in the concentrations of glutamate and glutamine in the striatum of animal models of PD described in previous ^{1}H MRS works seem to argue in favor of a disturbance in this cycle in PD.

Interestingly, the number of GS-positive astrocytes defined by immunohistochemical analysis is significantly higher in the dorsal striatum of MPTP-intoxicated mice than that of controls (Chassain et al. 2013) (Figure 9.7). These results are indirect evidence of changes in glutamate metabolism after dopaminergic denervation.

After infusion of [2-^{13}C] acetate in a rat model of PD, animals with a unilateral lesion of the dopaminergic nigrostriatal pathway, ^{13}C MRS is used to detect *in vivo* labeling in neosynthesized molecules (Chassain et al. 2005). The resonance of glutamine and glutamate C2 is detected at about 55 ppm (Figure 9.8a). Glutamate C4 (34.16 ppm) and glutamate/glutamine C3 (near 27 ppm) emerge, respectively, under the resonances of carbon methylene groups ($-CH_2-COO$) and $-CH_2$ moiety of fatty acids ($-CH_2-CH = CH$). The [2-^{13}C] acetate appears at 24.4 ppm. Spectral resolution is not sufficient to distinguish between the relative contribution of glutamate and glutamine to the C2 and C3 signals. Hence, only the glutamate C4 resonance is analyzed. In the parkinsonian group, glutamate C4 expressed as the percentage of lipid peak is significantly higher than in the control group (Figure 9.8b). Once again, increased glutamate metabolism is observed in dopamine-depleted striata and is restored by administration of the anti-parkinsonian drug, the levodopa (Chassain et al. 2005).

A lack of sensitivity is the main limiting feature of ^{13}C NMR spectroscopy. The intrinsic low sensitivity of NMR is linked to the low degree of polarization of the nuclear spin by experimentally achievable magnetic field at thermal equilibrium. In addition, the low *in vivo* abundance of ^{13}C and its lower magnetogyric ratio further limit the sensitivity of ^{13}C NMR. Thus, powerful new techniques to enhance weak NMR signals from metabolites have recently been developed (Golman

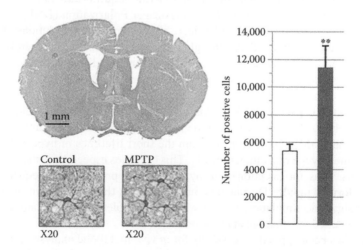

FIGURE 9.7 (See color insert.) The effect of 1-methyl-4-phenyl-1,2,3,6-tetrahydropyridine (MPTP) intoxication on glutamine synthetase (GS) labeling in the dorsal striatum of mice. Visualization of GS immunolabeling in coronal slice of the dorsal striatum. Typical labeling is shown (arrows) in the insets (X20). Scale bar, 1 mm. Quantitative analysis of the effect of dopaminergic (DA) denervation on the number of GS-positive cells in the dorsal striatum. Data are expressed as the mean number of immunoreactive cells ± standard deviation (SD) for 5 animals per group. Statistical comparisons were performed by two-way ANOVA, followed by Dunnett's test. **$p < 0.01$ versus the control group.

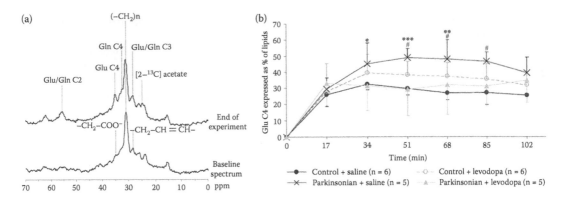

FIGURE 9.8 (a) *In vivo* ^{13}C NMR spectra of the cerebral hemisphere of a control rat using a ^{13}C acquisition sequence at 4.7 T with ^{1}H decoupling during acquisition. The baseline spectrum is an accumulation of 512 acquisition scans (17 min) during NaCl 9% infusion. The spectrum obtained at the end of the experiment is an accumulation of 512 scans (17 min) during $[2-^{13}C]$ sodium acetate infusion. Resonances present in the baseline spectrum are $-CH_2-CH = CH$ at 27 ppm, $(-CH_2)n$ of lipids at 30.3 ppm, $-CH_2-COO^-$ at 34 ppm, and PCr/Cr at 55 ppm. Other peaks present in the spectrum at the end of the experiment include $[2-^{13}C]$ acetate at 24.4 ppm, Glu/Gln C3 near 27 ppm, Gln C4 at 31.6 ppm, Glu C4 at 34.16 ppm, and Glu/Gln C2 near 55 ppm. (b) *In vivo* time courses of Glu C4 labeling. Peak areas are expressed as the percentage of the lipid peak. Before the start of $[2-^{13}C]$ acetate infusion, the ratio Glu C4/lipids was constant for each group. The value from baseline spectrum was subtracted from spectra obtained at different times. Data represent the mean ± SEM for the control + saline (n = 6), control + levodopa (50 mg/kg i.v.) (n = 6), parkinsonian + saline (n = 5), and parkinsonian + levodopa (50 mg/kg i.v.) (n = 5) groups. Zero time represents the start of $[2-^{13}C]$ acetate infusion. $*p < 0.05$, $**p < 0.01$, $***p < 0.001$ versus control + saline group and $\#p < 0.05$ versus parkinsonian + levodopa group.

et al. 2003). These techniques, referred to as hyperpolarization methods, increase the signal-to-noise ratio. The technique using ^{13}C, incorporated into small molecules, has produced polarization levels several orders of magnitude higher than thermal equilibrium values. The most versatile hyperpolarization technique is based on Dynamic Nuclear Polarization (DNP) (Ardenkjær-Larsen et al. 2003). To use the DNP for liquid probes (e.g., aqueous injectable solutions of molecular tracers), the probe is doped with free radicals in a glass-forming solvent (e.g., glycerol), frozen to a very low temperature (about 1 K) inside a magnetic field (3 T), and irradiated with microwaves to transfer a high polarization of electron spins residing in low-concentrated free radicals to the surrounding nuclear spins. After creating a "hyperpolarized" nuclear spin state in a frozen probe, the molecular sample is quickly dissolved in water (Ardenkjaer-Larsen et al. 2003). The liquid probe can then be administered in the body and used as a tracer to visualize its biodistribution and metabolism *in vivo*. The major limitation of the technique arises from the short lifetimes of hyperpolarized spin states in liquids, determined by the relaxation times T_1. This becomes especially critical when considering *in vivo* applications. Thus, the injection of the hyperpolarized probe and subsequent NMR examination has to be performed rapidly. Despite this time limitation, the huge gain in signal-to-noise obviates the need for signal accumulation, thereby allowing complete dynamic data acquisitions within the time window needed for imaging applications.

The technique has been applied successfully for *in vivo* metabolic analyses using stable isotope-enriched natural compounds. Studies with hyperpolarized compounds provide information on the physical state of tissue (MRI Magnetic Imaging) and on the metabolism of biomolecules (MRS) (Mansson et al. 2005; Golman et al. 2006a; Gallagher et al. 2008). Most of these investigations dealt with cardiac metabolism (Golman et al. 2008), metabolism in muscle (Golman et al. 2006a), and tumor diagnosis (Golman et al. 2006b; Day et al. 2007), using ^{13}C-pyruvate as a molecular probe. The great potential of the ^{13}C DNP-MRS method for metabolic imaging has also been demonstrated with other molecules (Gallagher et al. 2008). The recent hyperpolarization of endogenous molecules such as [1-^{13}C] glutamate (Gallagher et al. 2011) and [5-^{13}C] glutamine (Cabella et al. 2013) shows that ^{13}C DNP-MRS has potential use in the study of brain metabolism.

Thus, according to the choice of precursor, the application of ^{13}C metabolic imaging using hyperpolarized ^{13}C-labeled substrates to neurochemistry opens up a promising new avenue of research.

9.4 CONCLUSION

The studies reviewed in this chapter focused on alterations in the glutamate, glutamine, and GABA levels in the striatum after dopaminergic denervation. Higher concentrations of glutamate, glutamine, and GABA were observed in the striatum of animal models of PD. These changes may be associated with an increase in glutamatergic and GABAergic neurotransmission in the striatum after dopaminergic denervation. These modifications suggest that alterations in the metabolism, particularly the astroglial neurotransmitter cycling of glutamate and glutamine, may be involved in the pathophysiology of PD.

REFERENCES

Albrecht, J. The role of glutamine in brain pathology. In: *Glutamine, the Brain and Neurological Diseases*. 2016. Boca Raton, FL: CRC Press.

Andres, R., A. Ducray, U. Schlattner et al. 2008. Functions and effects of creatine in the central nervous system. *Brain Res. Bull.* 76:329–343.

Anglade, P., A. Mouatt-Prigent, Y. Agid et al. 1996. Synaptic plasticity in the caudate nucleus of patients with Parkinson's Disease. *Neurodegeneration* 5:121–128.

Ardenkjaer-Larsen, J.H., B. Fridlind, A. Gram et al. 2003. Increase in signal-to-noise ratio of >10,000 times in liquid-state NMR. *Proc. Natl. Acad. Sci. USA.* 100:10158–10163.

Bagga, P., A. Chugani, K. Varadarajan et al. 2013. *In vivo* NMR studies of regional cerebral energetics in MPTP model of Parkinson's disease: Recovery of cerebral metabolism with acute levodopa treatment. *J Neurochem.* 127:365–377.

Beitz, J.M. 2014. Parkinson's disease: A review. *Front Biosci. (Schol Ed).* 6:65–74.

Benarroch, E. 2008. N-acetylaspartate and N-acetylaspartylglutamate: Neurobiology and clinical significance. *Neurology* 70:1353–1357.

Bergman, H., T. Wichmann, B. Karmon et al. 1994. The primate subthalamic nucleus. II. Neuronal activity in the MPTP model of parkinsonism. *J Neurophysiol.* 72:507–520.

Bevan, M.D., P.J. Magill, D. Terman et al. 2002. Move to the rhythm: Oscillations in the subthalamic nucleus-external globus pallidus network. *Trends Neurosci.* 25:525–531.

Blandini, F., G. Nappi, C. Tassorelli et al. 2000. Functional changes of the basal ganglia circuitry in Parkinson's disease. *Prog. Neurobiol.* 62:63–88.

Braak, H., K. Del Tredici, U. Rüb et al. 2003. Staging of brain pathology related to sporadic Parkinson's disease. *Neurobiol. Aging* 24:197–211.

Brand, A., C. Richter-Landsberg, and D. Leibfritz. 1993. Multinuclear NMR studies on the energy metabolism of glial and neuronal cells. *Developmental Neuroscience* 15:289–298.

Butterworth, R.F. and Bemeur, C. 2016. *Brain Glutamine and Hepatic Encephalopathy. Glutamine, the Brain and Neurological Diseases*. Boca Raton, FL: CRC Press.

Cabella, C., M. Karlsson, C. Canapè et al. 2013. *In vivo* and *in vitro* liver cancer metabolism observed with hyperpolarized [5-13C] glutamine. *JMR* 232:45–52.

Calabresi, P., N.B. Mercuri, G. Sancesario et al. 1993. Electrophysiology of dopamine-denervated striatal neurons. Implications for Parkinson's disease. *Brain* 116:433–452.

Carta, A.R., S. Fenu, P. Pala et al. 2003. Selective modification in GAD67 mRNA levels in striatonigral and striatopallidal pathways correlate to dopamine agonist priming in 6-hydroxydopamine-lesioned rats. *Eur. J. Neurosci.* 18:2563–2572.

Centonze, D., P. Calabresi, P. Giacomini et al. 1999. Neurophysiology of Parkinson's disease: From basic research to clinical correlates. *Clin. Neurophysiol* 110:2006–2013.

Chassain, C., G. Bielicki, J.P. Donnat et al. 2005. Cerebral glutamate metabolism in Parkinson's disease: An *in vivo* dynamic 13C MRS study in the rat. *Exp. Neurol.* 191:276–284.

Chassain, C., G. Bielicki, E. Durand et al. 2008. Metabolic changes detected by proton magnetic resonance spectroscopy *in vivo* and *in vitro* in a Murin model of Parkinson's disease, the MPTP-intoxicated mice. *J Neurochem.* 105:874–882.

Chassain, C., G. Bielicki, C. Keller et al. 2010. Metabolic changes detected *in vivo* by 1H MRS in the MPTP-intoxicated mice. *NMR Biomed* 23:547–553.

Chassain, C., G. Bielicki, C. Carcenac et al. 2013. Does MPTP intoxication in mice induce metabolite changes in the nucleus accumbens? A ^{1}H nuclear MRS study. *NMR Biomed* 26(3):336–347.

Chassain, C., C. Melon, P. Salin et al. 2016. Metabolic, synaptic and behavioral impact of 5-week chronic deep brain stimulation in hemiparkinsonian rats. *J Neurochem*. 136(5):1004–1016.

Choe, B.X., J.W. Park, K.S. Lee et al. 1998. Neuronal laterality in Parkinson's disease with unilateral symptom by *in vivo* 1H magnetic resonance. *Invest Radiol*. 33:450–455.

Coune, P.G., M. Craveiro, M.N. Gaugler et al. 2013. An *in vivo* ultrahigh field 14.1 T (1) H-MRS study on 6-OHDA and alpha-synuclein-based rat models of Parkinson's disease: GABA as an early disease marker. *NMR Biomed* 26: 43–50. doi: 10.1002/nbm.2817.

Ciurleo, R., G. Di Lorenzo, P. Bramati, and S. Marino. 2014. Magnetic resonance spectroscopy: An *in vivo* molecular imaging biomarker for Parkinson's disease? *BioMed. Research Int*. 2014:Article ID 519816, 10 pages. doi: 10.1155/2014/519816.

Danbolt, N.C. 2001. Glutamate uptake. *Prog. Neurobiol*. 65:1–105.

Day, S.E., M.I. Kettunen, F.A. Gallagher et al. 2007. Detecting tumor response to treatment using hyperpolarized ^{13}C magnetic resonance imaging and spectroscopy. *Nat. Med*. 13:1382–1387.

Deelchand, D.K., A.A. Shestov, D.M. Koski et al. 2009. Acetate transport and utilization in the rat brain. *J. Neurochem*. 109:46–54.

De Graaf, R.A., P.B. Brown, G.F. Mason et al. 2003. Detection of [1,6-^{13}C$_2$]-glucose metabolism in rat brain by *in vivo* ^{1}H-[^{13}C]-NMR spectroscopy. *Magn. Res. Med*. 49:37–46.

De Graaf, R.A., D.L. Rothman, and K.L. Behar. 2011. State of the art direct ^{13}C and indirect ^{1}H-[^{13}C] NMR spectroscopy *in vivo*. A practical guide. *NMR Biomed* 24:958–972.

Emir, U.E., P.J. Tuite, and G. Öz. 2012. Elevated pontine and putamenal GABA levels in mild-moderate Parkinson disease detected by 7 Tesla proton MRS. *PloSONE* 7:1–7.

Firbank, M.J., R.M. Harrison, and J.T. O'Brien. 2002. A comprehensive review of proton magnetic resonance spectroscopy studies in dementia and Parkinson's disease. *Dement. Geriatr. Cogn. Disord*. 14:64–76.

Fremeau, R.T. Jr., S. Voglmaier, R.P. Seal et al. 2004. VGLUTs define subsets of excitatory neurons and suggest novel roles for glutamate. *Trends Neurosci*. 27:98–103.

Gallagher, F.A., M.I. Kettunen, S.E. Day et al. 2008. Magnetic resonance imaging of pH *in vivo* using hyperpolarized ^{13}C-labelled bicarbonate. *Nature* 453:940–943.

Gallagher, F.A., M.I. Kettunen, S.E. Day et al. 2011. Detection of tumor glutamate metabolism *in vivo* using 13C magnetic resonance spectroscopy and hyperpolarized [1–13C]glutamate. *Magn. Res. Med*. 66:18–23.

Goergen, S.K., H. Ang, F. Wong et al. 2014. Early MRI in term infants with perinatal hypoxic-ischaemic brain injury: Interobserver agreement and MRI predictors of outcome at 2 years. *Clin. Radiol*. 69:72–81.

Goldstein, D.S., C. Holmes, O. Bentho et al. 2008. Biomarkers to detect central dopaminergic deficiency and distinguish from multiple system atrophy. *Parkinsonism Relat. Disord*. 14:600–607.

Golman, K., L.E. Olsson, O. Axelsson et al. 2003. Molecular imaging using hyperpolarized ^{13}C. *Br. J. Radiol*. 76:S118–S127.

Golman, K., R.I. Zandt, and M. Thaning. 2006a. Real-time metabolic imaging. *Proc. Natl. Acad. Sci. USA*. 103:11270–11275.

Golman, K., R.I. Zandt, M. Lerche et al. 2006b. Metabolic imaging by hyperpolarized ^{13}C magnetic resonance imaging for *in vivo* tumor diagnosis. *Cancer Res*. 66:10855–10860.

Golman, K., J.S. Petersson, P. Magnusson et al. 2008. Cardiac metabolism measured noninvasively by hyperpolarized ^{13}C MRI. *Magn. Reson. Med*. 59:1005–1013.

Gruetter, R., E.J. Novotny, S.D. Boulware et al. 1994. Localized ^{13}C NMR spectroscopy in the human brain of amino acid labeling from D-[1-^{13}C]glucose. *J. Neurochem*. 63:1377–1385.

Hollerman, J.R. and A.A. Grace. 1992. Subthalamic nucleus cell firing in the 6-OHDA-treated rat: Basal activity and response to haloperidol. *Brain Res*. 590:291–299.

Hornykiewicz, O. 1998. Biochemical aspects of Parkinson's disease. *Neurology* 51:S2–S9.

Ingham, C.A., S.H. Hood, P. Taggart et al. 1998. Plasticity of synapses in the rat neostriatum after unilateral lesion of the nigrostriatal dopaminergic pathway. *J Neurosci*. 18:4732–4743.

Jonkers, N., S. Sarre, G. Ebinger et al. 2002. MK801 suppresses the L-DOPA-induced increase of glutamate in striatum of hemi-Parkinson rats. *Brain Res*. 926:149–155.

Kickler, N., P. Krack, V. Fraix et al. 2007. Glutamate measurement in Parkinson's disease using MRS at 3 T field strength. *NMR Biomed* 20:757–762.

Kickler, N., E. Lacombe, C. Chassain et al. 2009. Assessment of metabolic changes in the striatum of a rat model of parkinsonism: An *in vivo* (1)H MRS study. *NMR Biomed* 22:207–212.

Kish, S.J., A. Rajput, J. Gilbert et al. 1986. Elevated gamma-aminobutyric acid level in striatal but not extrastriatal brain regions in Parkinson's disease: Correlation with striatal dopamine loss. *Ann. Neurol.* 20:26–31.

Lebon, V., K.F. Petersen, G.W. Cline et al. 2002. Astroglial contribution to brain energy metabolism in humans revealed by ^{13}C nuclear magnetic resonance spectroscopy: Elucidation of the dominant pathway for neurotransmitter glutamate repletion and measurement of astrocytic oxidative metabolism. *J. Neurosci.* 22:1523–1531.

Lin, A.P., F. Shic, C. Enriquez, and B.D. Ross. 2003. Reduced glutamate neurotransmission in patients with Alzheimer's disease—An *in vivo* 13C magnetic resonance spectroscopy study. *Magn. Reson. Mater. Phys. Biol. Med.* 16:29–42.

Lindefors, N. and U. Ungerstedt. 1990. Bilateral regulation of glutamate tissue and extracellular levels in caudate-putamen by midbrain dopamine neurons. *Neurosci Lett.* 115:248–252.

Mackenzie, B. and J.D. Erickson. 2004. Sodium-coupled neutral amino acid (system N/A) transporters of the SLC38 gene family. *Pflugers Arch.* 447:784–795.

Månsson, S., E. Johansson, P. Magnusson et al. 2005. ^{13}C imaging a new diagnostic platform. *Eur. Radiol.* 16:57–67.

Martin, W.R.W. 2007. MR spectroscopy in neurodegenerative disease. *Mol. Imaging Biol.* 9:196–203.

Mazuel, L., C. Chassain, B. Jean et al. 2016. MRS for diagnosis and evaluation of treatment efficiency in Parkinson's disease. *Radiology* 278:505–513.

Meara, J., B.K. Bhowmick, and P. Hobson. 1999. Accuracy of diagnosis in patients with presumed Parkinson's disease. *Age Ageing* 28:99–102.

Melon, C., C. Chassain, G. Bielicki et al. 2015. Progressive metabolic changes under subthalamic nucleus DBS in parkinsonian rat. *J. Neurochem.* 132:703–712.

Meshul, C.K., N. Emre, C.M. Nakamura et al. 1999. Time-dependent changes in striatal glutamate synapses following a 6-hydroxydopamine lesion. *Neuroscience* 88:1–16.

Meshul, C.K., J.P. Cogen, H.W. Cheng et al. 2000. Alterations in rat striatal glutamate synapses following a lesion of the cortico- and/or nigrostriatal pathway. *Exp. Neurol.* 165:191–206.

Moffett, J.R., B. Ross, P. Arun et al. 2007. N-acetylaspartate in the CNS: From neurodiagnostics to neurobiology. *Prog. Neurobiol.* 81(2):89–131.

Nagatsu, T. and M. Sawada. 2007. Biochemistry of postmortem brains in Parkinson's disease: Historical overview and future prospects. *J. Neural. Transm. Suppl.* 72:113–120.

Obeso, J.A., C. Marin, C. Rodriguez-Oroz et al. 2008. The basal ganglia in Parkinson's disease: Current concepts and unexplained observations. *Ann. Neurol.* 64:S30–S46. doi: 10.1002/ana.21481.

Obeso, J.A., M.C. Rodriguez-Oroz, C.G. Goetz et al. 2010. Missing pieces in the Parkinson's disease puzzle. *Nature Med.* 16:653–661.

Obeso, J.A. and J.L. Lanciego. 2011. Past, present, and future of the pathophysiological model of the basal ganglia. *Front. Neuroanat.* 5:1–6, doi: 10.3389/fnana.2011.00039.

Pfeuffer, J., I. Tkac, S.W. Provencher et al. 1999. Toward an *in vivo* neurochemical profile: Quantification of 18 metabolites in short-echo-time 1H NMR spectra of the rat brain. *J. Magn. Reson.* 141:104–120.

Ramadan, S., A. Lin, and P. Stanwell. 2013. Glutamate and glutamine: A review of *in vivo* MRS in the human brain. *NMR Biomed* 26:1630–1646.

Ross, B.D. 1991. Biochemical considerations in ^{1}H spectroscopy. Glutamate and glutamine; myo-inositol and related metabolites. *NMR Biomed* 4:59–63.

Rothman, D.L., E.J. Novotny, G.I. Shulman et al. 1992. 1H-[13C] NMR measurements of [4–13C] glutamate turnover in human brain. *Proc. Natl. Acad. Sci. USA* 89:9603–9606.

Schousboe, A. 2003. Role of astrocytes in the maintenance and modulation of glutamatergic and GABAergic neurotransmission. *Neurochem. Res.* 28:347–352.

Schousboe, A. and H.S. Waagepetersen. 2005. Role of astrocytes in glutamate homeostasis: Implications for excitotoxicity. *Neurotox Res.* 8:221–225.

Shults, C.W. 2006. Lewy bodies. *Proc. Natl. Acad. Sci. USA* 103:1661–1668.

Soghomonian, J.J. and N. Laprade. 1997. Glutamate decarboxylase (GAD67 and GAD65) gene expression is increased in a subpopulation of neurons in the putamen of Parkinsonian monkeys. *Synapse* 27:122–132.

Sterling N.W., G. Du, M.M. Lewis et al. 2013. Striatal shape in Parkinson's disease. *Neurobiol. Aging* 34:2510–2516. doi: 10.1016/j.neurobiolaging.2013.05.017

Tanaka, Y., K. Niijima, Y. Mizuno et al. 1986. Changes in gamma-aminobutyric, glutamate, aspartate, glycine, and taurine contents in the striatum after unilateral lesions in rats. *Exp. Neurol.* 91:259–268.

Villalba, R.M. and Y. Smith. 2011. Neuroglial plasticity at striatal glutamatergic synapses in Parkinson's disease. *Front. Syst. Neurosci.* 5:68.

Section V

Glutamine and the Intestinal Tract

10 Glutamine and Intestinal Physiology and Pathology

François Blachier, Moïse Coeffier, Wei-Yun Zhu, Chunlong Mu, Yuxiang Yang, Guoyao Wu, Xiangfeng Kong, Antonio Lancha Jr., Mireille Andriamihaja, Daniel Tomé, and Yulong Yin

CONTENTS

10.1 INTRODUCTION

The metabolism and functions of glutamine in healthy intestine or in pathological situations cannot be dissociated from those of glutamate since these two nonessential amino acids possess a partially common metabolic fate (Blachier et al. 2009). In cells equipped with the enzymatic activity glutaminase (like enterocytes in which the catalytic activity is high), glutamine can be converted to glutamate and ammonia. Conversely, in cells equipped with glutamine synthetase (GS) activity (like colonocytes that are characterized by a high GS activity in comparison with enterocytes) (Andriamihaja et al. 2010), glutamate can be condensed with ammonia to form glutamine (Eklou-Lawson et al. 2009). However, glutamine, but not glutamate, can be used for the synthesis of several compounds, including purine and pyrimidine (Newsholme and Carrie 1994), N-acetylglucosamine and N-acetylgalactosamine; these latter two being involved in intestinal mucin synthesis (Reeds and Burrin 2001). If one considers the circulating concentrations of the 20 amino acids used for the synthesis of body protein measured in the plasma of healthy subjects, there is a striking difference between glutamate that is present at a very low concentration and glutamine that is present at the highest concentration among all amino acids (Cynober 2002). In food products like milk, the sum of glutamine and glutamate represents the highest protein-bound amino acids (Wu and Knabe 1994), and more generally glutamate by itself is one of the most abundant amino acid in alimentary protein (Beyreuther et al. 2007).

To document the effects of glutamine on intestine in physiological situation, one has to consider whether glutamine is acting by itself and/or through its metabolism and on what cell type in the intestinal mucosa the amino acid is active. In addition, the intestinal microbiota both in the small and large intestine may impact the metabolism of glutamine released in the process of protein digestion from alimentary and endogenous proteins. In various pathological situations, like those presented in this chapter, there are some indications that glutamine supplementation may benefit the intestinal mucosa. The aim of this chapter is then to focus on the metabolic and physiological effects of glutamine on the intestine in both healthy and several pathological situations in which the intestinal mucosa integrity is altered.

10.2 GLUTAMINE AND INTESTINAL PHYSIOLOGY

10.2.1 GLUTAMINE AND INTESTINAL FUNCTIONS

Glutamine is the preferential substrate of rapidly dividing cells such as epithelial cells and immune cells, that is, lymphocytes. Approximately 60% of absorbed glutamine is oxidized in the small intestine to provide energy (Windmueller and Spaeth 1978; Blachier et al. 2009). In the colon, glutamine can be provided from blood to the epithelial cells through the basolateral side. In addition, colonocytes can use the short-chain fatty acids acetate, propionate, and butyrate as fuel substrates. These short-chain fatty acids are produced by the microbiota from glutamate and from other amino acids released from undigested alimentary and endogenous proteins and from indigestible polysaccharides and oligosaccharides (Blachier et al. 2007).

Glutamine transport is coupled to sodium, and glutamine has an additive effect on sodium absorption compared with glucose, which suggests that glutamine may be beneficial in different intestinal injured conditions associated with diarrhea. Indeed, glutamine enters into enterocytes through amino acid transporter ATB0/ASCT2, a major sodium-dependent transporter (Avissar et al. 2004). During hypersecretion conditions, glutamine supply is associated with improved absorption (Lima et al. 2002; Coeffier et al. 2005).

Glutamine seems to be also involved in the regulation of other intestinal functions, that is, gut barrier and immunoinflammatory response, by acting on several metabolic pathways. Glutamine appears as the preferential fuel of immune cells and may regulate not only lymphocyte proliferation but also cytokine release (Yaryura-Tobias et al. 1970; Yaqoob and Calder 1998). Glutamine deficiency leads to a decrease of immune response in different pathophysiological conditions (Wernerman 2008). As reviewed (Rhoads and Wu 2009), glutamine may regulate gut barrier function by acting on proliferation/apoptosis balance and/or on protein synthesis/degradation and/or by acting on specific signalling pathways such as MAPKs. Proliferation rate of small intestinal epithelial cells is dependent on glutamine availability (Rhoads et al. 1997) as well as on apoptosis rate (Evans et al. 2003). Protein metabolism in the intestinal mucosa is also improved by glutamine (Higashiguchi et al. 1993; Coeffier et al. 2003). Particularly, glutamine stimulates protein synthesis in intestinal epithelial cells through the mTOR pathway (Boukhettala et al. 2012), whereas glutamine depletion induces GCN2 pathway leading to arrest of protein synthesis (Boukhettala et al. 2012). In addition, glutamine depletion is associated with increased intestinal permeability *in vitro* (Le Bacquer et al. 2003; Boukhettala et al. 2012) associated with a decreased expression of tight junction proteins, occludin, claudin-1, and ZO-1 (Li et al. 2004). Finally, glutamine has cytoprotective effects in the intestine, mainly related to its capacity to induce the heat shock proteins (HSP).

10.2.2 GLUTAMINE METABOLISM IN INTESTINAL CELLS

Although the Na^+-independent carriers (system L and B° transporters) are associated with the brush-border membranes of jejunal enterocytes (Fan et al. 1998), the Na^+-dependent B° transport system represents the major route of luminal glutamine absorption. It has to be kept in mind that glutamine can be also provided to epithelial intestinal cells from the circulating blood plasma. This is particularly true when considering colonic epithelial cells that cannot, except for a short period of time following birth, transfer amino acids to any significant extent from the lumen to the portal blood (Darragh et al. 1994) and thus depend on the blood plasma glutamine as one oxidative substrate for their energy supply (Darcy-Vrillon et al. 1993). As stated above, L-glutamate and

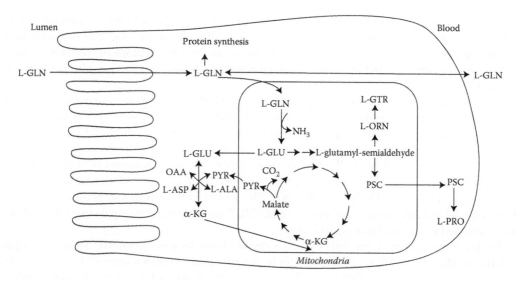

FIGURE 10.1 Schematic view of the metabolism of L-glutamine in enterocytes.

L-glutamine are extensively metabolized in enterocytes (Windmueller and Spaeth 1974; Ardawi and Newsholme 1985). L-glutamine originating from lumen or blood is degraded into L-glutamate and ammonia by the mitochondrial phosphate-dependent glutaminase activity (Wu et al. 1994; Wu et al. 1995) (Figure 10.1). Then, L-glutamate is exported into the cytosol and transaminated with oxaloacetate to produce alpha-ketoglutarate and L-aspartate (Blachier et al. 1999; Blachier et al. 2009). L-glutamate can also be transaminated in the presence of pyruvate to produce L-alanine and alpha-ketoglutarate (Wu et al. 1995). L-aspartate, either produced endogenously from glutamine/glutamate or originating from the luminal content, can enter the mitochondria for oxidative purpose (Windmueller and Spaeth 1976). Transamination is the principal pathway by which L-glutamate is converted to alpha-ketoglutarate in enterocytes since these cells have little capacity for the conversion of L-glutamate into alpha-ketoglutarate (and ammonia) through glutamate dehydrogenase (Madej et al. 2002). Alpha-ketoglutarate then reenters into the mitochondria and is used in the Krebs cycle (Duee et al. 1995) (Figure 10.1). L-glutamine and L-glutamate can be converted to other amino acids, including L-ornithine (Blachier et al. 1992), L-citrulline, and L-proline (Wu et al. 1994). Together with L-cysteine and glycine, L-glutamate is the precursor for the synthesis of glutathione in enterocytes (Reeds et al. 1997). The ratio of reduced/oxidized glutathione is an important parameter for the determination of intracellular concentrations of both oxygen-reactive and nitrogen-reactive species (Chakravarthi et al. 2006). Colonic epithelial cells are also able to metabolize glutamine and glutamate in metabolic pathways not vastly different from those in enterocytes (Darcy-Vrillon et al. 1994). The L-glutamine-degrading enzyme glutaminase is also highly expressed in colonocytes, but the GS activity appears to be much higher in colonocytes than in enterocytes (Eklou-Lawson et al. 2009), and this capacity to condense L-glutamate and ammonia is likely related to the high ammonia concentration in the large intestine (Mouille et al. 2004) and to the inhibitory effect of excessive concentration of ammonia toward colonocyte respiration (Mouille et al. 2004; Andriamihaja et al. 2010).

10.2.3 GLUTAMINE AND GASTROINTESTINAL BACTERIA

Dietary and host-derived proteins and amino acids are used for the growth and survival of bacteria in the digestive tract (Libao-Mercado et al. 2009). The conditionally essential amino acid glutamine, either synthesized by the cells or taken up from the luminal environment of the gastrointestinal tract, plays an important role in nitrogen balance and protein synthesis in bacteria (Forchhammer 2007) and small intestine (Wu et al. 2010a,b; Xi et al. 2010). Glutamine, together with glutamate, not only provides nitrogen for purines, pyrimidines, asparagine, tryptophan, histidine, glucosamine, p-aminobenzoate, and arginine in most bacteria but can also serve as key nitrogen donor for biosynthetic reactions.

The first step of glutamine metabolism in the bacterial cells is glutamine incorporation. Sodium-dependent transport and facilitated diffusion play an important role in most amino acid transport by some of the dominant amino acid-fermenting bacteria (Chen and Russell 1989; Chen and Russell 1990). However, transport of glutamine in *Streptococcus bovis* is likely driven by phosphate-bond energy (Chen and Russell 1989). Dashper confirmed that glutamine transport is likely to be energized by ATP hydrolysis (Dashper et al. 1995). The rate of glutamate and glutamine transport is related to cytoplasmic pH (Poolman et al. 1987). The activity of the transporter is maximal between pH 6.0 and 7.0 and can decrease rapidly above pH 7.0. Thus, glutamine transport into bacterial cells can be affected by extracellular environment.

Glutamine incorporated into bacterial cells derives from *de novo* synthesis. Studies with pure bacteria cultures showed that ammonia might be the preferred nitrogen source and support the fast growth for *Escherichia coli* (Reitzer 2003). The most important pathway for glutamine synthesis is the glutamine synthetase/glutamate synthetase (GS/GOGAT) pathway, which is ubiquitous and catalyzes the only reaction of glutamine formation in bacteria (Merrick and Edwards 1995; Reitzer 2003). Glutamine synthetase (GS) converts glutamate to glutamine and assimilate ammonia at the same time. Glutamate synthetase (GOGAT) transfers the amide group from glutamine to 2-ketoglutarate to produce two glutamate molecules.

As one of the metabolic fates, quantitatively significant amounts of dietary glutamine are catabolized by enterocytes during first-pass intestinal metabolism (Bergen and Wu 2009). *In vitro* studies also showed that the net utilization of glutamine by jejunal and ileal bacteria is about 22% and 40% (Dai et al. 2011), respectively, suggesting a considerable contribution of intestinal bacteria to the first-pass intestinal amino acid metabolism. Among the glutamine utilized by bacteria, about 10% are recovered in proteins, while 1% is oxidized. The remaining 89% glutamine is utilized in other metabolic routes, including pathways like deamination, transamination, and decarboxylation (Metges et al. 1999; Dai et al. 2010). The rapid utilization and metabolism of glutamine by small-intestinal bacteria may also suggest its role in the survival and growth of bacteria in the intestine through the regulation of the bacterial metabolism of nitrogenous compounds, particularly amino acids (Forchhammer 2007).

Glutamine may also affect amino acid utilization and metabolism by the small-intestinal bacteria, thereby modulating the production and profile of nitrogenous compounds in the lumen of small-intestine and whole-body amino acid homeostasis. *In vitro* bacterial culture studies (Dai et al. 2013) show that glutamine supplementation may regulate the utilization and metabolism of the arginine family of amino acid in pig small-intestinal bacteria. In jejunal mixed bacteria, net utilization of ornithine decreases while net utilization of citrulline increases in the presence of glutamine. In ileum mixed bacteria, net utilization of arginine increases while the net utilization of ornithine decreases with the addition of glutamine. The reduction in the net utilization of ornithine in the small-intestinal bacteria might result from the decreased flux of ornithine into citrulline in jejunal microbiota and increased fluxes of arginine into ornithine in the ileal microbiota. Glutamine supplementation also influences the metabolism of serine and aspartate by pig small-intestinal bacteria. The utilization of asparagine and serine by jejunal mixed bacteria is reduced while the net production is increased with the increasing doses of glutamine. Thus, the metabolism of glutamine and asparagine in small-intestinal bacteria might be closely related to each other.

In summary, glutamine can be synthesized in bacteria through GS/GOGAT pathway. The metabolism of glutamine by small intestinal bacteria may contribute considerably to the first-pass intestinal amino acid metabolism. The metabolic routes of glutamine include protein synthesis, oxidization into CO_2, and other metabolic pathways. In the small intestine, glutamine can also regulate other amino acid metabolism by luminal bacteria, especially arginine metabolism. Thus, the glutamine metabolism by intestinal bacteria is likely to be important among other amino acids and, consequently, the luminal homeostasis in the small intestine (Wang et al. 2008).

10.3 GLUTAMINE AND INTESTINAL PATHOLOGY

10.3.1 GLUTAMINE AND INTESTINAL INFLAMMATION AND MUCOSAL HEALING

In LPS-treated mice, Manhart et al. reported that glutamine supplementation is associated with an increase of lymphocyte population in Peyer's patch (Manhart et al. 2001). Interestingly, this glutamine effect is mediated by an enhanced content of intestinal gluthatione, a major antioxidant player. In malnourished rats, glutamine supplementation also increases intestinal gluthatione content (Belmonte et al. 2007). Several studies have also suggested that glutamine is able to regulate intestinal inflammatory response in experimental models. While glutamine depletion is associated with exacerbated inflammatory response (Liboni et al. 2005), and since a decrease of mucosal glutamine content has been reported during inflammatory bowel diseases (IBD) (Sido et al. 2006), glutamine supplementation is able to limit the inflammatory response in intestinal epithelial cells (Marion et al. 2004; Hubert-Buron et al. 2006). Interestingly, glutamine reduced inflammatory response not only by limiting proinflammatory cytokines but also by increasing anti-inflammatory cytokines (Aosasa et al. 2003; Coeffier et al. 2003). Similar data have been obtained in experimental models of colitis in rats (Ameho et al. 1997). By using a culture model of colonic biopsies obtained from patients with Crohn's disease, Lecleire et al. reported that glutamine is able to limit interleukin-8 and interleukin-6 release (Lecleire et al. 2008). Similar to the glutamine effects on gut barrier function, several signaling pathways have been proposed to contribute to the anti-inflammatory effects of glutamine, including the MAPK pathways (Rhoads and Wu 2009), Stat proteins (Kretzmann et al. 2008), and NF-κB pathways (Hubert-Buron et al. 2006; Lecleire et al. 2008). However, clinical trials evaluating glutamine supplementation in patients with IBD gave controversial results (Scheppach et al. 1996; Den Hond et al. 1999; Akobeng et al. 2000; Ockenga et al. 2005) and do not permit to conclude on the efficiency of glutamine supplementation in patients with IBD.

Glutamine supplementation for mucosal healing following an episode of intestinal mucosal inflammation has shown some efficiency in animal models. Indeed, oral glutamine supplementation (3%) is able to improve the healing of the small intestine mucosa after radiation-induced enteritis (Klimberg et al. 1990). In a model of anastomosis in rats, early enteral feeding with glutamine (12.5% given through an orogastric tube) was found to improve the microscopic aspect of the healing (Guven et al. 2007). Regarding supplementation with glutamate, it has been shown that supplementation with 5% monosodium glutamate for 5 days promotes small intestine mucosal healing after chemically-induced enteropathy in rats (Amagase et al. 2012). Recently, it has been shown that a mixture of glutamate (a major oxidative substrate in colonocytes and a precursor of glutathione, 0.57 g/day in the form of monosodium glutamate), methionine (a precursor of cysteine for glutathione synthesis, 0.31 g/day), and threonine (an amino acid highly used for mucin synthesis, 0.50 g/day) given in the mucosal healing phase after chemical induction of colitis in rats improves colonic mucosal regeneration/re-epithelialization after 10-day supplementation without affecting the spontaneous resolution of inflammation (Liu et al. 2013). Future studies should test dietary compounds (including glutamine and glutamate) individually or in combination for their capacity to improve mucosal healing after an active phase of intestinal mucosal inflammation in clinical trials. If successful, such an approach would be beneficial for patients by allowing a better definition of the most effective adjuvant nutritional supplementation for intestinal mucosal healing (Lan et al. 2015).

10.3.2 GLUTAMINE AND ENDOTOXEMIA AND SEPSIS

Endotoxemia is defined as the presence of endotoxin in blood and may result from a massive transfer of endotoxin (also currently called lipopolysaccharide [LPS]) from the intestinal lumen to the bloodstream due to impaired gut selective barrier function in the small and/or large intestine. Major endotoxemia may lead to sepsis defined as a medical condition characterized by a whole-body inflammatory state (also called Systemic Inflammatory Response Syndrome [SIRS]) (Tsiotou et al. 2005). In critically ill patients, the gastrointestinal tract is believed to play a central role in the pathogenesis of septic shock (Swank and Deitch 1996; Hassoun et al. 2001). Indeed, increased gut permeability and bacterial translocation play an active role in multiple organ failure by inducing a vicious cycle of increased intestinal permeability, leading to increased transfer of luminal compounds to the bloodstream. In this way, the gut may be seen as both an instigator and a victim of post-injury multiple organ failure (Hassoun et al. 2001). This idea was already proposed in the pioneering work of Deitch et al. (1987) showing that intraperitoneal injection of endotoxin to mice is able to promote the translocation of bacteria from the gut. Sepsis considerably alters the intestinal barrier functions, which in turn modifies the absorption and bioavailability of nutrients (Elwafi et al. 2012). In septic patients, sodium-dependent glutamine transport is decreased in both jejunum and ileum when compared to control healthy patients (Salloum et al. 1991). In the rat model, intraperitoneal injection of LPS resulted in a decrease of the sodium-dependent jejunal glutamine uptake and glutaminase activity (Souba et al. 1990; Salloum et al. 1991; Haque et al. 1997). In another experimental model of sepsis induced by cecal ligation and puncture, the capacity of enterocytes for glutamine oxidation and the intestinal mucosa glutaminase activity are also decreased (Ardawi et al. 1990; Ardawi and Majzoub 1991) with a concomitant negative nitrogen balance. However, the effect of endotoxemia and sepsis on glutamine metabolism in the intestinal mucosa is not specific for this amino acid, since absorption of other amino acids, including leucine, proline, glutamic acid, and arginine, is also affected (Salloum et al. 1991; Gardiner and Barbul 1993; Gardiner et al. 1995; Abad et al. 2001). Indeed, following endotoxemia, almost all circulating amino acids are markedly decreased, suggesting an overall decrease of the intestinal mucosa capacity for amino acid absorption (Boutry et al. 2012). In addition, endotoxemia affects the morphology of the intestinal mucosa (Chambon-Savanovitch et al. 1999; Crouser et al. 2000) and decreases the mucosal oxygen consumption (King et al. 1999). All these results reinforce the view that endotoxemia affects the intestinal functions and metabolism, including glutamine metabolism (Figure 10.2).

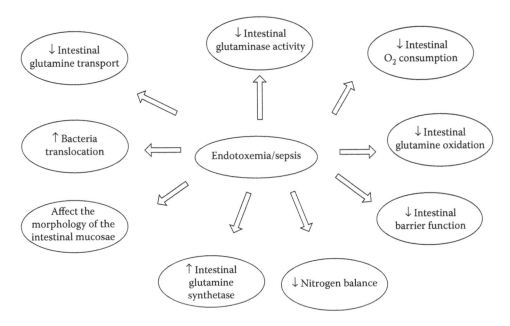

FIGURE 10.2 Schematic view of the effects of endotoxemia/sepsis on intestinal metabolism and physiology.

10.3.3 GLUTAMINE AND BACTERIAL TRANSLOCATION

The gut microflora is a complex mixture of autochthonous bacteria that have developed mutualistic relationship with their hosts. The gut epithelium forms an essential element of the mucosal barrier. The structural and functional integrity of mucosa confers efficient protection for intestinal and systemic homeostasis as a vast diversity of microbes and food antigens cover the luminal surface of the mucosa (Garrett et al. 2010). The disruption of gut barrier function may be involved in the pathogenesis of numerous gastrointestinal diseases such as IBD, irritable bowel syndrome (IBS), and infectious enterocolitis (Rao and Samak 2012). When the gut barrier function disrupts, the bacterial translocation may happen. The term bacterial translocation was first addressed by Berg and Garlington (1979). Under conditions of impaired intestinal barrier, both viable and nonviable microbes and microbial products, such as endotoxin, may spread to other tissues and organs through the epithelial mucosa into the mesenteric lymph nodes (MLNs) and blood vessels of the mesenteric circulation (Wiest and Rath 2003; Louis et al. 2013). The mechanisms of bacterial translocation include alteration in the normal gastrointestinal microflora and bacterial overgrowth, physical disruption of the gut mucosal barrier, and impaired host defense (Wiest and Rath 2003). Using mice infused with lipopolysaccharide and zymozan as an experimental model, it has been shown that these animals developed multiple organ dysfunction syndrome due to bacterial translocation from the intestine (Louis et al. 2013). Thus, the bacterial translocation may disrupt the homeostasis of gut or even whole body.

Dietary factors such as protein malnutrition may impair the antibacterial host defense and the gut–microbiota balance, while enteral or parenteral administration of glucose and amino acid solution is associated with modification of bacterial translocation (Deitch et al. 1987). Glutamine serves as a fuel source for cells such as intestine epithelial cells and plays a vital role in the maintenance of mucosal integrity (Brewster et al. 1998). The protective effects of glutamine against intestinal damage and bacterial translocation have been widely demonstrated. Earlier research conducted in rats with cerulein-induced acute pancreatitis showed that glutamine substitution may contribute to the reduction of bacterial translocation by improving gut barrier function (Foitzik et al. 1999). Glutamine availability plays a key role in the enterocytes for the modulation of bacterial translocation. Glutamine administration inhibits the tumor necrosis factor α-induced *Escherichia coli* translocation in Caco-2 epithelial cells, while under glutamine depletion the cytokine-induced bacterial translocation may be enhanced (Clark et al. 2003). Deprivation of dietary glutamine in infant rats by inhibiting glutamine synthase resulted in the increase of bacterial translocation (Potsic et al. 2002). In jaundiced rats, oral glutamine administration (20 mg/100 g body weight) has been shown to reduce bacterial translocation in blood and hepatocellular damage, to protect ileal epithelium and to reduce villus atrophy, suggesting an effective protection of glutamine in preventing or reducing bacterial translocation and oxidative damage (Karatepe et al. 2010). Glutamine treatment decreases the bacterial translocation by inhibiting the spread of *Escherichia coli* to organs such as liver, lung, and spleen in rats with intestinal obstruction (de Oliveira et al. 2006). Glutamine administration in LPS-challenged rats improves the intestinal microcirculation by increasing the functional capillary density of the intestine and decreasing the submucosal leukocyte activation, paralleled with the improvement of endotoxemia symptoms (Lehmann et al. 2012). Thus, glutamine may serve as an efficient protectant against bacterial translocation.

Although the mechanisms of glutamine against bacterial translocation remain unknown, the protective role of glutamine on intestine may possibly explain the phenomenon. Glutamine intake (0.5 g/kg ideal body weight) can significantly improve the intestinal permeability and the mucosal architecture in Crohn's disease patients (Benjamin et al. 2012), although in this study, the lack of a control group made the interpretation of the results difficult. Restoration of intestinal permeability and tight junctions has been reported after glutamine supplementation in different models both *in vitro* (Seth et al. 2004; Rao 2009; Beutheu et al. 2013) and *in vivo* (Beutheu et al. 2014). Pretreatment of Caco-2 cells with L-glutamine attenuated acetaldehyde-induced permeability to

LPS, which was associated with the prevention of acetaldehyde-induced redistribution of tight junction proteins, such as occludin, ZO-1 (Rao 2009). Conversion of glutamine into glutamate has been shown to be necessary in some studies (Vermeulen et al. 2011; Beutheu et al. 2013) while Seth et al. reported that inhibitor of glutaminase did not blunt glutamine effects (Seth et al. 2004).

It appears that the protective effect of L-glutamine is likely to be mediated by the transactivation of EGF receptor leading to activation of PKC and MAPK, which could induce the expression of tight junction proteins (Basuroy et al. 2005; Rao and Samak 2012). Other signaling pathways have also been proposed (Beutheu et al. 2014).

In summary, glutamine could mediate multiple protections against bacterial translocation and intestinal integrity. Although the molecular mechanisms of glutamine function are gradually uncovered, the clinical application of glutamine supplementation remains elusive and needs further future research since most studies performed have been experimental.

10.4 CONCLUSION AND PERSPECTIVES

Glutamine is highly metabolized in the small- and large-intestinal mucosa. In enterocytes and colonocytes, glutamine is converted into glutamate and ammonia, glutamate being a fuel substrate and a precursor of various compounds, including glutathione. Glutamine is also a precursor of several amino acids, including aspartate, alanine, proline, ornithine, and citrulline, which are released in the portal blood.

In animal models, glutamine is involved in numerous intestinal functions, including the maintenance of the gut barrier function through a regulating effect of this amino acid on the proliferation/apoptosis balance of intestinal epithelial cells through specific signaling pathways.

A significant part of glutamine released from alimentary and endogenous protein in the digestion process is used by the intestinal microbiota in various metabolic pathways, including deamination, transamination, decarboxylation, and protein synthesis. In addition, luminal glutamine interferes with the metabolism of several other amino acids by the intestinal bacteria.

Although studies with animal models of intestinal inflammation, mucosal healing, and endotoxemia suggest that glutamine supplementation is beneficial for the recovery of intestinal mucosal integrity and protection against bacterial translocation, the efficiency of such supplementation in clinical application remains presently elusive. Additional human studies are then required, in which glutamine, used individually and in combination with other deficient compounds from dietary origin, would be tested in supplements.

REFERENCES

Abad, B., J.E. Mesonero, M.T. Salvador et al. 2001. Effect of lipopolysaccharide on small intestinal L-leucine transport in rabbit. *Dig Dis Sci* 46(5):1113–9.
Akobeng, A.K., V. Miller, J. Stanton et al. 2000. Double-blind randomized controlled trial of glutamine-enriched polymeric diet in the treatment of active Crohn's disease. *J Pediatr Gastroenterol Nutr* 30(1):78–84.
Amagase, K., A. Ochi, A. Kojo et al. 2012. New therapeutic strategy for amino acid medicine: Prophylactic and healing promoting effect of monosodium glutamate against NSAID-induced enteropathy. *J Pharmacol Sci* 118(2):131–7.
Ameho, C.K., A.A. Adjei, E.K. Harrison et al. 1997. Prophylactic effect of dietary glutamine supplementation on interleukin 8 and tumour necrosis factor alpha production in trinitrobenzene sulphonic acid induced colitis. *Gut* 41(4):487–93.
Andriamihaja, M., A.M. Davila, M. Eklou-Lawson et al. 2010. Colon luminal content and epithelial cell morphology are markedly modified in rats fed with a high-protein diet. *Am J Physiol Gastrointest Liver Physiol* 299(5):G1030–7.
Aosasa, S., D. Wells-Byrum, J.W. Alexander et al. 2003. Influence of glutamine-supplemented Caco-2 cells on cytokine production of mononuclear cells. *JPEN J Parenter Enteral Nutr* 27(5):333–9.

Ardawi, M.S., Y.S. Jamal, A.A. Ashy et al. 1990. Glucose and glutamine metabolism in the small intestine of septic rats. *J Lab Clin Med* 115(6):660–8.

Ardawi, M.S. and M.F. Majzoub. 1991. Glutamine metabolism in skeletal muscle of septic rats. *Metabolism* 40(2):155–64.

Ardawi, M.S. and E.A. Newsholme. 1985. Fuel utilization in colonocytes of the rat. *Biochem J* 231(3):713–9.

Avissar, N.E., T.R. Ziegler, L. Toia et al. 2004. ATB0/ASCT2 expression in residual rabbit bowel is decreased after massive enterectomy and is restored by growth hormone treatment. *J Nutr* 134(9):2173–7.

Basuroy, S., P. Sheth, C.M. Mansbach et al. 2005. Acetaldehyde disrupts tight junctions and adherens junctions in human colonic mucosa: Protection by EGF and L-glutamine. *American Journal of Physiology-Gastrointestinal and Liver Physiology* 289(2):G367–G75.

Belmonte, L., M. Coeffier, F. Le Pessot et al. 2007. Effects of glutamine supplementation on gut barrier, glutathione content and acute phase response in malnourished rats during inflammatory shock. *World J Gastroenterol* 13(20):2833–40.

Benjamin, J., G. Makharia, V. Ahuja et al. 2012. Glutamine and whey protein improve intestinal permeability and morphology in patients with Crohn's disease: A randomized controlled trial. *Dig Dis Sci* 57(4):1000–12.

Berg, R.D. and A.W. Garlington. 1979. Translocation of certain indigenous bacteria from the gastrointestinal tract to the mesenteric lymph nodes and other organs in a gnotobiotic mouse model. *Infect Immun* 23(2):403–11.

Bergen, W.G. and G. Wu. 2009. Intestinal nitrogen recycling and utilization in health and disease. *J Nutr* 139(5):821–5.

Beutheu, S., I. Ghouzali, L. Galas et al. 2013. Glutamine and arginine improve permeability and tight junction protein expression in methotrexate-treated Caco-2 cells. *Clin Nutr* 32(5):863–9.

Beutheu, S., W. Ouelaa, C. Guerin et al. 2014. Glutamine supplementation, but not combined glutamine and arginine supplementation, improves gut barrier function during chemotherapy-induced intestinal mucositis in rats. *Clin Nutr* 33:694–701.

Beyreuther, K., H.K. Biesalski, J.D. Fernstrom et al. 2007. Consensus meeting: Monosodium glutamate—An update. *Eur J Clin Nutr* 61(3):304–13.

Blachier, F., C. Boutry, C. Bos et al. 2009. Metabolism and functions of L-glutamate in the epithelial cells of the small and large intestines. *Am J Clin Nutr* 90(3):814S–21S.

Blachier, F., G. Guihot-Joubrel, P. Vaugelade et al. 1999. Portal hyperglutamatemia after dietary supplementation with monosodium glutamate in pigs. *Digestion* 60(4):349–57.

Blachier, F., H. M'Rabet-Touil, L. Posho et al. 1992. Polyamine metabolism in enterocytes isolated from newborn pigs. *Biochim Biophys Acta* 1175(1):21–6.

Blachier, F., F. Mariotti, J.F. Huneau et al. 2007. Effects of amino acid-derived luminal metabolites on the colonic epithelium and physiopathological consequences. *Amino Acids* 33(4):547–62.

Boukhettala, N., S. Claeyssens, M. Bensifi et al. 2012. Effects of essential amino acids or glutamine deprivation on intestinal permeability and protein synthesis in HCT-8 cells: Involvement of GCN2 and mTOR pathways. *Amino Acids* 42:375–83.

Boutry, C., H. Matsumoto, C. Bos et al. 2012. Decreased glutamate, glutamine and citrulline concentrations in plasma and muscle in endotoxemia cannot be reversed by glutamate or glutamine supplementation: A primary intestinal defect? *Amino Acids* 43(4):1485–98.

Brewster, D., R. Kukuruzovic, and A. Haase. 1998. Short bowel syndrome, intestinal permeability and glutamine. *J Pediatr Gastroenterol Nutr* 27(5):614–6.

Chakravarthi, S., C.E. Jessop, and N.J. Bulleid. 2006. The role of glutathione in disulphide bond formation and endoplasmic-reticulum-generated oxidative stress. *EMBO Rep* 7(3):271–5.

Chambon-Savanovitch, C., M.C. Farges, F. Raul et al. 1999. Can a glutamate-enriched diet counteract glutamine depletion in endotoxemic rats? *J Nutr Biochem* 10(6):331–7.

Chen, G. and J.B. Russell. 1990. Transport and deamination of amino acids by a gram-positive, monensin-sensitive ruminal bacterium. *Applied and Environmental Microbiology* 56(7):2186–92.

Chen, G.J. and J.B. Russell. 1989. Sodium-dependent transport of branched-chain amino acids by a monensin-sensitive ruminal peptostreptococcus. *Appl Environ Microbiol* 55(10):2658–63.

Clark, E.C., S.D. Patel, P.R. Chadwick et al. 2003. Glutamine deprivation facilitates tumour necrosis factor induced bacterial translocation in Caco-2 cells by depletion of enterocyte fuel substrate. *Gut* 52(2):224–30.

Coeffier, M., B. Hecketsweiler, P. Hecketsweiler et al. 2005. Effect of glutamine on water and sodium absorption in human jejunum at baseline and during PGE1-induced secretion. *J Appl Physiol (1985)* 98(6):2163–8.

Coeffier, M., R. Marion, P. Ducrotte et al. 2003. Modulating effect of glutamine on IL-1beta-induced cytokine production by human gut. *Clin Nutr* 22(4):407–13.

Crouser, E.D., M.W. Julian, D.M. Weinstein et al. 2000. Endotoxin-induced ileal mucosal injury and nitric oxide dysregulation are temporally dissociated. *Am J Respir Crit Care Med* 161(5):1705–12.

Cynober, L.A. 2002. Plasma amino acid levels with a note on membrane transport: Characteristics, regulation, and metabolic significance. *Nutrition* 18(9):761–6.

Dai, Z.L., X.L. Li, P.B. Xi et al. 2013. L-Glutamine regulates amino acid utilization by intestinal bacteria. *Amino Acids* 45(3):501–12.

Dai, Z.L., J. Zhang, G. Wu et al. 2010. Utilization of amino acids by bacteria from the pig small intestine. *Amino Acids* 39(5):1201–15.

Dai, Z.L., G. Wu, and W.Y. Zhu. 2011. Amino acid metabolism in intestinal bacteria: Links between gut ecology and host health. *Front Biosci* 16:1768–86.

Darcy-Vrillon, B., M.T. Morel, C. Cherbuy et al. 1993. Metabolic characteristics of pig colonocytes after adaptation to a high fiber diet. *J Nutr* 123(2):234–43.

Darcy-Vrillon, B., L. Posho, M.T. Morel et al. 1994. Glucose, galactose, and glutamine metabolism in pig isolated enterocytes during development. *Pediatr Res* 36(2):175–81.

Darragh, A.J., P.D. Cranwell, and P.J. Moughan. 1994. Absorption of lysine and methionine from the proximal colon of the piglet. *Br J Nutr* 71(5):739–52.

Dashper, S.G., P.F. Riley, and E.C. Reynolds. 1995. Characterization of glutamine transport in *Streptococcus mutans*. *Oral Microbiol Immun* 10(3):183–87.

de Oliveira, M.A., D.S. Lemos, S.O.F. Diniz et al. 2006. Prevention of bacterial translocation using glutamine: A new strategy of investigation. *Nutrition* 22(4):419–24.

Deitch, E.A., J. Winterton, and R. Berg. 1987. Effect of starvation, malnutrition, and trauma on the gastrointestinal tract flora and bacterial translocation. *Arch Surg* 122(9):1019–24.

Den Hond, E., M. Hiele, M. Peeters et al. 1999. Effect of long-term oral glutamine supplements on small intestinal permeability in patients with Crohn's disease. *JPEN J Parenter Enteral Nutr* 23(1):7–11.

Duee, P.H., B. Darcy-Vrillon, F. Blachier et al. 1995. Fuel selection in intestinal cells. *Proc Nutr Soc* 54(1):83–94.

Eklou-Lawson, M., F. Bernard, N. Neveux et al. 2009. Colonic luminal ammonia and portal blood L-glutamine and L-arginine concentrations: A possible link between colon mucosa and liver ureagenesis. *Amino Acids* 37(4):751–60.

Elwafi, F., E. Curis, N. Zerrouk et al. 2012. Endotoxemia affects citrulline, arginine and glutamine bioavailability. *Eur J Clin Invest* 42(3):282–9.

Evans, M.E., D.P. Jones, and T.R. Ziegler. 2003. Glutamine prevents cytokine-induced apoptosis in human colonic epithelial cells. *J Nutr* 133(10):3065–71.

Fan, M.Z., O. Adeola, M.I. McBurney et al. 1998. Kinetic analysis of L-glutamine transport into porcine jejunal enterocyte brush-border membrane vesicles. *Comp Biochem Physiol A Mol Integr Physiol* 121(4):411–22.

Foitzik, T., M. Kruschewski, A.J. Kroesen et al. 1999. Does glutamine reduce bacterial translocation? A study in two animal models with impaired gut barrier. *Int J Colorectal Dis* 14(3):143–49.

Forchhammer, K. 2007. Glutamine signalling in bacteria. *Front Biosci* 12:358–70.

Gardiner, K. and A. Barbul. 1993. The role of the imino transporter protein in sepsis-impaired intestinal proline absorption. *JPEN J Parenter Enteral Nutr* 17(6):507–12.

Gardiner, K.R., G.M. Ahrendt, R.E. Gardiner et al. 1995. Failure of intestinal amino acid absorptive mechanisms in sepsis. *J Am Coll Surg* 181(5):431–6.

Garrett, W.S., J.I. Gordon, and L.H. Glimcher. 2010. Homeostasis and inflammation in the intestine. *Cell* 140(6):859–70.

Guven, A., M. Pehlivan, I. Gokpinar et al. 2007. Early glutamine-enriched enteral feeding facilitates colonic anastomosis healing: Light microscopic and immunohistochemical evaluation. *Acta Histochem* 109(2):122–9.

Haque, S.M., K. Chen, N. Usui et al. 1997. Effects of endotoxin on intestinal hemodynamics, glutamine metabolism, and function. *Surg Today* 27(6):500–5.

Hassoun, H.T., B.C. Kone, D.W. Mercer et al. 2001. Post-injury multiple organ failure: The role of the gut. *Shock* 15(1):1–10.

Higashiguchi, T., P.O. Hasselgren, K. Wagner et al. 1993. Effect of glutamine on protein synthesis in isolated intestinal epithelial cells. *JPEN J Parenter Enteral Nutr* 17(4):307–14.

Hubert-Buron, A., J. Leblond, A. Jacquot et al. 2006. Glutamine pretreatment reduces IL-8 production in human intestinal epithelial cells by limiting IkappaBalpha ubiquitination. *J Nutr* 136(6):1461–5.

Karatepe, O., E. Acet, M. Battal et al. 2010. Effects of glutamine and curcumin on bacterial translocation in jaundiced rats. *World J Gastroenterol* 16(34):4313.

King, C.J., S. Tytgat, R.L. Delude et al. 1999. Ileal mucosal oxygen consumption is decreased in endotoxemic rats but is restored toward normal by treatment with aminoguanidine. *Crit Care Med* 27(11):2518–24.

Klimberg, V.S., R.M. Salloum, M. Kasper et al. 1990. Oral glutamine accelerates healing of the small intestine and improves outcome after whole abdominal radiation. *Arch Surg* 125(8):1040–5.

Kretzmann, N.A., H. Fillmann, J.L. Mauriz et al. 2008. Effects of glutamine on proinflammatory gene expression and activation of nuclear factor kappa B and signal transducers and activators of transcription in TNBS-induced colitis. *Inflamm Bowel Dis* 14(11):1504–13.

Lan, A., F. Blachier, R. Benamouzig et al. 2015. Mucosal healing in inflammatory bowel diseases: Is there a place for nutritional supplementation? *Inflamm Bowel Dis* 21(1):198–207.

Le Bacquer, O., C. Laboisse, and D. Darmaun. 2003. Glutamine preserves protein synthesis and paracellular permeability in Caco-2 cells submitted to "luminal fasting." *Am J Physiol Gastrointest Liver Physiol* 285(1):G128–36.

Lecleire, S., A. Hassan, R. Marion-Letellier et al. 2008. Combined glutamine and arginine decrease proinflammatory cytokine production by biopsies from Crohn's patients in association with changes in nuclear factor-kappaB and p38 mitogen-activated protein kinase pathways. *J Nutr* 138(12):2481–6.

Lehmann, C., D. Pavlovic, J. Zhou et al. 2012. Intravenous free and dipeptide-bound glutamine maintains intestinal microcirculation in experimental endotoxemia. *Nutrition* 28(5):588–93.

Li, N., P. Lewis, D. Samuelson et al. 2004. Glutamine regulates Caco-2 cell tight junction proteins. *Am J Physiol Gastrointest Liver Physiol* 287(3):G726–33.

Libao-Mercado, A.J., C.L. Zhu, J.P. Cant et al. 2009. Dietary and endogenous amino acids are the main contributors to microbial protein in the upper gut of normally nourished pigs. *J Nutr* 139(6):1088–94.

Liboni, K.C., N. Li, P.O. Scumpia et al. 2005. Glutamine modulates LPS-induced IL-8 production through IkappaB/NF-kappaB in human fetal and adult intestinal epithelium. *J Nutr* 135(2):245–51.

Lima, A.A., G.H. Carvalho, A.A. Figueiredo et al. 2002. Effects of an alanyl-glutamine-based oral rehydration and nutrition therapy solution on electrolyte and water absorption in a rat model of secretory diarrhea induced by cholera toxin. *Nutrition* 18(6):458–62.

Liu, X., M. Beaumont, F. Walker et al. 2013. Beneficial effects of an amino acid mixture on colonic mucosal healing in rats. *Inflamm Bowel Dis* 19(13):2895–905.

Louis, K., M.G. Netea, D.-P. Carrer et al. 2013. Bacterial translocation in an experimental model of multiple organ dysfunctions. *J Surg Res* 183(2):686–94.

Madej, M., T. Lundh, and J.E. Lindberg. 2002. Activity of enzymes involved in energy production in the small intestine during suckling-weaning transition of pigs. *Biol Neonate* 82(1):53–60.

Manhart, N., K. Vierlinger, A. Spittler et al. 2001. Oral feeding with glutamine prevents lymphocyte and glutathione depletion of Peyer's patches in endotoxemic mice. *Ann Surg* 234(1):92–7.

Marc Rhoads, J. and G. Wu. 2009. Glutamine, arginine, and leucine signaling in the intestine. *Amino Acids* 37(1):111–22.

Marion, R., M.M. Coeffier, G. Gargala et al. 2004. Glutamine and CXC chemokines IL-8, Mig, IP-10 and I-TAC in human intestinal epithelial cells. *Clin Nutr* 23(4):579–85.

Merrick, M.J. and R.A. Edwards. 1995. Nitrogen control in bacteria. *Microbiological Reviews* 59(4):604–22.

Metges, C.C., K.J. Petzke, A.E. El-Khoury et al. 1999. Incorporation of urea and ammonia nitrogen into ileal and fecal microbial proteins and plasma free amino acids in normal men and ileostomates. *Am J Clin Nutr* 70(6):1046–58.

Mouille, B., V. Robert, and F. Blachier. 2004. Adaptative increase of ornithine production and decrease of ammonia metabolism in rat colonocytes after hyperproteic diet ingestion. *Am J Physiol Gastrointest Liver Physiol* 287(2):G344–51.

Newsholme, E.A. and A.L. Carrie. 1994. Quantitative aspects of glucose and glutamine metabolism by intestinal cells. *Gut* 35(1 Suppl):S13–7.

Ockenga, J., K. Borchert, E. Stuber et al. 2005. Glutamine-enriched total parenteral nutrition in patients with inflammatory bowel disease. *Eur J Clin Nutr* 59(11):1302–9.

Poolman, B., K.J. Hellingwerf, and W.N. Konings. 1987. Regulation of the glutamate-glutamine transport system by intracellular pH in *Streptococcus lactis*. *J Bacteriol* 169(5):2272–6.

Potsic, B., N. Holliday, P. Lewis et al. 2002. Glutamine supplementation and deprivation: Effect on artificially reared rat small intestinal morphology. *Pediatric Research* 52(3):430–6.

Rao, R. 2009. Occludin phosphorylation in regulation of epithelial tight junctions. *Ann N Y Acad Sci* 1165:62–8.

Rao, R.K. and G. Samak. 2012. Role of glutamine in protection of intestinal epithelial tight junctions. *J Epithelial Biol Pharmacol* 5:47–54.

Reeds, P.J. and D.G. Burrin. 2001. Glutamine and the bowel. *J Nutr* 131(9 Suppl):2505S–8S; discussion 23S–4S.

Reeds, P.J., D.G. Burrin, B. Stoll et al. 1997. Enteral glutamate is the preferential source for mucosal glutathione synthesis in fed piglets. *Am J Physiol* 273(2 Pt 1):E408–15.

Reitzer, L. 2003. Nitrogen assimilation and global regulation in *Escherichia coli*. *Annu Rev Microbiol* 57(1):155–76.

Rhoads, J.M., R.A. Argenzio, W. Chen et al. 1997. L-glutamine stimulates intestinal cell proliferation and activates mitogen-activated protein kinases. *Am J Physiol* 272(5 Pt 1):G943–53.

Salloum, R.M., E.M. Copeland, and W.W. Souba. 1991. Brush border transport of glutamine and other substrates during sepsis and endotoxemia. *Ann Surg* 213(5):401–9; discussion 09–10.

Scheppach, W., G. Dusel, T. Kuhn et al. 1996. Effect of L-glutamine and n-butyrate on the restitution of rat colonic mucosa after acid induced injury. *Gut* 38(6):878–85.

Seth, A., S. Basuroy, P. Sheth et al. 2004. L-Glutamine ameliorates acetaldehyde-induced increase in paracellular permeability in Caco-2 cell monolayer. *Am J Physiol Gastrointest Liver Physiol* 287(3):G510–7.

Sido, B., C. Seel, A. Hochlehnert et al. 2006. Low intestinal glutamine level and low glutaminase activity in Crohn's disease: A rational for glutamine supplementation? *Dig Dis Sci* 51(12):2170–9.

Souba, W.W., K. Herskowitz, V.S. Klimberg et al. 1990. The effects of sepsis and endotoxemia on gut glutamine metabolism. *Ann Surg* 211(5):543–9; discussion 49–51.

Swank, G.M. and E.A. Deitch. 1996. Role of the gut in multiple organ failure: Bacterial translocation and permeability changes. *World J Surg* 20(4):411–7.

Tsiotou, A.G., G.H. Sakorafas, G. Anagnostopoulos et al. 2005. Septic shock: Current pathogenetic concepts from a clinical perspective. *Med Sci Monit* 11(3):RA76–85.

Vermeulen, M.A., J. de Jong, M.J. Vaessen et al. 2011. Glutamate reduces experimental intestinal hyperpermeability and facilitates glutamine support of gut integrity. *World J Gastroenterol* 17(12):1569–73.

Wang, J., L. Chen, P. Li et al. 2008. Gene expression is altered in piglet small intestine by weaning and dietary glutamine supplementation. *J Nutr* 138(6):1025–32.

Wernerman, J. 2008. Clinical use of glutamine supplementation. *J Nutr* 138(10):2040S–44S.

Wiest, R. and H.C. Rath. 2003. Bacterial translocation in the gut. *Best Pract Res Clin Gastroenterol* 17(3):397–425.

Windmueller, H.G. and A.E. Spaeth. 1974. Uptake and metabolism of plasma glutamine by the small intestine. *J Biol Chem* 249(16):5070–9.

Windmueller, H.G. and A.E. Spaeth. 1976. Metabolism of absorbed aspartate, asparagine, and arginine by rat small intestine *in vivo*. *Arch Biochem Biophys* 175(2):670–6.

Windmueller, H.G. and A.E. Spaeth. 1978. Identification of ketone bodies and glutamine as the major respiratory fuels *in vivo* for postabsorptive rat small intestine. *J Biol Chem* 253(1):69–76.

Wu, G., F.W. Bazer, G.A. Johnson et al. 2010a. Important roles for L-glutamine in swine nutrition and production. *J Anim Sci*, 1: 2010–3614.

Wu, G., A.G. Borbolla, and D.A. Knabe. 1994. The uptake of glutamine and release of arginine, citrulline and proline by the small intestine of developing pigs. *J Nutr* 124(12):2437–44.

Wu, G., N.E. Flynn, W. Yan et al. 1995. Glutamine metabolism in chick enterocytes: Absence of pyrroline-5-carboxylase synthase and citrulline synthesis. *Biochem J* 306(Pt 3):717–21.

Wu, G. and D.A. Knabe. 1994. Free and protein-bound amino acids in sow's colostrum and milk. *J Nutr* 124(3):415–24.

Wu, X., C. Ma, L. Han et al. 2010b. Molecular characterisation of the faecal microbiota in patients with type II diabetes. *Curr Microbiol.* 61(1):69–78.

Xi, P., Z. Jiang, C. Zheng et al. 2010. Regulation of protein metabolism by glutamine: Implications for nutrition and health. *Front Biosci* 16:578–97.

Yaqoob, P. and P.C. Calder. 1998. Cytokine production by human peripheral blood mononuclear cells: Differential sensitivity to glutamine availability. *Cytokine* 10(10):790–4.

Yaryura-Tobias, J.A., A. Wolpert, L. White et al. 1970. A clinical evaluation of clopenthixol. *Curr Ther Res Clin Exp* 12(5):271–9.

11 Glutamine
General Facilitator of Gut Absorption and Repair

Essam Imseis, Yuying Liu, and J. Marc Rhoads

CONTENTS

11.1 INTRODUCTION

Glutamine (Gln) is the most abundant α-amino acid in human plasma and muscle tissue. It is also the primary metabolic fuel for the small intestine. Gln has been traditionally viewed as nonessential, inasmuch as the glutamate contained in the diet or intravenous blood can be converted in the liver and skeletal muscle to Gln. Gln is currently available for oral and parenteral use. In humans, it is used by bodybuilders to inhibit muscle breakdown and has been studied in infants with short bowel syndrome (SBS) and other types of diarrhea. Seminal work of Windmueller and Spaeth in the 1970s (Windmueller and Spaeth 1978, 1980) provided the observations leading to an explosion of Gln research in the 1980s and 1990s. This work showed that Gln was a major metabolic fuel of the small intestinal mucosa, significantly surpassing glucose and fatty acids.

In this review, we will discuss studies of our group and others relevant the effects of glutamine in the intestine. This chapter contains subsections as noted in the Table of Contents. We will discuss the effect of this important amino acid on Na^+ and fluid absorption; its impact on intestinal recovery from injury; and its unique signaling characteristics in the intestinal epithelium. Finally, its potential uses in human diseases will be outlined.

11.2   HISTORICAL OBSERVATIONS

Gln levels were found to be regulated by complex pathways within the bloodstream, liver, and intestine by elaborate interorgan metabolism and transport mechanisms. The clinical ramifications of Gln depletion were therefore difficult to study, because of the action of the enzyme Gln synthase, localized primarily in skeletal muscle, and, to a lesser extent, in liver, which maintains Gln levels by the conversion of glutamate to Gln (Watford et al. 2002). Similarly, administration of Gln enterally altered not only serum Gln level, but also the levels of several other amino acids, because of the action of specific enzymes, including phosphate-dependent glutaminase in the intestine, liver, kidneys, and immune system. A complex system of enzymes yielded critical levels of amino acids, including aspartate, proline, arginine, citrulline, ornithine, pyruvate, and other products (e.g., branched-chain α-ketoacids) into the portal circulation in a tissue-specific manner (Wu 1998).

By the 1990s, virtually all clinicians and investigators recognized that a certain level of Gln (> 0.5 mM) not only was desirable, but also was necessary for the health and function of the intestine. Others, mainly intensive care unit physicians, surgeons, gastroenterologists, and oncologists, wondered whether higher (supraphysiologic) levels could have therapeutic effects to enhance intestinal absorption and barrier function in various disease states. The 1990s witnessed international fervor in defining the role of Gln—in cancer-associated diarrhea syndromes, SBS, multiorgan system failure, oral rehydration solutions (ORSs) for acute diarrheal dehydration, chronic diarrhea, and inflammatory bowel disease.

11.3   GLUTAMINE STIMULATES INTESTINAL SALT AND WATER ABSORPTION

Our laboratory studied the effects of Gln on intestinal fluid and electrolyte absorption in piglets and calves for more than 15 years, with the aim being to determine whether Gln would be a useful addition to ORSs for humans with diarrhea (Rhoads et al. 1990; Rhoads 2004). The research by our group and others has consistently shown that Gln stimulates Na^+ absorption by electrogenic or Na^+-coupled absorption analogous to but distinct from glucose-Na^+ cotransport (Rhoads et al. 1991). In addition, Gln was found to stimulate electroneutral NaCl absorption (which is a coupled exchange at the brush border of Na^+ for H^+ and Cl^- for HCO_3^-) (Rhoads et al. 1990). Gln stimulates absorption in the jejunum or ileum of every mammalian species studied, including humans, chickens, pigs, rats, and cows, and is effective in newborn as well as older animals (Rhoads et al. 1990).

11.3.1   STUDIES IN MAMMALIAN SPECIES

We studied Gln in intestinal infectious enteropathies because of its potential as a therapeutic addition to ORS. Gln stimulated electrolyte absorption in rotavirus diarrhea (Rhoads et al. 1991) and in the enteritis produced by infection with *Cryptosporidium parvum* (Argenzio et al. 1994). Gln was additive to glucose in promoting Na^+ absorption (Rhoads et al. 1992; Grondahl and Skadhauge 1997). Gln was uniquely (and unexpectedly) capable of stimulating NaCl absorption when administered to the serosal (mesentery-facing) surface of the intestine (Rhoads et al. 1992). We postulated that the absorptive response to "blood-side" addition of Gln to the intestine was related to intracellular metabolism of Gln. Supporting this theory, we found that chemical blockade of

Gln-metabolizing enzymes such as phosphate-dependent glutaminase (with 6-diazo-5-oxo norleucine) or alanine aminotransferase (with amino (oxy)acetate) blocked the stimulation by Gln of electroneutral NaCl absorption (Rhoads et al. 1992). Our data were most consistent with a model in which the CO_2 produced by Gln metabolism yielded carbonic acid, which dissociated into H^+ and HCO_3^-, subsequently stimulating parallel exchanges in the gut brush border membrane (BBM) of Na^+ for H^+ and Cl^- for HCO_3^- (Rhoads et al. 1992) (Figure 11.1).

Subsequent research in other laboratories has identified three Na^+-dependent Gln transport mechanisms in the BBM: system B(o)AT1 (the dominant transporter), system A (ASCT2), and SN2 (Bode 2001; Saha et al. 2012). Recent work by Sundaram's group has shown that B(o)AT1 and SN2 transporters are differentially affected by intestinal chemotherapy injury in rabbits. In this intestinal disease, B(o)AT1 (localized to villus cell BBM) decreases while SN2 (localized to crypt cell BBM) increases (Saha et al. 2012). These findings could be relevant to infectious diarrhea, in which the epithelium is characterized by a crypt-dominant epithelium (Rhoads et al. 1990).

Other groups garnered similar evidence for the concept that Gln plus glucose could maximally enhance sodium absorption in the gut. Dechelotte et al. (1989) first showed that Gln and glucose have additive effects on Na^+ absorption in rabbit ileum, and (as mentioned) we found that this

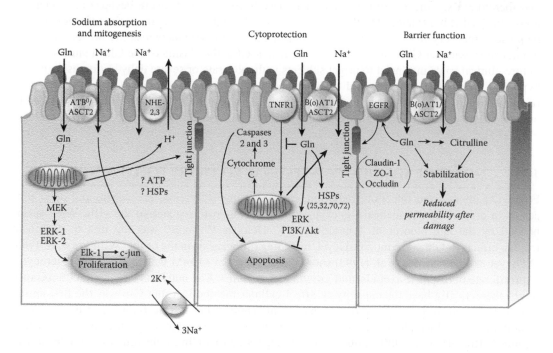

FIGURE 11.1 The figure summarizes the effects of Gln at the intestinal epithelial level. Gln enters the apical brush border membrane coupled to Na^+ across the B(o)AT1 or ASCT2 transporter. Its metabolism is linked to H^+ generation, which stimulates apical Na^+/H^+ exchange, across NHE2 or NHE3. Both processes contribute to transepithelial sodium absorption. Concomitantly, there is an enhancement of tight junction stability, leading to improved barrier function. Gln metabolism is also linked to mitogen-activated protein kinase (ERK) activation, leading to mitogenesis, and coupled with breast-milk components, Gln leads to more rapid villous repair. The middle cells shows pathways linked to Gln-enhanced cytoprotection. These include a block in the TNF-alpha receptor-mediated activation of caspases 2 and 3 via cytochrome c, which leaks out following the mitochondrial permeability transition. Additionally, Gln stimulates intestinal levels of heat shock proteins 25, 32, 70, and 72. The functions, along with ERK activation and PI-3 kinase activation also inhibit apoptosis during intestinal stress. Finally, Gln-mediated barrier stabilization is associated with increased levels of tight-junction-associated claudin-1, zonula-occludens-1, and occludin, all dependent on the activation of the epidermal growth factor receptor by Gln. Citrulline derived from Gln may also contribute to this effect, based on *in vitro* studies of epithelial cell membrane hypoxic damage.

additivity persists even in intestines infected with cryptosporidium and rotavirus (Rhoads et al. 1991; Argenzio et al. 1994). Desjeux et al. (1994) showed that Gln augments glucose in enhancing Na^+ absorption in a rabbit model of enteroadherent *Escherichia coli* diarrhea. Finally, Islam et al. in Bangladesh (Islam et al. 1997) and Silva et al. in Charlottesville, VA, USA (Silva et al. 1998) showed that Gln stimulates more Na^+ absorption than glucose in normal and cholera toxin-exposed rabbit intestine.

11.3.2 HUMAN STUDIES OF GLN IN ORAL REHYDRATION

In human volunteers, Van Loon et al. showed that Gln and glucose had comparable proabsorptive effects on intestinal Na^+ and water absorption (van Loon et al. 1996). Although separate absorption mechanisms were postulated, a clinical trial in Brazil comparing Gln-supplemented ORS with standard ORS in infants with diarrhea showed no difference in efficacy of the two preparations (Ribeiro et al. 1994). One criticism of this otherwise well-designed study was that the ORS supplemented with Gln was hypertonic, which could have drawn water into the intestinal lumen. Additionally, the study subjects were only mildly dehydrated (weight ~2% below rehydrated weight) at admission, and therefore a significant clinical effect may have been hard to measure because of "signal-to-noise" problems. If a trophic effect of Gln following villus injury secondary to the infection were to be present, recovery from diarrhea could occur by this additional mechanism. However, this study did not show whether Gln concentrations were increased in the plasma of the Gln-treated subjects. Future clinical trials may need to target subjects with moderate or severe dehydration using iso- or hypotonic rehydration solutions and to determine if the supplemental dose of Gln is sufficient to raise its concentration in the circulation. A review discussing the potential for Gln to be added to oral treatment solutions for infants with diarrhea was published by Guerrant's group (Carneiro-Filho et al. 2003).

11.4 GLUTAMINE STIMULATES INTESTINAL RECOVERY FOLLOWING INJURY

Following injury from infection, radiation, chemotherapy, starvation, endotoxin, and other processes, a critical step in recovery is crypt cell proliferation to regenerate the villi. Work spearheaded by the late pioneer of "glutaminology," Douglas Wilmore, was the first to document trophic effects of Gln at the mucosal level, including mitogenesis in the crypt (Wilmore et al. 1988; O'Dwyer et al. 1989). Ko et al. (1993) showed that a level of ~1 mM was required for enterocytes to proliferate in response to epidermal growth factor (EGF). Any nutrient of such vital importance might theoretically have the capacity to affect cellular metabolism, but Gln was the first amino acid to be found to not only improve oxidative metabolism but also to target specific mitogenic protein kinases, which phosphorylated their downstream targets (signaling which occurred within minutes) (Rhoads et al. 2000). Thus, Wilmore suggested that Gln might function as a "primitive hormone" for the gut.

During the past 20 years, more than 2000 scientific articles focusing on Gln have been published. However, the clinical research on Gln has not consistently shown beneficial effects. The most convincing studies showing Gln efficacy have been in severe stress models. These include multiorgan system failure, endotoxemia, skin burns, and cancer. Findings in rodent and pig models have been relatively consistent. Some examples of animal studies relevant to human disease from recent research will be summarized.

11.4.1 COLITIS

In a model of colitis in rats induced by dextran sodium sulfate (DSS), Wischmeyer's group showed that oral gavage feeding of Gln reduced diarrhea and blood in the stool, and induced protective levels of heat shock protein (HSP)25 and HSP70 in the colon (Xue et al. 2011). Studies in humans with Crohn's disease have not shown benefit of Gln with respect to induction of remission (Akobeng et al. 2000) or gut permeability (Den et al. 1999; Benjamin et al. 2012). However, in adults with ulcerative colitis, a Chinese trial of a Gln enterosoluble capsule added to a retention enema with glucocorticoid and metronidazole was superior to the steroid-metronidazole enema without Gln in producing remission of symptoms (Tan et al. 2008).

11.4.2 ENDOTOXIC GUT INJURY

Li et al. showed that in a "pup-in-a-cup" model of newborn intestinal inflammation, in which lipopolysaccharide (LPS) was fed orally, Gln-feeding reduced cytokine-induced neutrophil chemoatrractant (CINC) levels and oxidative injury (Li et al. 2004). Wischmeyer's group showed that endotoxic injury in septic rats was prevented by Gln feeding, and HSP25 and HSP70 were induced by Gln in the gut and lung (Wischmeyer 2002). In another sepsis model produced by cecal ligation and puncture, single-dose intravenous Gln improved survival and oxygenation, and reduced lung mechanical injury (Oliveira et al. 2009). In the intestine, enterocyte apoptosis and villus tip necrosis were largely prevented.

11.4.3 HYPOXIC INJURY

We aimed to determine the best way to promote villus regrowth after hypoxic injury, using a model of ischemia/reperfusion (I/R) injury in pigs with Thiry-Vella loops. In these loops, the villi were destroyed consistently by transient mesenteric arterial ligation; the technique allowed 100% animal survival despite severe gut injury. Gln and growth factors could then be instilled in the lumen. The procedure allowed several treatments to be compared simultaneously. We found that regrowth of villi was rapid and was not stimulated individually by Gln or transforming growth factor-alpha (TGF-α, a trophic component of breast milk), but was optimally stimulated by both together (Blikslager et al. 1999). An early event during the recovery process in response to Gln and TGF-α was recovery of two triglyceride-synthesizing enzymes in the mucosa mono- and diacylglycerol acyltransferases (Ahdieh et al. 1998).

Others have found beneficial effects of Gln given individually in oxidant injury models. For example, after ischemia reperfusion injury, a single dose of intravenous Gln reduced histological injury while reducing plasma levels of tumor necrosis factor (TNF)-α, inhibiting nitrotyrosylation of gut tissues, blocking gut nuclear factor-kappa B (NF-κB) activation, and reducing intestinal cell apoptosis, as measured by terminal deoxynucleotidyl transferase dUTP nick end labeling (TUNEL) assay and Bax/Bcl-2 levels (Mondello et al. 2010). In a rat model of high-altitude hypoxia, bacterial and endotoxin translocation as well as intestinal villus exfoliation were largely prevented by Gln administration (Zhou et al. 2011).

11.4.4 WEANLING DIARRHEA

One condition leading to perinatal mortality in the swine and beef industries is "weanling scours," a diarrheal condition associated with bacterial and viral infection (Lecce et al. 1982). Feeding 0.5% Gln during the weaning period reduced the incidence of diarrhea, and at the gut level, normalized villus and crypt height in the gut while reducing apoptosis (Jagust and Budinger 1992).

11.4.5 INTESTINAL INJURY ASSOCIATED WITH CANCER AND IMMUNOSUPPRESSANT THERAPY

In clinical practice, some of the most severe cases of diarrhea occur in patients receiving treatment for cancer. Very strong evidence has been presented for Gln in the preservation and recovery of intestinal structure following radiation injury. Both the villi and crypts are longer with oral Gln (Klimberg et al. 1990; Nambu et al. 1992; Campos et al. 1996), and the effect may be mediated by induction of heme oxygenase-1 (HO-1) (Giris et al. 2006). In a model of radiation-induced intestinal damage, inhibition of HO-1 with zinc protoporphyrin (Giris et al. 2006) or tin mesoporphyrin (Uehara et al. 2005) blocked the protective effect of Gln.

In one of the many studies looking at drug-induced gut injury, Gln reduced injury produced by the immunosuppressant methotrexate, while reducing membrane lipid peroxidation (Gulgun et al. 2010). Arginyl-glutamine dipeptide had similar protective effects (Li et al. 2012).

One intestinal-toxic agent is methionine sulfoximine, an inhibitor of glutamine synthase. Neu's group was able to produce villous atrophy in artificially fed rat pups via inhibition of Gln synthesis plus withdrawal from luminal Gln. Their procedures resulted in shorter ileal villi and sloughing of microvilli with degeneration of the terminal web (Potsic et al. 2002), and the effects could be reversed with Gln. Note that elevated concentrations of methionine sulfoximine may have other toxic effects than to act as an inhibitor of glutamine synthetase. Results from the rat and pig small intestines indicate the near absence of this enzyme from their mucosae.

11.4.6 OTHER MODELS

Other animal models of injury ameliorated or prevented by Gln include traumatic brain injury-associated intestinal damage (Feng et al. 2007), indomethacin injury (Basivireddy et al. 2004), and surgical manipulation injury (Prabhu et al. 2003).

11.5 MECHANISTIC CONSIDERATIONS REGARDING GLN IN MUCOSAL RECOVERY

Before discussing human trials of Gln in systemically ill patients, it is important to consider that Gln may protect the epithelium *from* injury as well as facilitate mucosal regeneration *following* damage.

11.5.1 GLN IS A SIGNAL TO ENHANCE EPITHELIAL INTEGRITY AND CELL SURVIVAL IN THE INTESTINE AND OTHER CRITICAL ORGANS

One way that Gln benefits the intestine is by stimulating its crypt-residing stem cells to proliferate, predominantly via mitogen-activated protein kinases (MAPKs) or extracellular signal-regulated kinases (ERKs). Gln also enhances cell survival in the intestine via HSPs and by inhibiting enterocyte apoptosis. A paradigm that we proposed was that the intestinal cell is like a Ferrari, with the fuel (Gln) when at high levels "pumping" a rapid start, and subsequently burning smoothly during the cruise. If the car were to run out of fuel, the car would drift into neutral and then become idle. Using this paradigm, acceleration would be analogous to Gln activating mitosis via the MAPKs (ERK-1 and ERK-2) (Rhoads et al. 1997), coasting analogous to maintaining physiological serum Gln levels for gut homeostasis (including crypt cell proliferation and migration up toward the villus tip), and braking analogous to causing a reduction in ambient Gln (Rhoads et al. 2000), which activates stress pathways, including Jun nuclear kinases (JNKs) (Beutheu et al. 2013), HSPs (Wischmeyer et al. 2001), leading to a "stop": intestinal cellular apoptosis (Larson et al. 2007).

11.5.1.1 Activation of Protective HSPs

Gln-mediated activation of the HSP pathway is responsible for cellular protection which has been tested in fibroblasts (Morrison et al. 2006) and intestinal epithelial cells (Wischmeyer et al. 1997). In-depth investigation of the mechanism by which Gln induces HSPs in intestinal cell lines has shown that luminal physiological Gln doses (1–5 mM), when applied to Gln-starved cells, increased their resistance to oxidant-mediated cell death, while nonmetabolizable analogue D-Gln was ineffective (Wischmeyer et al. 1997). To confirm Gln cytoprotection *in vivo*, rats were injected with Gln intravenously, resulting in supraphysiological serum levels (3–5 mM) transiently. Moreover, the Gln "blast" activated HSP25 (another smaller molecular weight HSP) in multiple organs, including the lung, heart, liver, and colon (Wischmeyer et al. 2001). This induction provided protection of the rats from a subsequent systemic challenge with bacterial endotoxin that was lethal in control rats (Wischmeyer et al. 2001). Gln treatment of intestinal and other epithelial cells also induces HSP70 (Wischmeyer et al. 1997) and 72 (Ropeleski et al. 2005) levels.

Another member of the HSP family is HO-1, a 32-kDa HSP. In several disease models, Gln protection requires HO-1 induction. For example, as mentioned, inhibition of HO-1 with zinc protoporphyrin blocked the protective effect of Gln in a model of radiation-induced intestinal damage (Giris et al. 2006). Similar findings were observed in rats injected with endotoxin. Uehara et al. showed that Gln treatment markedly induced HO-1 messenger RNA and protein in colonic epithelial cells as well as in the lamina propria cells in the ileum and the colon. If given before LPS administration, Gln significantly ameliorated LPS-induced mucosal injury, inflammation, and apoptotic cell death in the ileum and the colon, while reducing mortality (Uehara et al. 2005). Support for Gln induction of HSP is now strong; and even in critically ill humans, intravenous Gln increases circulating HSP70 expression (Ziegler et al. 2005).

11.5.1.2 Antiapoptotic Effects

Gln starvation induces apoptosis in enterocytes (Papaconstantinou et al. 1998). Evans et al. showed that tumor necrosis factor-alpha-related apoptosis-inducing ligand (TRAIL)-induced apoptosis was completely prevented by Gln, but was not inhibited by other amino acids, including the glutathione (GSH) constituents, glutamate, cysteine, and glycine. Cellular GSH was oxidized during TRAIL-induced apoptosis, an effect which was completely blocked by Gln. However, inhibition of GSH synthesis did not alter antiapoptotic effects of Gln. Thus, the concept was proposed that Gln specifically protects intestinal epithelial cells against cytokine-induced apoptosis, and that this occurs by a mechanism that is distinct from the protection against oxidative stress mediated by cellular GSH (Evans et al. 2003).

11.5.1.3 ERK and PI3K Pathway

Extracellular-signal-related kinase (ERK) and phosphatidylinositol-3 kinase (PI3K) signaling pathways play critical roles in regulating the effects of Gln on intestinal cell growth and survival (Larson et al. 2007). Recent studies on apoptosis and its relationship to the ERK pathway indicated that apoptosis was significantly increased following an ERK inhibition. Addition of Gln activated ERK and prevented cell apoptosis. The studies suggested a critical role for the ERK-signaling pathways in Gln-mediated cytoprotection. Furthermore, the activation of PI3K/Akt, the important pathways in cell growth and survival, was also assessed. The results showed that Gln starvation increased phosphorylated Akt levels; inhibition of Akt enhanced intestinal cell DNA fragmentation. Thus, the activation of PI3K/Akt during periods of Gln deprivation likely occurs as a protective mechanism to limit apoptosis associated with cellular stress (Larson et al. 2007).

11.5.2 Barrier Function: Gln Is Necessary for Tight Junction Stabilization

Tight junctions containing proteins such as occludin, zonula occludens-1 (ZO-1), and claudins anchor the intestinal epithelial cells together, much in the way that the plastic rings hold together a six pack of soda. Studies of intestinal cell monolayers have provided a mechanistic explanation for how Gln levels may impact the ability of the intestinal barrier to withstand injury. Li et al. showed that Gln deprivation caused dissolution of membrane-bound components of the tight junction claudin-1 and ZO-1 in Caco-2 cell monolayers (Li et al. 2004). Additionally, electron microscopic evaluation of Gln-deprived tissues showed a reduction in electron-dense material at the zonula occludens, rescued by 0.6 mM Gln. Simultaneous work from Seth et al. showed that enterocyte monolayer damage produced by acetaldehyde produced a dissolving effect on tight junction ZO-1, E-cadherin, and beta-catenin, which was completely rescued by 2 mM Gln. Interestingly, the tight junction-stabilizing effect was not inhibited by inhibiting Gln metabolism (Seth et al. 2004). In the setting of barrier disruption with intestinal monolayer exposure to acetaldehyde, Gln induced a rapid increase in the tyrosine phosphorylation of EGF receptor, and the protective effect of diglutamine (GlnGln) was prevented by AG1478, an EGF-receptor tyrosine kinase inhibitor. Gln protection of tight junctions in other models appears to require intact glutaminase function, essential to its oxidation (Beutheu et al. 2013); however, at least some of the protective effect may be shared with two of its alternative metabolites, citrulline and arginine (Chapman et al. 2012; Beutheu et al. 2013).

11.6 HUMAN STUDIES OF GLN IN GUT INJURY

There have been a number of relatively small human trials determining if Gln has benefit in certain diseases. None of these trials have conclusively shown benefit in a human disease, although most likely issues of statistical power and an ineffective dosage may have masked potential benefits.

11.6.1 *In Vitro* Studies of Human Biopsy Materials

The studies have supported a role of Gln in reducing proinflammatory IL-6 and IL-8 production by intestinal biopsies, while increasing anti-inflammatory IL-10 levels in the intestinal cells and circulating mononuclear cells (Coeffier et al. 2001, 2003). When extended to *in vivo* randomized, controlled trials, Gln appeared to reduce morbidity and gut permeability in patients with multiorgan system trauma (Houdijk et al. 1998). A number of subsequent studies confirmed beneficial findings in critically ill patients (Avenell 2006; Coeffier et al. 2008; Sevastiadou et al. 2011). Gln has been added to total parenteral nutrition (TPN) but is rarely given orally, except in experimental studies. In practice, Gln is rarely added to parenteral nutrition (PN) solutions, largely because PN with a small amount of Gln is spontaneously cyclized at room temperature to form pyroglutamic acid (a neurotoxic substance).

11.6.2 Gln and Nosocomial Infections

Yarandi et al. (2011) in Ziegler's group in a recent review of PN summarized a large number of clinical trials. The broad picture is that Gln indeed decreases nosocomial infections in critically ill patients and in bone marrow transplant patients (Yarandi et al. 2011); however, it has not been shown that Gln reduces length of hospital stay or mortality. Currently, we use Gln on an ad hoc basis; for example, in children with chronic diarrhea after bone marrow transplantation (BMT).

11.6.3 Gln in Cancer

The requirement of Gln in cell growth and survival has led to debate regarding its role in tumor biology. The high metabolic demands of rapidly growing tumors and the observation that Gln-supplemented cancer cells may have increased proliferation have led some investigators to target this pathway as an avenue for pharmacologic therapy in cancer (Eagle et al. 1956). Such efforts have been unsuccessful to date but continue to be pursued. In contrast to these earlier observations, some studies appear to show benefit of Gln supplementation in certain types of cancers (Hensley et al. 2013).

The role of Gln in treatment of recipients of BMT has been extensively studied. Individuals receiving BMT are often susceptible to complications often associated with injury to rapidly dividing cells, including enterocytes and immune cells. Gastrointestinal toxicity resulting in mucositis and diarrhea can be noted in up to three-fourths of BMT recipients (Woo et al. 1993; van Kraaij et al. 2000). Infectious complications are also common in these individuals and may be the result of bacterial, fungal, or viral infections, and this risk of infection may be due to increased translocation of infectious pathogens from the injured gut into the bloodstream. Protection from Gln could result from barrier stabilization or from direct immune-stimulating effects on cytokine production and immune cell proliferation (Soeters and Grecu 2012).

Because Gln is fuel for the enterocyte and because it is utilized by rapidly growing enterocytes and immune cells, there is some rationale for its use in cancer treatment following the BMT. In Gln-fed mice, Gln was noted to reduce intestinal damage, bloody diarrhea, and mortality following administration of radiation or methotrexate (Fox et al. 1988; Klimberg et al. 1990). Use of Gln in humans has produced conflicting results. To date, there are over 25 studies utilizing Gln in BMT recipients of varying methodological quality and study heterogeneity. A number of reviews of these studies reveal that benefits of Gln supplementation in these patients are inconclusive. A recent Cochrane review demonstrated a reduced incidence of positive blood cultures in BMT patients receiving PN supplemented with Gln but no clear effect on hospital length of stay (Tubman et al. 2008). A subsequent meta-analysis of 17 trials revealed a decreased incidence of mucositis and opioid use with oral Gln supplementation and a reduced incidence of positive blood cultures in BMT patients receiving intravenous Gln. This meta-analysis also noted a potential increased risk of disease tumor relapse noted in two small studies (Crowther et al. 2009). The European Society for Clinical Nutrition and Metabolism (ESPEN) guidelines concluded that there is potential benefit for Gln supplementation in doses of 0.6 g/kg/day, based on their review of the available literature (Bozzetti et al. 2009).

One reason for equivocal clinical results in the face of overwhelming preclinical evidence for efficacy is that Gln could be beneficial in only certain subgroups of patients, such as those with low serum Gln levels. Alternatively, the patients are deficient not only in Gln but also in other amino acids (e.g., arginine). Review of the animal studies shows that often higher than physiological luminal concentrations (2–3 mM) were often used. Consider the effects of three levels of administration: "*serum* physiological" (mimicking normal levels of 600–800 micromolar (μM) in serum); "*lumen physiological levels*" (mimicking postprandial levels as measured in the intestine of suckling pigs by Wu and Knabe (95% confidence interval = 1–4 mM) (Wu and Knabe 1994); or *pharmacological* levels (>4 mM). Suboptimal dosing may have affected results in human trials.

11.6.4 GLN IN THE PREVENTION OF NECROTIZING ENTEROCOLITIS

As an example of the importance of considering Gln levels, a well-designed and well-powered, multicenter, placebo-controlled trial aimed to determine if premature infants would achieve feeding tolerance earlier if Gln were administered in TPN. This study, conducted by the multicenter Neonatal Network, was designed in such a way that the protocol required the removal of 25% of the essential and nonessential amino acids from the PN, to be replaced with Gln, rather than supplementation of the standard solution with Gln or alternative amino acids (Poindexter et al. 2004). This is a questionable experimental design. Consequently, serum Gln levels increased only from a mean value of 291 to 381 μM (Poindexter et al. 2003), which is inadequate. In the adult studies that have shown beneficial effects of Gln in patients with multiple traumas or in surgical patients, serum Gln levels have always exceeded 530 μM (Houdijk et al. 1998; Novak et al. 2002; Beale et al. 2008). This level is well below the level of ~1 mM that has been shown to protect from apoptosis and stabilize tight junctions *in vitro* (Ko et al. 2001). Note that levels in human milk are ~600 μM compared with about 50 μM in formula, with glutamate values about twice this high (Baldeon et al. 2014).

A number of subsequent neonatal studies in more than 2700 premature infants appear to have the same conclusion of lack of Gln efficacy. The most recent review had a total of five studies that reported that Gln was "added to parenteral nutrition," but in at least the above-mentioned study, it was actually subtracted from total amino acid nutrition; in only five smaller studies was it used as a supplement, given enterally. Serum Gln levels were not measured in most of the studies and were low in those in which it was reported (Moe-Byrne et al. 2012). Recently, a Cochrane Database systematic review analyzed 12 studies of 2877 preterm infants that were investigated in randomized controlled trials or quasi-randomized trials. Half the studies looked at effects of enteral Gln and half determined the results of intravenous Gln (Moe-Byrne et al. 2012). Results showed no change in mortality, incidence of infectious complications, or incidence of NEC. However, in this and previous Cochrane reviews, there is no mention of which studies added Gln to standard amino acid requirements and compared with an isonitrogenous control, and which studies subtracted required amino acids and replaced with Gln, and even more importantly which determined whether Gln serum levels were restored to normal (Moe-Byrne et al. 2012). There have been only three trials looking at neurodevelopmental outcomes in Gln-treated premature babies (with inconclusive results). One study of 65 preterm infants showed that the head circumference and white and gray matter volumes were increased in children who received Gln (de Kieviet et al. 2014).

11.6.5   GLN IN SHORT BOWEL SYNDROME

Use of Gln supplementation has also been studied in individuals with SBS following massive small bowel resection. Individuals with SBS may experience a period of intestinal adaptation following massive bowel resection, a time when need for PN support decreases and enteral tolerance increases as a result of structural or functional changes in the intestinal mucosa. These individuals are susceptible to systemic infections, often from gut-derived bacteria that may translocate through the bowel wall through a disrupted intestinal mucosa. Glutamine supplementation in those with SBS may therefore be helpful, given the trophic effects of Gln. Glutamine's immunomodulatory effects may also be helpful in management of SBS, inasmuch as there may be an increased risk for bacterial gut translocation and subsequent systemic bacterial infection.

In animals, results of studies in which Gln was used to stimulate intestinal adaptation are conflicting, with some studies revealing improvement in mucosal mass and others revealing no improvement in intestinal mass with Gln supplementation (Tamada et al. 1992; Vanderhoof et al. 1992). Nevertheless, there may be immunoprotective effects attributable to Gln in animal models of SBS. In a rat model of SBS, the replacement of 20% of the dietary casein with Gln appeared to result in increased total serum antibodies, decreased serum antibody to bacterial LPS, and increased stool intestinal immunoglobulin A (Tian et al. 2009).

Despite these observations, human studies utilizing Gln in conjunction with conventional PN support have been disappointing. Scolapio et al. (2001) performed a randomized placebo controlled trial in eight adult patients with SBS with 8 weeks of oral Gln supplementation and noted no improvement in intestinal morphology, gastrointestinal transit, D-xylose absorption, or stool output with Gln. A recent Cochrane review in neonates with severe gastrointestinal disease found no obvious benefit with intravenous or enteral Gln supplementation although only two studies were deemed to be of methodologic quality for inclusion in this analysis (Wagner et al. 2012).

Glutamine has also been used in conjunction with growth hormone (GH) in patients with SBS (Ziegler et al. 2003). A pilot unblended study by Byrne et al. (1995) in patients with PN-dependent SBS showed that a 3-week regimen of GH administration, intravenous or oral Gln (30 g/day), and a high-carbohydrate/low-fat diet significantly improved intestinal sodium, fluid, nitrogen, and energy absorption and improved lean body mass. In a larger group of chronic SBS patients undergoing the same protocol of GH+Gln+diet modification for three weeks followed by maintenance on the modified diet and Gln supplementation alone, PN requirements were either eliminated or markedly decreased in a large proportion of the patients at follow-up 1 year later (Byrne et al. 1995). Later, a prospective, double-blind, randomized, placebo-controlled clinical trial performed in 41 adults dependent on PN with SBS indicated that only subjects receiving GH+Gln+diet maintained significant reductions in PN for at least 3 months (Byrne et al. 1995). However, both a Cochrane review as well as a statement by the European Society for Clinical Nutrition and Metabolism does not recommend GH with or without Gln use for routine use because there is no clear beneficial effect of this treatment (Van et al. 2009; Wales et al. 2010).

In summary, based on the available literature, there does not appear to be good evidence for recommending Gln for routine use in individuals with SBS, particularly in those receiving some enteral feedings. One possible explanation for the lack of efficacy of Gln in short bowel syndrome is that its serum levels are higher in these subjects because less Gln is metabolized by the intestine.

11.7 CONCLUSIONS

It is an enigma that the major popular use today for Gln appears to be for bodybuilders who consume Gln powder to enhance muscle mass. However, it should be noted that guidelines published by the European Society for Clinical Nutrition and Metabolism and the German Association for Nutritional Medicine recommended that patients in the intensive care unit receive 0.2–0.4 g/kg/day Gln intravenously daily. In the United States, it has been recommended that "use should be considered if a product is available" (Yarandi et al. 2011). Clearly, interest in Gln has faded from its high glory in the late twentieth century, but Gln remains of considerable widespread interest in the medical-surgical-intensive care community and particularly among those interested in optimizing intestinal function—for example, those who treat diarrheal diseases and patients receiving chemotherapy and radiation therapy.

REFERENCES

Ahdieh N, Blikslager AT, Bhat BG, Coleman RA, Argenzio RA, and Rhoads JM. 1998. L-glutamine and transforming growth factor-alpha enhance recovery of monoacylglycerol acyltransferase and diacylglycerol acyltransferase activity in porcine postischemic ileum. *Pediatr Res* 43(2):227–233.

Akobeng AK, Miller V, Stanton J, Elbadri AM, and Thomas AG. 2000. Double-blind randomized controlled trial of glutamine-enriched polymeric diet in the treatment of active Crohn's disease. *J Pediatr Gastroenterol Nutr* 30(1):78–84.

Argenzio RA, Rhoads JM, Armstrong M, and Gomez G. 1994. Glutamine stimulates prostaglandin-sensitive Na(+)-H+ exchange in experimental porcine cryptosporidiosis. *Gastroenterology* 106(6):1418–1428.

Avenell A. 2006. Glutamine in critical care: Current evidence from systematic reviews. *Proc Nutr Soc* 65(3):236–241.

Baldeon ME, Mennella JA, Flores N, Fornasini M, and San GA. 2014. Free amino acid content in breast milk of adolescent and adult mothers in Ecuador. *Springerplus* 3:104.

Basivireddy J, Jacob M, and Balasubramanian KA. 2004. Oral glutamine attenuates indomethacin-induced small intestinal damage. *Clin Sci (Lond)* 107(3):281–289.

Beale RJ, Sherry T, Lei K, Campbell-Stephen L, McCook J, Smith J, Venetz W, Alteheld B, Stehle P, and Schneider H. 2008. Early enteral supplementation with key pharmaconutrients improves Sequential Organ Failure Assessment score in critically ill patients with sepsis: Outcome of a randomized, controlled, double-blind trial. *Crit Care Med* 36(1):131–144.

Benjamin J, Makharia G, Ahuja V, Anand Rajan KD, Kalaivani M, Gupta SD, and Joshi YK. 2012. Glutamine and whey protein improve intestinal permeability and morphology in patients with Crohn's disease: A randomized controlled trial. *Dig Dis Sci* 57(4):1000–1012.

Beutheu S, Ghouzali I, Galas L, Dechelotte P, and Coeffier M. 2013. Glutamine and arginine improve permeability and tight junction protein expression in methotrexate-treated Caco-2 cells. *Clin Nutr* 32(5):863–869.

Blikslager AT, Rhoads JM, Bristol DG, Roberts MC, and Argenzio RA. 1999. Glutamine and transforming growth factor-alpha stimulate extracellular regulated kinases and enhance recovery of villous surface area in porcine ischemic-injured intestine. *Surgery* 125(2):186–194.

Bode BP. 2001. Recent molecular advances in mammalian glutamine transport. *J Nutr* 131(9 Suppl):2475S–2485S.

Bozzetti F, Arends J, Lundholm K, Micklewright A, Zurcher G, and Muscaritoli M. 2009. ESPEN Guidelines on Parenteral Nutrition: Non-surgical oncology. *Clin Nutr* 28(4):445–454.

Byrne TA, Morrissey TB, Nattakom TV, Ziegler TR, and Wilmore DW. 1995. Growth hormone, glutamine, and a modified diet enhance nutrient absorption in patients with severe short bowel syndrome. *JPEN J Parenter Enteral Nutr* 19(4):296–302.

Byrne TA, Persinger RL, Young LS, Ziegler TR, and Wilmore DW. 1995. A new treatment for patients with short-bowel syndrome. Growth hormone, glutamine, and a modified diet. *Ann Surg* 222(3):243–254.

Campos FG, Waitzberg DL, Mucerino DR, Goncalves EL, Logulo AF, Habr-Gama A, and Rombeau JL. 1996. Protective effects of glutamine enriched diets on acute actinic enteritis. *Nutr Hosp* 11(3):167–177.

Carneiro-Filho BA, Bushen OY, Brito GA, Lima AA, and Guerrant RL. 2003. Glutamine analogues as adjunctive therapy for infectious diarrhea. *Curr Infect Dis Rep* 5(2):114–119.

Chapman JC, Liu Y, Zhu L, and Rhoads JM. 2012. Arginine and citrulline protect intestinal cell monolayer tight junctions from hypoxia-induced injury in piglets. *Pediatr Res* 72(6):576–582.

Coeffier M, Claeyssens S, Lecleire S, Leblond J, Coquard A, Bole-Feysot C, Lavoinne A, Ducrotte P, and Dechelotte P. 2008. Combined enteral infusion of glutamine, carbohydrates, and antioxidants modulates gut protein metabolism in humans. *Am J Clin Nutr* 88(5):1284–1290.

Coeffier M, Marion R, Ducrotte P, and Dechelotte P. 2003. Modulating effect of glutamine on IL-1beta-induced cytokine production by human gut. *Clin Nutr* 22(4):407–413.

Coeffier M, Miralles-Barrachina O, Le PF, Lalaude O, Daveau M, Lavoinne A, Lerebours E, and Dechelotte P. 2001. Influence of glutamine on cytokine production by human gut *in vitro*. *Cytokine* 13(3):148–154.

Crowther M, Avenell A, and Culligan DJ. 2009. Systematic review and meta-analyses of studies of glutamine supplementation in haematopoietic stem cell transplantation. *Bone Marrow Transplant* 44(7):413–425.

de Kieviet JF, Vuijk PJ, van den Berg A, Lafeber HN, Oosterlaan J, and van Elburg RM. 2014. Glutamine effects on brain growth in very preterm children in the first year of life. *Clin Nutr* 33(1):69–74.

Dechelotte P, Darmaun D, Rongier M, and Desjeux JF. 1989. Glutamine transport in isolated rabbit ileal epithelium. *Gastroenterol Clin Biol* 13(10):816–821.

Den HE, Hiele M, Peeters M, Ghoos Y, and Rutgeerts P. 1999. Effect of long-term oral glutamine supplements on small intestinal permeability in patients with Crohn's disease. *JPEN J Parenter Enteral Nutr* 23(1):7–11.

Desjeux JF, Nath SK, and Taminiau J. 1994. Organic substrate and electrolyte solutions for oral rehydration in diarrhea. *Annu Rev Nutr* 14:321–342.

Eagle H, Oyama VI, Levy M, Horton CL, and Fleischman R. 1956. The growth response of mammalian cells in tissue culture to L-glutamine and L-glutamic acid. *J Biol Chem* 218(2):607–616.

Evans ME, Jones DP, and Ziegler TR. 2003. Glutamine prevents cytokine-induced apoptosis in human colonic epithelial cells. *J Nutr* 133(10):3065–3071.

Feng D, Xu W, Chen G, Hang C, Gao H, and Yin H. 2007. Influence of glutamine on intestinal inflammatory response, mucosa structure alterations and apoptosis following traumatic brain injury in rats. *J Int Med Res* 35(5):644–656.

Fox AD, Kripke SA, De PJ, Berman JM, Settle RG, and Rombeau JL. 1988. Effect of a glutamine-supplemented enteral diet on methotrexate-induced enterocolitis. *JPEN J Parenter Enteral Nutr* 12(4):325–331.

Giris M, Erbil Y, Oztezcan S, Olgac V, Barbaros U, Deveci U, Kirgiz B, Uysal M, and Toker GA. 2006. The effect of heme oxygenase-1 induction by glutamine on radiation-induced intestinal damage: The effect of heme oxygenase-1 on radiation enteritis. *Am J Surg* 191(4):503–509.

Grondahl ML, and Skadhauge E. 1997. Effect of mucosal amino acids on SCC and Na and Cl fluxes in the porcine small intestine. *Comp Biochem. Physiol A Physiol* 118(2):233–237.

Gulgun M, Karaoglu A, Kesik V, Kurt B, Erdem O, Tok D, Kismet E, Koseoglu V, and Ozcan O. 2010. Effect of proanthocyanidin, arginine and glutamine supplementation on methotrexate-induced gastrointestinal toxicity in rats. *Methods Find Exp Clin Pharmacol* 32(9):657–661.

Hensley CT, Wasti AT, and DeBerardinis RJ. 2013. Glutamine and cancer: Cell biology, physiology, and clinical opportunities. *J Clin Invest* 123(9):3678–3684.

Houdijk AP, Rijnsburger ER, Jansen J, Wesdorp RI, Weiss JK, McCamish MA, Teerlink T, Meuwissen SG, Haarman HJ, Thijs LG, and van Leeuwen PA. 1998. Randomised trial of glutamine-enriched enteral nutrition on infectious morbidity in patients with multiple trauma. *Lancet* 352(9130):772–776.

Islam S, Mahalanabis D, Chowdhury AK, Wahed MA, and Rahman AS. 1997. Glutamine is superior to glucose in stimulating water and electrolyte absorption across rabbit ileum. *Dig Dis Sci* 42(2):420–423.

Jagust WJ, and Budinger TF. 1992. New neuroimaging techniques for investigating of brain-behavior relationships. *NIDA Res Monogr* 124:95–115.

Klimberg VS, Salloum RM, Kasper M, Plumley DA, Dolson DJ, Hautamaki RD, Mendenhall WR, Bova FC, Bland KI, Copeland EM, III. 1990. Oral glutamine accelerates healing of the small intestine and improves outcome after whole abdominal radiation. *Arch Surg* 125(8):1040–1045.

Ko TC, Beauchamp RD, Townsend CM, Jr., and Thompson JC. 1993. Glutamine is essential for epidermal growth factor-stimulated intestinal cell proliferation. *Surgery* 114(2):147–153.

Ko YG, Kim EY, Kim T, Park H, Park HS, Choi EJ, and Kim S. 2001. Glutamine-dependent antiapoptotic interaction of human glutaminyl-tRNA synthetase with apoptosis signal-regulating kinase 1. *J Biol Chem* 276(8):6030–6036.

Larson SD, Li J, Chung DH, and Evers BM. 2007. Molecular mechanisms contributing to glutamine-mediated intestinal cell survival. *Am J Physiol Gastrointest Liver Physiol* 293(6):G1262–G1271.

Lecce JG, Balsbaugh RK, Clare DA, and King MW. 1982. Rotavirus and hemolytic enteropathogenic *Escherichia coli* in weanling diarrhea of pigs. *J Clin Microbiol* 16(4):715–723.

Li N, Lewis P, Samuelson D, Liboni K, and Neu J. 2004. Glutamine regulates Caco-2 cell tight junction proteins. *Am J Physiol Gastrointest Liver Physiol* 287(3):G726–G733.

Li N, Liboni K, Fang MZ, Samuelson D, Lewis P, Patel R, and Neu J. 2004. Glutamine decreases lipo-polysaccharide-induced intestinal inflammation in infant rats. *Am J Physiol Gastrointest Liver Physiol* 286(6):G914–G921.

Li N, Ma L, Liu X, Shaw L, Li CS, Grant MB, and Neu J. 2012. Arginyl-glutamine dipeptide or docosahexae-noic acid attenuates hyperoxia-induced small intestinal injury in neonatal mice. *J Pediatr Gastroenterol Nutr* 54(4):499–504.

Moe-Byrne T, Wagner JV, and McGuire W. 2012. Glutamine supplementation to prevent morbidity and mor-tality in preterm infants. *Cochrane Database Syst Rev* 3:CD001457.

Mondello S, Galuppo M, Mazzon E, Domenico I, Mondello P, Carmela A, and Cuzzocrea S. 2010. Glutamine treatment attenuates the development of ischaemia/reperfusion injury of the gut. *Eur J Pharmacol* 643(2–3):304–315.

Morrison AL, Dinges M, Singleton KD, Odoms K, Wong HR, and Wischmeyer PE. 2006. Glutamine's protection against cellular injury is dependent on heat shock factor-1. *Am J Physiol Cell Physiol* 290(6):C1625–C1632.

Nambu T, Bamba T, and Hosoda S. 1992. Promotion of healing by orally administered glutamine in elemental diet after small intestinal injury by X-ray radiation. *Asia Pac J Clin Nutr* 1(3):175–182.

Novak F, Heyland DK, Avenell A, Drover JW, and Su X. 2002. Glutamine supplementation in serious illness: A systematic review of the evidence. *Crit Care Med* 30(9):2022–2029.

O'Dwyer ST, Smith RJ, Hwang TL, and Wilmore DW. 1989. Maintenance of small bowel mucosa with gluta-mine-enriched parenteral nutrition. *JPEN J Parenter Enteral Nutr* 13(6):579–585.

Oliveira GP, Oliveira MB, Santos RS et al. 2009. Intravenous glutamine decreases lung and distal organ injury in an experimental model of abdominal sepsis. *Crit Care* 13(3):R74.

Papaconstantinou HT, Hwang KO, Rajaraman S, Hellmich MR, Townsend CM, Jr., and Ko TC. 1998. Glutamine deprivation induces apoptosis in intestinal epithelial cells. *Surgery* 124(2):152–159.

Poindexter BB, Ehrenkranz RA, Stoll BJ et al. 2003. Effect of parenteral glutamine supplementa-tion on plasma amino acid concentrations in extremely low-birth-weight infants. *Am J Clin Nutr* 77(3):737–743.

Poindexter BB, Ehrenkranz RA, Stoll BJ et al. 2004. Parenteral glutamine supplementation does not reduce the risk of mortality or late-onset sepsis in extremely low birth weight infants. *Pediatrics* 113(5):1209–1215.

Potsic B, Holliday N, Lewis P, Samuelson D, DeMarco V, and Neu J. 2002. Glutamine supplementation and deprivation: Effect on artificially reared rat small intestinal morphology. *Pediatr Res* 52(3):430–436.

Prabhu R, Thomas S, and Balasubramanian KA. 2003. Oral glutamine attenuates surgical manipulation-induced alterations in the intestinal brush border membrane. *J Surg Res* 115(1):148–156.

Rhoads JM, Argenzio RA, Chen W, Graves LM, Licato LL, Blikslager AT, Smith J, Gatzy J, and Brenner DA. 2000. Glutamine metabolism stimulates intestinal cell MAPKs by a cAMP-inhibitable, Raf-independent mechanism. *Gastroenterology* 118(1):90–100.

Rhoads JM, Argenzio RA, Chen W, Rippe RA, Westwick JK, Cox AD, Berschneider HM, and Brenner DA. 1997. L-glutamine stimulates intestinal cell proliferation and activates mitogen-activated protein kinases. *Am J Physiol* 272(5 Pt 1):G943–G953.

Rhoads JM, Keku EO, Bennett LE, Quinn J, and Lecce JG. 1990. Development of L-glutamine-stimulated electroneutral sodium absorption in piglet jejunum. *Am J Physiol* 259(1 Pt 1):G99–G107.

Rhoads JM, Keku EO, Quinn J, Woosely J, and Lecce JG. 1991. L-glutamine stimulates jejunal sodium and chloride absorption in pig rotavirus enteritis. *Gastroenterology* 100(3):683–691.

Rhoads JM, Keku EO, Woodard JP, Bangdiwala SI, Lecce JG, and Gatzy JT. 1992. L-glutamine with D-glucose stimulates oxidative metabolism and NaCl absorption in piglet jejunum. *Am J Physiol* 263(6 Pt 1):G960–G966.

Rhoads M. 2004. Glutamine is the gas pedal but not the ferrari. *J Pediatr Gastroenterol Nutr* 38(5):474–476.

Ribeiro JH, Ribeiro T, Mattos A, Palmeira C, Fernandez D, Sant'Ana I, Rodrigues I, Bendicho MT, and Fontaine O. 1994. Treatment of acute diarrhea with oral rehydration solutions containing glutamine. *J Am Coll Nutr* 13(3):251–255.

Ropeleski MJ, Riehm J, Baer KA, Musch MW, and Chang EB. 2005. Anti-apoptotic effects of L-glutamine-mediated transcriptional modulation of the heat shock protein 72 during heat shock. *Gastroenterology* 129(1):170–184.

Saha P, Arthur S, Kekuda R, and Sundaram U. 2012. Na-glutamine co-transporters B(0)AT1 in villus and SN2 in crypts are differentially altered in chronically inflamed rabbit intestine. *Biochim Biophys Acta* 1818(3):434–442.

Scolapio JS, McGreevy K, Tennyson GS, and Burnett OL. 2001. Effect of glutamine in short-bowel syndrome. *Clin Nutr* 20(4):319–323.

Seth A, Basuroy S, Sheth P, and Rao RK. 2004. L-Glutamine ameliorates acetaldehyde-induced increase in paracellular permeability in Caco-2 cell monolayer. *Am J Physiol Gastrointest Liver Physiol* 287(3):G510–G517.

Sevastiadou S, Malamitsi-Puchner A, Costalos C, Skouroliakou M, Briana DD, Antsaklis A, and Roma-Giannikou E. 2011. The impact of oral glutamine supplementation on the intestinal permeability and incidence of necrotizing enterocolitis/septicemia in premature neonates. *J Matern Fetal Neonatal Med* 24(10):1294–1300.

Silva AC, Santos-Neto MS, Soares AM, Fonteles MC, Guerrant RL, and Lima AA. 1998. Efficacy of a glutamine-based oral rehydration solution on the electrolyte and water absorption in a rabbit model of secretory diarrhea induced by cholera toxin. *J Pediatr Gastroenterol Nutr* 26(5):513–519.

Soeters PB, and Grecu I. 2012. Have we enough glutamine and how does it work? A clinician's view. *Ann Nutr Metab* 60(1):17–26.

Tamada H, Nezu R, Imamura I, Matsuo Y, Takagi Y, Kamata S, and Okada A. 1992. The dipeptide alanyl-glutamine prevents intestinal mucosal atrophy in parenterally fed rats. *JPEN J. Parenter Enteral Nutr* 16(2):110–116.

Tan H, Sun MY, and Yang J. 2008. [Effect of retention enema with combination of compound glutamine entero-soluble capsule and glucocorticoids for treatment of ulcerative colitis]. *Zhongguo Zhong Xi Yi Jie He Za Zhi* 28(7):645–647.

Tian J, Hao L, Chandra P, Jones DP, Willams IR, Gewirtz AT, and Ziegler TR. 2009. Dietary glutamine and oral antibiotics each improve indexes of gut barrier function in rat short bowel syndrome. *Am J Physiol Gastrointest Liver Physiol* 296(2):G348–G355.

Tubman TR, Thompson SW, and McGuire W. 2008. Glutamine supplementation to prevent morbidity and mortality in preterm infants. *Cochrane Database Syst Rev* (1):CD001457.

Uehara K, Takahashi T, Fujii H, Shimizu H, Omori E, Matsumi M, Yokoyama M, Morita K, Akagi R, and Sassa S. 2005. The lower intestinal tract-specific induction of heme oxygenase-1 by glutamine protects against endotoxemic intestinal injury. *Crit Care Med* 33(2):381–390.

van Kraaij MG, Dekker AW, Verdonck LF, van Loon AM, Vinje J, Koopmans MP, and Rozenberg-Arska M. 2000. Infectious gastro-enteritis: An uncommon cause of diarrhoea in adult allogeneic and autologous stem cell transplant recipients. *Bone Marrow Transplant* 26(3):299–303.

van Loon FP, Banik AK, Nath SK, Patra FC, Wahed MA, Darmaun D, Desjeux JF, and Mahalanabis D. 1996. The effect of L-glutamine on salt and water absorption: A jejunal perfusion study in cholera in humans. *Eur J Gastroenterol Hepatol* 8(5):443–448.

Van GA, Cabre E, Hebuterne X, Jeppesen P, Krznaric Z, Messing B, Powell-Tuck J, Staun M, and Nightingale J. 2009. ESPEN Guidelines on Parenteral Nutrition: Gastroenterology. *Clin Nutr* 28(4):415–427.

Vanderhoof JA, Blackwood DJ, Mohammadpour H, and Park JH. 1992. Effects of oral supplementation of glutamine on small intestinal mucosal mass following resection. *J Am Coll Nutr* 11(2):223–227.

Wagner JV, Moe-Byrne T, Grover Z, and McGuire W. 2012. Glutamine supplementation for young infants with severe gastrointestinal disease. *Cochrane Database Syst Rev* 7:CD005947.

Wales PW, Nasr A, de SN, and Yamada J. 2010. Human growth hormone and glutamine for patients with short bowel syndrome. *Cochrane Database Syst Rev* (6):CD006321.

Watford M, Chellaraj V, Ismat A, Brown P, and Raman P. 2002. Hepatic glutamine metabolism. *Nutrition* 18(4):301–303.

Wilmore DW, Smith RJ, O'Dwyer ST, Jacobs DO, Ziegler TR, and Wang XD. 1988. The gut: A central organ after surgical stress. *Surgery* 104(5):917–923.

Windmueller HG and Spaeth AE. 1978. Identification of ketone bodies and glutamine as the major respiratory fuels *in vivo* for postabsorptive rat small intestine. *J Biol Chem* 253(1):69–76.

Windmueller HG and Spaeth AE. 1980. Respiratory fuels and nitrogen metabolism *in vivo* in small intestine of fed rats. Quantitative importance of glutamine, glutamate, and aspartate. *J Biol Chem* 255(1):107–112.

Wischmeyer PE. 2002. Glutamine and heat shock protein expression. *Nutrition* 18(3):225–228.

Wischmeyer PE, Kahana M, Wolfson R, Ren H, Musch MM, and Chang EB. 2001. Glutamine induces heat shock protein and protects against endotoxin shock in the rat. *J Appl Physiol (1985)* 90(6):2403–2410.

Wischmeyer PE, Musch MW, Madonna MB, Thisted R, and Chang EB. 1997. Glutamine protects intestinal epithelial cells: Role of inducible HSP70. *Am J Physiol* 272(4 Pt 1):G879–G884.

Woo SB, Sonis ST, Monopoli MM, and Sonis AL. 1993. A longitudinal study of oral ulcerative mucositis in bone marrow transplant recipients. *Cancer* 72(5):1612–1617.

Wu G. 1998. Intestinal mucosal amino acid catabolism. *J Nutr* 128(8):1249–1252.

Wu G, and Knabe DA. 1994. Free and protein-bound amino acids in sow's colostrum and milk. *J Nutr* 124(3):415–424.

Xue H, Sufit AJ, and Wischmeyer PE. 2011. Glutamine therapy improves outcome of *in vitro* and *in vivo* experimental colitis models. *JPEN J Parenter Enteral Nutr* 35(2):188–197.

Yarandi SS, Zhao VM, Hebbar G, and Ziegler TR. 2011. Amino acid composition in parenteral nutrition: What is the evidence? *Curr Opin Clin Nutr Metab Care* 14(1): 75–82.

Zhou QQ, Yang DZ, Luo YJ, Li SZ, Liu FY, and Wang GS. 2011. Over-starvation aggravates intestinal injury and promotes bacterial and endotoxin translocation under high-altitude hypoxic environment. *World J Gastroenterol* 17(12):1584–1593.

Ziegler TR, Evans ME, Fernandez-Estivariz C, and Jones DP. 2003. Trophic and cytoprotective nutrition for intestinal adaptation, mucosal repair, and barrier function. *Annu Rev Nutr* 23:229–261.

Ziegler TR, Ogden LG, Singleton KD, Luo M, Fernandez-Estivariz C, Griffith DP, Galloway JR, and Wischmeyer PE. 2005. Parenteral glutamine increases serum heat shock protein 70 in critically ill patients. *Intensive Care Med* 31(8):1079–1086.

12 Therapeutic Role of Glutamine in Inflammatory Bowel Disease

Hongyu Xue and Paul Wischmeyer

CONTENTS

12.1 INTRODUCTION

The concept that dietary elements may serve as modulators of intestinal physiology and the gut's response to stress or injury has been hypothesized for many years. The gut is an attractive target for dietary modulation, owing to its direct exposure to nutritional elements orally/enterally delivered, participation in cellular uptake and metabolism of nutrients, and high plasticity in response to nutritional stimuli. Many physiological and pathological states affecting the gut are suggested to be sensitive to nutritional modulation, including intestinal adaptation during the life cycle (e.g., growth, weaning, old age), following nutritional stresses (e.g., re-feeding after malnutrition, intravenous feeding), inflammatory injuries (e.g., inflammatory bowel disease [IBD]) and a variety of chronic or acute insults (e.g., cancer chemotherapy/radiotherapy, surgical resection, ischemia–reperfusion injury).

Inflammatory bowel disease (IBD) is characterized by an idiopathic, chronic, and recurrent inflammation of the gastrointestinal (GI) tract. It comprises two major forms, that is, Crohn's disease (CD) and ulcerative colitis (UC), with distinct clinical and histopathological features. A widely accepted hypothesis accentuates the contributory role of genetic, enteric microbiota, and immunological factors in IBD pathogenesis (Sartor 2006). IBD is believed to be caused by an exaggerated immune response toward commensal bacteria in genetically susceptible individuals (Sartor 2006). Based on this understanding, the conventional treatment of IBD includes the use of corticosteroids, immunosuppressants, antibiotics, and biologic agents (e.g., anti-tumor necrosis factor [TNF]-α). However, the use of these chemical and biologic agents is often accompanied by significant side effects, which are of clinical concern (Triantafillidis and Stanciu 2012). Growing evidence suggests that a variety of dietary elements, which are generally affordable and safe, may extensively influence the intestinal immune-microbial axis. This creates a unique niche for potential use of these nutrients as therapeutics for IBD.

Glutamine has been shown to be a prominent gut-trophic factor with a versatile function in the GI tract via modulating intestinal immunity and promoting GI cytoprotective mechanisms in a variety of settings of inflammatory stress and injury (Calder 2007). The aim of this review is to investigate the therapeutic potential of glutamine in *in vitro* and *in vivo* IBD models.

12.2   MULTIFACTORIAL NATURE OF IBD PATHOGENESIS

It is widely hypothesized that the intestinal inflammation and mucosal damage characterized of IBD is triggered and perpetuated by excessive host immune responses to a subset of commensal enteric bacteria in genetically susceptible hosts.

Tremendous interest in IBD pathogenesis research has been directed toward understanding the role of the intestinal immune-microbial axis, which is characterized by a dynamic balance between enteric microbes, particularly commensal flora, and host mucosal defense, in the initiation and development of chronic IBD.

A disrupted compositional balance between beneficial and aggressive species of the enteric flora could create a proinflammatory milieu in the intestinal lumen of a susceptible host (Sartor 2009).

Nonetheless, colitis can be induced in a genetically susceptible host with normal commensal bacteria species (Sartor 2009). These findings indicate that the nature of the host defensive response, rather than the biological properties of an enteric bacterial species per se, may more crucially determine the role of microbe/host interaction in the initiation of IBD. The sustained and exaggerated mucosal immune response serves as primary trigger of chronic intestinal inflammation and tissue damage that are manifested in IBD patients (Sartor 2006).

Compromised intestinal barrier function may lead to increased uptake of antigens, thus constantly priming the immune activation and turning the mucosal immune homeostasis toward a proimmune milieu. Increased gut permeability has been found in families with CD, indicating a role of gut barrier function in IBD predisposition.

An excessive innate and adaptive immune response is a more common feature in human IBD (Sartor 2006). Sustained immune activation is arguably the driver of tissue damage and has been a primary target that a large body of therapeutic endeavors has been focusing on (Sartor 2006; Xavier and Podolsky 2007). The innate immune system constitutes the first line of immune defense and provides immediate defense against infection. Macrophages and dendritic cells in the lamina propria are activated and increased in quantities in human and experimental IBD. Functionally, monocyte and polymorphonuclear cell-derived production of proinflammatory cytokines is also augmented in IBD.

NFκB is the master transcriptional regulator of a variety of proinflammatory mediators including cytokines (e.g., IL-1β, tumor necrosis factors [TNF], IL-6, and IL-8), adhesion molecules (e.g., intercellular adhesion molecule 1) and costimulatory molecules (e.g., CD40, CD80, CD86). Enhanced expression and activation of NFκB is strongly induced in the inflamed mucosal tissue of IBD patients (Rogler et al. 1998). Biologic and pharmacological targeting therapeutics to block NFκB activation has been shown to ameliorate the spontaneous colitis in IL-10-deficient mice (Dave et al. 2007).

The mucosal tissue damage characterized in IBD is more attributable to the excessive activation of adaptive immunity, which is primed by the innate immune responses (Sartor and Hoentjen 2005). The effectors of adaptive immune responses include a variety of lymphocyte populations, that is, T cells polarized with a T_H1, T_H17, or T_H2 phenotype, immunoglobulin-secreting B cells, regulatory T (T_{reg}) and B (B_{reg}) cells. CD and UC have distinct T-cell cytokine profiles with the former exhibiting a T_H1 polarization and the latter dominated by a T_H2 phenotype (Sartor and Hoentjen 2005).

In addition to activated innate and acquired immune responses, loss of tolerance to commensals is a common feature to both CD and UC. It's a vital task for the intestinal immune system to mount protective immune responses against harmful intestinal pathogens while preventing excessive responses to innocuous commensal microbiome. Tolerance is an active physiological mechanism to sustain immune "unresponsiveness" to commensal bacterial antigens and is crucial for preventing harmful hypersensitivity responses in the intestine. Regulatory T cells (T_{reg}) are the primary executors for maintaining tolerance to commensal microbes. Recent research has shown that these T_{reg} cells are crucial in preventing intestinal inflammation and even have a key role in reverse established colitis (Mottet et al. 2003).

Given the multifactorial nature of IBD pathogenesis, much of the current understanding of IBD pathogenesis is based upon the studies of a variety of animal and cell models that resemble several key immunological and histopathological aspects of human IBD. Examples of animal IBD models are listed in Table 12.1 representing a multifold of targeting mechanistic points of pathobiology.

12.3 EVIDENCE FOR NUTRITIONAL MODULATION OF IBD BY GLUTAMINE

Glutamine is proposed to become conditionally essential during stress states where demand for glutamine outstrips its synthesis from endogenous precursors. In patients with CD during remission, splanchnic glutamine utilization does not seem to be altered, and there is no glutamine deficiency at the whole-body level as reflected by the plasma level of glutamine (Bourreille et al. 2004). However, local intestinal glutamine deficiency has been reported in active CD and UC lesions of human biopsies (Balasubramanian et al. 2009). The latter findings also furnish a theoretical niche for glutamine supplementation in IBD, which may potentially improve the outcomes by correcting the local intestinal glutamine deficiency.

12.3.1 CLINICAL EVIDENCE

Results from a limited body of clinical trials are considerably mixed (Table 12.2). In a pilot study, in which topical administration of glutamine and butyrate was compared on pouchitis secondary to ileal pouch-anal anastomosis, 6 of the 10 patients receiving glutamine suppository had no recurrence of pouchitis, whereas only 3 of the 9 patients receiving butyrate suppository had no recurrence (Wischmeyer et al. 1993). Compromised gut barrier function as manifested by increased intestinal permeability (IP) is a common feature of IBD. In a randomized controlled trial, patients with CD in the remission phase with an abnormal IP received oral glutamine treatment at 0.5 g/kg/day. At the

---

TABLE 12.1

Examples of Experimental Animal Inflammatory Bowel Disease Models

Chemically induced colitis
Trinitrobenzene sulfonic acid-induced colitis
Dextran sulfate sodium-induced colitis
Iodoacetamide-induced colitis
Acetic-acid-induced colitis
Spontaneously occurring
C3H/HeJBir mice
SAMP1/Yit mice
Compromised intestinal barrier function
Mutated multidrug-resistant gene mice
Intestinal trefoil factor knockout mice
Altered cytokine balance
IL-10 knockout mice
Interleukin-2 knockout/IL-2 receptor (R)α knockout mice
TNF-3′ untranslated region knockout mice
STAT-4 transgenic mice
Altered T-cell function
T-cell receptor mutant mice
HLA-B27 transgenic rat

TABLE 12.2

Clinical Trials of Glutamine Supplementation in Inflammatory Bowel Disease

Total Number of Subjects	Subject Features	Design	Form of Glutamine	Dose of Glutamine	Route of Glutamine Administration	Duration of Glutamine Treatment	Control	Glutamine's Effects on Examined Endpoints	Reference
28 (n = 14 for each group)	Patients with CD in the remission phase with an abnormal IP	Randomized, controlled	Free glutamine	0.5 g/kg/day	Oral	2 months	Whey protein at 0.5 g/kg/day via oral administration	Glutamine increased IP and villous crypt ratio compared to pretreatment values; whey protein equally improved these endpoints.	Benjamin et al. (2012)
19 (n = 10 for glutamine; n = 9 for butyrate)	Patients with pouchitis secondary to ileal pouch	Pilot, controlled	Free glutamine		Topical via suppository	21 days	Butyrate administered via suppository	Six of the 10 patients receiving glutamine treatment showing no recurrence of pouchitis vs. 3 of the 9 patients receiving butyrate suppository having no recurrence.	Wischmeyer et al. (1993)

(Continued)

TABLE 12.2 (*Continued*)
Clinical Trials of Glutamine Supplementation in Inflammatory Bowel Disease

Total Number of Subjects	Subject Features	Design	Form of Glutamine	Dose of Glutamine	Route of Glutamine Administration	Duration of Glutamine Treatment	Control	Glutamine's Effects on Examined Endpoints	Reference
11 (all receiving glutamine treatment)	Patients with inactive or moderate CD	Uncontrolled	Free glutamine	6 g/day (3 g twice a day)	Oral	Not known	No control	Glutamine improved IP and nutritional status compared to pretreatment values.	Zoli et al. (1995)
16 (n = 7 for glutamine treatment, n = 9 for control)	Pediatric patients with active CD	Randomized, double-blind, controlled	Not specified (free glutamine or protein-bound)	Approximately 8.5 g/day	Glutamine-enriched polymeric diet (42% of amino acid composition)	4 weeks	Isocaloric, isonitrogenous, standard polymeric diet with a low glutamine content (4% of its amino acid content as glutamine, the amount naturally occurring in foods)	Glutamine-enriched diet was less effective than the standard low-glutamine polymeric diet in improving disease activity index.	Akobeng et al. (2000)

(*Continued*)

TABLE 12.2 (Continued)
Clinical Trials of Glutamine Supplementation in Inflammatory Bowel Disease

Total Number of Subjects	Subject Features	Design	Form of Glutamine	Dose of Glutamine	Route of Glutamine Administration	Duration of Glutamine Treatment	Control	Glutamine's Effects on Examined Endpoints	Reference
14 (n = 7 for glutamine, n = 7 for placebo)	Patients with CD with increased IP	Randomized, double-blind, placebo-controlled	Free glutamine	Oral: 21 g/day (7 g three times a day)	Oral or given in TPN when TPN became necessary	4 weeks	Glycine as placebo at 21 g/day (7 g three times a day)	Neither glutamine nor placebo treatment improved IP, CD activity index, C-reactive protein, or nutritional status; plasma levels of glutamine, glutamate and ammonia were not changed after glutamine treatment.	Den Hond et al. (1999)
24 (n = 12 for glutamine +, and n = 12 for glutamine−)	Patients with active IBD (19 CD; five ulcerative colitis) who needed to be on TPN for at least a week	Randomized, double-blind, controlled	Alanyl-glutamine	0.3 g/kg/day, equivalent to 0.2 g/kg/day glutamine	0.3 g/kg/day alanyl-glutamine added to 1.2 g/kg/day of a glutamine-free standard amino-acid solution.	≥ 7 days	Isonitrogenous, isocaloric TPN with 1.5 g/kg/day of a glutamine-free standard amino acid mixture	Glutamine treatment did not change glutamine plasma levels, IP, disease activity, length of TPN, hospital stay.	Ockenga et al. (2005)

CD: Crohn's disease; IBD: inflammatory bowel disease; IP: intestinal permeability; TPN: total parenteral nutrition.

end of the 2-month study, glutamine treatment significantly improved IP and intestinal morphormetry (Benjamin et al. 2012). In another uncontrolled pilot study, oral glutamine treatment at 6 g/day significantly improved IP and overall nutritional status compared to pretreatment values in patients with inactive or moderate CD (Zoli et al. 1995).

Nonetheless, a number of clinical trials also show an absence of clear benefits by glutamine supplementation in IBD outcomes. Compared to a standard polymeric diet with a low glutamine content (4% of amino acid composition), a glutamine-enriched polymeric diet (42% of amino acid composition, ~8.5 g/day glutamine delivered) given to pediatric patients with active CD for 4 weeks offered no benefits in disease activity index, weight and acute-phase reactants (Akobeng et al. 2000). Another trial showed that oral supplementation of glutamine in single form at 21 g/day (7 g, three times a day) was not able to improve the IP or other endpoints such as CD activity index and C-reactive protein in patients with CD (Den Hond et al. 1999). Of note, plasma levels of glutamine and glutamate were not changed after glutamine treatment, which may suggest that glutamine administration as factored by dose, administration schedule and duration, could be insufficient (Den Hond et al. 1999). Compared to glutamine-free standard total parenteral nutrition (TPN), glutamine-enriched (0.2 g/kg/day) TPN was also found unable to improve the IP or other outcomes examined in patients with active IBD, although parenteral glutamine treatment was also found unable to change glutamine plasma levels (Ockenga et al. 2005).

12.3.2 PRECLINICAL EVIDENCE FROM EXPERIMENTAL IBD MODELS

Although limited, the preclinical studies are generally supportive of a positive role in a variety of experimental IBD models (Table 12.3). Multiple interrelated key players in IBD pathogenesis could be potentially modulated by glutamine treatments (Figure 12.1).

12.3.2.1 Improving Intestinal Barrier Integrity

Compromised gut barrier function plays a pivotal role in the initiation and progression of intestinal inflammation characteristic of IBD (Sartor 2009). In a guinea pig model of carrageenan-induced UC-like colitis, glutamine-enriched elemental diet at 2% (w/v) was shown to reduce gut-derived endotoxin translocation compared to a standard elemental diet with low glutamine content (0.64% [w/v]) (Fujita and Sakurai 1995). In an *ex vivo* study using isolated rat colonic mucosa, glutamine supplied from only serosal side reduced the permeability of the colonic mucosa injured by hydrochloric acid (HCl). A greater benefit was achieved with glutamine added to both luminal and serosal sides. A beneficial effect with glutamine-supplemented parenteral nutrition is indicated (Scheppach et al. 1996). Dugan et al. (Dugan and McBurney 1995) studied effects of luminal glutamine on IP using isolated ileum loops perfused with or without glutamine. Ileal perfusion with a glutamine solution effectively prevents endotoxin-induced increases in mucosal permeability (Dugan and McBurney 1995).

Glutamine may potentially modulate a multitude of key mechanistic players in upholding intestinal epithelial homeostasis. *Splanchnic perfusion and intestinal microcirculation* are essential for preservation of mucosal structural integrity. Glutamine, either administered enterally or parenterally, can modulate intestinal microcirculation, which has been shown to be compromised in intestinal segments in colitis models (Flynn et al. 1992; Kruschewski et al. 1998; Foitzik et al. 1999). Glutamine luminal perfusions helped to reestablish microvascular circulation after hemorrhagic shock in a rat model (Flynn et al. 1992). In a trinitrobenzene sulfonic acid (TNBS) colitis model, glutamine-supplemented TPN increased colonic capillary blood flow (Kruschewski et al. 1998; Foitzik et al. 1999), indicating a protection in the intestinal microcirculation.

Gut barrier is also dependent on epithelial homeostasis determined by the dynamic balance between *epithelial proliferation and death*. Glutamine has long been proposed as a gut-trophic factor that stimulates enterocyte proliferation, prevents excessive apoptosis, and thus promotes epithelial homeostasis recovery during a variety of acute and chronic stresses/injuries (Reeds and

TABLE 12.3

Preclinical Studies of Glutamine Supplementation in Inflammatory Bowel Disease Models

Animal/Cell Line/Tissue	Glutamine Dose	Administration Route	Form of Glutamine	Duration of Treatment	Control Treatment	Results	Reference
Guinea-pig model of carrageenan-induced UC-like colitis	The same elemental control diet supplemented with 2% (w/v) glutamine	Oral	Free glutamine	5 days	Chemically defined elemental diet containing 0.644% (w/v) glutamine	Glutamine-enriched elemental diet reduced endotoxin level of portal vein.	Fujita and Sakurai (1995)
Isolated distal ileum loops in piglets *in vivo*	Ringer's lactate solution supplemented with 2% glutamine	Luminal perfusion	Free glutamine	280 min	Ringer's lactate solution without glutamine	Glutamine perfusion prevented endotoxin-induced increases in mucosal permeability, but did not alter intestinal myeloperoxidase (MPO) activity.	Dugan and McBurney (1995)
TNBS-induced colitis in Sprague-Dawley rats	Glutamine at 0.5 g/kg/day	Via TPN	Alanyl-glutamine	48 h	Alanyl-glycine-enriched isocaloric and isonitrogenous standard TPN solution	Glutamine treatment increased colonic capillary blood flow, but had no effect on IP or bacterial translocation.	Foitzik et al. (1999)
Ex vivo isolated rat colonic injured by luminal hydrochloric acid and resealing was studied with or without added glutamine or butyrate	Glutamine 2 mM added to incubation medium (Krebs-Ringer solution)	*Ex vivo*, both luminal and serosal exposure as compared to single serosal exposure	Free glutamine	4 h	Equimolar NaCl added to Krebs-Ringer solution	Glutamine supplied from both luminal and serosal sides decreased IP and permeation of *Escherichia coli*.	

(Continued)

TABLE 12.3 (*Continued*)
Preclinical Studies of Glutamine Supplementation in Inflammatory Bowel Disease Models

Animal/Cell Line/Tissue	Glutamine Dose	Administration Route	Form of Glutamine	Duration of Treatment	Control Treatment	Results	Reference
						Glutamine supplied from serosal side alone diminished IP. Both glutamine treatments promoted colonocyte proliferation.	Scheppach et al. (1996)
Sprague-Dawley rat model of DSS-induced colitis (via oral 5% DSS) for 7 days)	Concurrent glutamine (0.75 g/kg/day) treatment throughout the 7-day DSS treatment	Oral gavage	Free glutamine	7 days	Sham (water)	Glutamine-attenuated DSS-induced colitis by decreasing area under curve for bleeding and diarrhea, associated with enhanced HSP25 and HSP70 in colonic mucosa.	Xue et al. (2011)
TNBS-induced colitis in Sabra rats	Glutamine enemas (50 mg in 1 mL saline, once a day)	Topical	Free glutamine	[a]Schedule 1: day −2 to day +7 ; Schedule 2: day −2 to day +3; Schedule 3: day 0 to day +7	Saline enemas	Only prophylactic topical glutamine treatment (Schedule 1 and 2, but not Schedule 3) reduced macroscopic inflammation, histological index, and MPO activity, reduced tissue oxidative injury, increased ascorbic acid and energy-rich phosphates in colonic mucosa.	Israeli et al. (2004)

(*Continued*)

TABLE 12.3 (*Continued*)

Preclinical Studies of Glutamine Supplementation in Inflammatory Bowel Disease Models

Animal/Cell Line/Tissue	Glutamine Dose	Administration Route	Form of Glutamine	Duration of Treatment	Control Treatment	Results	Reference
TNBS-induced colitis in Wistar-Albino rats	1 g/kg/day	Intragastric gavage	Free glutamine	Day −3 to day 15	Saline	Glutamine treatment preserved mucosal structural integrity, increased GSH store and HO-1 expression and decreased oxidative injury, apoptosis and NFκB p50 expression.	Giris et al. (2007)
TNBS-induced colitis in Wistar rats	25 mg/kg/day	Rectal administration	Free glutamine	4 h after the induction of colitis till day 7	Receiving TNBS treatment alone	Glutamine preserved structural and functional integrity, reduced colonic myeloperoxidase activity, tissue TNF-α and IFN-γ levels, and NFκB activation.	Kretzmann et al. (2008)
Acetic acid-induced colitis in Wistar rats	25 mg/kg/day	Rectal administration	Free glutamine	48 and 24 before acetic acid instillation	Receiving acetic acid alone	Glutamine preserved structural and functional integrity, decreased tissue oxidative injury, and NFκB activation.	Fillmann et al. (2007)
TNBS-induced colitis in Sprague-Dawley rats	2% and 4% glutamine-enriched (w/w) casein-based (20%, w/w) semipurified diet	Glutamine-enriched diet	Free glutamine	[a]Day −14 till the end of study (day +14)	Isonitrogenous and isocaloric diet with glutamine substituted by glycine	Both glutamine-enriched diets attenuated weight loss, improved intestinal histological integrity, prevented bacterial translocation and reduced IL-8 and TNF-α levels in inflamed tissue. Four percent glutamine-diet was associated with better benefits compared to 2% glutamine-diet.	Ameho et al. (1997)

(Continued)

TABLE 12.3 (*Continued*)
Preclinical Studies of Glutamine Supplementation in Inflammatory Bowel Disease Models

Animal/Cell Line/Tissue	Glutamine Dose	Administration Route	Form of Glutamine	Duration of Treatment	Control Treatment	Results	Reference
Endotoxemia in Sprague-Dawley rats induced by LPS injections on two consecutive days	Glutamine in drinking water (2%)	Glutamine-contained drinking water	Free glutamine	Starting 2 days before LPS injection till 1 day after the 2nd dose of LPS	Rats receiving LPS alone	Glutamine treatment protected endotoxemia-induced intestinal mucosal injury, reduced expression of TLR4 and MyD88.	Kessel et al. (2008)
DSS-induced colitis in C57BL/6 mice	Alanyl-glutamine at 0.75 g/kg/day, which provided 0.5 g glutamine/kg/day	Intraperitoneal injection	Alanyl-glutamine	Preventive schedule: glutamine (day −3 to day 0) then saline (day 0 to day +2); interventional schedule: saline (day −3 to day 0) then glutamine (day 0 to day +2)	Isovolumic saline	Either pre- or post-DSS Glutamine treatment diminished structural destruction, reduced expression of TLR4 and IL-17A expression, increased IκB/NFκB ratio. Compared to the post-DSS schedule, pre-DSS glutamine better preserved structural integrity associated with increased expression of mucin 2, trefoil factor 3, and Hsp70.	Hou et al. (2013)

Day 0 designated as the day when DSS treatment was initiated.
DSS: dextran sulfate sodium; **HSP:** heat shock protein; **IP:** intestinal permeability; **LPS:** lipopolysaccharides; **TNBS:** trinitrobenzene sulfonic acid; **TPN:** total parenteral nutrition; **UC:** ulcerative colitis.
[a] Day −*n* and +*n* designated as *n* days before or after TNBS instillation, respectively.

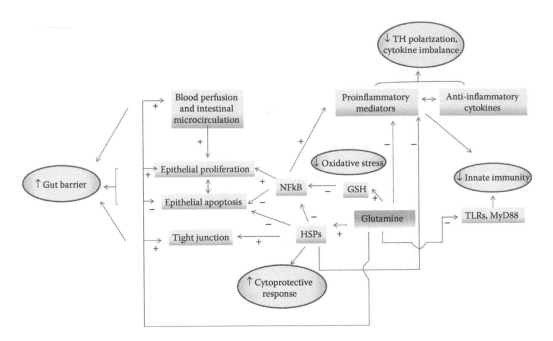

FIGURE 12.1 Glutamine modulates multiple interrelated key players in inflammatory bowel disease pathogenesis, which may overall favor an ameliorated functional, structural, and immune homeostasis in the intestinal mucosa. HSP: heat shock protein; MyD88: myeloid differentiation primary response gene 88; T_H: T-helper lymphocyte; TLR: toll-like receptor.

Burrin 2001). In Scheppach et al.'s *ex vivo* study using isolated rat colonic mucosa injured by HCl, glutamine exposure at the serosal side with and without luminal glutamine exposure increased in crypt cell proliferation, associated with an improved IP (Scheppach et al. 1996). In cultured non-transformed young adult mouse colonic epithelial cells (YAMC) exposed to concurrent cytokine (IFN-γ + TNF-α) and glutamine treatment, glutamine deprivation, or insufficient glutamine supply (glutamine supplanted at 0 or 0.25 mM) renders the cells more vulnerable to cytokine injury with increased apoptosis and diminished cell proliferation, whereas this effect can be blunted with adequate glutamine supply at 0.5 mM or higher (Xue et al. 2011). Likewise, in cultured human colon carcinoma, HT-29 cells injured with a combination of IFN-γ + TNF-α or a single cytokine, tumor necrosis factor-alpha-related apoptosis-inducing ligand (TRAIL), cytokine-induced apoptosis was attenuated by glutamine treatment in a dose-dependent manner and was completely blocked when glutamine was supplied at 0.5 mM (Evans et al. 2003).

Tight junctions (TJ), which are multiprotein complexes composed of integral membrane proteins (i.e., occludin, claudins, and zonula occludens [ZO]-1, ZO-2, and ZO-3), serve as a vital cellular component of mucosal barrier and are the principal determinant of mucosal permeability. Compromised TJs, for example, a loss of occluding and other TJ proteins such as ZO-1, JAM-A, and claudin-1, contribute to the barrier defects in IBD (Kucharzik et al. 2001). Disrupted integrity of TJ may result in paracellular transport of bacterial lipopolysaccharides (LPS) and luminal antigens, which may culminate in a constantly stimulated proinflammatory milieu in intestinal mucosal tissue (Sartor and Muehlbauer 2007). Glutamine is essential to TJ protein expression and cellular localization (Li et al. 2004; Li and Neu 2009). Deprivation of glutamine from cell culture medium or inhibition of glutamine synthetase (GS) resulted in a reduced expression of claudin-1, occludin, and ZO-1, abnormal subcellular re-localization of claudin-1 and irregular junctional complexes formation (Li et al. 2004) and an increased permeability of Caco-2 cell monolayers (DeMarco et al. 2003). Given the glutamine deficiency commonly found in the local intestinal mucosal tissue of

IBD patients, which may jeopardize the mucosal tissue into a condition that renders an altered TJ protein expression and/or localization, exogenous glutamine supplementation may conceivably help to preserve TJ integrity and thus maintain mucosal homeostasis.

The notion that oxidative stress has a key role in triggering and propagating and/or propagation of IBD leads to theoretical basis for using antioxidants or compounds that can evoke or boost antioxidant defense during IBD conditions (Zhu and Li 2012). Glutamine (via glutamate) is a precursor for glutathione synthesis and has been suggested to be rate limiting for glutathione synthesis during stress (Welbourne 1979). Enteral or topical glutamine supplementation has been consistently shown to preserve the glutathione (GSH) store in models of TNBS and acetic acid-induced colitis (Fillmann et al. 2007; Giris et al. 2007; Kretzmann et al. 2008). Interestingly, glutamine treatment seems to increase other players of host antioxidant defense in addition to GSH store. Topical use of glutamine enemas reduced tissue oxidative damage in TNBS-induced colitis and increased tissue ascorbic acid levels in olonic mucosa (Israeli et al. 2004).

NFκB pathway plays a pivotal role in the pathogenesis of IBD via activating proinflammatory mediator expression. It is noteworthy that activation of NFκB pathway is sensitive to the intracellular redox state. The activation of NFκB by most of the extracellular inducers is dependent on the phosphorylation and subsequent degradation of IκB, inhibitor of NFκB, which results in release of p65/p50 complex and its rapid nuclear translocation where it activates the target gene transcription. The increase in intracellular GSH by glutamine can reduce the activity of the redox-sensitive IκB kinases (IKK), which subsequently stabilizes IκB and downregulates activation of NFκB (Sen and Packer 1996). This pinpoints a mechanistic target point by which glutamine may potentially affect inflammatory mediator network. In TNBS or acetic acid-induced colitis, glutamine administered via rectal route was shown to reduce oxidative stress and inhibited NFκB signaling (Fillmann et al. 2007; Kretzmann et al. 2008). Glutamine treatment at 1 g/kg/day via intragastric gavage could also reduce tissue oxidative stress, increase GSH store and reduce colonic p50 expression in rats with TNBS-induced colitis (Giris et al. 2007). We also show that in cultured YAMC cells, exogenous glutamine could reduce cytokine-induced nuclear translocation of NFκB p65 subunit and inducible nitric oxide synthase (iNOS) expression (Xue et al. 2011).

12.3.2.2 Regulating Intestinal Innate Immunity

A defective suppression of innate immunity is implicated in IBD initiation and progression (Xavier and Podolsky 2007). Toll-like receptors (TLRs) have emerged as a central point in innate immunity (Medzhitov 2001). Activation of these receptors via binding to their microbial ligands such as LPS or double-stranded RNA initiates an inflammatory cascade that attempts to clear the offending pathogen and further helps shaping specific adaptive immune response (Medzhitov 2001). Expression of TLRs, especially TLR4 and TLR2, is upregulated on intestinal epithelial cells and the intestinal macrophages of patients with IBD (Hausmann et al. 2002). Kessel et al. demonstrated that oral glutamine treatment protected endotoxemia-induced intestinal mucosal injury, associated with downregulation of expression of TLR4 and myeloid differentiation primary response gene 88 (MyD88), a key adaptor protein recruiting downstream kinase that leads to NFκB activation (Kessel et al. 2008). Intraperitoneal administration of alanyl-glutamine was also shown to reduce colonic TLR4 expression and attenuated DSS-induced colitis (Hou et al. 2013).

12.3.2.3 Modulating Cytokine Balance and T Cell Polarization

The immune homeostasis of intestinal mucosa is regulated by a delicate balance of proinflammatory and anti-inflammatory cytokines. This cytokine network profoundly affects the nature of the response by effector immune cells to intestinal microbes and their products (Chahine and Bahna). In both CD and UC, the cytokine balance is severely disrupted and shifted toward the proinflammatory side (Sartor and Hoentjen 2005).

Coeffier et al. investigated how glutamine affected the cytokine network in cultured biopsies from human duodenum or colon *ex vivo* (Coeffier et al. 2002; Lecleire et al. 2008). Glutamine treatment at a physiological dose of 0.5 mM could effectively decrease the basal spontaneous production of IL-6 and IL-8 of cultured biopsies as compared to an isonitrogenous amino acid mixture (Coeffier et al. 2002). Further, glutamine at supraphysiological doses up to 10 mM suppressed IL-1β induced production of IL-6 and IL-8 and at the same time increased production of the anti-inflammatory cytokine IL-10 compared to physiological dose at 0.5 mM (Coeffier et al. 2003). Further, glutamine at the supraphysiological dose decreased IL-6 and IL-8 spontaneous production and NFκB p65 subunit expression, as compared to the physiological dose at 0.6 mM, in cultured inflamed colonic biopsies from patients with active CD (Lecleire et al. 2008). These *ex vivo* models allow a mechanistic pursue of glutamine's action on cytokine-related signaling pathways in human gut tissue (Lecleire et al. 2008). In a TNBS model, pretreatment with semipurified diet enriched with 2% and 4% glutamine (w/w) for two weeks before TNBS induction reduced the levels of proinflammatory cytokines IL-8 and TNF-α in inflamed tissue and attenuated the disease activity (Ameho et al. 1997). IL-17A expression in the colonic tissue could be reduced by glutamine treatment in the same model (Hou et al. 2013).

12.3.2.4 Enhancing Intestinal Cytoprotective Heat Shock Response

Induction of heat shock proteins (HSPs) is a key innate mechanism to protect cells against stress/injury, and adequate expression of HSPs (e.g., HSP25, HSP70, heme oxygenase [HO]-1) is essential to upholding the structural and functional integrity of the intestinal mucosa. Multiple lines of evidence reveal a key protective role of HSPs against inflammatory injury in IBD. Chang et al. (Hu et al. 2007) have shown that the HSP expression is markedly suppressed in human IBD lesions, which may contribute to the dysregulated proinflammatory response seen in IBD patients. During a variety of stress conditions, HSPs preserve intestinal epithelial cytoskeletal integrity, maintain integrity of intestinal TJ (Liu et al. 2003) and preventing permeability changes (Liu et al. 2003), which ultimately leads to better preserved intestinal barrier function. Further, activation of intestinal HSP expression has been shown to be a potent anti-inflammatory signal through downregulation of NFκB pathway (Voegeli et al. 2008). Thus, HSPs potentially modulate a gamut of interrelated processes or factors contributing to IBD pathogenesis, suggesting a multiplicity of HSPs' action.

Mucosal injury associated with IBD is in nature a result from the unbalanced interplays between cytotoxic factors/conditions and cell inherent defense capacity. Therapeutic strategies to promote cellular protection of the inflamed mucosa have been inadequately explored. Promoting HSP expression appears to be a promising therapeutic target for preventing intestinal inflammatory injury. However, laboratory approaches using chemical or hyperthermia are not practical for clinical application due to their inherent toxicities. We demonstrated for the first time that oral bolus glutamine administration in pharmacological dose (0.75 g/kg/day) enhanced colonic epithelial expression of inducible HSPs in DSS-induced colitis model associated with mitigated disease activity (Xue et al. 2011). Further, in cultured YAMC cells, glutamine increased cellular HSP25 and HSP70 in a dose-dependent manner and attenuated cytokine-induced injury (Xue et al. 2011). Echoed with our study, Hou et al. (2013) also showed that parenteral administration (intraperitoneal) of glutamine at 0.5 g/kg/day also enhanced colonic epithelial HSP70 expression and attenuated DSS-induced colitis. Thus, given the safe profile of its clinical use, glutamine has the potential to be developed as the first clinically relevant enhancer of heat shock response and may further elicit benefits in improving outcomes in IBD. Heat shock transcription factor (HSF)1 serves as the master regulator of HSP expression. Modulation of HSF1 transactivation activity is generally thought to be the main point of control for HSF1 activation of Hsp expression. How HSF1 expression as a transcription factor per se is largely unknown. With a further pursuit on the mechanisms underlying glutamine-mediated HSP expression upregulation, we for the first time demonstrated that glutamine not only can stimulate HSF1 transactivation, but also intriguingly can act as a competent inducer of HSF1 expression per se (Xue et al. 2012). This conceptual advance provides a novel mechanistic frame for regulation of HSF1-HSP axis.

12.4 CONCLUSIONS

In experimental IBD models, glutamine seems to be a promising nutrient that may serve therapeutic roles to modulate a multitude of interrelated mechanistic factors, for example, intestinal barrier integrity, tissue oxidative burden/stress, cytokine network, and innate cytoprotective mechanisms (i.e., HSP). Overall, this may lead to prevention or attenuation of intestinal inflammatory injury related to IBD. Despite significant clinical data supporting its use in conditions such as trauma, sepsis, burns, and cancer chemotherapies, its therapeutic use in the setting of IBD has been inadequately explored because the importance of basic pharmacologic principles (i.e., route, dose, and schedule) have not been considered. Basic questions on how to administer this nutrient in a clinically relevant and effective paradigm, which have been defined in conditions such as critical illness, still remain poorly answered in IBD settings.

Topical administration of glutamine, which conceivably ensures a great bioavailability of glutamine to local inflamed tissue, is associated with relatively consistent positive results in both clinical and experimental settings (Wischmeyer et al. 1993; Israeli et al. 2004; Kretzmann et al. 2008; Fillmann et al. 2007). Considerable debate has taken place regarding whether enteral or parenteral administration of glutamine provides greater benefits. Direct communication between gut mucosa and enteral glutamine has irreplaceable benefits to the GI tract as a whole via preferential use as fuel source or precursors of important biomolecules via direct luminal absorption of upper small intestine, modifying mucosal immunity, and stimulating splanchnic blood perfusion and intestinal blood microcirculation. Compared to the enteral route, parenteral administration of glutamine would presumably result in a greater bioavailability to lower small intestine and large intestine, which are most frequently involved in IBD, as enteral glutamine supply is subject to a great deal of first-pass metabolism in the upper small bowel. Available evidence is not adequate to support one route as opposed to the other.

In *in vitro* cytokine-induced injury models, we and others demonstrated that insufficient glutamine supply at concentrations less than 0.5 mM in the media, which mimics tissue glutamine deficiency *in vivo*, renders the cells more sensitive to cytokine-induced cell death (Evans et al. 2003; Xue et al. 2011). In light of this, large pharmacological doses of glutamine (at or approaching 0.5 g/kg/day), when supplied enterally *in vivo*, may thus pharmacokinetically lead to an adequate and sustained elevation of tissue glutamine level in lower small intestine and large intestine, which is likely essential for correcting glutamine deficiency and overcoming the threshold to elicit benefits (e.g., HSR). Markedly insufficient (or nonpharmacologic) doses of glutamine used in some of these clinical trials, which is evidenced by the failure to increase plasma glutamine concentrations, may thus not able to result in an adequate increase in tissue-free glutamine pool size. Of note, in conditions such as Gln supplementation of TPN in critical illness or in various dosing/route studies of bone marrow transplant, glutamine doses that may exceed the usual physiological requirements can consistently produce positive results in terms of clinical and mechanistic outcomes (Ziegler et al. 2005; Wischmeyer 2008). Although, reasonable doses ($\leq$0.5 g/kg/day i.v. or orally/enterally) should be utilized as a maximal dose as risk may occur at larger does (Heyland et al. 2013). The newly emerged conception of administering glutamine as "therapeutic nutrient" warrants more experimental and clinical trials in the settings of IBD.

REFERENCES

Akobeng, A. K., V. Miller, J. Stanton, A. M. Elbadri, and A. G. Thomas. 2000. Double-blind randomized controlled trial of glutamine-enriched polymeric diet in the treatment of active Crohn's disease. *J Pediatr Gastroenterol Nutr* 30 (1):78–84.

Ameho, C. K., A. A. Adjei, E. K. Harrison, K. Takeshita, T. Morioka, Y. Arakaki, E. Ito et al. 1997. Prophylactic effect of dietary glutamine supplementation on interleukin 8 and tumour necrosis factor alpha production in trinitrobenzene sulphonic acid induced colitis. *Gut* 41 (4):487–493.

Balasubramanian, K., S. Kumar, R. R. Singh, U. Sharma, G. Ahuja, G. K. Makharia, and N. R. Jagannathan. 2009. Metabolism of the colonic mucosa in patients with inflammatory bowel diseases: An *in vitro* proton magnetic resonance spectroscopy study. *Magn Reson Imaging* 27 (1):79–86.

Benjamin, J., G. Makharia, V. Ahuja, K. D. Anand Rajan, M. Kalaivani, S. D. Gupta, and Y. K. Joshi. 2012. Glutamine and whey protein improve intestinal permeability and morphology in patients with Crohn's disease: A randomized controlled trial. *Dig Dis Sci* 57 (4):1000–1012.

Bourreille, A., B. Humbert, P. Maugere, J. P. Galmiche, and D. Darmaun. 2004. Glutamine metabolism in Crohn's disease: A stable isotope study. *Clin Nutr* 23 (5):1167–1175.

Calder, P. C. 2007. Immunonutrition in surgical and critically ill patients. *Br J Nutr* 98 (Suppl 1):S133–S139.

Chahine, B. G. and S. L. Bahna. The role of the gut mucosal immunity in the development of tolerance against allergy to food. *Curr Opin Allergy Clin Immunol* 10 (3):220–225.

Coeffier, M., R. Marion, P. Ducrotte, and P. Dechelotte. 2003. Modulating effect of glutamine on IL-1beta-induced cytokine production by human gut. *Clin Nutr* 22 (4):407–413.

Coeffier, M., R. Marion, A. Leplingard, E. Lerebours, P. Ducrotte, and P. Dechelotte. 2002. Glutamine decreases interleukin-8 and interleukin-6 but not nitric oxide and prostaglandins e(2) production by human gut in-vitro. *Cytokine* 18 (2):92–97.

Dave, S. H., J. S. Tilstra, K. Matsuoka, F. Li, T. Karrasch, J. K. Uno, A. R. Sepulveda et al. 2007. Amelioration of chronic murine colitis by peptide-mediated transduction of the IkappaB kinase inhibitor NEMO binding domain peptide. *J Immunol* 179 (11):7852–7859.

DeMarco, V. G., N. Li, J. Thomas, C. M. West, and J. Neu. 2003. Glutamine and barrier function in cultured Caco-2 epithelial cell monolayers. *J Nutr* 133 (7):2176–2179.

Den Hond, E., M. Hiele, M. Peeters, Y. Ghoos, and P. Rutgeerts. 1999. Effect of long-term oral glutamine supplements on small intestinal permeability in patients with Crohn's disease. *JPEN J Parenter Enteral Nutr* 23 (1):7–11.

Dugan, M. E. and M. I. McBurney. 1995. Luminal glutamine perfusion alters endotoxin-related changes in ileal permeability of the piglet. *JPEN J Parenter Enteral Nutr* 19 (1):83–87.

Evans, M. E., D. P. Jones, and T. R. Ziegler. 2003. Glutamine prevents cytokine-induced apoptosis in human colonic epithelial cells. *J Nutr* 133 (10):3065–3071.

Fillmann, H., N. A. Kretzmann, B. San-Miguel, S. Llesuy, N. Marroni, J. Gonzalez-Gallego, and M. J. Tunon. 2007. Glutamine inhibits over-expression of pro-inflammatory genes and down-regulates the nuclear factor kappaB pathway in an experimental model of colitis in the rat. *Toxicology* 236 (3):217–226.

Flynn, W. J., Jr., J. R. Gosche, and R. N. Garrison. 1992. Intestinal blood flow is restored with glutamine or glucose suffusion after hemorrhage. *J Surg Res* 52 (5):499–504.

Foitzik, T., M. Kruschewski, A. J. Kroesen, H. G. Hotz, G. Eibl, and H. J. Buhr. 1999. Does glutamine reduce bacterial translocation? A study in two animal models with impaired gut barrier. *Int J Colorectal Dis* 14 (3):143–149.

Fujita, T. and K. Sakurai. 1995. Efficacy of glutamine-enriched enteral nutrition in an experimental model of mucosal ulcerative colitis. *Br J Surg* 82 (6):749–751.

Giris, M., Y. Erbil, S. Dogru-Abbasoglu, B. T. Yanik, H. Alis, V. Olgac, and G. A. Toker. 2007. The effect of heme oxygenase-1 induction by glutamine on TNBS-induced colitis. The effect of glutamine on TNBS colitis. *Int J Colorectal Dis* 22 (6):591–599.

Hausmann, M., S. Kiessling, S. Mestermann, G. Webb, T. Spottl, T. Andus, J. Scholmerich et al. 2002. Toll-like receptors 2 and 4 are up-regulated during intestinal inflammation. *Gastroenterology* 122 (7):1987–2000.

Heyland, D., J. Muscedere, P. E. Wischmeyer, D. Cook, G. Jones, M. Albert, G. Elke, M. M. Berger, and A. G. Day. 2013. A randomized trial of glutamine and antioxidants in critically ill patients. *N Engl J Med* 368 (16):1489–1497.

Hou, Y. C., C. C. Chu, T. L. Ko, C. L. Yeh, and S. L. Yeh. 2013. Effects of alanyl-glutamine dipeptide on the expression of colon-inflammatory mediators during the recovery phase of colitis induced by dextran sulfate sodium. *Eur J Nutr* 52 (3):1089–1098.

Hu, S., M. J. Ciancio, M. Lahav, M. Fujiya, L. Lichtenstein, S. Anant, M. W. Musch, and E. B. Chang. 2007. Translational inhibition of colonic epithelial heat shock proteins by IFN-gamma and TNF-alpha in intestinal inflammation. *Gastroenterology* 133 (6):1893–1904.

Israeli, E., E. Berenshtein, D. Wengrower, L. Aptekar, R. Kohen, G. Zajicek, and E. Goldin. 2004. Prophylactic administration of topical glutamine enhances the capability of the rat colon to resist inflammatory damage. *Dig Dis Sci* 49 (10):1705–1712.

Kessel, A., E. Toubi, E. Pavlotzky, J. Mogilner, A. G. Coran, M. Lurie, R. Karry, and I. Sukhotnik. 2008. Treatment with glutamine is associated with down-regulation of Toll-like receptor-4 and myeloid differentiation factor 88 expression and decrease in intestinal mucosal injury caused by lipopolysaccharide endotoxaemia in a rat. *Clin Exp Immunol* 151 (2):341–347.

Kretzmann, N. A., H. Fillmann, J. L. Mauriz, C. A. Marroni, N. Marroni, J. Gonzalez-Gallego, and M. J. Tunon. 2008. Effects of glutamine on proinflammatory gene expression and activation of nuclear factor kappa B and signal transducers and activators of transcription in TNBS-induced colitis. *Inflamm Bowel Dis* 14 (11):1504–1513.

Kruschewski, M., S. Perez-Canto, A. Hubotter, T. Foitzik, and H. J. Buhr. 1998. Protective effect of glutamine on microcirculation of the intestine in experimental colitis. *Langenbecks Arch Chir Suppl Kongressbd* 115 (Suppl I):229–231.

Kucharzik, T., S. V. Walsh, J. Chen, C. A. Parkos, and A. Nusrat. 2001. Neutrophil transmigration in inflammatory bowel disease is associated with differential expression of epithelial intercellular junction proteins. *Am J Pathol* 159 (6):2001–2009.

Lecleire, S., A. Hassan, R. Marion-Letellier, M. Antonietti, G. Savoye, C. Bole-Feysot, E. Lerebours, P. Ducrotte, P. Dechelotte, and M. Coeffier. 2008. Combined glutamine and arginine decrease proinflammatory cytokine production by biopsies from Crohn's patients in association with changes in nuclear factor-kappaB and p38 mitogen-activated protein kinase pathways. *J Nutr* 138 (12):2481–2486.

Li, N., P. Lewis, D. Samuelson, K. Liboni, and J. Neu. 2004. Glutamine regulates Caco-2 cell tight junction proteins. *Am J Physiol Gastrointest Liver Physiol* 287 (3):G726–G733.

Li, N. and J. Neu. 2009. Glutamine deprivation alters intestinal tight junctions via a PI3-K/Akt mediated pathway in Caco-2 cells. *J Nutr* 139 (4):710–714.

Liu, T. S., M. W. Musch, K. Sugi, M. M. Walsh-Reitz, M. J. Ropeleski, B. A. Hendrickson, C. Pothoulakis, J. T. Lamont, and E. B. Chang. 2003. Protective role of HSP72 against Clostridium difficile toxin A-induced intestinal epithelial cell dysfunction. *Am J Physiol Cell Physiol* 284 (4):C1073–C1082.

Medzhitov, R. 2001. Toll-like receptors and innate immunity. *Nat Rev Immunol* 1 (2):135–145.

Mottet, C., H. H. Uhlig, and F. Powrie. 2003. Cutting edge: Cure of colitis by CD4 + CD25+ regulatory T cells. *J Immunol* 170 (8):3939–3943.

Ockenga, J., K. Borchert, E. Stuber, H. Lochs, M. P. Manns, and S. C. Bischoff. 2005. Glutamine-enriched total parenteral nutrition in patients with inflammatory bowel disease. *Eur J Clin Nutr* 59 (11):1302–1309.

Reeds, P. J. and D. G. Burrin. 2001. Glutamine and the bowel. *J Nutr* 131 (9 Suppl):2505S–2508S; discussion 2523S–2504S.

Rogler, G., K. Brand, D. Vogl, S. Page, R. Hofmeister, T. Andus, R. Knuechel, P. A. Baeuerle, J. Scholmerich, and V. Gross. 1998. Nuclear factor kappaB is activated in macrophages and epithelial cells of inflamed intestinal mucosa. *Gastroenterology* 115 (2):357–369.

Sartor, R. B. 2006. Mechanisms of disease: Pathogenesis of Crohn's disease and ulcerative colitis. *Nat Clin Pract Gastroenterol Hepatol* 3 (7):390–407.

Sartor, R. B. 2009. Microbial-host interactions in inflammatory bowel diseases and experimental colitis. *Nestle Nutr Workshop Ser Pediatr Program* 64:121–132; discussion 132–127, 251–127.

Sartor, R. B. and F. Hoentjen. 2005. Proinflammatory cytokines and signaling pathways in intestinal innate immune cells. In: *Mucosal Immunol*, edited by Mestecky J., Lamm M. E., McGhee J. R., Bienenstock J., Mayer L. and Strober W., 681–701. Philadelphia: Elsevier.

Sartor, R. B. and M. Muehlbauer. 2007. Microbial host interactions in IBD: Implications for pathogenesis and therapy. *Curr Gastroenterol Rep* 9 (6):497–507.

Scheppach, W., G. Dusel, T. Kuhn, C. Loges, H. Karch, H. P. Bartram, F. Richter, S. U. Christl, and H. Kasper. 1996. Effect of L-glutamine and n-butyrate on the restitution of rat colonic mucosa after acid induced injury. *Gut* 38 (6):878–885.

Sen, C. K. and L. Packer. 1996. Antioxidant and redox regulation of gene transcription. *Faseb J* 10 (7):709–720.

Triantafillidis, J. K. and C. Stanciu. 2012. *Inflammatory Bowel Disease: Etiopathogenesis, Diagnosis, Treatment*, 4th Edition. Athens, Greece: Technogramma.

Voegeli, T. S., A. J. Wintink, Y. Chen, and R. W. Currie. 2008. Heat shock proteins 27 and 70 regulating angiotensin II-induced NF-kappaB: A possible connection to blood pressure control? *Appl Physiol Nutr Metab* 33 (5):1042–1049.

Welbourne, T. C. 1979. Ammonia production and glutamine incorporation into glutathione in the functioning rat kidney. *Can J Biochem* 57 (3):233–237.

Wischmeyer, P., J. H. Pemberton, and S. F. Phillips. 1993. Chronic pouchitis after ileal pouch-anal anastomosis: Responses to butyrate and glutamine suppositories in a pilot study. *Mayo Clin Proc* 68 (10):978–981.

Wischmeyer, P. E. 2008. Glutamine: Role in critical illness and ongoing clinical trials. *Curr Opin Gastroenterol* 24 (2):190–197.

Xavier, R. J. and D. K. Podolsky. 2007. Unravelling the pathogenesis of inflammatory bowel disease. *Nature* 448 (7152):427–434.

Xue, H., D. Slavov, and P. E. Wischmeyer. 2012. Glutamine-mediated dual regulation of heat shock transcription factor-1 activation and expression. *J Biol Chem* 287 (48):40400–40413.

Xue, H., A. J. Sufit, and P. E. Wischmeyer. 2011. Glutamine therapy improves outcome of *in vitro* and *in vivo* experimental colitis models. *JPEN J Parenter Enteral Nutr* 35 (2):188–197.

Zhu, H. and Y. R. Li. 2012. Oxidative stress and redox signaling mechanisms of inflammatory bowel disease: Updated experimental and clinical evidence. *Exp Biol Med (Maywood)* 237 (5):474–480.

Ziegler, T. R., L. G. Ogden, K. D. Singleton, M. Luo, C. Fernandez-Estivariz, D. P. Griffith, J. R. Galloway, and P. E. Wischmeyer. 2005. Parenteral glutamine increases serum heat shock protein 70 in critically ill patients. *Intensive Care Med* 31 (8):1079–1086.

Zoli, G., M. Care, F. Falco, C. Spano, R. Bernardi, and G. Gasbamini. 1995. Effect of oral glutamine on intestinal permeability and nutritional status in Crohn's disease. *Gastroenterology* 108:A766.

Section VI

*Glutamine and the Catabolic State:
Role of Glutamine in Critical
Illness During Childhood*

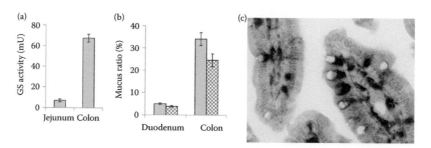

FIGURE 2.1 (a) GS enzyme activity in jejunum and colon. GS activity was measured in tissue homogenates. Activity was determined spectrophotometrically with the γ-glutamyltransferase assay and expressed as nmoles/min mg total protein (mU) at 37°C. (b) Percentage of intestinal epithelial surface occupied by mucus in jejunum and colon of control (homogeneous gray) and GS-KO/I mice (cross-hatched). The "stained surface" of Alcian blue-stained sections was determined in four random pictures with ImageJ. (c) Ileal villus stained for the presence of GS in a wild-type mouse. The presence of GS was demonstrated with mouse monoclonal antibodies (clone GS-6, R&D Systems, UK). Antibody binding was visualized with the appropriate alkaline phosphatase-coupled secondary antisera. Specific staining is seen in the goblet cells only. Positive cells in the submucosa represent immune cells containing immunoglobulins that are recognized by the second antibody (see also Figures 2.3 and 2.4).

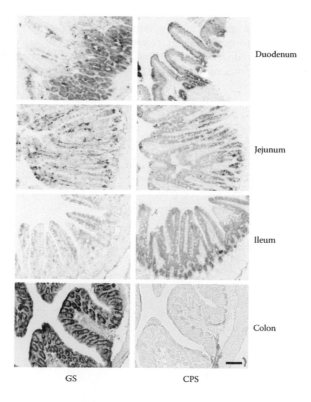

FIGURE 2.2 Serial sections of the intestine in fed control mice were stained for the presence of GS or carbamoyl-phosphate synthetase (CPS). The presence of CPS was visualized with a rabbit antiserum (Charles et al. 1983) and an alkaline phosphatase-coupled secondary antiserum. Note the roughly reciprocal staining pattern of GS and CPS. The staining intensity of GS is relatively low in the small intestine, except for Brunner's glands in the duodenum, whereas its staining in the colon is intense. CPS is present in the epithelium of the small intestine, except for Brunner's glands and the colon, where it is nearly absent. Magnification: 10× (bar: 0.1 mm).

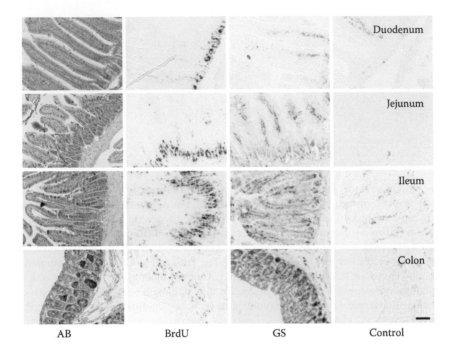

Duodenum

Jejunum

Ileum

Colon

AB　　　　　BrdU　　　　　GS　　　　　Control

FIGURE 2.3 Serial sections of the intestine of fed control females were stained for the presence of mucus (Alcian Blue with nuclear fast red counter staining), bromodeoxyuridine (BrdU), or GS; 32.5 µmol (10 mg) BrdU per 10 g body weight dissolved in 50 µL 0.9% NaCl was injected intraperitoneally 150 and 30 min before sacrifice. The control represents a section without first antibody. Magnification: 10× (bar: 0.1 mm).

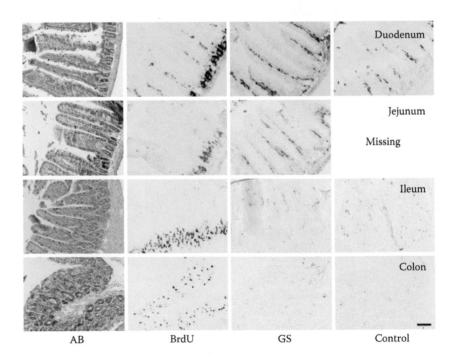

Duodenum

Jejunum

Missing

Ileum

Colon

AB　　　　　BrdU　　　　　GS　　　　　Control

FIGURE 2.4 Serial sections of the intestine of fed GS-KO/I females were stained for the presence of mucus, BrdU, or GS. Note that the stain in the duodenum and jejunum after incubation with the GS antibody is present in the stem of the villus and not in the epithelium. This staining pattern is also seen in the section incubated with the secondary antiserum only. The jejunal control section ("missing") was lost in the course of the immunohistochemical procedure. Bar: 0.1 mm.

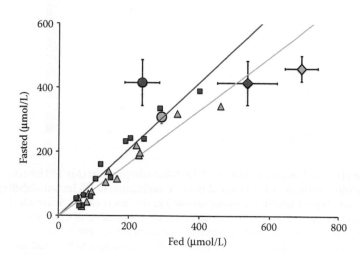

FIGURE 2.5 Correlation between fed and 24-h-fasted portal-vein amino acid concentrations in control and GS/KO/I mice. Amino acid concentrations in deproteinized plasma samples were determined by HPLC (van Eijk et al. 1993). Control mice are represented by red symbols (regression line in red as well) and GS-KO/I mice by blue symbols (regression line: blue). Circles represent glutamine and diamonds alanine. Please note that amino acids, except for glutamine and alanine, are not identified by name.

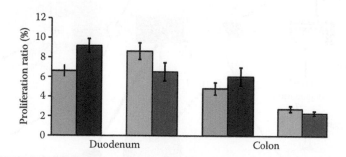

FIGURE 2.6 BrdU incorporation into epithelial cells of the duodenum or colon. Control (red columns) or GS-KO/I (blue columns) mice were either fed (light columns) or 24-h-fasted (dark columns) when they were treated with BrdU. BrdU incorporation in the colon was ~70% of that in the duodenum and sensitive to fasting (~2-fold decrease), irrespective of whether the animal was or was not GS-deficient in the intestinal epithelium. The effect of fasting was most prominent in GS-KO/I mice and may also have decreased incorporation in the duodenum.

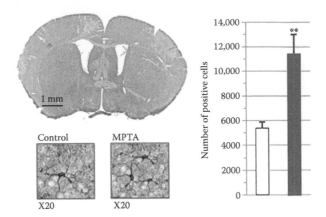

FIGURE 9.7 The effect of 1-methyl-4-phenyl-1,2,3,6-tetrahydropyridine (MPTP) intoxication on glutamine synthetase (GS) labeling in the dorsal striatum of mice. Visualization of GS immunolabeling in coronal slice of the dorsal striatum. Typical labeling is shown (arrows) in the insets (X20). Scale bar, 1 mm. Quantitative analysis of the effect of dopaminergic (DA) denervation on the number of GS-positive cells in the dorsal striatum. Data are expressed as the mean number of immunoreactive cells ± standard deviation (SD) for 5 animals per group. Statistical comparisons were performed by two-way ANOVA, followed by Dunnett's test. **$p < 0.01$ versus the control group.

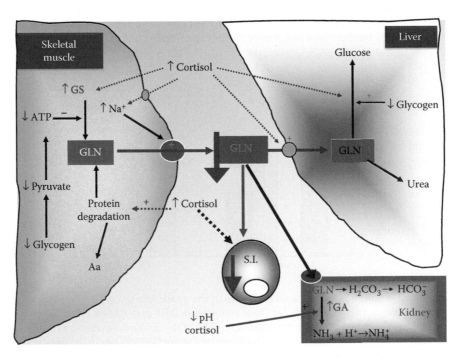

FIGURE 22.1 Alteration in the kinetics of transport of glutamine (GLN) in muscle tissue, resulting in decreased release of GLN during and after exercise.

13 Glutamine in the Critically Ill Neonate

Nan Li, Liya Ma, and Josef Neu

CONTENTS

13.1 INTRODUCTION

Glutamine (Gln), the most abundant amino acid in the body, serves as an important metabolic intermediate, signaling molecule, and nutrient. Gln is considered to be a conditionally essential amino acid. Under stress conditions, such as trauma, infection, or sepsis, cells and tissues in the immune system increase the consumption of Gln (Newsholme 2001). However, the body may not be able to produce adequate amounts of Gln to meet the increased demands. Therefore, supplementation of Gln is important during stress.

Premature infants appear to have a particular need for the supplementation of Gln. Premature birth leads to an abrupt cessation of a special combination of nutrients required for the rapidly developing fetus, including Gln (Neu et al. 2002). In the first weeks after birth, these infants frequently lack luminal nutrients containing Gln, but obtain most of their nutrition from the parenteral route containing no Gln. In addition, premature infants are exposed to various perinatal stresses, including hypotension, hypoxia, hyperoxia, hypothermia, and anemia. These highly stressed infants have increased consumption of Gln during their first several weeks after birth (Neu and Li 2007). Moreover, other precursors involved in the Gln synthesis pathway may not be adequately provided during this highly vulnerable period.

Over the past decades, the importance of Gln has been studied extensively, both in animals and humans. In critically ill adults, studies have demonstrated that Gln supplementation is safe and reduces mortality and improve outcomes in seriously ill patients (Griffiths et al. 1997; Novak et al. 2002; Kreymann et al. 2006; Wischmeyer 2006). In very-low-birth-weight (VLBW) infants, studies have been done to evaluate the effect of parenteral or enteral Gln supplementation on morbidity, mortality, and other outcomes in the neonatal period (Roig et al. 1996; Neu et al. 1997; Vaughn et al. 2003; Poindexter et al. 2004; van den Berg et al. 2005a,b; Sevastiadou et al. 2011; Moe-Byrne et al. 2012). Some studies have demonstrated benefits with Gln supplementation (Neu et al. 1997; Vaughn et al. 2003; van den Berg et al. 2005a,b). However, other studies showed no benefits (Lacey et al. 1996; Poindexter et al. 2004). In this review, we will focus on Gln effects on gut, provide a summary of recent studies and applications of Gln supplementation including long-term observations in neonates, and also discuss studies of Gln dipeptides.

13.2   GUT AND GLN IN NEONATES

Gastrointestinal diseases are among the highest causes of neonatal morbidity and mortality (American Gastroenterological Association Medical 2000). Several defense layers against bacterial invasion comprise the intestinal barrier, including the mucus layer, the epithelium, and the under-lying mucosal immune system. Intestinal epithelial cells produce proinflammatory cytokines and other mediators when stimulated, acting as both antigen processing and immune effector cells. In premature infants, the intestinal epithelium is constantly exposed to various microbes and antigens that may disrupt tight junctions, and impair intestinal cellular function by increasing monolayer permeability (Xu et al. 1999). The intestinal barrier dysfunction may cause further small intesti-nal injury. This intestinal injury may occur in a variety of severe pathophysiologic conditions in pediatric patients, which can result in systemic inflammatory response syndrome (SIRS), bacte-rial translocation, distal organ damage, and even multiple organ failure. Among them, necrotiz-ing enterocolitis (NEC) is one of the most common and devastating diseases found in premature infants in neonatal intensive care units (NICUs) with high mortality, long hospitalization, and high financial cost (Neu and Walker 2011). It can also affect distant organs such as the brain and place affected infants at substantially increased risk for neurodevelopmental delays. Intestinal inflam-matory mediators such as TNF-α, interleukin (IL)-1, IL-6, IL-8, IL-12, and IL-18, PAF produced by enterocytes, and inflammatory cells contribute to the pathogenesis of NEC (Caplan et al. 1990; Markel et al. 2006). In addition, intestinal vascular dysfunction associated with hypoxia-reoxygen-ation (H/R) may also be involved in the pathophysiology of NEC (Gellen et al. 2003; Richir et al. 2007; Nankervis et al. 2008).

As a predominant amino acid, Gln is provided to the fetus through the placenta (Battaglia and Regnault 2001). For the critically ill or VLBW infants especially for those with intestinal injury, Gln deficiency may become a serious problem. Free Gln is not a component of parenteral amino acid solutions because of low solubility and instability (Verbruggen et al. 2010). Premature infants in the first weeks of life and infants with gut problems will receive most of their nutrients from Gln-free parenteral nutrition solution (Neu 2003), making them vulnerable to Gln deficiency and related dis-eases. During catabolic stress, Gln consumption may exceed the supply, and both plasma and skeletal muscle pools of free Gln are severely reduced (Oliveira et al. 2010). In addition, under stress condi-tions, premature and ill infants are not able to synthesize sufficient Gln to meet demand. Low plasma concentrations of Gln have been associated with a higher incidence of NEC (Becker et al. 2000).

Gln has been proved to maintain mucosal integrity (Li et al. 1994) and intestinal barrier functions (Li, Lewis et al. 2004; Li and Neu 2009). *In vitro* studies of Gln deprivation in intestinal epithelial cells show decreased transepithilial resistance and reduced tight junction proteins, including clau-din 1, occluding ad ZO-1 (Li et al. 1994; Li, Lewis et al. 2004). The Gln effect on maintenance of intestinal barrier function is associated with the PI3 kinase pathway. These findings suggested that integrity of intestinal monolayer and tight junctions rely on Gln, especially under stress condition.

Previous studies have reported the role of Gln in anti-inflammation (Akisu et al. 2003) and regulating the immune response (Wischmeyer et al. 2001a,b) and indicated the ability of Gln to attenuate the inflammatory response via IκB/NF-κB signaling pathway (Singleton et al. 2005; Yeh et al. 2005), Gln significantly decreased lipopolysaccharide-induced inflammatory mediators in the intestine, liver and lung in an infant rodent pup-in-the-cup model (Li, Liboni et al. 2004). Therefore, there appears to be a strong relationship between gut-derived systemic inflammation and Gln. The ability of Gln to decrease gut-derived systemic inflammation has especially significant implications for premature infants.

The other mechanisms of Gln intestinal protective action include tissue protection (Neu and Li 2007), preservation of antioxidant capacity (Neu and Li 2007), decrease of intestinal apoptosis by increasing Bcl-2 expression (Ban and Kozar 2010; Yuan et al. 2010), and increase of heat shock proteins (Wischmeyer et al. 1997). Gln protects intestinal epithelial cells against H/R-induced apop-tosis through increasing Bcl-2 expression (Yuan et al. 2010). Oral supplementation of Gln reduced the histologic evidence of intestinal injury in young mice by inhibiting intestinal cytokine release in an H/R-induced experimental NEC model (Koc et al. 1998). Gln also has protective effects on ischemia-/reperfusion-induced intestinal injury in animal models through attenuating neutrophil infiltration, P-selectin and ICAM-1 upregulation in the ileum, tyrosine residues nitration, PARP activation, NF-κB expression, apoptosis, and Bax and Bcl-2 expression (Mondello et al. 2010).

13.3 CLINICAL STUDIES OF GLN

Clinical studies in premature infants have proved the safety of both enteral and parenteral Gln supplementations. One of the first randomized studies was in 44 VLBW infants in the presence and absence of Gln supplementation via total parenteral nutrition (TPN) (Lacey et al. 1996). The results indicated that Gln supplementation reduced days of TPN, shortened length of time to full enteral feedings, and decreased periods of ventilator support in the infants less than 800 g body weight. The length of stay in the NICU also tends to be shorter. This study suggests that Gln was safe and probably conditionally essential in extremely low-birth-weights (ELBW) premature infants. A large multicenter, randomized, double-masked clinical trial in 1433 ELBW infants was conducted to evaluate the safety and efficacy of early PN supplemented with Gln in decreasing the risk of death or late-onset sepsis (Poindexter et al. 2004). No significant adverse events were observed with Gln supplementation. However, Gln showed no effect on tolerance of enteral feeds, NEC, or growth (Poindexter et al. 2004). The methods used in this study have been questioned (Neu 2003), but because of the largely negative results, it will be unlikely that a similar study with more appropriate controls will be repeated.

In premature BW infants, Gln supplementation enterally administered has been reported to reduce hospital costs (Dallas et al. 1998), decrease morbidity (Neu et al. 1997), be well tolerated in critically ill infants and tended to be associated with less infectious morbidity and mortality in this high-risk population (Barbosa et al. 1999). An early study of enteral Gln supplementation in VLBW infants showed a decrease in hospital-acquired sepsis with evidence of a blunted inflammatory response secondary to decrease translocation of proinflammatory antigens (Neu et al. 1997). A clinical trial of enteral Gln supplementation in low-birthweight infants showed decreased sepsis in the Gln-supplemented group (van den Berg et al. 2005a,b). In this study, Gln-enriched enteral nutrition did not improve feeding tolerance. However, infectious morbidity was significantly lowered in infants who received Gln-enriched enteral nutrition (van den Berg et al. 2005a,b). In a multicenter trial in 649 VLBW infants less than 7 days of age were randomized to Gln supplementation or standard of care control feedings; Neonates in the Gln group were provided Gln at a dose of 0.3 g/kg/day enterally for the first 28 days (Vaughn et al. 2003). Enteral Gln did not show differences in primary outcome, sepsis, but showed significant improvement on secondary outcomes, which included intestinal function and a decrease in grades 3–4 intraventricular hemorrhages or periventricular leukomalacia in survivors (Vaughn et al. 2003). Inflammatory mediators were not measured in this large trial of enteral supplementation. Recently a study reported a placebo-controlled randomized trial of the impact of oral Gln supplementation on the intestinal permeability and incidence of NEC/septicemia in premature neonates (Sevastiadou et al. 2011). One hundred and one preterm neonates with gestational age <34 weeks and birth weight <2000 g were involved. Oral Gln supplementation with 0.3 g/kg/day for no more than 30 days results in decreased intestinal permeability and less NEC/septicemia (Sevastiadou et al. 2011).

The benefit of using the enteral route is that more Gln can be delivered directly to the intestine when exposed to stress agents and can be rapidly used by the intestinal epithelium. Intravenous infusions rarely result in plasma concentration of more than 1 mM, which is also supported by a study in which no differences were shown between groups for plasma concentrations of Gln during the enteral supplementation of Gln (van den Berg et al. 2005a,b). Panigrahi et al. reported that Gln decreased bacterial translocation when supplied by the apical versus the basolateral route using Caco-2 monolayers (Panigrahi et al. 1997). It is not clear if the enteral route offers a greater capability to modulate inflammation. However, enteral supplementation could reduce the amount taken up from the arterial supply by the intestine, therefore leaving more substrates, including essential amino acids for nonsplanchnic organs.

A recent Cochrane review identified 11 randomized and a total of 2771 preterm infants participated in controlled trials (Moe-Byrne et al. 2012). Five of them evaluated enteral Gln supplementation and six of them evaluated parenteral Gln supplementation. Gln supplementation did not show a significant effect on mortality or major neonatal morbidities including the incidence of invasive infection or NEC by meta-analysis. It was concluded that the available trial data do not provide evidence that Gln supplementation provides significant benefits for preterm infants. In another review related to Gln randomized studies in early life, the author also concluded that "although apparently safe in animal models (pups), premature infants, and critically ill children, Gln supplementation does not reduce mortality or late onset sepsis, and its routine use cannot be recommended in these sensitive populations. Large prospectively stratified trials are needed" (Briassouli and Briassoulis 2012). Based on the controversial results, some investigators suggest that further study in this area is no longer necessary. However, in a recent review, more recent research in the area of Gln supplementation is described and the authors suggest additional studies are still warranted (van Zwol, Neu et al. 2011), especially with a suggestion for neurodevelopmental benefits.

In summary, studies done so far have suggested that in infants Gln supplementation is safe both enterally and parenterally. However, the results for efficacy on a limited number of outcomes have been controversial. The use of Gln alone has not become routine. In infants and critically ill children, the effects are unknown since less data are available during childhood.

13.4   LONG-TERM FOLLOW-UP STUDY OF GLN-SUPPLEMENTED INFANTS

A follow-up study administration in preterm infants from the Amsterdam group showed that enteral Gln-enriched nutrition decreased the risk of allergic and infectious disease at 6 years of age (van Zwol, Moll et al. 2011). A decreased risk of gastrointestinal tract infections was also found in the Gln-supplemented group. Using the same cohort, a follow-up study utilized MRI volumetric measures of brain structures as well as fractional anisotropy of major white matter tracts when these children reached school age (de Kieviet et al. 2012). In addition, another study by the same group in 65 very-preterm (<32 weeks gestation) children indicates a specific increase in head circumference growth in very-preterm children that received neonatal Gln supplementation, and suggests that group differences in brain structure volumes at school age may have emerged during the first year of life (de Kieviet et al. 2014).

13.5   EFFECTS OF ARGININE-GLN DIPEPTIDE

Arginine is the substrate for nitric oxide synthesis, a potent vasodilator and anti-inflammatory (Moncada et al. 1991). Arginine also serves as a precursor for the synthesis of Gln and other amino acids. Hospitalized premature infants often experience various stresses that increase the utilization of critical amino acids beyond the endogenous biosynthetic ability. Arginine requirements are higher in infants who are stressed due to higher utilization in conditions such as NEC or pulmonary hypertension. Therefore, in addition to deprivation of Gln, those infants also have low blood arginine levels (Wu et al. 2004). Just as with Gln, plasma arginine concentrations are associated with NEC (Zamora et al. 1997; Becker et al. 2000; Richir et al. 2007). Although arginine is supplied in parenteral amino acid solutions, it still may not be sufficient to meet the needs of critically ill premature and VLBW infants. Previous studies indicated that arginine can protect intestinal epithelial integrity via a mechanism dependent on NO donation (Chapman et al. 2012). In a newborn mouse model, supplementing L-arginine increased tissue levels of NO and reduced morphologic intestinal injury among mice undergoing hypoxia/reoxygenation (Cintra et al. 2008). Other animal studies also supported the protective effects of arginine on hypoxic intestinal injuries (Akisu et al. 2002; Kabaroglu et al. 2005). Arginine supplementation has been reported to decrease the incidence of NEC and did not increase neurodevelopmental disability in later life in several clinical studies (Amin et al. 2002, 2009; Shah and Shah 2004, 2007; Polycarpou et al. 2013). No adverse effects were observed in neonates receiving L-arginine supplementation. The incidence of NEC stage III was significantly lower in the arginine-supplemented group (Polycarpou et al. 2013).

However, providing Gln or arginine as an individual amino acid has limitations. Low solubility and instability during heat sterilization and prolonged storage limit the use of free Gln in the routine clinical setting. The concept of combining amino acids to improve stability and solubility of Gln has been raised and utilized the combination of alanine and Gln (Furst et al. 1989, 1990; Furst 2001). There is the theoretical benefit of enhanced absorption of the dipeptide compared with single amino acid by virtue of oligopeptide transporters located in the intestinal brush border membrane in both the small and large intestines (Adibi 1997). Several Gln dipeptides such as alanyl-Gln (Tazuke et al. 2003) and glycyl-Gln (Jiang et al. 2006) have been used to study various diseases in animal models and in human trials that supported its safety and efficacy (Furst et al. 1990; Bober-Olesinska and Kornacka 2005). It has been demonstrated that Gln dipeptide added to a standard amino acid solution increased blood levels of Gln and decreased the incidence of NEC compared with control group in VLBW neonates (Bober-Olesinska and Kornacka 2005). In other clinical studies, nitrogen balance was shown to be more positive in catabolic patients receiving L-alanyl-L-Gln solution than in control patients receiving isonitrogenous, isoenergetic total parenteral nutrition (Furst et al. 1990).

In recent years, combination of arginine and Gln as a dipeptide (Arg-Gln) has been used to take advantage of both amino acids and overcome the drawbacks of free Gln. Studies in a neonatal mouse model showed that intraperitoneal or enteral administration of Arg-Gln dipeptide reduced abnormal retinal neovascularization and vascular leakage, pulmonary or intestinal injury induced by hyperoxia (Neu et al. 2006; Li et al. 2012; Ma et al. 2012). Premature newborns often need high concentrations of oxygen. However, hyperoxia could be considered as an oxidative stress condition that affects the development of the intestine (Giannone et al. 2007). In a study using a hyperoxia-induced retinopathy mouse model, Arg-Gln significantly reduced retinal neovascularization in the oxygen-induced retinopathy compared with the control dipeptide Ala-Gln (Neu et al. 2006). This effect was associated with decreased retinal VEGF mRNA levels. Dipeptide Arg-Gln appears to be safe and may prove beneficial in the prevention of retinopathy of prematurity with future human infant studies (Neu et al. 2006). In a mouse hyperoxic intestinal injury study (Li et al. 2012), Arg-Gln inhibited hyperoxia-induced myeloperoxidase activity and returned LDH activity to levels of control. In addition, Arg-Gln reversed hyperoxia-induced apoptotic cell death in distal small intestine (Li et al. 2012). In the same animal model, Arg-Gln prevented the development of important indicators of hyperoxia-induced lung injury, including histologic changes, myeloperoxidase, lactate dehydrogenase, and inflammatory cytokines associated with restoration of levels of nuclear factor-kappaB inhibitor (Ma et al. 2012). These studies demonstrated the protective effects of Arg-Gln supplementation. With the positive animal studies, it is tempting to carry out clinical studies in humans.

13.6 CONCLUSIONS

Gln has been shown to provide benefit in several models of intestinal injury and is safe in infants. However, the use of Gln alone has not become routine since the results for efficacy on a limited number of outcomes have been controversial. The long-term effects of Gln on neurodevelopment in preterm infants should prompt additional investigation. Using the dipeptide Arg-Gln appears to have several benefits and preliminary studies support that it is safe and effective in a rodent model of hyperoxia-induced retinopathy, lung and intestinal damage. With the positive animal studies, it would be tempting to carry out control clinical studies in the future.

REFERENCES

Adibi, S A. 1997. The oligopeptide transporter (Pept-1) in human intestine: Biology and function. *Gastroenterology* 113(1): 332–340.

Akisu, M, Baka, M, Huseyinov, A et al. 2003. The role of dietary supplementation with L-glutamine in inflammatory mediator release and intestinal injury in hypoxia/reoxygenation-induced experimental necrotizing enterocolitis. *Ann Nutr Metab* 47(6): 262–266.

Akisu, M, Ozmen, D, Baka, M et al. 2002. Protective effect of dietary supplementation with L-arginine and L-carnitine on hypoxia/reoxygenation-induced necrotizing enterocolitis in young mice. *Biol Neonate* 81(4): 260–265.

American Gastroenterological Association Medical. 2000. American Gastroenterological Association Medical Position Statement: Guidelines on intestinal ischemia. *Gastroenterology* 118(5): 951–953.

Amin, H J, Soraisham, A S and Sauve, R S. 2009. Neurodevelopmental outcomes of premature infants treated with l-arginine for prevention of necrotising enterocolitis. *J Paediatr Child Health* 45(4): 219–223.

Amin, H J, Zamora, S A, McMillan, D D et al. 2002. Arginine supplementation prevents necrotizing enterocolitis in the premature infant. *J Pediatr* 140(4): 425–431.

Ban, K and Kozar, R A. 2010. Glutamine protects against apoptosis via downregulation of Sp3 in intestinal epithelial cells. *Am J Physiol Gastrointest Liver Physiol* 299(6): G1344–G1353.

Barbosa, E, Moreira, E A, Goes, J E et al. 1999. Pilot study with a glutamine-supplemented enteral formula in critically ill infants. *Rev Hosp Clin Fac Med Sao Paulo* 54(1): 21–24.

Battaglia, F C and Regnault, T R. 2001. Placental transport and metabolism of amino acids. *Placenta* 22(2–3): 145–161.

Becker, R M, Wu, G, Galanko, J A et al. 2000. Reduced serum amino acid concentrations in infants with necrotizing enterocolitis. *J Pediatr* 137(6): 785–793.

Bober-Olesinska, K and Kornacka, M K. 2005. Effects of glutamine supplemented parenteral nutrition on the incidence of necrotizing enterocolitis, nosocomial sepsis and length of hospital stay in very low birth weight infants. *Med Wieku Rozwoj* 9(3 Pt 1): 325–333.

Briassouli, E and Briassoulis, G. 2012. Glutamine randomized studies in early life: The unsolved riddle of experimental and clinical studies. *Clin Dev Immunol* 2012: 749189.

Caplan, M S, Sun, X M, Hseuh, W et al. 1990. Role of platelet activating factor and tumor necrosis factor-alpha in neonatal necrotizing enterocolitis. *J Pediatr* 116(6): 960–964.

Chapman, J C, Liu, Y, Zhu, L et al. 2012. Arginine and citrulline protect intestinal cell monolayer tight junctions from hypoxia-induced injury in piglets. *Pediatr Res* 72(6): 576–582.

Cintra, A E, Martins, J L, Patricio, F R et al. 2008. Nitric oxide levels in the intestines of mice submitted to ischemia and reperfusion: L-arginine effects. *Transplant Proc* 40(3): 830–835.

Dallas, M J, Bowling, D, Roig, J C et al. 1998. Enteral glutamine supplementation for very-low-birth-weight infants decreases hospital costs. *JPEN J Parenter Enteral Nutr* 22(6): 352–356.

de Kieviet, J F, Oosterlaan, J, Vermeulen, R J et al. 2012. Effects of glutamine on brain development in very preterm children at school age. *Pediatrics* 130(23071202): 1121–1127.

de Kieviet, J F, Vuijk, P J, van den Berg, A et al. 2014. Glutamine effects on brain growth in very preterm children in the first year of life. *Clin Nutr* 33(1): 69–74.

Furst, P. 2001. New developments in glutamine delivery. *J Nutr* 131(9 Suppl): 2562S–2568S.

Furst, P, Albers, S and Stehle, P. 1989. Availability of glutamine supplied intravenously as alanylglutamine. *Metabolism* 38(8 Suppl 1): 67–72.

Furst, P, Albers, S and Stehle, P. 1990. Glutamine-containing dipeptides in parenteral nutrition. *JPEN J Parenter Enteral Nutr* 14(4 Suppl): 118S–124S.

Gellen, B, Kovacs, J, Nemeth, L et al. 2003. Vascular changes play a role in the pathogenesis of necrotizing enterocolitis in asphyxiated newborn pigs. *Pediatr Surg Int* 19(5): 380–384.

Giannone, P J, Bauer, J A, Schanbacher, B L et al. 2007. Effects of hyperoxia on postnatal intestinal development. *Biotech Histochem* 82(1): 17–22.

Griffiths, R D, Jones, C and Palmer, T E. 1997. Six-month outcome of critically ill patients given glutamine-supplemented parenteral nutrition. *Nutrition* 13(4): 295–302.

Jiang, J W, Zheng, S S, Xue, F et al. 2006. Enteral feeding of glycyl-glutamine dipeptide improves the structure and absorptive function of the small intestine after allogenetic liver transplantation in rats. *Hepatobiliary Pancreat Dis Int* 5(2): 199–204.

Kabaroglu, C, Akisu, M, Habif, S et al. 2005. Effects of L-arginine and L-carnitine in hypoxia/reoxygenation-induced intestinal injury. *Pediatr Int* 47(1): 10–14.

Koc, E, Arsan, S, Ozcan, H et al. 1998. The effect of asphyxia on gut blood flow in term neonates. *Indian J Pediatr* 65(2): 297–302.

Kreymann, K G, Berger, M M, Deutz, N E et al. 2006. ESPEN Guidelines on Enteral Nutrition: Intensive care. *Clin Nutr* 25(2): 210–223.

Lacey, J M, Crouch, J B, Benfell, K et al. 1996. The effects of glutamine-supplemented parenteral nutrition in premature infants. *JPEN J Parenter Enteral Nutr* 20(1): 74–80. PMID: 8788268.

Li, J, Langkamp-Henken, B, Suzuki, K et al. 1994. Glutamine prevents parenteral nutrition-induced increases in intestinal permeability. *JPEN J Parenter Enteral Nutr* 18(4): 303–307.

Li, N, Lewis, P, Samuelson, D et al. 2004. Glutamine regulates Caco-2 cell tight junction proteins. *Am J Physiol Gastrointest Liver Physiol* 287(3): G726–733.

Li, N, Liboni, K, Fang, M Z et al. 2004. Glutamine decreases lipopolysaccharide-induced intestinal inflammation in infant rats. *Am J Physiol Gastrointest Liver Physiol* 286(6): G914–921.

Li, N, Ma, L, Liu, X et al. 2012. Arginyl-glutamine dipeptide or docosahexaenoic acid attenuates hyperoxia-induced small intestinal injury in neonatal mice. *J Pediatr Gastroenterol Nutr* 54(4): 499–504.

Li, N and Neu, J. 2009. Glutamine deprivation alters intestinal tight junctions via a PI3-K/Akt mediated pathway in Caco-2 cells. *J Nutr* 139(4): 710–714.

Ma, L, Li, N, Liu, X et al. 2012. Arginyl-glutamine dipeptide or docosahexaenoic acid attenuate hyperoxia-induced lung injury in neonatal mice. *Nutrition* 28(11–12): 1186–1191.

Markel, T A, Crisostomo, P R, Wairiuko, G M et al. 2006. Cytokines in necrotizing enterocolitis. *Shock* 25(4): 329–337.

Moe-Byrne, T, Wagner, J V and McGuire, W. 2012. Glutamine supplementation to prevent morbidity and mortality in preterm infants. *Cochrane Database Syst Rev* 3: CD001457.

Moncada, S, Palmer, R M and Higgs, E A. 1991. Nitric oxide: Physiology, pathophysiology, and pharmacology. *Pharmacol Rev* 43(2): 109–142.

Mondello, S, Galuppo, M, Mazzon, E et al. 2010. Glutamine treatment attenuates the development of ischaemia/reperfusion injury of the gut. *Eur J Pharmacol* 643(2–3): 304–315.

Nankervis, C A, Giannone, P J and Reber, K M. 2008. The neonatal intestinal vasculature: Contributing factors to necrotizing enterocolitis. *Semin Perinatol* 32(2): 83–91.

Neu, J. 2003. Glutamine supplements in premature infants: Why and how. *J Pediatr Gastroenterol Nutr* 37(5): 533–535.

Neu, J, Afzal, A, Pan, H et al. 2006. The dipeptide Arg-Gln inhibits retinal neovascularization in the mouse model of oxygen-induced retinopathy. *Invest Ophthalmol Vis Sci* 47(7): 3151–3155.

Neu, J, Auestad, N and DeMarco, V G. 2002. Glutamine metabolism in the fetus and critically ill low birth weight neonate. *Adv Pediatr* 49: 203–226.

Neu, J and Li, N. 2007. Pathophysiology of glutamine and glutamate metabolism in premature infants. *Curr Opin Clin Nutr Metab Care* 10(1): 75–79.

Neu, J, Roig, J C, Meetze, W H et al. 1997. Enteral glutamine supplementation for very low birth weight infants decreases morbidity. *J Pediatr* 131(5): 691–699.

Neu, J and Walker, W A. 2011. Necrotizing enterocolitis. *N Engl J Med* 364(3): 255–264.

Newsholme, P. 2001. Why is L-glutamine metabolism important to cells of the immune system in health, postinjury, surgery or infection? *J Nutr* 131(9 Suppl): 2515S–2522S; discussion 2523S–2514S.

Novak, F, Heyland, D K, Avenell, A et al. 2002. Glutamine supplementation in serious illness: A systematic review of the evidence. *Crit Care Med* 30(9): 2022–2029.

Oliveira, G P, Dias, C M, Pelosi, P et al. 2010. Understanding the mechanisms of glutamine action in critically ill patients. *An Acad Bras Cienc* 82(2): 417–430.

Panigrahi, P, Gewolb, I H, Bamford, P et al. 1997. Role of glutamine in bacterial transcytosis and epithelial cell injury. *JPEN J Parenter Enteral Nutr* 21(2): 75–80.

Poindexter, B B, Ehrenkranz, R A, Stoll, B J et al. 2004. Parenteral glutamine supplementation does not reduce the risk of mortality or late-onset sepsis in extremely low birth weight infants. *Pediatrics* 113(5): 1209–1215.

Polycarpou, E, Zachaki, S, Tsolia, M et al. 2013. Enteral L-arginine supplementation for prevention of necrotizing enterocolitis in very low birth weight neonates: A double-blind randomized pilot study of efficacy and safety. *JPEN J Parenter Enteral Nutr* 37(5): 617–622.

Richir, M C, Siroen, M P, van Elburg, R M et al. 2007. Low plasma concentrations of arginine and asymmetric dimethylarginine in premature infants with necrotizing enterocolitis. *Br J Nutr* 97(5): 906–911.

Roig, J C, Meetze, W H, Auestad, N et al. 1996. Enteral glutamine supplementation for the very low birthweight infant: plasma amino acid concentrations. *J Nutr* 126(4 Suppl): 1115S–1120S.

Sevastiadou, S, Malamitsi-Puchner, A, Costalos, C et al. 2011. The impact of oral glutamine supplementation on the intestinal permeability and incidence of necrotizing enterocolitis/septicemia in premature neonates. *J Matern Fetal Neonatal Med* 24(21463215): 1294–1300.

Shah, P and Shah, V. 2004. Arginine supplementation for prevention of necrotising enterocolitis in preterm infants. *Cochrane Database Syst Rev*(4): CD004339.

Shah, P and Shah, V. 2007. Arginine supplementation for prevention of necrotising enterocolitis in preterm infants. *Cochrane Database Syst Rev*(3): CD004339.

Singleton, K D, Beckey, V E and Wischmeyer, P E. 2005. Glutamine prevents activation of NF-kappaB and stress kinase pathways, attenuates inflammatory cytokine release, and prevents acute respiratory distress syndrome (ARDS) following sepsis. *Shock* 24(6): 583–589.

Tazuke, Y, Wasa, M, Shimizu, Y et al. 2003. Alanyl-glutamine-supplemented parenteral nutrition prevents intestinal ischemia-reperfusion injury in rats. *JPEN J Parenter Enteral Nutr* 27(2): 110–115.

van den Berg, A, van Elburg, R M, Teerlink, T et al. 2005a. A randomized controlled trial of enteral glutamine supplementation in very low birth weight infants: plasma amino acid concentrations. *J Pediatr Gastroenterol Nutr* 41(1): 66–71.

van den Berg, A, van Elburg, R M, Westerbeek, E A et al. 2005b. Glutamine-enriched enteral nutrition in very-low-birth-weight infants and effects on feeding tolerance and infectious morbidity: a randomized controlled trial. *Am J Clin Nutr* 81(6): 1397–1404.

van Zwol, A, Moll, H A, Fetter, W P F et al. 2011. Glutamine-enriched enteral nutrition in very low birthweight infants and allergic and infectious diseases at 6 years of age. *Paediatr Perinat Epidemiol* 25(21133970): 60–66.

van Zwol, A, Neu, J and van Elburg, R M. 2011. Long-term effects of neonatal glutamine-enriched nutrition in very-low-birth-weight infants. *Nutr Rev* 69(1): 2–8.

Vaughn, P, Thomas, P, Clark, R et al. 2003. Enteral glutamine supplementation and morbidity in low birth weight infants. *J Pediatr* 142(6): 662–668.

Verbruggen, S, Sy, J, Arrivillaga, A et al. 2010. Parenteral amino acid intakes in critically ill children: a matter of convenience. *JPEN J Parenter Enteral Nutr* 34(3): 329–340.

Wischmeyer, P E. 2006. The glutamine story: Where are we now? *Curr Opin Crit Care* 12(2): 142–148.

Wischmeyer, P E, Kahana, M, Wolfson, R et al. 2001a. Glutamine induces heat shock protein and protects against endotoxin shock in the rat. *J Appl Physiol (1985)* 90(6): 2403–2410.

Wischmeyer, P E, Kahana, M, Wolfson, R et al. 2001b. Glutamine reduces cytokine release, organ damage, and mortality in a rat model of endotoxemia. *Shock* 16(5): 398–402.

Wischmeyer, P E, Musch, M W, Madonna, M B et al. 1997. Glutamine protects intestinal epithelial cells: role of inducible HSP70. *Am J Physiol* 272(4 Pt 1): G879–884.

Wu, G, Jaeger, L A, Bazer, F W et al. 2004. Arginine deficiency in preterm infants: biochemical mechanisms and nutritional implications. *J Nutr Biochem* 15(8): 442–451.

Xu, D Z, Lu, Q, Kubicka, R et al. 1999. The effect of hypoxia/reoxygenation on the cellular function of intestinal epithelial cells. *J Trauma* 46(2): 280–285.

Yeh, C L, Hsu, C S, Yeh, S L et al. 2005. Dietary glutamine supplementation modulates Th1/Th2 cytokine and interleukin-6 expressions in septic mice. *Cytokine* 31(5): 329–334.

Yuan, Z Q, Zhang, Y, Li, X L et al. 2010. HSP70 protects intestinal epithelial cells from hypoxia/reoxygenation injury via a mechanism that involves the mitochondrial pathways. *Eur J Pharmacol* 643(2–3): 282–288.

Zamora, S A, Amin, H J, McMillan, D D et al. 1997. Plasma L-arginine concentrations in premature infants with necrotizing enterocolitis. *J Pediatr* 131(2): 226–232.

Section VII

Glutamine and the Catabolic State: Role of Glutamine in Critical Illness from Adulthood

14 Rationale for and Efficacy of Glutamine Supplementation in Critical Illness

Christina C. Kao and Farook Jahoor

CONTENTS

14.1 METABOLIC AND PHYSIOLOGIC ROLES OF GLUTAMINE RELEVANT TO CRITICAL ILLNESS

Glutamine, the most abundant free amino acid in the human body, is present in the highest concentration in both plasma and skeletal muscle (Xi et al. 2011), and contributes more than 50% of the free amino acid pool in the body (Young and Ajami 2001). The majority of glutamine entering the plasma is derived from skeletal muscle (Biolo et al. 1995), and approximately one-third of all nitrogen derived from protein metabolism is transported in the form of glutamine (Biolo et al. 2005). Healthy adults have an endogenous glutamine production of 50–80 g/day (Wernerman 2011). Stable isotope tracer studies have determined that 40%–60% of plasma glutamine is oxidized, 10%–20% is used for gluconeogenesis, and the remainder is used for protein synthesis and production of other macromolecules (Biolo et al. 2005). Glutamine has numerous physiologic roles that make it very important during conditions of stress, such as critical illness, as shown in Table 14.1.

TABLE 14.1

Glutamine Mechanisms of Action on Different Organs

Organ	Actions
Intestinal tract	Fuel for proliferating enterocytes
	Precursor for formation of citrulline
	Maintenance of gut barrier function
Lung	Increase heat shock protein expression
Immune cells	Fuel for proliferating immune cells
	Maintain oxidant–antioxidant balance
	Control of apoptosis
	Synthesis of NAD
	Support of neutrophil function
Liver	Substrate for gluconeogenesis
	Regulation of PEPCK
	Supply of Krebs cycle intermediates
	Modulator of cell signaling through cellular osmolarity/hydration
Skeletal muscle	Nitrogen transport
	Control of protein synthesis and degradation
	Detoxification of ammonia
Kidney	Ammoniagenesis
	Regulation of acid–base status
	Gluconeogenesis
Central nervous system	Precursor for GABA synthesis
Pancreas	Enhances glucose-stimulated insulin secretion
All body tissues	Precursor for glutathione synthesis

NADPH = nicotinamide adenine dinucleotide phosphate; PEPCK = phosphoenolpyruvate carboxykinase; GABA = gamma-aminobutyric acid.

14.1.1 GLUTAMINE SYNTHESIS AND CARBON METABOLISM

Glutamine is synthesized in most tissues and organs from glutamate and ammonia by the enzyme glutamine synthetase. Glutamate is produced ubiquitously by the transamination of several amino acids, which react with α-ketoglutarate to produce glutamate and α-ketoacids. In skeletal muscle, the branched chain amino acids (BCAAs) leucine, isoleucine, and valine are the primary amino donors. Therefore, glutamine synthesis requires a sufficient supply of transaminating amino acids, in particular BCAAs, as well as pyruvate, acetyl CoA, and other Krebs cycle intermediates needed to maintain α-ketoglutarate availability. In fact, the carbon skeleton of glutamine is mainly derived from pyruvate. At the same time, glutamine is responsible for replenishing Krebs cycle intermediates via its deamidation to glutamate and subsequent conversion to α-ketoglutarate, especially in rapidly proliferating tissues (Soeters and Grecu 2012).

14.1.2 GLUTAMINE AND GLUCOSE METABOLISM

Stable isotope studies demonstrate that 10%–20% of administered glutamine tracer is utilized for gluconeogenesis and that glutamine is a major glucose precursor in humans in the postabsorptive state (Hankard et al. 1997). In addition to serving as a substrate for gluconeogenesis, glutamine also controls the expression and activity of the enzyme phosphoenolpyruvate carboxykinase (PEPCK), an important regulator of gluconeogenesis (Lavoinne et al. 1996). Glutamine may also affect glucose uptake and utilization by enhancing glucose-stimulated insulin secretion by the pancreatic β-cell as well as modulating insulin's action at the cellular level (Curi et al. 2005).

14.1.3 GLUTAMINE AS A PRECURSOR FOR KEY COMPOUNDS

Glutamine is a precursor for many compounds essential for proliferating cells. As a precursor of glutamate, glutamine is important for the synthesis of glutathione, a tripeptide synthesized from glutamate, cysteine, and glycine. Glutathione is the most abundant antioxidant in the body and the major intracellular detoxification agent (Zhang and Forman 2012). Glutamine also provides the amide moiety for the synthesis of nicotamine adenine dinucleotide (NAD+), which serves many roles in proliferating tissues. For example, it is utilized by enzymes involved in the production of free radicals, superoxide, and nitric oxide (NO), which in turn are needed for immune cell function (Newsholme 2001) as well as reduction of other molecules such as glutathione. Glutamine is also used for the synthesis of purine and pyrimidine nucleotide, *N*-acetylglucosamine-6-phosphate (a substrate needed for the synthesis of glycoproteins), and the imidazole ring of histidine.

14.1.4 SPLANCHNIC METABOLISM OF DIETARY GLUTAMINE

Glutamine normally constitutes 8%–12% of total amino acid content of dietary proteins. In the gut, glutamine is the major source of energy for proliferating enterocytes, and in health, the gastrointestinal tract is the major organ of glutamine utilization (Souba et al. 1990). Stable isotope studies have demonstrated that approximately 40%–75% of enterally administered glutamine undergoes first-pass extraction within the splanchnic bed in healthy humans (Matthews et al. 1993; Hankard et al. 1995; Thibault et al. 2008; Kao et al. 2013), where its major fate is oxidation (Haisch et al. 2000). Along with its use by the gut for energy production and protein synthesis, another metabolic fate of glutamine in the gut is its conversion to citrulline in enterocytes (Curis et al. 2005). Citrulline, in turn, is the only precursor for *de novo* synthesis of arginine in the kidney.

14.1.5 GLUTAMINE AS A NONTOXIC NITROGEN CARRIER

Glutamine plays an important role in the storage and transport of ammonia in the body. Normally, the concentration of free ammonia in blood and tissues is low. Although the majority of nitrogen is excreted as urea, only hepatic cells contain all the enzymes of the urea cycle in significant quantities. Therefore, organs other than the liver must rely upon the glutamine synthetic pathway for ammonia detoxification and maintenance of nontoxic ammonia levels (Meister 1956). In the kidney, regulation of excretion of the ammonia formed from glutamine via glutaminase is also essential for maintaining the body's acid–base status (Meister 1956; Biolo et al. 1995).

14.1.6 ADDITIONAL ROLES OF GLUTAMINE

Glutamine has other physiologic roles that may become important in the critically ill patient. Heat shock proteins (HSPs) render cells more resistant to extreme stress through prevention of cell damage and death. In the laboratory, glutamine is a potent enhancer of HSP expression in multiple organs of the intact animal and in multiple cell types (Wischmeyer 2002). Modulated by HSP-70, glutamine administration decreases levels of circulating interleukin-6 (IL-6), tumor necrosis factor-α (TNF-α), and decreases activity of nuclear factor-κB (NF-κB) in models of sepsis and lung injury (Singleton et al. 2005; Singleton and Wischmeyer 2007). Critically ill patients with severe sepsis have impaired endotoxin- or LPS-induced expression of HSP in their blood lymphocytes and mononuclear cells (Schroeder et al. 1999; Schroeder et al. 1999).

There is evidence that glutamine may also be a regulator of muscle protein turnover. Addition of glutamine to chick muscle cells increased the rate of muscle protein synthesis and decreased protein degradation (Wu and Thompson 1990). Enteral glutamine supplementation stimulates gut mucosal protein fractional synthesis rate and attenuates ubiquitin-dependent proteolysis, thus improving gut protein balance (Coeffier et al. 2003). Glutamine is a significant contributor to total-cell osmolarity and hydration. Transport of glutamine into cells causes osmotic swelling (Lavoinne et al. 1998), and cell swelling and shrinkage may in turn be important for the regulation of protein synthesis (Haussinger et al. 1994).

14.2 CHANGES IN GLUTAMINE METABOLISM IN CRITICAL ILLNESS

Although under normal conditions glutamine is a dietary nonessential amino acid, in critical illness, glutamine supply is insufficient to meet its demand, making it conditionally essential. This mismatch between demand and availability occurs because glutamine uptake by tissues and organs exceeds its rate of synthesis and release from skeletal muscle. In conditions of stress or severe injury, there is a net breakdown of skeletal muscle protein with increased release of amino acids into the circulation and uptake of these amino acids by the splanchnic bed and kidney. However, this is accompanied by increased amino acid oxidation and a net loss of nitrogen, the source of which is mainly skeletal muscle protein (Wolfe et al. 1989). Further, because glutamine may constitute up to 50% of the amino acids released from skeletal muscle (Kapadia et al. 1985), this can lead to its intracellular depletion in muscle cells. In support of this, free glutamine concentrations in the muscle are decreased in critical illness (Gamrin et al. 1996; Biolo et al. 2005) and do not improve over time (Gamrin et al. 1997). Intramuscular glutamine depletion may subsequently contribute to loss of muscle mass (Biolo et al. 2005).

Critically ill patients have low plasma glutamine concentrations, and low glutamine concentrations are associated with increased mortality (Oudemans-van Straaten et al. 2001; Rodas et al. 2012). One reason that plasma glutamine concentrations are decreased may be because there is increased uptake of glutamine by other organs. Tissues that may be removing glutamine at an increased rate include the liver, spleen, and particularly the gut (Wolfe et al. 1989; Kao et al. 2013). Besides its numerous anabolic roles, glutamine taken up by the liver and kidney is used for gluconeogenesis and ureagenesis.

In critical illness, the depletion of both intramuscular and circulating glutamine concentrations points toward an inability to increase intramuscular glutamine synthesis to match its rate of uptake. In support of this, stable isotope studies have found that in critical illness, glutamine rate of appearance in plasma is unchanged (Jackson et al. 1999; Kao et al. 2013) despite increased protein breakdown, indicating a potential defect in *de novo* glutamine synthesis. Muscle glutamine synthesis requires the availability of BCAAs as well as adequate sources of carbon skeletons for α-ketoglutarate synthesis. A deficiency of any of these precursors may therefore contribute to inadequate glutamine synthesis. Because of the glutamine deficiency found in critically ill patients, there has been increasing interest in glutamine supplementation in these patients.

14.3 GLUTAMINE ROUTES OF SUPPLEMENTATION AND PHARMACOKINETICS

14.3.1 PARENTERAL GLUTAMINE SUPPLEMENTATION

Glutamine supplementation can be provided via either oral or intravenous administration. Conventional parenteral nutrition formulas do not contain glutamine, because glutamine is not stable in aqueous solution. At room temperature, there is significant hydrolysis of glutamine to glutamic acid and ammonia. However, use of glutamine-containing dipeptides can overcome this problem (Furst et al. 1997), and these dipeptides can also be safely administered through a peripheral vein (Berg et al. 2002). The bioavailability of glutamine administered intravenously is 100%, and even with peripheral administration, there is uniform uptake by splanchnic tissues. Intravenous glutamine administration restores plasma glutamine concentration in a dose-dependent fashion but does not change muscle glutamine concentration (Flaring et al. 2003; Berg et al. 2005). Glutamine given intravenously is rapidly cleared from the plasma (Berg et al. 2005).

14.3.2 Enteral Glutamine Supplementation

Standard enteral formulas also contain little glutamine. When glutamine is given as part of commercially available immuno-modulating formulas, the glutamine concentration is variable, ranging from 5 g/L to 13.4 g/L (Marik and Zaloga 2008). The pharmacokinetics of enterally administered glutamine are not as clear as those of parenterally administered glutamine. The majority of enterally administered glutamine is absorbed by the upper jejunum (Dechelotte et al. 1991) and thus may not reach the distal intestines. In healthy humans, 40%–75% of dietary glutamine undergoes first-pass splanchnic extraction, and this is also true in critically ill, fasting adults (Kao et al. 2013). Nevertheless, administration of enteral glutamine does significantly increase plasma glutamine concentration in a dose-dependent manner (Dechelotte et al. 1991) and improves plasma glutamine concentrations in critically ill patients (Zhou et al. 2003). However, it does not alter muscle glutamine concentration or muscle glutamine kinetics in critical illness (Gore and Wolfe 2002). Although both parenteral and enteral glutamine administration lead to significant increases in plasma glutamine concentration, there is a greater increase in glutamine concentration via the parenteral route (Melis et al. 2005).

14.4 PHYSIOLOGIC EFFECTS OF GLUTAMINE SUPPLEMENTATION IN HUMANS

14.4.1 Glutamine Supplementation and Glucose Metabolism

The potential clinical benefits of glutamine are derived from glutamine's physiologic and metabolic roles as shown in Table 14.2. Because critical illness is associated with increased glucose production, hyperglycemia, and insulin resistance and glutamine is an important precursor for glucose production, it was hypothesized that glutamine could attenuate these alterations in glucose metabolism. In one study of 114 patients with multiple trauma, postsurgical complications, or pancreatitis randomized to either intravenous alanyl-glutamine (Ala-Gln) or intravenous alanine and proline (Ala + Pro), patients receiving Ala-Gln had significantly less hyperglycemia, less requirement for insulin therapy, and fewer nosocomial infections when compared with the Ala + Pro group

---

TABLE 14.2

Clinical Outcomes Demonstrating Improvements in Patients Supplemented with Glutamine

Glucose metabolism
   Prevent hyperglycemia
   Reduce requirement for insulin therapy
   Decrease insulin resistance
   Improve insulin-mediated glucose disposal
Gut function
   Prevent increase in intestinal permeability
   Maintain mucosal integrity
Oxidant–antioxidant balance
   Maintain muscle glutathione concentrations
Cellular protection
   Enhance expression of heat shock protein 70
Infectious complications[a]
Mortality[a]

[a] In some studies.

(Dechelotte et al. 2006). The reduction in infections was mainly a result of decreased incidence of pneumonia. In a smaller study of patients with multiple trauma, supplementation with parenteral Ala-Gln led to a decrease in endogenous insulin secretion, less insulin resistance in the fasting state, and better insulin-mediated glucose disposal (Bakalar et al. 2006). In a Spanish multicenter study, administration of Ala-Gln dipeptide-supplemented total parenteral nutrition (TPN) led to statistically though not clinically significant decreases in plasma glucose concentration (149 ± 46 mg/dL with supplementation vs. 155 ± 51 mg/dL without, $p < 0.04$) and hourly insulin dose (4.3 ± 3.3 IU with supplementation vs. 4.7 ± 3.7 IU without, $p < 0.001$) when compared with TPN alone (Grau et al. 2011). In addition, insulin administration for the same level of glycemia was 54% less in the Ala-Gln supplemented group.

14.4.2 GLUTAMINE SUPPLEMENTATION AND GUT FUNCTION

Because glutamine is the major energy source for enterocytes, glutamine may be necessary to maintain gut barrier function, restrict translocation of bacteria, and consequently help to prevent the development of multisystem organ failure. In postsurgical patients receiving TPN, addition of Ala-Gln prevented a worsening of intestinal permeability and maintained duodenal villus height, indicating that glutamine helps to maintain the gut barrier and preserve mucosal integrity (van der Hulst et al. 1993). Similarly, in patients with severe burns who received enteral feeding, gut permeability as measured by the lactulose/mannitol ratio was less in those patients who received Ala-Gln supplementation as compared with those who did not (Zhou et al. 2003), again demonstrating that glutamine may help to maintain gut integrity.

14.4.3 GLUTAMINE SUPPLEMENTATION AND HEAT SHOCK PROTEINS

The induction of HSPs is a key mechanism, which provides cellular protection against systemic inflammation and renders cells more resistant to extreme stress. Because glutamine upregulates the expression of HSP-70 in animal models (Wischmeyer et al. 2001), its effect on HSP in critically ill patients was studied in a small group of patients admitted to the surgical intensive care unit with an anticipated 7-day requirement for parenteral nutrition. Supplementation with parenteral glutamine compared with placebo led to a greater rise in serum HSP-70 concentrations over time, and the magnitude of increase in HSP-70 concentrations was associated with improved clinical outcomes, including decreased intensive care unit (ICU) and ventilator days (Ziegler et al. 2005).

14.4.4 GLUTAMINE SUPPLEMENTATION AND GLUTATHIONE

In critically ill patients, both reduced and total glutathione concentrations in the skeletal muscle are decreased, and the ratio of reduced to total glutathione is also decreased, demonstrating an environment of increased oxidative stress (Hammarqvist et al. 1997). Supplementation of TPN with parenteral glutamine prevented the depletion of muscle glutathione (Flaring et al. 2003) in patients undergoing abdominal surgery. Similarly, patients admitted to the surgical ICU after non-pancreatic surgery who received Ala-Gln-supplemented TPN had improvement in plasma-reduced glutathione after 7 days (Luo et al. 2008).

14.5 EFFECTS OF GLUTAMINE ON INFECTIOUS COMPLICATIONS AND MORTALITY IN CRITICAL ILLNESS

14.5.1 ENTERAL GLUTAMINE SUPPLEMENTATION

There are few high-quality trials investigating the clinical benefit of enteral glutamine supplementation. In one small study, burn patients receiving enteral glutamine supplementation had a significant decrease in mortality compared with patients who did not receive supplementation (Garrel et al. 2003). However, in the largest study of a heterogeneous group of 363 Australian ICU patients receiving enteral nutrition supplemented with either glutamine or glycine (Hall et al. 2003), glutamine supplementation had no effect on 6-month mortality or incidence of severe sepsis. When data from 8 trials examining the effect of glutamine-supplemented enteral nutrition in critically ill patients were pooled in a meta-analysis, there was no overall difference in mortality (RR = 0.81, 95% confidence interval 0.48–1.34) or infectious complications (RR = 0.83, 95% confidence interval 0.64–1.08) between groups who received glutamine and those who did not (*Composition of Enteral Nutrition: Glutamine* 2013). As a result, there is insufficient evidence to recommend routine use of enteral glutamine in critically ill patients (*Composition of Enteral Nutrition: Glutamine* 2013).

14.5.2 PARENTERAL GLUTAMINE SUPPLEMENTATION

The majority of clinical studies of parenteral glutamine in critically ill patients are small or also include noncritical patients. A summary of key clinical studies is presented in Table 14.3. Prior recommendation for using intravenous glutamine supplementation in critically ill patients (Heyland et al. 2003) was based mainly on two single-center studies. In one of the first studies of parenteral glutamine supplementation, 84 patients admitted to a general ICU with an Acute Physiological and Chronic Health Evaluation (APACHE) II score of ≥11 were randomized in a double-blind fashion to receive TPN with or without glutamine supplementation. Patients who received glutamine supplementation had significantly lower 6-month mortality than those who did not (33% vs. 57%), with the major cause of death in both groups being multisystem organ failure (Griffiths et al. 1997). Interestingly, this difference in mortality occurred late, as survival curves in the two groups were similar at 20 days. In another study, 144 ICU patients were

TABLE 14.3
Select Key Trials of Parenteral Glutamine Supplementation in Critical Illness

Study	Number of Participants	Route of Nutrition	Length of Supplementation	Primary Outcome	Findings
Griffiths et al. (1997)	84	Parenteral	Until death or as long as clinically required	Survival at 6 months	Gln supplementation decreased 6-month mortality
Goeters et al. (2002)	95	Parenteral and enteral	As long as central venous access was required	Multiple	Gln supplementation improved 6-month survival in patients treated ≥9 days
Scandinavian glutamine study (Wernerman et al. 2011)	413	Parenteral or enteral	Throughout ICU stay	Change in SOFA score from day 1 to 7	Decreased ICU mortality with GLN supplementation
SIGNET Trial (Andrews et al. 2011)	502	Parenteral	7 days	New infections at 14 days and mortality	No effect on new infections or mortality
REDOX (Heyland et al. 2013)	1223	Parenteral and enteral	Maximum 28 days	28-Day mortality	Trend toward increased 28-day mortality in GLN-supplemented group

randomized to receive either supplementation with parenteral Ala-Gln or no supplementation, but only 95 patients who completed 5 days of nutritional support were analyzed (Goeters et al. 2002). There was no difference between the groups in ICU or hospital mortality, but in a subgroup of 68 patients who stayed in the ICU at least 9 days, 6-month mortality was lower in the glutamine supplemented group.

In the last few years, three large trials of parenteral glutamine supplementation have been published. The Scandinavian glutamine trial (Wernerman et al. 2011) was a multicenter trial of 413 ICU patients receiving either parenteral or enteral nutrition who were randomized to also receive either parenteral Ala-Gln or placebo. In the per-protocol but not the intention-to-treat analysis, ICU mortality was improved with glutamine supplementation; however, there was no difference in 6-month mortality. In the SIGNET trial (Andrews et al. 2011), 502 ICU patients were randomized to either glutamine-supplemented TPN or standard TPN. Glutamine supplementation had no effect on the incidence of new infections or mortality. A systematic review of parenteral glutamine trials that included these two trials found that parenteral glutamine was associated with only a trend toward reduction in mortality (RR = 0.88, p = 0.10) and a trend toward a reduction in infectious complications (RR 0.86, p = 0.09) (Dhaliwal et al. 2014). As a result of the weaker overall effect after the addition of these two trials, the *Canadian Clinical Practice Guidelines* downgraded its recommendation for parenteral glutamine in critically ill patients in 2013. Therefore, the current recommendation states that parenteral glutamine supplementation should be considered in critically ill patients, rather than strongly recommended (Dhaliwal et al. 2014).

The REDOX study was a very large multicenter study in 40 ICUs, which randomized 1223 critically ill patients with multiorgan failure and on mechanical ventilation to receive either a combination of parenteral and enteral glutamine supplementation or placebo (Heyland et al. 2013). Contrary to the hypothesis, there was actually a trend toward increased 28-day mortality (32.4% in patients who received glutamine vs. 27.2% in patients who did not receive glutamine, p = 0.05) as well as a significantly increased in-hospital and 6-month mortality in patients who received glutamine compared to those who did not. The REDOX authors subsequently conducted a post hoc analysis in an attempt to identify potential subgroups of patients that might benefit from glutamine supplementation, but there was no subgroup that was associated with a positive treatment effect (Heyland et al. 2015). However, the greatest potential for harm was found in patients with renal dysfunction, and approximately one-third of included patients had renal dysfunction at baseline.

14.6   CONTROVERSIES IN GLUTAMINE SUPPLEMENTATION

The REDOX trial unexpectedly demonstrated potential harm from glutamine supplementation in critically ill patients. However, methodological differences between the REDOX study and prior studies may help to explain the conflicting results. First, the study population in the REDOX study was composed of a heterogeneous group of patients with multisystem organ failure of whom more than 75% were medical and were older (mean age 63.3 years) and sicker (mean APACHE II score of 26.3) than in patients in previous studies. Glutamine supplementation in the REDOX study was administered both enterally and parenterally, with the patients mainly receiving enteral feeding, whereas in prior studies, the majority of patients received TPN with parenteral glutamine supplementation. Perhaps the most significant factor influencing the results of the REDOX study was that not all the REDOX patients were glutamine-deficient. In a subgroup of 66 patients, plasma glutamine concentrations were measured, and median plasma glutamine concentrations were normal. Only 31% of patients had a low baseline glutamine concentration (<420 μmol/L) and 15% had levels that were high (Heyland and Dhaliwal 2013). Because high plasma glutamine concentrations have been associated with increased mortality (Gottschalk et al. 2013), glutamine supplementation in those patients with high baseline glutamine concentrations may be contributed to it leading to potential harm.

14.7 CONCLUSIONS

Glutamine plays many key physiologic and metabolic roles, and its production and utilization are altered in critically ill patients. In critical illness, uptake of glutamine by tissues and organs exceeds its rate of release from the periphery, leading to glutamine deficiency manifested by a decreased plasma concentration. This glutamine depletion is the basis for numerous clinical trials investigating the effects of glutamine supplementation in critically ill patients. However, the studies are varied in terms of patient population, dose, route, and duration of glutamine administration, and route and amount of nutrition given to patients. Based on the results of the REDOX study, neither parenteral nor enteral glutamine supplementation should be given to critically ill patients with multisystem organ failure. However, because only a portion of patients in the REDOX study were glutamine deficient, future studies will need to identify patients who are glutamine-deficient in order to appropriately target those patients with a potential need for glutamine supplementation.

REFERENCES

Andrews, P. J., A. Avenell, D. W. Noble et al. 2011. Randomised trial of glutamine, selenium, or both, to supplement parenteral nutrition for critically ill patients. *BMJ* 342:d1542.
Bakalar, B., F. Duska, J. Pachl et al. 2006. Parenterally administered dipeptide alanyl-glutamine prevents worsening of insulin sensitivity in multiple-trauma patients. *Crit Care Med* 34 (2):381–6.
Berg, A., E. Forsberg, and J. Wernerman. 2002. The local vascular tolerance to an intravenous infusion of a concentrated glutamine solution in ICU patients. *Clin Nutr* 21 (2):135–9.
Berg, A., O. Rooyackers, A. Norberg, and J. Wernerman. 2005. Elimination kinetics of L-alanyl-L-glutamine in ICU patients. *Amino Acids* 29 (3):221–8.
Biolo, G., R. Y. Fleming, S. P. Maggi, and R. R. Wolfe. 1995. Transmembrane transport and intracellular kinetics of amino acids in human skeletal muscle. *Am J Physiol* 268 (1 Pt 1):E75–84.
Biolo, G., F. Zorat, R. Antonione, and B. Ciocchi. 2005. Muscle glutamine depletion in the intensive care unit. *Int J Biochem Cell Biol* 37 (10):2169–79.
Coeffier, M., S. Claeyssens, B. Hecketsweiler, A. Lavoinne, P. Ducrotte, and P. Dechelotte. 2003. Enteral glutamine stimulates protein synthesis and decreases ubiquitin mRNA level in human gut mucosa. *Am J Physiol Gastrointest Liver Physiol* 285 (2):G266–73.
Composition of Enteral Nutrition: Glutamine. 2013 [cited December 16, 2014]. Available from www.critical-carenutrition.com.
Curi, R., C. J. Lagranha, S. Q. Doi et al. 2005. Molecular mechanisms of glutamine action. *J Cell Physiol* 204 (2):392–401.
Curis, E., I. Nicolis, C. Moinard et al. 2005. Almost all about citrulline in mammals. *Amino Acids* 29 (3):177–205.
Dechelotte, P., D. Darmaun, M. Rongier, B. Hecketsweiler, O. Rigal, and J. F. Desjeux. 1991. Absorption and metabolic effects of enterally administered glutamine in humans. *Am J Physiol* 260 (5 Pt 1):G677–82.
Dechelotte, P., M. Hasselmann, L. Cynober et al. 2006. L-alanyl-L-glutamine dipeptide-supplemented total parenteral nutrition reduces infectious complications and glucose intolerance in critically ill patients: The French controlled, randomized, double-blind, multicenter study. *Crit Care Med* 34 (3):598–604.
Dhaliwal, R., N. Cahill, M. Lemieux, and D. K. Heyland. 2014. The Canadian critical care nutrition guidelines in 2013: An update on current recommendations and implementation strategies. *Nutr Clin Pract* 29 (1):29–43.
Flaring, U. B., O. E. Rooyackers, J. Wernerman, and F. Hammarqvist. 2003. Glutamine attenuates post-traumatic glutathione depletion in human muscle. *Clin Sci (Lond)* 104 (3):275–82.
Furst, P., K. Pogan, and P. Stehle. 1997. Glutamine dipeptides in clinical nutrition. *Nutrition* 13 (7–8):731–7.
Gamrin, L., K. Andersson, E. Hultman, E. Nilsson, P. Essen, and J. Wernerman. 1997. Longitudinal changes of biochemical parameters in muscle during critical illness. *Metabolism* 46 (7):756–62.
Gamrin, L., P. Essen, A. M. Forsberg, E. Hultman, and J. Wernerman. 1996. A descriptive study of skeletal muscle metabolism in critically ill patients: Free amino acids, energy-rich phosphates, protein, nucleic acids, fat, water, and electrolytes. *Crit Care Med* 24 (4):575–83.
Garrel, D., J. Patenaude, B. Nedelec et al. 2003. Decreased mortality and infectious morbidity in adult burn patients given enteral glutamine supplements: A prospective, controlled, randomized clinical trial. *Crit Care Med* 31 (10):2444–9.

Goeters, C., A. Wenn, N. Mertes et al. 2002. Parenteral L-alanyl-L-glutamine improves 6-month outcome in critically ill patients. *Crit Care Med* 30 (9):2032–7.

Gore, D. C. and R. R. Wolfe. 2002. Glutamine supplementation fails to affect muscle protein kinetics in critically ill patients. *JPEN J Parenter Enteral Nutr* 26 (6):342–9; discussion 349–50.

Gottschalk, A., C. Wempe, and C. Goeters. 2013. Glutamine in the ICU: Who needs supply? *Clin Nutr* 32 (4):668–9.

Grau, T., A. Bonet, E. Minambres et al. 2011. The effect of L-alanyl-L-glutamine dipeptide supplemented total parenteral nutrition on infectious morbidity and insulin sensitivity in critically ill patients. *Crit Care Med* 39 (6):1263–8.

Griffiths, R. D., C. Jones, and T. E. Palmer. 1997. Six-month outcome of critically ill patients given glutamine-supplemented parenteral nutrition. *Nutrition* 13 (4):295–302.

Haisch, M., N. K. Fukagawa, and D. E. Matthews. 2000. Oxidation of glutamine by the splanchnic bed in humans. *Am J Physiol Endocrinol Metab* 278 (4):E593–602.

Hall, J. C., G. Dobb, J. Hall, R. de Sousa, L. Brennan, and R. McCauley. 2003. A prospective randomized trial of enteral glutamine in critical illness. *Intensive Care Med* 29 (10):1710–6.

Hammarqvist, F., J. L. Luo, I. A. Cotgreave, K. Andersson, and J. Wernerman. 1997. Skeletal muscle glutathione is depleted in critically ill patients. *Crit Care Med* 25 (1):78–84.

Hankard, R. G., D. Darmaun, B. K. Sager, D. D'Amore, W. R. Parsons, and M. Haymond. 1995. Response of glutamine metabolism to exogenous glutamine in humans. *Am J Physiol* 269 (4 Pt 1):E663–70.

Hankard, R. G., M. W. Haymond, and D. Darmaun. 1997. Role of glutamine as a glucose precursor in fasting humans. *Diabetes* 46 (10):1535–41.

Haussinger, D., F. Lang, and W. Gerok. 1994. Regulation of cell function by the cellular hydration state. *Am J Physiol* 267 (3 Pt 1):E343–55.

Heyland, D. K. and R. Dhaliwal. 2013. Role of glutamine supplementation in critical illness given the results of the REDOXS study. *JPEN J Parenter Enteral Nutr* 37 (4):442–3.

Heyland, D. K., R. Dhaliwal, J. W. Drover, L. Gramlich, and P. Dodek. 2003. Canadian clinical practice guidelines for nutrition support in mechanically ventilated, critically ill adult patients. *JPEN J Parenter Enteral Nutr* 27 (5):355–73.

Heyland, D. K., G. Elke, D. Cook et al. 2015. Glutamine and antioxidants in the critically ill patient: A post hoc analysis of a large-scale randomized trial. *JPEN J Parenter Enteral Nutr* 39 (4):401–9.

Heyland, D., J. Muscedere, P. E. Wischmeyer et al. 2013. A randomized trial of glutamine and antioxidants in critically ill patients. *N Engl J Med* 368 (16):1489–97.

Jackson, N. C., P. V. Carroll, D. L. Russell-Jones, P. H. Sonksen, D. F. Treacher, and A. M. Umpleby. 1999. The metabolic consequences of critical illness: Acute effects on glutamine and protein metabolism. *Am J Physiol* 276 (1 Pt 1):E163–70.

Kao, C., J. Hsu, V. Bandi, and F. Jahoor. 2013. Alterations in glutamine metabolism and its conversion to citrulline in sepsis. *Am J Physiol Endocrinol Metab* 304 (12):E1359–64.

Kapadia, C. R., M. F. Colpoys, Z. M. Jiang, D. J. Johnson, R. J. Smith, and D. W. Wilmore. 1985. Maintenance of skeletal muscle intracellular glutamine during standard surgical trauma. *JPEN J Parenter Enteral Nutr* 9 (5):583–9.

Lavoinne, A., A. Husson, M. Quillard, A. Chedeville, and A. Fairand. 1996. Glutamine inhibits the lowering effect of glucose on the level of phosphoenolpyruvate carboxykinase mRNA in isolated rat hepatocytes. *Eur J Biochem* 242 (3):537–43.

Lavoinne, A., D. Meisse, M. Quillard, A. Husson, S. Renouf, and A. Yassad. 1998. Glutamine and regulation of gene expression in rat hepatocytes: The role of cell swelling. *Biochimie* 80 (10):807–11.

Luo, M., C. Fernandez-Estivariz, D. P. Jones et al. 2008. Depletion of plasma antioxidants in surgical intensive care unit patients requiring parenteral feeding: Effects of parenteral nutrition with or without alanyl-glutamine dipeptide supplementation. *Nutrition* 24 (1):37–44.

Marik, P. E. and G. P. Zaloga. 2008. Immunonutrition in critically ill patients: A systematic review and analysis of the literature. *Intensive Care Med* 34 (11):1980–90.

Matthews, D. E., M. A. Marano, and R. G. Campbell. 1993. Splanchnic bed utilization of glutamine and glutamic acid in humans. *Am J Physiol* 264 (6 Pt 1):E848–54.

Meister, A. 1956. Metabolism of glutamine. *Physiol Rev* 36 (1):103–27.

Melis, G. C., P. G. Boelens, J. R. van der Sijp et al. 2005. The feeding route (enteral or parenteral) affects the plasma response of the dipetide Ala-Gln and the amino acids glutamine, citrulline and arginine, with the administration of Ala-Gln in preoperative patients. *Br J Nutr* 94 (1):19–26.

Newsholme, P. 2001. Why is L-glutamine metabolism important to cells of the immune system in health, postinjury, surgery or infection? *J Nutr* 131 (9 Suppl):2515S–22S; discussion 2523S–4S.

Oudemans-van Straaten, H. M., R. J. Bosman, M. Treskes, H. J. van der Spoel, and D. F. Zandstra. 2001. Plasma glutamine depletion and patient outcome in acute ICU admissions. *Intensive Care Med* 27 (1):84–90.

Rodas, P. C., O. Rooyackers, C. Hebert, A. Norberg, and J. Wernerman. 2012. Glutamine and glutathione at ICU admission in relation to outcome. *Clin Sci (Lond)* 122 (12):591–7.

Schroeder, S., J. Bischoff, L. E. Lehmann et al. 1999. Endotoxin inhibits heat shock protein 70 (HSP70) expression in peripheral blood mononuclear cells of patients with severe sepsis. *Intensive Care Med* 25 (1):52–7.

Schroeder, S., C. Lindemann, A. Hoeft et al. 1999. Impaired inducibility of heat shock protein 70 in peripheral blood lymphocytes of patients with severe sepsis. *Crit Care Med* 27 (6):1080–4.

Singleton, K. D., V. E. Beckey, and P. E. Wischmeyer. 2005. Glutamine prevents activation of NF-kappaB and stress kinase pathways, attenuates inflammatory cytokine release, and prevents acute respiratory distress syndrome (ARDS) following sepsis. *Shock* 24 (6):583–9.

Singleton, K. D. and P. E. Wischmeyer. 2007. Glutamine's protection against sepsis and lung injury is dependent on heat shock protein 70 expression. *Am J Physiol Regul Integr Comp Physiol* 292 (5):R1839–45.

Soeters, P. B. and I. Grecu. 2012. Have we enough glutamine and how does it work? A clinician's view. *Ann Nutr Metab* 60 (1):17–26.

Souba, W. W., K. Herskowitz, R. M. Salloum, M. K. Chen, and T. R. Austgen. 1990. Gut glutamine metabolism. *JPEN J Parenter Enteral Nutr* 14 (4 Suppl):45S–50S.

Thibault, R., S. Welch, N. Mauras et al. 2008. Corticosteroids increase glutamine utilization in human splanchnic bed. *Am J Physiol Gastrointest Liver Physiol* 294 (2):G548–53.

van der Hulst, R. R., B. K. van Kreel, M. F. von Meyenfeldt et al. 1993. Glutamine and the preservation of gut integrity. *Lancet* 341 (8857):1363–5.

Wernerman, J. 2011. Glutamine supplementation. *Ann Intensive Care* 1 (1):25.

Wernerman, J., T. Kirketeig, B. Andersson et al. 2011. Scandinavian glutamine trial: A pragmatic multi-centre randomised clinical trial of intensive care unit patients. *Acta Anaesthesiol Scand* 55 (7):812–8.

Wischmeyer, P. E. 2002. Glutamine and heat shock protein expression. *Nutrition* 18 (3):225–8.

Wischmeyer, P. E., M. Kahana, R. Wolfson, H. Ren, M. M. Musch, and E. B. Chang. 2001. Glutamine induces heat shock protein and protects against endotoxin shock in the rat. *J Appl Physiol (1985)* 90 (6):2403–10.

Wolfe, R. R., F. Jahoor, and W. H. Hartl. 1989. Protein and amino acid metabolism after injury. *Diabetes Metab Rev* 5 (2):149–64.

Wu, G. Y. and J. R. Thompson. 1990. The effect of glutamine on protein turnover in chick skeletal muscle *in vitro*. *Biochem J* 265 (2):593–8.

Xi, P., Z. Jiang, C. Zheng, Y. Lin, and G. Wu. 2011. Regulation of protein metabolism by glutamine: Implications for nutrition and health. *Front Biosci (Landmark Ed)* 16:578–97.

Young, V. R. and A. M. Ajami. 2001. Glutamine: The emperor or his clothes? *J Nutr* 131 (9 Suppl):2449S–59S; discussion 2486S–7S.

Zhang, H. and H. J. Forman. 2012. Glutathione synthesis and its role in redox signaling. *Semin Cell Dev Biol* 23: 722–8.

Zhou, Y. P., Z. M. Jiang, Y. H. Sun, X. R. Wang, E. L. Ma, and D. Wilmore. 2003. The effect of supplemental enteral glutamine on plasma levels, gut function, and outcome in severe burns: A randomized, double-blind, controlled clinical trial. *JPEN J Parenter Enteral Nutr* 27 (4):241–5.

Ziegler, T. R., L. G. Ogden, K. D. Singleton et al. 2005. Parenteral glutamine increases serum heat shock protein 70 in critically ill patients. *Intensive Care Med* 31 (8):1079–86.

15 Role of Glutamine Oxidative Injury Pathways in Critically Ill Patients

Kaushik Mukherjee, Addison K. May, and Naji N. Abumrad

CONTENTS

15.1 INTRODUCTION

Glutamine is a *conditionally essential* amino acid that helps maintain the cellular oxidation–reduction state, immune and gut barrier function, nitrogen transport, protein synthesis, glucose metabolism, and insulin sensitivity following stress (Labow and Souba 2000; Melis et al. 2004; Bakalar et al. 2006; Dechelotte et al. 2006; Galera et al. 2010; Grau et al. 2011). It is the most abundant free amino acid but consumption exceeds production and levels may fall rapidly following severe stress (Roth et al. 1982; Parry-Billings et al. 1990; Oudemans-van Straaten et al. 2001; Fläring et al. 2003b; Coster, McCauley, and Hall 2004; Melis et al. 2004; Eroglu 2009). Low serum glutamine levels are associated with immune dysfunction and increased mortality (Robinson et al. 1992; Luo et al. 1996; Labow and Souba 2000; Melis et al. 2004; Fläring et al. 2005; Singleton et al. 2005; Luo et al. 2008; Eroglu 2009; Grau et al. 2011) while high levels may also be associated with mortality (Labow and Souba 2000; Melis et al. 2004; Bakalar et al. 2006; Dechelotte et al. 2006; Galera et al. 2010; Grau et al. 2011).

Glutamine is the precursor for the important cellular antioxidant glutathione (GSH), and systemic and skeletal muscle GSH levels correlate with organ failure and mortality (Roth et al. 1982; Parry-Billings et al. 1990; Oudemans-van Straaten et al. 2001; Fläring et al. 2003b; Coster, McCauley, and Hall 2004; Melis et al. 2004; Eroglu 2009). The reduction potential of the GSH/glutathione disulfide (GSSG) redox couple plays an important role in cell signaling and may be altered by glutamine supplementation. Glutamine helps maintain nitrogen and acid–base balance and provides energy for high-turnover cell populations, such as enterocytes and some immune cells (Vermeulen et al. 2007). Enteral glutamine prevents TNF-α-induced transcellular bacterial translocation and inhibitors of glutamine's metabolism to α-ketoglutarate, such as amino-oxyacetate, limit this effect (Melis et al.

2004; Vermeulen et al. 2007). Glutamine may also ameliorate the inflammatory milieu by altering the balance of pro- and anti-inflammatory cytokines, at least partially mediated by increasing heat shock protein expression (Melis et al. 2004). Glutamine increases expression of the cytoprotective heat shock protein (HSP-70) and decreases serum TNF and IL-6 levels following severe stress (Robinson et al. 1992; Luo et al. 1996, 2008; Labow and Souba 2000; Melis et al. 2004; Fläring et al. 2005; Singleton et al. 2005; Eroglu 2009; Grau et al. 2011).

Glutamine also influences glycemic control during critical illness. Stress-induced insulin resistance (IR) correlates with the severity of illness and mortality independent of blood glucose levels (Wischmeyer 2006). Insulin resistance may be altered by several factors including nutritional provision, glycemic control, adiponectin, and infection (Ziegler et al. 2005; Wischmeyer 2007, 2008; Dungan, Braithwaite, and Preiser 2009; Venkatesh et al. 2009; Mukherjee et al. 2014). Glutamine has been shown to reduce IR following severe illness, and thus, it may improve outcomes via this mechanism (Bakalar et al. 2006; Dechelotte et al. 2006; Langouche et al. 2007; Grau et al. 2011).

The evidence relating to glutamine supplementation has spanned more than 20 years of research and thousands of patients, but without a clear understanding about the risks and benefits of glutamine supplementation in critical illness. This review summarizes basic and clinical research related to glutamine's role in critical illness.

15.2 BASIC SCIENCE STUDIES

15.2.1 SIGNIFICANCE OF GLUTAMINE LEVELS

The supply of glutamine from skeletal muscle is constantly balanced against numerous demands. In times of high demand, such as starvation, sepsis, multisystem trauma, and postsurgical stress, glutamine may be depleted, making it *conditionally* essential. The literature supporting this assertion is fairly robust, extending from rodent to canine to human models after polytrauma and sepsis (Askanazi et al. 1980; Roth et al. 1982; Meinz et al. 1998; Olde Damink et al. 1999; Lavery and Glover 2000; O'Leary et al. 2001; Hammarqvist et al. 2005; Soeters and Grecu 2012). For example, glutamine levels in patients with severe abdominal sepsis after laparotomy were 362 ± 117 µmol/L (survivors) and 384 ± 194 µmol/L (nonsurvivors) versus 526 ± 101 µmol/L in healthy controls (Roth et al. 1982).

On the other hand, dramatic increases in plasma glutamine levels occur in patients with hepatic failure (Deutz 2008; Holecek 2013) and renal dysfunction (Divino Filho et al. 1997), particularly in the elderly (Galera et al. 2010) and children (Broyer et al. 1980). Sixty-nine percent of critically ill patients with multiple organ failures had a normal or elevated serum glutamine level (Heyland and Dhaliwal 2013). After adjustment for age and Acute Physiology and Chronic Health Evaluation II (APACHE II) score, serum glutamine levels of <400 µM or >930 µM were associated with increased mortality (OR 2.95 [95% CI 1.38, 6.32], p = 0.005). Additionally, a ratio of reduced GSH to total GSH greater than 0.65 was also associated with increased 6-month mortality (OR 2.35 [95% CI 1.02, 5.41] p < 0.001) (Rodas et al. 2012). Therefore, the effects of critical illness, age, and organ function must be balanced when attempting to develop a clear relationship between serum glutamine levels and outcome.

15.2.2 REDOX FUNCTIONS OF GLUTAMINE

Glutamine also exerts an antioxidant effect via its conversion into glutamate and subsequently GSH, a key molecule in the regulation of intracellular redox potential (Melis et al. 2004; Vermeulen et al. 2007). Both glutamine and GSH levels are reduced in critical illness (Fläring et al. 2003a). Thus, decreased levels of glutamine available for GSH synthesis may exacerbate the decline in antioxidant potential. It is unclear whether the effects and putative benefits of glutamine derive more from its anti-inflammatory or antioxidant properties.

Physiologic insults such as trauma, aging, and cardiovascular disease may alter the balance between pro-oxidant and antioxidant species by *increasing pro-oxidants rather than decreasing antioxidants*; thus merely administering antioxidants may be insufficient to compensate for the insult. For example, with increasing age, there is a shift in the direction of increased GSSG (oxidized species) and decreased GSH (reduced species) (Jones 2006). GSSG levels are also increased in post-chemotherapy patients (Jonas et al. 2000) and smokers (Moriarty 2003). GSH depletion in rat models of hemorrhagic shock and resuscitation results in significant hepatic and renal dysfunction and increased mortality (Robinson et al. 1992).

Different redox pathways (e.g., GSH-GSSG and cysteine [Cys]/cystine [CySS]) are not in equilibrium, so that changes in one pathway are not necessarily reflected in others (Jones 2006). To address the vagaries of assessing the redox state, many researchers use prostaglandin-derived F2-isoprostane levels as biomarkers of oxidative stress, particularly *in vivo* (Milne, Musiek, and Morrow 2005). Levels of these arachidonic acid metabolites correlate with levels of lipid peroxidation and oxidative stress in numerous disease states, including atherosclerosis, diabetes, pulmonary disease, obesity, and smoking (Milne, Musiek, and Morrow 2005). To date, limited data exist using isoprostanes to assess glutamine's effect. Ongoing research using these tools may assist in clearly establishing the link between glutamine levels and the degree of oxidative insult.

15.2.3 IMMUNOMODULATORY EFFECTS OF GLUTAMINE

While glutamine's role in limiting oxidative injury remains unclear, its anti-inflammatory effects are well established and dependent on levels of heat shock proteins (HSP), acute phase reactants that assist in the refolding of proteins denatured by incipient insults (Wischmeyer et al. 2001a). Three members of the HSP family that play a vital role in cellular protection are HSP-70, HSP-72, and HSP-25 (rat equivalent of human HSP-27). Glutamine's attenuation of cellular metabolic dysfunction and cell death appear to be HSP-dependent, as heat shock transcription factor-1 (HSF-1) knockout models eliminate glutamine's effect (Peng et al. 2006). *In vitro* work suggests that glutamine induces a concentration-dependent increase in HSP-70 in intestinal epithelial cell lines, conferring a survival advantage against thermal and oxidative injury that is reversed by quercetin, an inhibitor of HSP-70 expression (Wischmeyer et al. 1997). Quercetin administration decreased HSP-70 expression and prevented glutamine-induced reduction of plasma TNF-α, chemokines, and neutrophil infiltration, and abolished glutamine's renal-protective effects in murine acute kidney injury models (Peng et al. 2013). Likewise, glutamine's protective effect against injury in a rodent model of smoke inhalation was associated with increased HSP-70 levels, increased levels of heme oxygenase 1, and decreased levels of NF-κB (Driks et al. 2013). Evidence also suggests that glutamine depletion results in decreased ability of human leukocytes to boost their HSP-70 expression in response to increased temperature. Glutamine also inhibits production of inducible nitric oxide synthetase (iNOS) and reduces nitric oxide (NO) levels, and these effects are abrogated in an HSF-1 knockout model incorporating murine embryonic fibroblast cells (Peng et al. 2006).

Rat endotoxemia models have helped shed light on the relationship between glutamine and both HSPs (Wischmeyer et al. 2001a). Wischmeyer and colleagues demonstrated that a single dose of glutamine significantly increased HSP-25 and HSP-72 levels in multiple organs, including the heart, lung, colon, kidney, liver, and ileum, in the unstressed rats. Sprague-Dawley rats injected with lipopolysaccharide (LPS) had reduced mortality when treated with glutamine and fluid resuscitation; rats receiving glutamine and fluid resuscitation had reduced cellular infiltrates and improved morphology in alveolar and ileal tissues (Wischmeyer et al. 2001a). In a rat model of sepsis involving a controlled cecal puncture, animals receiving glutamine had increased levels of HSF-1 phosphorylation, HSP-25, and HSP-70. Metabolic parameters including ATP/ADP ratio and nicotinamide adenine (NAD) levels were also improved in the group receiving glutamine. The glutamine group also had a lower mortality (33% vs. 78%); quercetin reversed the glutamine-induced increases in HSP levels and improvements in mortality. There was no effect observed on GSH, potentially indicating that the HSP-mediated effects were more significant than those mediated by oxidation and reduction pathways (Singleton et al. 2005).

Glutamine increased HSP-72 levels in human peripheral blood mononuclear cells in response to thermal injury and attenuated increases in TNF-α levels in response to LPS stimulation (Wischmeyer et al. 2003). Similar findings were demonstrated with glutamate treatment in intestinal epithelial cells; 6-diazo-5-oxo-L-norleucine (DON), an inhibitor of the glutaminase enzyme responsible for converting glutamine to glutamate (Phanvijhitsiri 2006), prevented the increase in HSP-25 levels. On the other hand, the administration of buthionine sulfoximine, an inhibitor of the transformation of glutamine and glutamate to GSH, had no effect; the authors inferred that the increase in HSP-25 levels was predominantly due to conversion of glutamate to glutamine and not via a redox pathway.

Rodent models of Gram-negative sepsis simulated by LPS administration have also proved instructive. Administration of glutamine in conjunction with fluid resuscitation resulted in attenuated release of TNF-α and IL-1β, and rats receiving glutamine had significantly decreased mortality (Wischmeyer et al. 2001b). The effect of glutamine was manifested by improvements in oxygenation and base deficit 6 h after LPS administration. Autopsy data indicated that the rats receiving glutamine had better preservation of tissue structure and decreased amounts of inflammatory cell infiltration into the lung and small intestine. Similarly, glutamine administration resulted in decreased serum levels of TNF-α and decreased leukocyte adherence and plasma extravasation compared to controls (Scheibe et al. 2009).

Taken together, the cellular and animal model data suggest that glutamine may exert significant protective effects during critical illness. The weight of the data suggests that beneficial effects are mediated through anti-inflammatory mechanisms rather than redox pathways.

15.3   CLINICAL STUDIES

Glutamine has been studied in multiple populations of critically ill patients, including burn, postsurgical, trauma, and mixed patients with mixed results. In the burn, trauma, and, to a lesser extent, postsurgical patient populations, some evidence supports glutamine depletion following stress and a resulting drop in the serum glutamine levels (Askanazi et al. 1980; Roth et al. 1982; Meinz et al. 1998; Olde Damink et al. 1999; Lavery and Glover 2000; O'Leary et al. 2001; Hammarqvist et al. 2005; Soeters and Grecu 2012). Thus, a theoretical benefit of glutamine administration to correct a relative deficiency exists in these populations. In critically ill populations with large proportions of medical patients, data to support glutamine consumption are more variable, with a significant proportion of patients with high levels that might contribute to increased mortality (Rodas et al. 2012; Heyland et al. 2013). Medical patients lack acute injury or surgical stress to acutely deplete glutamine and thus have less rationale to support a state of glutamine deficiency. The difference in medical versus surgical populations may have a role in the varied outcomes among the various studies. Infection has been studied as an endpoint with more consistent results, but unacceptably high infection rates in the control populations limit the interpretation of these findings. While individual studies have suggested a potential mortality benefit, these studies have been underpowered. The largest available study demonstrated an increase in mortality with glutamine administration in a predominately medical population with established organ failure at study entry.

15.3.1   BURNS

Severe burn injury results in profound stress, catabolism, nutritional depletion, and high mortality. Due to the stress-related glutamine consumption following burn injury, this population may benefit from glutamine supplementation. Four randomized single-center clinical trials have been conducted, one of which studied parenteral glutamine administration. Two studies evaluated infection, two studied wound healing, and two studied hospital length of stay. Two studies evaluated glutamine levels, so it was possible to make a determination regarding the effectiveness of gluta-mine administration. These studies suggest positive influences on infection, nutritional parameters, and possibly mortality. Unfortunately, these studies are sufficiently heterogeneous with limited power so that they do not provide a clear treatment directive (Table 15.1).

Wischmeyer and colleagues were the first to study the effect of glutamine administration in severely burned patients in a double-blind, randomized fashion (Wischmeyer et al. 2001c). They compared intravenous glutamine (0.57 g/kg/day) versus an isonitrogenous control in 26 patients with 25%–90% TBSA burns. The primary endpoint was incidence of Gram-negative bacteremia. Secondary endpoints included levels of acute phase reactants and nutritional data (transferrin, prealbumin, and C-reactive peptide). The glutamine arm had a significantly lower incidence of Gram-negative bacteremia (8% vs. 43%, p = 0.04) but there was no difference in the incidence of Gram-positive bacteremia. Prealbumin and transferrin were significantly higher in the glutamine arm, and CRP was lower. Although this small study was well designed, it was not powered to address mortality. The validity of the primary finding is called into question by the high incidence of bacteremia in both arms (58% Gram-positive bacteremia in the glutamine arm and 43% Gram-positive and Gram-negative bacteremia in the control arm). Despite these concerns, the observa-tion that the availability of glutamine assists with Gram-negative but not Gram-positive organisms deserves further investigation.

The remaining three major studies utilized enteral glutamine. Garrel and colleagues studied the enteral administration of 26 g/day of enteral glutamine in a 45-patient single-center double-blinded trial of severely burned patients with total body surface area (TBSA) of 20%–80% against

TABLE 15.1
Glutamine and Outcome in Burns

Study	Sample Size	Population	Route and Dosage	Outcomes in Glutamine Arm	Comparison (Glutamine vs. Control)	P Value
Peng (2005)	48	30%–75% TBSA	0.5 g/kg/day enteral	Glutamine level Hospital LOS	608 ± 147 vs. 447 ± 132 µmol/L 46.6 ± 13.0 vs. 55.7 ± 17.4 days	<0.01 <0.05
Zhou (2003)	40	50%–80% TBSA	0.35 g/kg/day enteral	Glutamine level Wound healing Hospital LOS Hospital cost	591 ± 74 vs. 400 ± 41 µmol/L 86 ± 2% vs. 72 ± 3% wound healed at 30 days 67 ± 4 vs. 73 ± 6 days $7593 ± $747 vs. $8343 ± $1042	0.048 0.041 0.026 0.031
Garrel (2003)	45	20%–80% TBSA	26 g/day enteral	Mortality Days of positive blood cultures *Pseudomonas* infections	2/19 (10.5%) vs. 12/22 (54.5%) 1.2 vs. 4.3 days/ patient 0/19 vs. 6/22 (27%)	<0.05 <0.05 <0.05
Wischmeyer (2001)	26	25%–90% TBSA	0.57 g/kg/day parenteral	Gram-negative bacteremia	1/13 (8%) vs. 6/13 (43%)	0.04

TBSA: Total body surface area; LOS: length of stay

an isocaloric isonitrogenous control (Garrel et al. 2003). Zhou and colleagues also studied enteral glutamine administration (0.35 mg/kg/day) for 40 burn patients with TBSA 50%–80%, with at least 20%–40% TBSA third-degree burns (Zhou et al. 2003). Peng and colleagues conducted a randomized controlled trial of 48 patients with TBSA 30%–75%, using 0.5 mg/kg/day of enteral glutamine (Peng et al. 2005). None of the studies was initially powered to address mortality, although Garrel's study did show a significant mortality difference (2/19 deaths in the glutamine group vs. 12/22 in the control group by intention-to-treat analysis). Garrel's study also was the only one designed to study an infectious endpoint. Patients in the glutamine group had fewer days of positive blood cultures (1.2 days per patient vs. 4.3 days per patient in the control group). No patients in the glutamine group grew *Pseudomonas aeruginosa* from their blood culture, as opposed to 6/22 patients in the control group. The authors speculated that, as glutamine was enterally administered without an associated significant change in serum glutamine, that glutamine was largely absorbed by the gut mucosa and resulted in decreased bacterial translocation of *Pseudomonas* organisms into the bloodstream. The 54.5% mortality in the control group was excessive for the level of burn injury, leading to concerns about other possible differences between the control and glutamine groups. The authors point out that additional multicenter trials are needed.

Zhou and Peng both evaluated plasma glutamine levels, wound healing, and hospital length of stay. Zhou found plasma glutamine levels were nearly identical between groups on the first post-injury day (381 ± 36.4 vs. 357 ± 55 M in the control vs. glutamine group) but increased in the glutamine group by post-injury day 12 (to 591 ± 74 μM). In the other study, the findings were similar, with baseline glutamine levels of 397.4 ± 169.4 in the control group and 407.1 ± 152.8 in the glutamine group and a significant increase after 14 days of treatment in the glutamine group (607.9 ± 147.2 vs. 447.4 ± 132.4, p < 0.01). Patients in the glutamine group in both studies had improved wound healing although Peng did not specify how this was measured; in the Zhou study, the glutamine group had more of their wound healed after 30 days (86 ± 2% vs. 72 ± 3% in the control group). Patients in the glutamine group had decreased length of stay in both studies and decreased hospital costs in the Zhou study. Peng measured intestinal permeability and endotoxin levels and found that both were lower in the glutamine group compared to burned controls, although not as low as in healthy controls.

After reviewing the available burn data, there are still a number of unanswered questions. Firstly, it is unclear what differences arise between enteral and parenteral glutamine. Secondly, the significance of plasma glutamine levels is also unclear. Thirdly, at least two of the studies have unusually poor outcomes, either with infection rates or mortality. Given the complexity of caring for burn patients, a multicenter trial may be warranted.

15.3.2 SURGICAL AND TRAUMA PATIENTS

Previous work has led investigators to believe that postsurgical critically ill and trauma patients might benefit from glutamine administration due to a drop in serum glutamine levels caused by their physiologic stress (Askanazi et al. 1980; Roth et al. 1982; Meinz et al. 1998; Olde Damink et al. 1999; Lavery and Glover 2000; O'Leary et al. 2001; Hammarqvist et al. 2005; Soeters and Grecu 2012). Askanazi noted that plasma glutamine levels were decreased by 50% from healthy controls in patients 3–4 days after multisystem trauma (Askanazi et al. 1980).

Trials with clinical endpoints in a surgical or trauma population are shown in Table 15.2. These published studies generally support a reduction in infectious complication and perhaps improvements in other outcome variables. However, all studies are small and have considerable variability in populations, delivery methods, dosing, and endpoints.

Three major studies have been performed of enteral glutamine supplementation in trauma and postsurgical critically ill patients. Schulman prospectively studied a surgical and trauma population without blinding in the intensive care unit (ICU) with the primary endpoint of in-hospital mortality (Schulman et al. 2005). The treatment groups received either immune-modulated tube feeds with

TABLE 15.2
Glutamine and Clinical Outcome in Surgery and Trauma

Study	Sample Size	Population	Route and Dosage	Outcomes in Glutamine Arm	Comparison (Glutamine vs. Control)	P Value
Perez-Barcena (2014)	142	Trauma (ISS > 10)	0.5 g/kg/day parenteral	Glutamine level New infections Length of stay Mortality	380 (IQR 302–476) vs. 322 (274–361) µmol/L No difference	<0.005
Soguel (2008)	86	Burn (40) Trauma (46)	30 g/day enteral (received 16–22 g)	SOFA scores	No difference	
Estivariz (2008)	59 (27 non-pancreatic surgery)	SICU	0.5 g/kg/day parenteral	*Non-pancreatic surgery* Overall infections Pneumonia Bloodstream infection *Pancreatic surgery*	13 vs. 36 infections 6 vs. 16 cases 0 vs. 7 cases No difference	<0.03 <0.05 <0.01
Spindler-Vesel (2007)	113 (32 in glutamine arm)	Trauma	1.55 g/day enteral	Intestinal permeability Ventilator days ICU days Organ failure	Increased at 7 days No difference	<0.02
Dechelotte (2006)	114	Trauma (38) SICU (65) Pancreatitis (11)	0.5 g/kg/day parenteral	Combination endpoint (infection + wound complication + death) Infections per patient Pneumonia Death ICU LOS	24/58 (41%) vs. 34/56 (61%) 0.45 vs. 0.71 10/58 (17%) vs. 19/56 (34%) No difference	<0.05 <0.05 <0.05
Schulman (2005)	185	Trauma (175) SICU (10)	0.4 g/kg/day enteral	Mortality	20/121 (16.6%) vs. 4/64 (6.3%)	0.0478
Falcao de Arruda (2004)	23	Traumatic brain injury	30 g/day enteral	Infections per patient Ventilator days ICU LOS	1 (range 0–3) vs. 3 (1–5) 7 (range 1–15) vs. 14 (3–53) day 10 (range 5–20) vs. 22 (7–57) day	<0.01 <0.01 0.04
Houdijk (1998)	60	Trauma (ISS > 20)	30.5 g/day enteral	Pneumonia Bacteremia Sepsis	6/35 (17%) vs. 16/37 (43%) 3/35 (9%) vs. 14/37 (38%) 1/35 (3%) vs. 8/37 (22%)	<0.02 <0.005 <0.02

ISS: Injury Severity Score; IQR: interquartile range; LOS: length of stay.

0.4 g/kg/day enteral glutamine or isocaloric and isonitrogenous control tube feeds. Mortality in the control group was 6.3% (4/64) versus 16.6% (20/121) in the pooled treatment groups (p = 0.048). In both of the regression models developed by the investigators, which controlled for disease severity and age, there was a possible association between glutamine administration and mortality (p values of 0.08 and 0.11).

Houdijk studied the enteral administration of 30.5 g/day of glutamine versus control in a cohort of 60 severely injured trauma patients with an injury severity score (ISS) greater than 20 (Houdijk et al. 1998). Falcao de Arruda studied the enteral administration of 30 g/day of glutamine with *Lactobacillus* as a probiotic in 23 patients with moderate to severe traumatic brain injury (Glasgow Coma Scale scores 5–12) (Falcão de Arruda and de Aguilar-Nascimento 2004). Both studies used an isocaloric isonitrogenous control and studied infection as their primary endpoints. Houdijk noted that patients in the glutamine cohort had lower rates of pneumonia (17% vs. 43%, p < 0.02), bacteremia (7% vs. 38%, p < 0.005), and sepsis (3% vs. 22%, p < 0.02), while Falcao de Arruda found that the infection rate was higher in the control group (100%) as opposed to the glutamine group (50%) and that the median number of infections per patient was higher in the control group than the study group (3 vs. 1). Both studies are plagued by high infection rates in the control group. Falcao de Arruda did not clarify the impairment of gas exchange, an indicator superior to radiographic infiltrate, secretions, fever, or leukocytosis, in his definition of pneumonia (Boots et al. 2005). The definition of wound infection used in this study is also unusual as it required an abscess to be present with purulent secretion with a positive culture.

Spindler-Vesel randomized 113 critically ill trauma patients to one of four groups: glutamine, fiber, peptide diet, and standard enteral formula, and fiber with symbiotic compounds (a combination of probiotics and prebiotics) (Spindler-Vesel et al. 2007). The dose of administered glutamine, 1.55 g/day, is much lower than in other studies and thus the study's lack of statistical significance could be due to this alone; glutamine levels were not measured so it was not possible to determine a dose–response relationship.

Three randomized trials of intravenous glutamine in critically ill trauma and postsurgical patients have all focused on incidence of infection as a primary endpoint. Dechelotte and colleagues performed a multicenter, double-blinded, randomized controlled trial of intravenous glutamine at 0.5 g/kg/day in ICU units in France (Dechelotte et al. 2006). The population in this study consisted of 38 trauma patients, 65 complex postsurgical patients, and 11 patients with severe pancreatitis (total n = 114). Estivariz and colleagues conducted a similar double-blinded randomized controlled trial of TPN with 0.5 g/kg/day glutamine supplementation in 59 postsurgical critically ill patients (Estivariz et al. 2008). Both studies used an isocaloric isonitrogenous control. Dechelotte found no differences in mortality but fewer infections per patient in the glutamine arm (0.45 vs. 0.71 in the placebo arm, p < 0.05). Estivariz noted a significantly decreased rate of overall infection, bloodstream infection, pneumonias, and infections with *Staphylococcus aureus*, fungi, and enteric Gram-negative organisms in the glutamine group after non-pancreatic operations. Both of these studies have high infection rates in the control group—almost one infection per patient in the Dechelotte study and almost a 100% rate of pneumonia and a 41% rate of bloodstream infections in the Estivariz study.

A recently published study by Pérez-Bárcena studied intravenous glutamine supplementation in 142 critically injured patients with an ISS of at least 10, expected ICU stay of at least 48 h, and need for enteral or parenteral nutrition (Pérez-Bárcena et al. 2014). Patients were randomized to either 5 days of glutamine (0.5 g/kg/day) or normal saline placebo given in addition to standard nutritional supplementation. The primary endpoint was the number of new infections in the first 14 days. Basal glutamine levels were similar in both groups (307 µM [IQR 238, 380] in the placebo group vs. 311 µM [243, 380] in the glutamine group), and glutamine supplementation resulted in significant increases in plasma glutamine levels (380 µM [302, 476] vs. 322 µM [274, 361] measured after 6 days of supplementation, p = 0.005). These changes did not result in any significant differences in the primary endpoints, including those with severe injuries as documented by an ISS > 24. This study was well designed but lacked an isocaloric isonitrogenous control group.

The available data for critically ill surgical patients have similar drawbacks to the data available for critically ill burned patients. First, multiple studies have unexpectedly high infection rates in the control group, calling into question the true effectiveness of glutamine. Secondly, questions regarding the effectiveness of enteral as compared to parenteral glutamine remain unanswered. Thirdly, the one study that addressed mortality found increased mortality in the group receiving glutamine supplementation. The limitations of existing studies emphasize the need for a well-controlled and well-randomized multicenter trial to address the numerous complexities involved in nutritional supplementation, infection, and outcomes in critically ill patients.

15.3.3 Mixed ICU Populations

Medical patients differ from postsurgical and trauma patients as the latter populations suffer a significant surgical or injury-related insult in addition to their baseline comorbidities. The studies that have been performed in medical or mixed populations have not demonstrated a significant benefit of glutamine supplementation and have suggested possible harm in patients with elevated serum glutamine levels.

Andrews conducted a randomized controlled trial in 10 ICUs in Scotland with 502 patients receiving parenteral glutamine (20.2 g/day) alone, selenium (500 mcg) alone, or both selenium and glutamine, for up to 7 days. Primary outcomes were 6-month mortality rates and the number of infections in a 14-day period. Secondary outcomes included ICU and hospital length of stay and organ failure as measured by SOFA scores. Glutamine had no effect on any of the primary or secondary outcomes (Andrews et al. 2011).

The *Reducing Deaths due to Oxidative Stress* (REDOXS) trial was powered to assess a mortality endpoint using a 2×2 factorial design with supplementation of glutamine, an antioxidant cocktail, placebo, and both glutamine and antioxidant cocktails. Glutamine was administered as 0.50 g/kg/day of intravenous alanyl-glutamine dipeptide and 30 g of enteral glutamine in the form of alanyl-glutamine and glycine-glutamine dipeptides (Heyland et al. 2013). The antioxidant cocktail was made of two components: (1) intravenous selenium, 500 µg with (2) enteral selenium, 300 µg; zinc, 20 mg; beta-carotene, 10 mg; vitamin E, 500 mg; and vitamin C, 1500 mg.

The study population consisted of 75% medical patients and 20% surgical patients, with approximately 4% of the population being trauma patients. Mean age in all groups was greater than 60 years, mean APACHE II score was 26, and most patients had one or more associated medical comorbidities. 97% of study patients presented with shock, approximately 2/3 of whom had septic shock and 1/3 of whom had cardiogenic shock. Approximately 95% of study patients had failure of at least two organ systems, with renal dysfunction in approximately 1/3 of cases. More than 90% of patients met criteria for acute lung injury and the vast majority of patients in the study were mechanically ventilated. This population was determined by the authors to be critically ill, likely glutamine deficient, and likely to benefit from glutamine administration.

The 28-day mortality rate was higher in the glutamine group (32.4% vs. 27.2%, adjusted OR 1.28 [95% CI 1.00, 1.64] (p = 0.05); hospital and 6-month mortality followed the same trend. Glutamine administration did not demonstrate a reduction in SOFA scores or infection rates. Patients with more than two failed organ systems or aged between 65 and 75 years had a more pronounced increase in mortality.

The authors attributed the difference in results to their high dose of prescribed glutamine, including both enteral and parenteral administrations. This is perhaps coupled with the high incidence of renal insufficiency in the study population, which has been associated with impaired glutamine excretion, particularly in the elderly (Galera et al. 2010). In addition, they cited the high proportion of patients in the study with multiorgan failure and shock, early administration of glutamine, and early enteral feeding as possible causes for poor outcome. Finally, they note that their initial assumption that the critically ill patients in their study would be glutamine-deficient might be incorrect. Glutamine levels were not low on the limited subset of patients tested; in fact approximately 15% of patients had supranormal levels that, as previously mentioned, have been associated with increased mortality. To complicate the picture further, the REDOXS study did not include a high number of trauma or burn patients, who have been shown to have low glutamine levels that respond to glutamine administration (Peng et al. 2005; Schulman et al. 2005). Also, the proportion of reduced to total GSH was not measured in the REDOXS study.

The findings in the REDOXS study have resulted in a re-evaluation in the field about the utility of glutamine in patients with critical illness. The senior investigators who led the REDOXS have recently published a putative algorithm for studying the efficacy of glutamine administration in the critically ill. They recommended avoiding glutamine in patients with shock or multiorgan failure. Further, they advocated the use of parenteral glutamine administration only for patients requiring parenteral nutrition and using enteral glutamine administration only for trauma and burn patients (Heyland and Dhaliwal 2013). It is difficult to ignore the findings of the REDOXS study, showing higher mortality with the use of glutamine. These would lead investigators to conclude that the REDOXS study's findings are definitive enough that performing a similar study is not warranted.

15.3.4 META-ANALYSES

Since sample size is limited in most of the randomized controlled trials, several authors have published meta-analyses of existing studies. These studies are summarized in Table 15.3.

Avenell reviewed a total of 31 studies of parenteral or enteral nutrition containing glutamine in postsurgical or critically ill patients through August 2008 (Avenell 2009). Of these, 22 trials were in critically ill patients (two in burns, nine in mixed ICU patients, three in trauma patients, four in pancreatitis, and four in surgical ICU patients). Eight trials were in elective gastrointestinal surgery patients, and one was in a mixed inpatient hospital population. The authors found that the administration of parenteral (RR 0.71 [95% CI 0.49, 1.03]) or enteral (RR 1.05 [0.71, 1.54]) glutamine in critical illness was not associated with a significant mortality benefit, except in patients with pancreatitis (RR 0.36 [0.13, 0.99]). The use of parenteral (RR 0.78 [0.63, 0.97]), but not enteral (RR 0.91 [0.74, 1.10]), glutamine in critical illness altered infection rates. Postsurgical patients receiving parenteral nutrition with glutamine had a lower risk of infection (RR 0.43 [0.27, 0.69]).

Novak performed a meta-analysis of 14 randomized controlled trials of glutamine in surgical and ICU patients in 2002 (Novak et al. 2002) and updated these data on www.criticalcarenutrition.com in 2009 (2009). The 2009 update contained data from 21 trials; however, eight of the studies in the 2002 paper were not carried over to the 2009 update, without explanation. The 2002 study reported a pooled relative risk of mortality of 0.78 [95% CI 0.58, 1.04]) for glutamine administration (enteral or parenteral) and a pooled relative risk of infectious complications of 0.81 [0.64, 1.00]. Both of these beneficial effects were also seen in 2009. Both meta-analyses showed a reduction in length of stay of 2.5 days. In addition, the authors reported a pooled reduction in hospital stay of 2.6 days [0.7, 4.5]. The 2009 update showed a mortality benefit with glutamine administration (RR 0.75 [0.61, 0.93]) for the first time in a meta-analysis. It also showed a benefit for infectious complications (RR 0.79 [0.68, 0.93]) and a reduction in length of stay of 2.6 days [0.74, 4.39]. The 2009 update indicates that, even with the chosen studies, there is a large amount of heterogeneity, with the meta-analysis outcomes potentially skewed by a single trial. The 2009 results were again reviewed in 2013, and in light of the outcome of the REDOXS trial, the study recommended enteral glutamine in patients with multitrauma and burns and critical illness *without* multiorgan failure (2009). However, the elimination of some studies between 2002 and 2009 could have affected the results.

Another meta-analysis by Wang studied glutamine supplementation of parenteral nutrition in elective surgical patients (Wang et al. 2010). The inclusion parameters of the analysis required an isonitrogenous isocaloric control and an endpoint involving clinical outcomes, length of stay, or cost. Fourteen trials were pooled and these demonstrated significant reduction in the risk of infectious complications (RR 0.69 [95% CI 0.50, 0.95]). Despite significant heterogeneity, the data demonstrated a reduction in hospital stay of 3.95 days [95% CI 1.60, 6.30] in the high-quality studies with alanine-glutamine dipeptide and 5.40 days [95% CI 8.46, 2.33] in the studies with glycine-glutamine dipeptide. There was no mortality benefit in elective general surgery patients.

TABLE 15.3

Meta-Analyses of Glutamine Trials

Meta-Analysis	Year	RCTs	Patients (n)	Population	Outcome	Odds/Risk	95% CI	p-Value	Other
Lin	2012	4	155	Burns	Mortality	OR 0.13	0.03–0.51	0.004	
					Gram-negative bacteremia	OR 0.27	0.08–0.92	0.04	
Wang Y	2010	14	587	Surgical	Mortality	RR 0.38	0.09–1.53	0.17	n = 87
					Infectious complications	RR 0.69	0.5–0.95	0.02	ALA-GLN group
					Hospital LOS	3.84 days less	(−5.4 to −2.28)	<0.001	ALA-GLN group
						5.4 days less	(−8.46 to −2.33)	<0.001	GLY-GLN group
Novak F (updated)	2009	21	1564	Critically ill	Mortality	RR 0.75	0.59–0.96	0.02	
					Infectious complications	RR 0.79	0.63–0.98	0.04	
					ICU LOS	4.5 days less	(−8.28 to −0.72)	**0.02**	
Avenell A	2006	24	1726	Critically ill + elective surgery	Mortality	RR 0.81	0.65–1.02	NS	
					Infectious complications	RR 0.76	0.64–0.9		
					MOF/RF	RR 0.82	0.61–1.1	NS	

RCT: randomized controlled trial, CI: confidence interval, RR: relative risk, ICU: intensive care unit, LOS: length of stay, ALA-GLN: alanyl-glutamine, GLY-GLN: glycyl-glutamine, NS: nonsignificant, MOF: multiorgan failure, RF: renal failure.

The existing meta-analyses suggest a mortality benefit, but only in specific subsets of patients. They consistently demonstrate a reduction in infectious complications with the administration of glutamine, but this effect depends on the infection rate in the control group, which is frequently quite high. Based on the quality and heterogeneity of existing studies, it is unlikely that additional meta-analyses will improve our understanding of the risks and benefits of glutamine administration in the critically ill population.

15.4 TRIALS CURRENTLY IN PROGRESS

Given the scale and outcome of the REDOXS study, it is unlikely that another large trial with a primary mortality endpoint will be undertaken in the near future. As previously mentioned, clinical equipoise may exist for smaller scale trials focused on the trauma and burn populations. One of these studies (PI: Addison May, MD) is currently being conducted at our institution (Figure 15.1). We hypothesized critically ill patients receiving intravenous glutamine would have (a) improved glucose metabolism and stress-induced IR, (b) increased plasma cytoprotective and antioxidant molecules, and (c) more rapid recovery of stress biomarkers. Our primary endpoint will be IR in trial subjects as measured by the euglycemic hyperinsulinemic clamp (EHC) (DeFronzo, Tobin, and Andres 1979); secondary endpoints include infection, organ failure as measured by SOFA score, and the levels of oxidative stress and heat shock proteins.

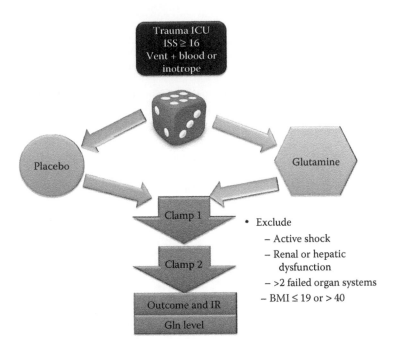

FIGURE 15.1 Schema for trial of parenteral glutamine in trauma patients. Adult patients with Injury Severity Score (ISS) ≥16, necessity for mechanical ventilation, and administration of blood transfusion, vasopressors, or both within the first 24 h after injury satisfy our inclusion criteria and are randomized. Extra emphasis is placed on ensuring patients are no longer in active shock and have adequate renal and hepatic function to be able to metabolize glutamine. Insulin resistance (IR) is directly calculated through the euglycemic hyperinsulinemic clamp technique, with adjunctive measures of antioxidant molecules.

We plan a double blind, randomized placebo-controlled trial of alanyl-glutamine dipeptide (Fresenius-Kabi, Inc.) dosed at 0.5 g/kg/day for 7 days or until discharge from the ICU. The target population is 18–75 years of age with an ISS ≥ 16 and need for mechanical ventilation and either blood or inotropic support prior to enrollment; these patients have an expected mortality of 26% and an expected 8.1-day mean ICU length of stay. Patients with a body mass index <19 or >40 kg/m² would be excluded, along with patients with multisystem organ failure, pregnancy, known insulin-dependent diabetes, corticosteroid administration prior to enrollment, head Abbreviated Injury Score >4 or intracranial pressure >20 mmHg despite therapy, or known disease or acute failure affecting the liver and kidneys. Specific lessons learned from the REDOXS trial include more careful assessment of renal and hepatic function and exclusion of patients who are obese or in multiorgan system failure.

By establishing a framework for the effects of glutamine on IR and oxidative injury markers in critically injured patients, we hope to create a foundation for a larger, perhaps multicenter effort focused on trauma and burn patients focused on clinical endpoints of mortality and infection.

15.5 CONCLUSIONS

Despite extensive *in vitro* and *in vivo* studies including a numerous randomized clinical trials, the risk to benefit ratio of glutamine remains uncertain. The REDOXS study certainly informs the design of new trials in areas of clinical equipoise such as trauma and burns. Based on results from the REDOXS study, glutamine administration to patients with existing multisystem organ failure, particularly renal failure, is contraindicated. A greater understanding of the patient populations that might benefit from glutamine supplementation and glutamines mechanisms of action in the critically ill may identify patients who would benefit from glutamine replacement.

REFERENCES

Andrews, P J D, A Avenell, D W Noble, M K Campbell, B L Croal, W G Simpson, L D Vale et al. 2011. Randomised trial of glutamine, selenium, or both, to supplement parenteral nutrition for critically ill patients. *BMJ* 342 (mar17 2): d1542–2. doi: 10.1136/bmj.d1542.

Askanazi, J, Y A Carpentier, C B Michelsen, D H Elwyn, P Fürst, L R Kantrowitz, F E Gump, and J M Kinney. 1980. Muscle and plasma amino acids following injury. Influence of intercurrent infection. *Annals of Surgery* 192 (1): 78–85.

Avenell, A. 2009. Symposium 4: Hot topics in parenteral nutrition current evidence and ongoing trials on the use of glutamine in critically-ill patients and patients undergoing surgery. *Proceedings of the Nutrition Society* 68 (03): 261. doi: 10.1017/S0029665109001372.

Bakalar, B, F Duška, J Pachl, M Fric, M Otahal, J Pažout, and M Anděl. 2006. Parenterally administered dipeptide alanyl-glutamine prevents worsening of insulin sensitivity in multiple-trauma patients. *Critical Care Medicine* 34 (2): 381–6. doi: 10.1097/01.CCM.0000196829.30741.D4.

Boots, R J, J Lipman, R Bellomo, D Stephens, and R E Heller. 2005. Predictors of physician confidence to diagnose pneumonia and determine illness severity in ventilated patients. Australian and New Zealand Practice in Intensive Care (ANZPIC II). *Anaesthesia Intensive Care* 33 (1): 112–9.

Broyer, M, G Jean, A M Dartois, and C Kleinknecht. 1980. Plasma and muscle free amino acids in children at the early stages of renal failure. *The American Journal of Clinical Nutrition* 33 (7): 1396–401.

Coster, J, R McCauley, and J Hall. 2004. Glutamine: Metabolism and application in nutrition support. *Asia Pacific Journal of Clinical Nutrition* 13 (1): 25–31.

Dechelotte, P, M Hasselmann, L Cynober, B Allaouchiche, M s Coffier, B Hecketsweiler, V Merle et al. 2006. L-alanyl-L-glutamine dipeptide supplemented total parenteral nutrition reduces infectious complications and glucose intolerance in critically ill patients: The French controlled, randomized, double-blind, multicenter study. *Critical Care Medicine* 34 (3): 598–604. doi: 10.1097/01.CCM.0000201004.30750.D1.

DeFronzo, R A, J D Tobin, and R Andres. 1979. Glucose clamp technique: A method for quantifying insulin secretion and resistance. *The American Journal of Physiology* 237 (3): E214–23.

Deutz, Nicolaas E P. 2008. The 2007 ESPEN Sir David Cuthbertson Lecture: Amino acids between and within organs. The glutamate-glutamine-citrulline-arginine pathway. *Clinical Nutrition* 27 (3): 321–7. doi: 10.1016/j.clnu.2008.03.010.

Divino Filho, J C, P Bárány, P Stehle, P Fürst, and J Bergström. 1997. Free amino-acid levels simultaneously collected in plasma, muscle, and erythrocytes of uraemic patients. *Nephrology, Dialysis, Transplantation: Official Publication of the European Dialysis and Transplant Association—European Renal Association* 12 (11): 2339–48.

Driks, M R, L Wuquan, D E Craven, X Qiu, B R Celli, J Wang, M Manning et al. 2013. The therapeutic efficacy of glutamine for rats with smoking inhalation injury. *International Immunopharmacology* 16 (2). Elsevier B.V.: 248–53. doi: 10.1016/j.intimp.2013.02.022.

Dungan, K M, S S Braithwaite, and J-C Preiser. 2009. Stress hyperglycaemia. *The Lancet* 373 (9677). Elsevier Ltd.: 1798–807. doi: 10.1016/S0140-6736(09)60553-5.

Eroglu A. 2009. The effect of intravenous alanyl-glutamine supplementation on plasma glutathione levels in intensive care unit trauma patients receiving enteral nutrition: The results of a randomized controlled trial. *Anesthesia & Analgesia* 109 (2): 502–5. doi: 10.1213/ane.0b013e3181a83178.

Estivariz, C F, D P Griffith, M Luo, E E Szeszycki, N Bazargan, N Dave, N M Daignault et al. 2008. Efficacy of parenteral nutrition supplemented with glutamine dipeptide to decrease hospital infections in critically ill surgical patients. *Journal of Parenteral and Enteral Nutrition* 32 (4): 389–402. doi: 10.1177/0148607108317880.

Falcão de Arruda I S and J E de Aguilar-Nascimento. 2004. Benefits of Early Enteral Nutrition with Glutamine and Probiotics in Brain Injury Patients. *Clinical Science (London, England:1979)* 106 (3): 287–92. doi: 10.1042/CS20030251.

Fläring, U B, O E Rooyackers, C Hebert, T Bratel, F Hammarqvist, and J Wernerman. 2005. Temporal changes in whole-blood and plasma glutathione in ICU patients with multiple organ failure. *Intensive Care Medicine* 31 (8): 1072–8. doi: 10.1007/s00134-005-2687-0.

Fläring, U B, O E Rooyackers, J Wernerman, and F Hammarqvist. 2003a. Glutamine attenuates post-traumatic glutathione depletion in human muscle. *Clinical Science (London, England: 1979)* 104 (3): 275–82. doi: 10.1042/CS20020198.

Fläring U B, O E Rooyackers, J Wernerman, and F Hammarqvist. 2003b. Temporal changes in muscle glutathione in ICU patients. *Intensive Care Medicine* 29 (12): 2193–8. doi: 10.1007/s00134-003-2031-5.

Galera, S C, F V Fechine, M J Teixeira, Z C B Coelho, R C de Vasconcelos, and P R L de Vasconcelos. 2010. The safety of oral use of L-glutamine in middle-aged and elderly individuals. *Nutrition* 26 (4). Elsevier Ltd.: 375–81. doi: 10.1016/j.nut.2009.05.013.

Garrel, D, J Patenaude, B Nedelec, L Samson, J Dorais, J Champoux, M D'Elia, and J Bernier. 2003. Decreased mortality and infectious morbidity in adult burn patients given enteral glutamine supplements: A prospective, controlled, randomized clinical trial. *Critical Care Medicine* 31 (10): 2444–9. doi: 10.1097/01. CCM.0000084848.63691.1E.

Grau, T, A Bonet, E Miñambres, L Piñeiro, J A Irles, A Robles, J Acosta et al. 2011. The effect of L-alanyl-L-glutamine dipeptide supplemented total parenteral nutrition on infectious morbidity and insulin sensitivity in critically ill patients*. *Critical Care Medicine* 39 (6): 1263–8. doi: 10.1097/ CCM.0b013e31820eb774.

Hammarqvist, F, K Andersson, J Luo, and J Wernerman. 2005. Free amino acid and glutathione concentrations in muscle during short-term starvation and refeeding. *Clinical Nutrition* 24 (2): 236–43. doi: 10.1016/j.clnu.2004.10.004.

Heyland, D, J Muscedere, P E Wischmeyer, D Cook, G Jones, M Albert, G Elke, M M Berger, and A G Day. 2013. A randomized trial of glutamine and antioxidants in critically ill patients. *New England Journal of Medicine* 368 (16): 1489–97. doi: 10.1056/NEJMoa1212722.

Heyland, D K and R Dhaliwal. 2013. Role of glutamine supplementation in critical illness given the results of the REDOXS study. *Journal of Parenteral and Enteral Nutrition*, May. doi: 10.1177/0148607113488421.

Holecek, M. 2013. Evidence of a vicious cycle in glutamine synthesis and breakdown in pathogenesis of hepatic encephalopathy–therapeutic perspectives. *Metabolic Brain Disease* 29 (1): 9–17. doi: 10.1007/ s11011-013-9428-9.

Houdijk, A P J, E R Rijnsburger, J Jansen, R C I Wesdorp, J K Weiss, M A McCamish, T Teerlink et al. 1998. Randomised trial of glutamine-enriched enteral nutrition on infectious morbidity in patients with multiple trauma. *The Lancet* 352 (9130): 772–6. doi: 10.1016/S0140-6736(98)02007-8.

Jonas, C R, A B Puckett, D P Jones, D P Griffith, E E Szeszycki, G F Bergman, C E Furr et al. 2000. Plasma antioxidant status after high-dose chemotherapy: A randomized trial of parenteral nutrition in bone marrow transplantation patients. *The American Journal of Clinical Nutrition* 72 (1): 181–9.

Jones D P. 2006. Redefining oxidative stress. *Antioxidants & Redox Signaling* 8 (9–10): 1865–79. doi: 10.1089/ ars.2006.8.1865.

Labow B I and W W Souba. 2000. Glutamine. *World Journal of Surgery* 24 (12): 1503–13. doi: 10.1007/ s002680010269.

Langouche, L, S Vander Perre, P J Wouters, A D'Hoore, T K Hansen, and G van den Berghe. 2007. Effect of intensive insulin therapy on insulin sensitivity in the critically ill. *Journal of Clinical Endocrinology & Metabolism* 92 (10): 3890–7. doi: 10.1210/jc.2007-0813.

Lavery, G G and P Glover. 2000. The metabolic and nutritional response to critical illness. *Current Opinion in Critical Care* 6 (4): 233–8.

Luo J L, F Hammarqvist, K Andersson, and J Wernerman. 1996. Skeletal muscle glutathione after surgical trauma. *Annals of Surgery* 223 (4): 420–7.

Luo M, N Bazargan, D P Griffith, C F Estívariz, L M Leader, K A Easley, N M Daignault et al. 2008. Metabolic effects of enteral versus parenteral alanyl-glutamine dipeptide administration in critically ill patients receiving enteral feeding: A pilot study. *Clinical Nutrition* 27 (2): 297–306. doi: 10.1016/j. clnu.2007.12.003.

Meinz, H, D B Lacy, J Ejiofor, and O P McGuinness. 1998. Alterations in hepatic gluconeogenic amino acid uptake and gluconeogenesis in the endotoxin treated conscious dog. *Shock* 9 (4): 296–303.

Melis, G C, N ter Wengel, P G Boelens, and P A M van Leeuwen. 2004. Glutamine: Recent developments in research on the clinical significance of glutamine. *Current Opinion in Clinical Nutrition and Metabolic Care* 7 (1): 59–70. doi: 10.1097/01.mco.0000109608.04238.25.

Milne, G L, E S Musiek, and J D Morrow. 2005. F 2-Isoprostanes as markers of oxidative stress in vivo: An overview. *Biomarkers* 10 (s1): 10–23. doi: 10.1080/13547500500216546.

Moriarty, S. 2003. Oxidation of glutathione and cysteine in human plasma associated with smoking. *Free Radical Biology and Medicine* 35 (12): 1582–8. doi: 10.1016/j.freeradbiomed.2003.09.006.

Mukherjee, K, K J Sowards, S E Brooks, P R Norris, J B Boord, and A K May. 2014. Insulin resistance increases before ventilator-associated pneumonia in euglycemic trauma patients. *Surgical Infections* 15 (6): 713–20. doi: 10.1089/sur.2013.164.

Novak F, D K Heyland, A Avenell, J W Drover, and X Su. 2002. Glutamine supplementation in serious illness: A systematic review of the evidence. *Critical Care Medicine* 30 (9): 2022–9. doi: 10.1097/01. CCM.0000026106.58241.95.

Olde Damink, S W, I de Blaauw, N E Deutz, and P B Soeters. 1999. Effects in vivo of decreased plasma and intracellular muscle glutamine concentration on whole-body and hindquarter protein kinetics in rats. *Clinical Science (London, England: 1979)* 96 (6): 639–46.

O'Leary, M J, C N Ferguson, M J Rennie, C J Hinds, J H Coakley, and V R Preedy. 2001. Sequential changes in in vivo muscle and liver protein synthesis and plasma and tissue glutamine levels in sepsis in the rat. *Clinical Science (London, England: 1979)* 101 (3): 295–304.

Oudemans-van Straaten H M, R J Bosman, M Treskes, H J I van der Spoel, and D F Zandstra. 2001. Plasma glutamine depletion and patient outcome in acute ICU admissions. *Intensive Care Medicine* 27 (1): 84–90. doi: 10.1007/s001340000703.

Parry-Billings M, J Evans, P C Calder, and E A Newsholme. 1990. Does glutamine contribute to immunosuppression after major burns?. *The Lancet* 336 (8714): 523–5.

Peng, X, H Yan, H You, P Wang, and S Wang. 2005. Clinical and protein metabolic efficacy of glutamine granules-supplemented enteral nutrition in severely burned patients. *Burns* 31 (3): 342–6. doi: 10.1016/j.burns.2004.10.027.

Peng, Z-Y, C R Hamiel, A Banerjee, and P E Wischmeyer. 2006. Glutamine attenuation of cell death and inducible nitric oxide synthase expression following inflammatory cytokine-induced injury is dependent on heat shock factor-1 expression. *JPEN Journal of Parenteral and Enteral Nutrition* 30 (5): 400–7. doi: 10.1177/0148607106030005400.

Peng, Z-Y, F Zhou, H-Z Wang, X-Y Wen, T D Nolin, J V Bishop, and J A Kellum. 2013. The anti-oxidant effects are not the main mechanism for glutamine's protective effects on acute kidney injury in mice. *European Journal of Pharmacology* 705 (1–3). Elsevier: 11–9. doi: 10.1016/j.ejphar.2013.02.028.

Pérez-Bárcena, J, P Marsé, A Zabalegui-Pérez, E Corral, R Herrán-Monge, M Gero-Escapa, M Cervera et al. 2014. A randomized trial of intravenous glutamine supplementation in trauma ICU patients. *Intensive Care Medicine* 40 (4): 539–47. doi: 10.1007/s00134-014-3230-y.

Phanvijhitsiri, K. 2006. Heat induction of heat shock protein 25 requires cellular glutamine in intestinal epithelial cells. *AJP: Cell Physiology* 291 (2): C290–9. doi: 10.1152/ajpcell.00225.2005.

Robinson, M K, J D Rounds, R W Hong, D O Jacobs, and D W Willmore. 1992. Glutamine deficiency increases organ dysfunction after hemorrhagic shock. *Surgery* 112 (2): 140–7.

Rodas, P C, O Rooyackers, C Hebert, Å Norberg, and J Wernerman. 2012. Glutamine and glutathione at ICU admission in relation to outcome. *Clinical Science (London, England: 1979)* 122 (12): 591–7. doi: 10.1007/s00134-008-1356-5.

Roth, E, J Funovics, F Mühlbacher, M Schemper, W Mauritz, P Sporn, and A Fritsch. 1982. Metabolic disorders in severe abdominal sepsis: Glutamine deficiency in skeletal muscle. *Clinical Nutrition* 1 (1): 25–41. doi: 10.1016/0261-5614(82)90004-8.

Scheibe R, M Schade, M Grundling, D Pavlovic, K Starke, M Wendt, S Retter et al. 2009. Glutamine and alanyl-glutamine dipeptide reduce mesenteric plasma extravasation, leukocyte adhesion and Tumor Necrosis Factor-A (TNF-A) release during experimental endotoxemia. *Journal of Physiology and Pharmacology: An Official Journal of the Polish Physiological Society* 60 (Suppl 8) (December): 19–24.

Schulman A S, K F Willcutts, J A Claridge, H L Evans, A E Radigan, K B O'Donnell, J R Camden et al. 2005. Does the addition of glutamine to enteral feeds affect patient mortality? *Critical Care Medicine* 33 (11): 2501–6. doi: 10.1097/01.CCM.0000185643.02676.D3.

Singleton, K D, N Serkova, V E Beckey, and P E Wischmeyer. 2005. Glutamine attenuates lung injury and improves survival after sepsis: Role of enhanced heat shock protein expression. *Critical Care Medicine* 33 (6): 1206–13. doi: 10.1097/01.CCM.0000166357.10996.8A.

Soeters, P B and I Grecu. 2012. Have we enough glutamine and how does it work a clinician's view. *Annals of Nutrition and Metabolism* 60 (1): 17–26. doi: 10.1159/000334880.

Spindler-Vesel, A, S Bengmark, I Vovk, O Cerovic, and L Kompan. 2007. Synbiotics, prebiotics, glutamine, or peptide in early enteral nutrition: A randomized study in trauma patients. *JPEN Journal of Parenteral and Enteral Nutrition* 31 (2): 119–26. doi: 10.1177/0148607107031002119.

Venkatesh B, I Hickman, J Nisbet, J Cohen, and J Prins. 2009. Changes in serum adiponectin concentrations in critical illness: A preliminary investigation. *Critical Care* 13 (4): R105. doi: 10.1186/cc7941.

Vermeulen M A R, M C G van de Poll, G C Ligthart-Melis, C H C Dejong, M P van den Tol, P G Boelens, and P A M van Leeuwen. 2007. Specific amino acids in the critically ill patient? exogenous glutamine/arginine: A common denominator? *Critical Care Medicine* 35 (Suppl): S568–76. doi: 10.1097/01.CCM.0000278600.14265.95.

Wang, Y, Z M Jiang, M T Nolan, H Jiang, H R Han, K Yu, H L Li, B Jie, and X K Liang. 2010. The impact of glutamine dipeptide-supplemented parenteral nutrition on outcomes of surgical patients: A meta-analysis of randomized clinical trials. *Journal of Parenteral and Enteral Nutrition* 34 (5): 521–9. doi: 10.1177/0148607110362587.

Wischmeyer, P E. 2006. Glutamine: The first clinically relevant pharmacological regulator of heat shock protein expression?. *Current Opinion in Clinical Nutrition and Metabolic Care* 9 (3): 201–6. doi: 10.1097/01.mco.0000222100.44256.6b.

Wischmeyer, P E. 2007. Glutamine: Mode of action in critical illness. *Critical Care Medicine* 35 (Suppl): S541–4. doi: 10.1097/01.CCM.0000278064.32780.D3.

Wischmeyer, P E. 2008. Glutamine: Role in critical illness and ongoing clinical trials. *Current Opinion in Gastroenterology* 24 (2): 190–7. doi: 10.1097/MOG.0b013e3282f4db94.

Wischmeyer, P E, M Kahana, R Wolfson, H Ren, M M Musch, and E B Chang. 2001a. Glutamine induces heat shock protein and protects against endotoxin shock in the rat. *Journal of Applied Physiology (Bethesda, MD: 1985)* 90 (6): 2403–10.

Wischmeyer, P E, M Kahana, R Wolfson, H Ren, M M Musch, and E B Chang. 2001b. Glutamine reduces cytokine release, organ damage, and mortality in a rat model of endotoxemia. *Shock* 16 (5): 398–402.

Wischmeyer, P E, J Lynch, J Liedel, R Wolfson, J Riehm, L Gottlieb, and M Kahana. 2001c. Glutamine administration reduces Gram-negative bacteremia in severely burned patients: A prospective, randomized, double-blind trial versus isonitrogenous control. *Critical Care Medicine* 29 (11): 2075–80.

Wischmeyer, P E, M M Musch, M B Madonna, R Thisted, and E B Chang. 1997. Glutamine protects intestinal epithelial cells: Role of inducible HSP70. *The American Journal of Physiology* 272 (4 Pt 1): G879–84.

Wischmeyer P E, J Riehm, K D Singleton, H Ren, M W Musch, M Kahana, and E B Chang. 2003. Glutamine attenuates tumor necrosis factor-alpha release and enhances heat shock protein 72 in human peripheral blood mononuclear cells. *Nutrition* 19 (1): 1–6.

Www.Criticalcarenutrition.com 2009. Clinical Practice Guidelines 4.1 (C) Composition of en: Glutamine: January 31, 2009. July 10. http://www.criticalcarenutrition.com/docs/cpg/4.1c_englu_FINAL.pdf.

Zhou, Y P, Z M Jiang, Y H Sun, X R Wang, E L Ma, and D Wilmore. 2003. The effect of supplemental enteral glutamine on plasma levels, gut function, and outcome in severe burns: A randomized, double-blind, controlled clinical trial. *JPEN. Journal of Parenteral and Enteral Nutrition* 27 (4): 241–5. doi: 10.1177/0148607103027004241.

Ziegler, T R, L G Ogden, K D Singleton, M Luo, C Fernandez-Estivariz, D P Griffith, J R Galloway, and P E Wischmeyer. 2005. Parenteral glutamine increases serum heat shock protein 70 in critically ill patients. *Intensive Care Medicine* 31 (8): 1079–86. doi: 10.1007/s00134-005-2690-5.

16 Glutamine Supplementation in Critical Illness
Clinical Endpoints

Marie Smedberg and Jan Wernerman

CONTENTS

16.1 INTRODUCTION

The use of glutamine supplementation in critical illness may have three different rationales: (i) to be a part of the amino acid content of an optimal protein supply; (ii) to aim at restoring a possible shortage or deficit as evidenced by low plasma and/or tissue concentrations; or (iii) to be given with the purpose of having pharmacological effects by itself or in combination with other substances. When evaluating the clinical outcomes related to glutamine supplementation, it is therefore important to differentiate between these three purposes. In a number of reviews and meta-analyses, this is not done, and consequently, mixing up these targets of therapy will add to the confusion perhaps connected to the task of supplementing the critically ill with glutamine.

For example, grouping studies related to the route of administration or the general dose will add little to the understanding of results if the purpose of the study is not scrutinized. Authors of published studies do not facilitate the reading of their publications, as this goal is very often not stated explicitly. Most often, patients with a potential deficit are mixed up with patients not associated with any indications of such a deficit. Furthermore, deficits may or may not be possible to compensate for using supplementation.

Until now, very few studies give plasma concentrations of glutamine as an indication of possible deficit and possible effect of treatment. This may be excused as long as no harm was associated with glutamine supplementation. The mixture of patients with and without a possible glutamine shortage, naturally, resulted in a mixture of results related to the case mix in the particular study; and in the end, an inability to answer the question was proposed, namely, is supplementation in a possibly glutamine-deficient state beneficial?

The absence of conclusive results led investigators to the unfortunate pharmaconutrition hypothesis. The doses given were thought to be inadequate and, therefore, the increase to supraphysiological levels without proper control of safety. The harm recently reported in a large study of very high supplementation combined with hypocaloric nutrition to patients in the acute phase of sepsis with two or more organ failures has put an end to the indiscriminative use of glutamine supplementation (Heyland et al. 2013). The harmful results are so far not explained, and epidemiologic exploration of the database associated with the study unfortunately provides very little hypothesis generation.

In this perspective, the clinical endpoints of glutamine supplementation to the critically ill are presented and discussed in the context of possible deficiency, underlying pathology, and case mix of patients in studies.

16.2   ROUTE OF ADMINISTRATION

Following intravenous glutamine administration, there is an immediate increase in plasma glutamine concentration, which returns back to the preadministration level quite rapidly when intravenous administration stops (Albers et al. 1988, 1989; Berg et al. 2005; Ligthart-Melis et al. 2007; Sodergren et al. 2010). As crystalline glutamine is not stable in aqueous solution, studies involving intravenous glutamine administration were done with newly prepared solutions only (Hammarqvist et al. 1989; Stehle et al. 1989). The invention to use glutamine-containing dipeptides made it possible to use intravenous glutamine more widely (Wernerman 2003). In healthy individuals, the dipeptide, usually L-alanyl-L-glutamine or L-glycyl-L-glutamine, is rapidly and completely hydrolyzed when administered intravenously as a bolus or as a constant infusion (Albers et al. 1988, 1989; Berg et al. 2005). Also, in critically ill patients with organ failures, the dipeptide is rapidly and completely hydrolyzed, even when administered in high doses (Berg et al. 2005). When administering high doses of glutamine-containing dipeptides to critically ill patients, the increase in plasma glutamine concentration is rapidly returning back to preadministration levels after cessation of the administration as illustrated in Figure 16.1 (Berg et al. 2005; Tjader et al. 2004).

When glutamine is administered by the enteral route, the effect on plasma concentration is different. After an ordinary meal including glutamine-containing proteins, for example, there is only a marginal increase of plasma glutamine concentration (Matthews and Campbell 1992). This is in contrast to the increase in other amino acids, like branched-chain amino acids, which show a more substantial response to feeding. When glutamine-containing dipeptides are administered enterally, a similar hydrolysis as when administered intravenously is seen, but the increase in plasma glutamine concentration is of much lower magnitude (Ligthart-Melis et al. 2007). This difference in the effect on plasma glutamine concentration is attributable to the so-called "first-pass elimination," where some of the glutamine taken up from the gut are utilized in cells of the intestine and the liver before reaching the general circulation. The extent of this "first-pass elimination" is related to dose and to whether or not other nutrients are administered in parallel to glutamine (Darmaun et al. 1994; Gelfand et al. 1986). Still the capacity of the gut to absorb glutamine already in the upper part of the jejunum is high (Dechelotte et al. 1991).

The different handling of glutamine related to the route of administration must of course be taken into consideration when the clinical effects of glutamine supplementation are discussed. For intravenously administered glutamine, there is a clear dose-response in terms of the effect on plasma concentration (Berg et al. 2005; Ligthart-Melis et al. 2007; Melis et al. 2005; Tjader et al. 2004), and for enterally administered glutamine, this is less clear (Ligthart-Melis et al. 2007; Melis et al. 2005). The result is that regardless if the rational of supplementation is to try to restore normal plasma glutamine levels, or just to provide glutamine in amounts similar to those of ordinary food, there will be a difference in terms of the effect on plasma glutamine concentration (Wernerman 2014). Also, regardless of the route of administration, the supplemented subject will restore the plasma glutamine concentration back to preadministration level. As there is no way to store glutamine, it will be metabolized, which puts a metabolic demand upon the organism, in particular, the kidneys. The handling

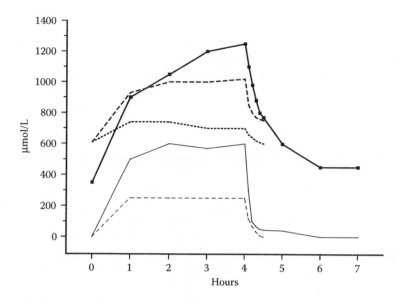

FIGURE 16.1 Illustration of the difference between intravenous and enteral administrations of glutamine. When given enterally, the response in plasma glutamine concentration is much lower. When given intravenously, there is a clear dose-response in terms of dipeptide concentration. After the end of infusion, concentrations are rapidly returning back to preinfusion levels. Plasma concentrations of glutamine (bold lines) and the dipeptide L-alanyl-L-glutamine (thin lines) during a 4-h infusion period in fully fed critically ill patients with multiple organ failure (solid lines), and postabsorptive patients scheduled for elective surgery (dotted and dashed lines). Dose to critically ill patients was 0.087 g/kg/h intravenously and to elective surgery patients was 0.040 g/kg/h intravenously (dashed line) and enterally (dotted line). (Figure drawn out of published data from Ligthart-Melis, G. C. et al. 2007 and Berg, A. et al. 2005).

of glutamine overdosing is not well characterized, not in healthy individuals, and definitely not in critically ill patients (Heyland et al. 2013). When overdosing is administered by the enteral route, the lower impact on plasma glutamine concentration will to some extent disguise this potential problem.

16.3 PATIENT GROUPS

16.3.1 Postoperative

Historically, observations of glutamine deficits were first reported in postoperative patients by a decrease of intracellular glutamine concentration to low values (Vinnars et al. 1975). This decrease was not obligatory accompanied by a decrease of plasma concentration to low values (Askanazi et al. 1980; Vinnars et al. 1975). The decrease develops during this initial postoperative period, and a nadir in muscle free glutamine concentration is seen on postoperative after 2 to 4 days. A larger operative trauma results in a greater decrease and a later nadir (Petersson et al. 1992). The low intracellular concentration of glutamine is restored slowly, with a return to normal after 2–4 weeks, related to the degree of decrease (Askanazi et al. 1980; Petersson et al. 1992). Provision of conventional parenteral nutrition does not alter the development of a drop in intracellular glutamine concentration (Vinnars et al. 1980). Addition of glutamine to postoperative parenteral nutrition, however, prevents the development of free glutamine depletion in skeletal muscle (Hammarqvist et al. 1989, 1990; Petersson et al. 1994; Stehle et al. 1989). If glutamine supplementation is discontinued, the decrease in muscle free glutamine is only delayed (Petersson et al. 1994). If intravenous supplementation is started when the decrease in muscle glutamine level is already established, it is not readily influenced (Tjader et al. 2004).

16.3.2 CRITICAL ILLNESS

In critically ill subjects, the degree of glutamine depletion in terms of low intracellular concentration in muscle is more pronounced as compared to postoperative patients (Gamrin et al. 1996, 1997; Roth et al. 1982; Tjader et al. 2004). The major difference is that the temporal pattern of development of the low concentration is not known. In an experimental system when healthy volunteers are given endotoxin, a period of decrease is seen over 24 h with an initial brief increase in muscle free glutamine (Vesali et al. 2005). Also, when healthy individuals are subjected to starvation only, a decrease in muscle free glutamine develops over 3 days, with the degree of decrease more marginal, however (Luo et al. 1997). Also, for critically ill patients, the low concentration of muscle glutamine is not influenced by exogenous intravenous supplementation even in high doses as illustrated in Figure 16.2 (Tjader et al. 2004). The possibility to prevent a decrease has not yet been explored.

In some contrast to the postoperative patients, critically ill patients may also have a low plasma glutamine concentration (Oudemans-van Straaten et al. 2001; Rodas et al. 2012). Approximately 35% of patients have such a low level and this group of patients have a higher 6-month mortality rate as compared to normoglutaminemic patients (Oudemans-van Straaten et al. 2001; Rodas et al. 2012). With multiple stepwise logistic regression, hypoglutaminemia at the intensive care unit (ICU) admission has been demonstrated to be an independent risk factor for mortality, which adds prediction to conventional risk scoring such as APACHE and SAPS (Rodas et al. 2012). Intravenous supplementation with glutamine or glutamine-containing dipeptides can normalize plasma concentration in critically ill patients although the decrease in muscle is unaffected (Tjader et al. 2004). There is also information over the efflux of endogenous glutamine from muscle during critical illness, which is increased as compared to healthy subjects but unaltered over time in the ICU despite the lower-than-normal plasma concentration in some patients (Vesali et al. 2002).

The splanchnic organs are the target for the export of free glutamine from muscle (Marliss et al. 1971; Matthews et al. 1993; Wernerman et al. 1985). In the muscles of a healthy subject versus a

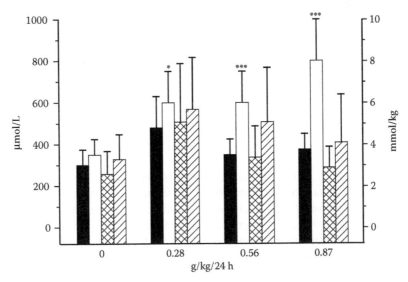

FIGURE 16.2 Illustration of the relation between plasma and tissue glutamine concentrations in a dose-finding study for 5 days in critically ill patients with multiple organ failures. Patients were fully fed according to energy expenditure and were supplemented with intravenous glutamine (crystalline) keeping the diet given. With increasing dose, plasma glutamine concentration increased into the normal range, while the concentration in muscle was not significantly increased. Solid and open bars represent plasma glutamine before and during supplementation, respectively (left y-axis). Cross-hatched and hatched bars represent muscle glutamine before and at the end of supplementation, respectively (right y-axis). Asterisks denote level of statistical significance as compared to basal. (Figure drawn out of published data from Tjader, I. et al. 2004.)

critically ill subject, there is a vast difference with a ratio of 1:30 compared to plasma glutamine for healthy subjects, decreasing to a ratio of 1:1.5 to 1.10 in the critically ill subjects (Gamrin et al. 1996; Roth et al. 1982). In the liver, the ratio is lower, approximately 1:10 in healthy subjects (Barle et al. 1996), and in the intestinal mucosa of the duodenum and colon, a ratio of 1:5 is seen in healthy subjects (Ahlman et al. 1993a; Ahlman et al. 1993b). Among critically ill patients, the free glutamine in intestinal mucosa decreases, but the relation to plasma concentration stays the same as in healthy subjects (Ahlman et al. 1995).

16.3.3 ONCOLOGY AND HEMATOLOGY

Several studies have reported beneficial effects on patients with hematological malignancies and bone marrow transplantations (Aquino et al. 2005; Brown et al. 1998; Jebb et al. 1995; Schloerb and Amare 1993, 1999; Wilmore et al. 1999; Ziegler et al. 1992). When mortality outcomes have been reported, it has been difficult to document the comparability between the groups (Pytlik et al. 2002; Schloerb and Amare 1993). Improved tolerance to oncological treatment is also reported, in particular, mucositis (Aquino et al. 2005; Ward et al. 2009). In parallel to the studies reporting beneficial effects, there are studies that report neutral results, but just singular studies that report possible harm (Pytlik et al. 2002). Eventually, Cochrane reports including meta-analyses have been presented (Murray and Pindoria 2009). Overall, the conclusions are that the evidence so far has been insufficient for solid recommendations; on the other hand, no statements over risk for harm are expressed. In general, there is no relation between possible glutamine depletion in terms of low plasma or tissue concentrations available in the publications, and furthermore, the reviews and meta-analyses do not consider hypoglutaminemia as a possible selection of patients in need of supplementation as well as in no need of the same.

16.3.4 GASTROINTESTINAL

The hypothesis that glutamine availability is crucial for regeneration of intestinal mucosa has emerged from animal experiments. The evidence for a similar role for glutamine in humans is less convincing. This goes in parallel with the difference in susceptibility to inactivity atrophy of the mucosa and the risk of microbial translocation, which is obviously different between species (MacFie 1997). Nevertheless, glutamine supplementation in states of gastrointestinal insufficiency has been reported to have positive effects on tolerance to feeding and infectious complications (Conejero et al. 2002; de Aguilar-Nascimento et al. 2007; Ong et al. 2012; Tremel et al. 1994); again in parallel, there are reports of neutral effects. Consequently, meta-analyses do not find convincing evidence that allows for recommendations of glutamine supplementation in relation to gastrointestinal insufficiency (Tremel et al. 1994; Tubman et al. 2005; Wagner et al. 2012). A special patient group in this category is the premature-born infants, which has attained particular interest (Duggan et al. 2004; Neu et al. 1997; Ong et al. 2012; Tubman et al. 2005). In summary, there are insufficient evidences for any general recommendations. However, the available studies have not been able to address the question over whether treatment to subjects with a possible deficit, suggested by a low plasma or tissue concentrations, may be beneficial.

16.4 OUTCOMES

16.4.1 PROXY MEASURES

In postoperative patients, nitrogen balance has been a common proxy endpoint. In postoperative patients fed parenterally, a better nitrogen balance is seen during intravenous glutamine supplementation (Hammarqvist et al. 1989, 1990; Stehle et al. 1989). There is also a statistical correlation between nitrogen balance and the attenuation of muscle free glutamine concentration (Wernerman et al. 1990).

16.4.2 MORBIDITY

As a possible shortage of glutamine may result in an impairment of the defense against infections, a reduction of infections has been a frequent endpoint in studies. This is also reported during enteral supplementation after traffic accidents, after pancreatitis, and in successfully fed ICU long-stayers (Conejero et al. 2002; Estivariz et al. 2008; Fuentes-Orozco et al. 2008; Houdijk et al. 1998; Jones et al. 1999; Oguz et al. 2007). Others have failed to detect such improvements after enteral gluta-mine supplementation in adequately fed general ICU patients (Hall et al. 2003). In most of these studies, plasma glutamine concentrations were not reported, not in the basal state and not as an effect of supplementation. When concentrations were obtained, few subjects were hypoglutamin-emic, and the effect of supplementation in plasma concentration is marginal (Beale et al. 2008; Heyland et al. 2013; Houdijk et al. 1998). The number of infections and colonization after condition-ing before bone marrow transplantation is improved after intravenous glutamine supplementation (Ziegler et al. 1992). General morbidity in ICU patients in terms of organ failure scoring is improved when enteral supplementation is added to fully fed ICU patients (Beale et al. 2008).

16.4.3 MORTALITY

Mortality rate is often regarded as the ultimate outcome measure, in particular, for critically ill patients. The difficulty in conjunction with glutamine supplementation is the absence of any direct connection between hypoglutaminemia or hyperglutaminemia, and mortality. The need for gluta-mine availability to manufacture nucleotides necessary for cell division (Newsholme and Calder 1997) may give a reasonable explanation for a lower infection rate, a better outcome after infections, a better gastrointestinal function, and so on, which would transfer into morbidity improvements and then secondarily into mortality advantages. In studies reporting a mortality advantage or disadvan-tage, this is not always the case.

For a mortality endpoint to be conclusive, the group of patients studied must represent a com-paratively high mortality risk. In two classic studies where intravenous glutamine supplementation in combination with full parenteral feeding during ICU stay gave a mortality advantage, the mortal-ity measure was 6-month all-cause mortality (Goeters et al. 2002; Griffiths et al. 1997). So, part of the mortality was post-ICU and postintervention, and therefore, the causality between intervention and endpoint has been questioned (Maratea et al. 2014). The same goes for a more recent study of enteral supplementation as a part of a multisupplementation during ICU stay in fully fed patients where 6-month all-cause mortality was elevated in a subgroup exposed to glutamine supplementa-tion in the ICU (van Zanten et al. 2014). In other studies of fully fed ICU patients given intrave-nous glutamine supplementation during ICU stay, no differences in 6-month mortalities have been detected (Andrews et al. 2011). One of these studies, namely, the Scandinavian glutamine study, showed a mortality benefit during ICU stay, which was not sustained at the 6-month follow-up (Wernerman et al. 2011). All these studies report of groups of patients given adequate nutrition and low or moderate doses of glutamine supplementation, regardless of the routes of administration. Only exceptionally have the plasma concentrations of glutamine been reported. When such report-ing is at hand, administration have been enteral, and the effect on plasma concentration therefore marginal (Barle et al. 1996; Houdijk et al. 1998). So, it may be concluded that the hypothesis that glutamine depleted critically ill patients, as represented by hypoglutaminemia at ICU admission, has not been adequately tested.

In a recent study of hypocalorically fed critically ill patients supplemented with pharmacological doses of glutamine using combined routes of administration, enterally and parenterally, a mortal-ity disadvantage is reported (Heyland et al. 2013). Included patients were not monitored for plasma glutamine concentration, except for a subgroup of subjects where approximately 30% were hypo-glutaminemic, in accord with reports from other studies (Oudemans-van Straaten et al. 2001; Rodas et al. 2012). Furthermore, a possible randomization bias may limit the generalizability of the results

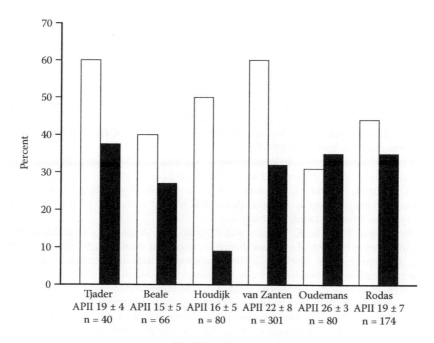

FIGURE 16.3 Illustration of variability in glutamine status in different studies in critically ill patients, underlining the need to characterize this variable in the outcome studies. Patient case-mix, frequency of admission hypoglutaminemia (% with <400 μmol/L, open bars), severity of illness scoring, and 6-month mortality outcome (solid bars) in published studies with these variables available. In some of the studies, a part of the patients were supplemented with glutamine during ICU stay. (Figure drawn out of published data from Tjader et al. 2004, Beale et al. 2008, Houdijk et al. 1998, van Zanten et al. 2014, Oudemans van Straaten et al. 2001, ands rodas et al. 2012 as indicated.)

(Buijs et al. 2013), and the extremely unbalanced supply of amino acids in itself causes a metabolic burden upon, in particular, kidneys and liver (van de Poll et al. 2007).

The absence of information over the frequency of hypoglutaminemia in the outcome studies makes interpretation difficult, in particular, as the admission plasma glutamine concentration is not at all reflected by the risk scoring at this time point [29]. It is possible that the case mix of patients in studies with conflicting results may be the major difference between the studies, and the comparability between groups in terms of admission plasma glutamine concentration, or in terms of plasma glutamine concentration during treatment (efficacy of treatment), may not actually allow for meaningful comparisons. This problem is illustrated in Figure 16.3.

16.5 CONCLUSIONS AND PERSPECTIVES

The agenda for future studies over glutamine supplementation in critical illness should presently not focus on outcomes. There are two other burning issues to be addressed: (i) is hypoglutaminemia in critical illness a sign of depletion or just limited to be a biomarker for poor outcome? and (ii) why is overadministration of a self-substance like glutamine associated with mortality risk?

Even though the hypotheses of pharmaconutrition should now be removed from the agenda, it remains to answer the question if a possible deficit, known to be associated with a poor outcome, may be an indication for supplementation. As outlined above, there are a number of publications reporting improved outcomes, although not specifically associated with glutamine depletion. It is frustrating that all these studies were performed without relating dose of supplementation to possible deficit. The enthusiasm for future studies is not on top, and it is unlikely that manufacturers of nutritional products will offer support for such studies. Still, it is a responsibility to our patients to explore whether there is a possible benefit for them, or to turn the question around whether there is a possible harm to withhold supplementation in cases of depletion.

REFERENCES

Ahlman, B., C. E. Leijonmarck, C. Lind, E. Vinnars, and J. Wernerman. 1993a. Free amino acids in biopsy specimens from the human colonic mucosa. *J Surg Res* 55(6):647–53.

Ahlman, B., C. E. Leijonmarck, and J. Wernerman. 1993b. The content of free amino acids in the human duodenal mucosa. *Clin Nutr* 12(5):266–71.

Ahlman, B., O. Ljungqvist, B. Persson, L. Bindslev, and J. Wernerman. 1995. Intestinal amino acid content in critically ill patients. *JPEN J Parenter Enteral Nutr* 19(4):272–8.

Albers, S., J. Wernerman, P. Stehle, E. Vinnars, and P. Furst. 1988. Availability of amino acids supplied intravenously in healthy man as synthetic dipeptides: Kinetic evaluation of L-alanyl-L-glutamine and glycyl-L-tyrosine. *Clin Sci (Lond)* 75(5):463–8.

Albers, S., J. Wernerman, P. Stehle, E. Vinnars, and P. Furst. 1989. Availability of amino acids supplied by constant intravenous infusion of synthetic dipeptides in healthy man. *Clin Sci (Lond)* 76(6):643–8.

Andrews, P. J., A. Avenell, D. W. Noble et al. 2011. Randomised trial of glutamine, selenium, or both, to supplement parenteral nutrition for critically ill patients. *BMJ* 342:d1542.

Aquino, V. M., A. R. Harvey, J. H. Garvin et al. 2005. A double-blind randomized placebo-controlled study of oral glutamine in the prevention of mucositis in children undergoing hematopoietic stem cell transplantation: A pediatric blood and marrow transplant consortium study. *Bone Marrow Transplant* 36(7):611–6.

Askanazi, J., Y. A. Carpentier, C. B. Michelsen et al. 1980. Muscle and plasma amino acids following injury. Influence of intercurrent infection. *Ann Surg* 192(1):78–85.

Barle, H., B. Ahlman, B. Nyberg, K. Andersson, P. Essen, and J. Wernerman. 1996. The concentrations of free amino acids in human liver tissue obtained during laparoscopic surgery. *Clin Physiol* 16(3):217–27.

Beale, R. J., T. Sherry, K. Lei et al. 2008. Early enteral supplementation with key pharmaconutrients improves sequential organ failure assessment score in critically ill patients with sepsis: Outcome of a randomized, controlled, double-blind trial. *Crit Care Med* 36(1):131–44.

Berg, A., O. Rooyackers, A. Norberg, and J. Wernerman. 2005. Elimination kinetics of L-alanyl-L-glutamine in ICU patients. *Amino Acids* 29(3):221–8.

Brown, S. A., A. Goringe, C. Fegan et al. 1998. Parenteral glutamine protects hepatic function during bone marrow transplantation. *Bone Marrow Transplant* 22(3):281–4.

Buijs, N., M. A. Vermeulen, and P. A. van Leeuwen. 2013. Glutamine and antioxidants in critically ill patients. *N Engl J Med* 369(5):484.

Conejero, R., A. Bonet, T. Grau et al. 2002. Effect of a glutamine-enriched enteral diet on intestinal permeability and infectious morbidity at 28 days in critically ill patients with systemic inflammatory response syndrome: A randomized, single-blind, prospective, multicenter study. *Nutrition* 18(9):716–21.

Darmaun, D., B. Just, B. Messing et al. 1994. Glutamine metabolism in healthy adult men: Response to enteral and intravenous feeding. *Am J Clin Nutr* 59(6):1395–402.

de Aguilar-Nascimento, J. E., C. Caporossi, D. B. Dock-Nascimento, I. S. de Arruda, K. Moreno, and W. Moreno. 2007. Oral glutamine in addition to parenteral nutrition improves mortality and the healing of high-output intestinal fistulas. *Nutr Hosp* 22(6):672–6.

Dechelotte, P., D. Darmaun, M. Rongier, B. Hecketsweiler, O. Rigal, and J. F. Desjeux. 1991. Absorption and metabolic effects of enterally administered glutamine in humans. *Am J Physiol* 260(5 Pt 1):G677–82.

Duggan, C., A. R. Stark, N. Auestad et al. 2004. Glutamine supplementation in infants with gastrointestinal disease: A randomized, placebo-controlled pilot trial. *Nutrition* 20(9):752–6.

Estivariz, C. F., D. P. Griffith, M. Luo et al. 2008. Efficacy of parenteral nutrition supplemented with glutamine dipeptide to decrease hospital infections in critically ill surgical patients. *JPEN J Parenter Enteral Nutr* 32(4):389–402.

Fuentes-Orozco, C., G. Cervantes-Guevara, I. Mucino-Hernandez et al. 2008. L-Alanyl-L-glutamine-supplemented parenteral nutrition decreases infectious morbidity rate in patients with severe acute pancreatitis. *JPEN J Parenter Enteral Nutr* 32(4):403–11.

Gamrin, L., K. Andersson, E. Hultman, E. Nilsson, P. Essen, and J. Wernerman. 1997. Longitudinal changes of biochemical parameters in muscle during critical illness. *Metabolism* 46(7):756–62.

Gamrin, L., P. Essen, A. M. Forsberg, E. Hultman, and J. Wernerman. 1996. A descriptive study of skeletal muscle metabolism in critically ill patients: Free amino acids, energy-rich phosphates, protein, nucleic acids, fat, water, and electrolytes. *Crit Care Med* 24(4):575–83.

Gelfand, R. A., M. G. Glickman, R. Jacob, R. S. Sherwin, and R. A. DeFronzo. 1986. Removal of infused amino acids by splanchnic and leg tissues in humans. *Am J Physiol* 250(4 Pt 1):E407–13.

Goeters, C., A. Wenn, N. Mertes et al. 2002. Parenteral L-alanyl-L-glutamine improves 6-month outcome in critically ill patients. *Crit Care Med* 30(9):2032–7.

Griffiths, R. D., C. Jones, and T. E. Palmer. 1997. Six-month outcome of critically ill patients given glutamine-supplemented parenteral nutrition. *Nutrition* 13(4):295–302.

Hall, J. C., G. Dobb, J. Hall, R. de Sousa, L. Brennan, and R. McCauley. 2003. A prospective randomized trial of enteral glutamine in critical illness. *Intensive Care Med* 29:1710–6.

Hammarqvist, F., J. Wernerman, R. Ali, A. von der Decken, and E. Vinnars. 1989. Addition of glutamine to total parenteral nutrition after elective abdominal surgery spares free glutamine in muscle, counteracts the fall in muscle protein synthesis, and improves nitrogen balance. *Ann Surg* 209(4):455–61.

Hammarqvist, F., J. Wernerman, A. von der Decken, and E. Vinnars. 1990. Alanyl-glutamine counteracts the depletion of free glutamine and the postoperative decline in protein synthesis in skeletal muscle. *Ann Surg* 212(5):637–44.

Heyland, D., J. Muscedere, P. E. Wischmeyer et al. 2013. A randomized trial of glutamine and antioxidants in critically ill patients. *N Engl J Med* 368(16):1489–97.

Houdijk, A. P., E. R. Rijnsburger, J. Jansen et al. 1998. Randomised trial of glutamine-enriched enteral nutrition on infectious morbidity in patients with multiple trauma. *Lancet* 352(9130):772–6.

Jebb, S. A., R. Marcus, and M. Elia. 1995. A pilot study of oral glutamine supplementation in patients receiving bone marrow transplants. *Clin Nutr* 14(3):162–5.

Jones, C., T. E. Palmer, and R. D. Griffiths. 1999. Randomized clinical outcome study of critically ill patients given glutamine-supplemented enteral nutrition. *Nutrition* 15(2):108–15.

Ligthart-Melis, G. C., M. C. van de Poll, C. H. Dejong, P. G. Boelens, N. E. Deutz, and P. A. van Leeuwen. 2007. The route of administration (enteral or parenteral) affects the conversion of isotopically labeled L-[2–15*N*]glutamine into citrulline and arginine in humans. *JPEN J Parenter Enteral Nutr* 31(5):343–48; discussion 349–50.

Luo, J. L., F. Hammarovist, K. Andersson, and J. Wernerman. 1997. Glutathione in human skeletal muscle: Effects of food intake, surgical trauma and critical illness. *Clin Nutr* 16(3):141–3.

MacFie, J. 1997. Bacterial translocation in surgical patients. *Ann R Coll Surg Engl* 79(3):183–9.

Maratea, D., V. Fadda, S. Trippoli, and A. Messori. 2014. Glutamine in critically ill patients: Trial-sequential analysis. *Clin Nutr* 33(4):735–6.

Marliss, E. B., T. T. Aoki, T. Pozefsky, A. S. Most, and G. F. Cahill, Jr. 1971. Muscle and splanchnic glutmine and glutamate metabolism in postabsorptive andstarved man. *J Clin Invest* 50(4):814–7.

Matthews, D. E. and R. G. Campbell. 1992. The effect of dietary protein intake on glutamine and glutamate nitrogen metabolism in humans. *Am J Clin Nutr* 55(5):963–70.

Matthews, D. E., M. A. Marano, and R. G. Campbell. 1993. Splanchnic bed utilization of glutamine and glutamic acid in humans. *Am J Physiol* 264(6 Pt 1):E848–54.

Melis, G. C., P. G. Boelens, J. R. van der Sijp et al. 2005. The feeding route (enteral or parenteral) affects the plasma response of the dipetide Ala-Gln and the amino acids glutamine, citrulline and arginine, with the administration of Ala-Gln in preoperative patients. *Br J Nutr* 94(1):19–26.

Murray, S. M. and S. Pindoria. 2009. Nutrition support for bone marrow transplant patients. *Cochrane Database Syst Rev* (1):CD002920.

Neu, J., J. C. Roig, W. H. Meetze et al. 1997. Enteral glutamine supplementation for very low birth weight infants decreases morbidity. *J Pediatr* 131(5):691–9.

Newsholme, E. A. and P. C. Calder. 1997. The proposed role of glutamine in some cells of the immune system and speculative consequences for the whole animal. *Nutrition* 13(7–8):728–30.

Oguz, M., M. Kerem, A. Bedirli et al. 2007. L-Alaninyl-L-glutamine supplementation improves the outcome after colorectal surgery for cancer. *Colorectal Dis* 9(6):515–20.

Ong, E. G., S. Eaton, A. M. Wade et al. 2012. Randomized clinical trial of glutamine-supplemented versus standard parenteral nutrition in infants with surgical gastrointestinal disease. *Br J Surg* 99(7):929–38.

Oudemans-van Straaten, H. M., R. J. Bosman, M. Treskes, H. J. van der Spoel, and D. F. Zandstra. 2001. Plasma glutamine depletion and patient outcome in acute ICU admissions. *Intensive Care Med* 27(1):84–90.

Petersson, B., E. Vinnars, S. O. Waller, and J. Wernerman. 1992. Long-term changes in muscle free amino acid levels after elective abdominal surgery. *Br J Surg* 79(3):212–6.

Petersson, B., S. O. Waller, E. Vinnars, and J. Wernerman. 1994. Long-term effect of glycyl-glutamine after elective surgery on free amino acids in muscle. *JPEN J Parenter Enteral Nutr* 18(4):320–5.

Pytlik, R., P. Benes, M. Patorkova et al. 2002. Standardized parenteral alanyl-glutamine dipeptide supplementation is not beneficial in autologous transplant patients: A randomized, double-blind, placebo-controlled study. *Bone Marrow Transplant* 30(12):953–61.

Rodas, P. C., O. Rooyackers, C. Hebert, A. Norberg, and J. Wernerman. 2012. Glutamine and glutathione at ICU admission in relation to outcome. *Clin Sci (Lond)* 122(12):591–7.

Roth, E., J. Funovics, F. Muhlbacher et al. 1982. Metabolic disorders in severe abdominal sepsis: Glutamine deficiency in skeletal muscle. *Clin Nutr* 1(1):25–41.

Schloerb, P. R. and M. Amare. 1993. Total parenteral nutrition with glutamine in bone marrow transplantation and other clinical applications (a randomized, double-blind study). *JPEN J Parenter Enteral Nutr* 17(5):407–13.

Schloerb, P. R. and B. S. Skikne. 1999. Oral and parenteral glutamine in bone marrow transplantation: A randomized, double-blind study. *JPEN J Parenter Enteral Nutr* 23(3):117–22.

Sodergren, M. H., P. Jethwa, S. Kumar, H. D. Duncan, T. Johns, and C. B. Pearce. 2010. Immunonutrition in patients undergoing major upper gastrointestinal surgery: A prospective double-blind randomised controlled study. *Scand J Surg* 99(3):153–61.

Stehle, P., J. Zander, N. Mertes et al. 1989. Effect of parenteral glutamine peptide supplements on muscle glutamine loss and nitrogen balance after major surgery. *Lancet* 1(8632):231–3.

Tjader, I., O. Rooyackers, A. M. Forsberg, R. F. Vesali, P. J. Garlick, and J. Wernerman. 2004. Effects on skeletal muscle of intravenous glutamine supplementation to ICU patients. *Intensive Care Med* 30(2):266–75.

Tremel, H., B. Kienle, L. S. Weilemann, P. Stehle, and P. Furst. 1994. Glutamine dipeptide-supplemented parenteral nutrition maintains intestinal function in the critically ill. *Gastroenterology* 107(6):1595–601.

Tubman, T. R., S. W. Thompson, and W. McGuire. 2005. Glutamine supplementation to prevent morbidity and mortality in preterm infants. *Cochrane Database Syst Rev* (1):CD001457.

van de Poll, M. C., G. C. Ligthart-Melis, P. G. Boelens, N. E. Deutz, P. A. van Leeuwen, and C. H. Dejong. 2007. Intestinal and hepatic metabolism of glutamine and citrulline in humans. *J Physiol* 581(Pt 2):819–27.

van Zanten, A. R., F. Sztark, U. X. Kaisers et al. 2014. High-protein enteral nutrition enriched with immune-modulating nutrients vs standard high-protein enteral nutrition and nosocomial infections in the ICU: A randomized clinical trial. *JAMA* 312(5):514–24.

Vesali, R. F., M. Klaude, O. E. Rooyackers, T. Jader I, H. Barle, and J. Wernerman. 2002. Longitudinal pattern of glutamine/glutamate balance across the leg in long-stay intensive care unit patients. *Clin Nutr* 21(6):505–14.

Vesali, R. F., M. Klaude, O. Rooyackers, and J. Wernerman. 2005. Amino acid metabolism in leg muscle after an endotoxin injection in healthy volunteers. *Am J Physiol Endocrinol Metab* 288(2):E360–4.

Vinnars, E., J. Bergstrom, and P. Furst. 1975. Influence of the postoperative state on the intracellular free amino acids in human muscle tissue. *Ann Surg* 182(6):665–71.

Vinnars, E., P. Furst, S. O. Liljedahl, J. Larsson, and B. Schildt. 1980. Effect of parenteral nutrition on intracellular free amino acid concentration. *JPEN J Parenter Enteral Nutr* 4(2):184–7.

Wagner, J. V., T. Moe-Byrne, Z. Grover, and W. McGuire. 2012. Glutamine supplementation for young infants with severe gastrointestinal disease. *Cochrane Database Syst Rev* 7:CD005947.

Ward, E., M. Smith, M. Henderson et al. 2009. The effect of high-dose enteral glutamine on the incidence and severity of mucositis in paediatric oncology patients. *Eur J Clin Nutr* 63 (1):134–40.

Wernerman, J. 2003. Glutamine to intensive care unit patients. *JPEN J Parenter Enteral Nutr* 27(4):302–3.

Wernerman, J. 2014. Glutamine supplementation to critically ill patients? *Crit Care* 18(2):214.

Wernerman, J., R. Brandt, T. Strandell, L. G. Allgen, and E. Vinnars. 1985. The effect of stress hormones on the interorgan flux of amino acids and on the concentration of free amino acids in skeletal muscle. *Clin Nutr* 4(4):207–16.

Wernerman, J., F. Hammarqvist, and E. Vinnars. 1990. Alpha-ketoglutarate and postoperative muscle catabolism. *Lancet* 335(8691):701–3.

Wernerman, J., T. Kirketeig, B. Andersson et al. 2011. Scandinavian glutamine trial: A pragmatic multi-centre randomised clinical trial of intensive care unit patients. *Acta Anaesthesiol Scand* 55(7):812–8.

Wilmore, D. W., P. R. Schloerb, and T. R. Ziegler. 1999. Glutamine in the support of patients following bone marrow transplantation. *Curr Opin Clin Nutr Metab Care* 2(4):323–7.

Ziegler, T. R., L. S. Young, K. Benfell et al. 1992. Clinical and metabolic efficacy of glutamine-supplemented parenteral nutrition after bone marrow transplantation. A randomized, double-blind, controlled study. *Ann Intern Med* 116(10):821–8.

17 Glutamine Supplementation in Critical Illness
Action Mechanisms

Moïse Coëffier and Pierre Déchelotte

CONTENTS

17.1 INTRODUCTION

Classified as a nonessential amino acid since it can be synthesized *de novo*, glutamine is now considered as conditionally essential in catabolic states (Souba 1997). Glutamine is the most abundant amino acid in the plasma and is involved in a large variety of metabolic and biochemical processes. In hypercatabolic conditions, low plasma glutamine levels have been reported and associated with a bad prognosis (Planas et al. 1993). Critically ill patients and patients after major surgery are at risk of malnutrition, bacterial translocation, and acquired infections. Up to 40% of patients in the intensive care unit (ICU) may be concerned by hospital- or ICU-acquired nosocomial infections (Vincent et al. 1995), leading to an increase of length of stay and mortality risks, as well as hospital costs. Several studies have shown the efficacy of glutamine parenteral supplementation to reduce complication rate and mortality in critically ill and postoperative patients (Wischmeyer et al. 2014). Based on the available evidence, European guidelines stated that intravenous glutamine should be added in critically ill patients receiving total parenteral nutrition (Singer et al. 2009). Griffiths et al. reported that parenteral glutamine improved the 6-month outcome (Griffiths et al. 1997) and that the severity and the in-ICU death rate linked to infectious complications was reduced in glutamine-treated patients (Griffiths et al. 2002). In a French randomized, controlled, double-blind multicenter trial, parenteral glutamine was evaluated in 114 critically ill patients admitted for multiple trauma, complicated surgery, pancreatitis, or sepsis and was associated with an improved clinical outcome (Dechelotte et al. 2006). Several other studies also reported beneficial effects of parenteral glutamine supplementation in critically ill patients (Estivariz et al. 2008; Fuentes-Orozco et al. 2008; Grau et al. 2011; Goeters et al. 2002). In addition, glutamine plasma level was depleted and restored after supplementation with parenteral glutamine (Boelens et al. 2002; Tjader et al. 2004). However, in another study (Andrews et al. 2011), glutamine supplementation did not influence outcome. Finally, a large recent study raised concerns about the potential deleterious effects of glutamine in very sick patients (Heyland et al. 2013), but in this latter study, the dose of glutamine was much higher than the recommended dose and nutritional intake was

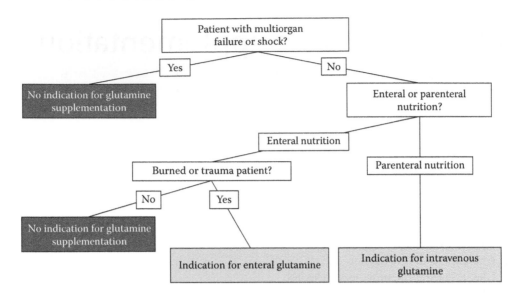

FIGURE 17.1   Algorithm proposed for the use of glutamine supplementation in critically ill patients. The recommended dose of glutamine for enteral supplementation is about 0.35–0.5 g.kg⁻¹.day⁻¹. For intravenous supplementation, the dose of glutamine should be about 0.35 g.kg⁻¹.day⁻¹ (or 0.5 g.kg⁻¹.day⁻¹ of glutamine dipeptide).

limited. Taking into account all these clinical data, an algorithm (Figure 17.1) has been proposed for glutamine supplementation in critically ill patients (Heyland and Dhaliwal 2013). Intravenous glutamine should be used in critically ill patients under total parenteral nutrition and without renal, hepatic, or persistent multiorgan failure.

A limited number of studies have evaluated the effects of glutamine enteral supplementation in critically ill patients (Conejero et al. 2002; Hall et al. 2003; Houdijk et al. 1998), in trauma patients (Boelens et al. 2002), or in burn patients (Garrel et al. 2003; Peng et al. 2004; Zhou et al. 2003). Based on these studies, the European Society for Clinical Nutrition and Metabolism stated that glutamine should be added to standard enteral nutrition in burned and trauma patients (Kreymann et al. 2006). However, there were insufficient data to support enteral glutamine supplementation in surgical or heterogeneous critically ill patients (Kreymann et al. 2006).

The mechanisms possibly contributing to the beneficial effects of glutamine in ICU patients are summarized and discussed below.

17.2   GLUTAMINE AND GUT BARRIER

van der Hulst et al. (1993) first reported that intravenous glutamine limited bacterial translocation across the gut barrier in critically ill patients. Then, it has been suggested that beneficial effects of glutamine on infectious complications in ICU patients may be related to an improved gut barrier function in patients receiving glutamine (De-Souza and Greene 2005). Indeed, gut barrier plays a critical role in the defense of the organism and an alteration of intestinal barrier may contribute to the occurrence of infections. Several factors are involved in the regulation of gut barrier such as intestinal microbiota, mucus, tight junctions between epithelial cells, and intestinal immune system. Glutamine appears to be a key factor to the regulation of tight junctions between epithelial cells. *In vitro* data underlined that glutamine deficiency induced loss of tight junctions by decreasing tight junctions proteins, that is, occludin, claudin-1, or zonula occludens-1 (ZO-1) (Li et al. 2004), which was associated with an increase of paracellular permeability (Boukhettala et al. 2012). Addition of glutamine was able to restore these alterations (Li et al. 2004). In other conditions of injury, glutamine supply also improved tight junctions and paracellular permeability (Beutheu et al. 2013; Seth et al. 2004; Vermeulen et al. 2011). Similar observations have been done in animal models (Beutheu et al. 2014; Wang et al. 2015; Xu et al. 2014). In addition, intestinal barrier function is also influenced by the balance between cell proliferation and apoptosis on the one hand and between protein synthesis and degradation on the other hand. Glutamine stimulated enterocyte proliferation (Rhoads et al. 1997) and decreased human intestinal epithelial cell apoptosis (Evans et al. 2003). Glutamine also stimulated intestinal protein synthesis in epithelial cell lines (Boukhettala et al. 2012; Le Bacquer et al. 2003), in animals (Higashiguchi et al. 1995), and in human duodenal mucosa (Coeffier et al. 2003). In addition, glutamine also regulates ubiquitin-ATP-dependent proteolytic pathway (Bertrand et al. 2014; Coeffier et al. 2003; Hubert-Buron et al. 2006) and autophagy (Liboni et al. 2005; Sakiyama et al. 2009).

In clinical studies, improvement of intestinal permeability after glutamine supplementation has been shown in burned patients (Zhou et al. 2003) or in critically ill patients (van der Hulst et al. 1993) but was not found by others (Hulsewe et al. 2004).

17.3 GLUTAMINE AND INFLAMMATORY RESPONSE

Experimental data suggest that glutamine has anti-inflammatory properties in various cell types. *In vitro*, glutamine deprivation was associated with an increase of proinflammatory response assessed by IL-8 (Huang et al. 2003) or chemokine (Marion et al. 2004) release in intestinal epithelial cell line Caco-2 through NF-κB pathway activation (Liboni et al. 2005). In contrast, increasing glutamine concentration was associated with a downregulation of inflammatory response by limiting proinflammatory cytokine IL-6 and IL-8 and by increasing anti-inflammatory cytokine IL-10 both in intestinal epithelial cells (Aosasa et al. 2003) and in human intestinal mucosa (Coeffier et al. 2001, 2002, 2003). In rats, intravenous glutamine supplementation prevented the reduction of intestinal IL-4 and IL-10 induced by total parenteral nutrition (Fukatsu et al. 2001). Similar results were observed for immunoglobulin A production (Kudsk et al. 2000). In endotoxemic rats, intravenous glutamine (0.75 g.kg^{-1}) reduced TNFα production and apoptosis, which was associated with improved survival rate (Uehara et al. 2005). This result has been confirmed in the cecal ligature and puncture model of sepsis (Singleton 2005). Finally, in hypoxic rats, glutamine also reduced pulmonary inflammatory response (Singleton and Wischmeyer 2008).

In clinical studies performed in patients with acute pancreatitis, glutamine-supplemented parenteral nutrition decreased the inflammatory response, as showed by a decrease of IL-8 (de Beaux et al. 1998) or a decrease of CRP (Ockenga et al. 2002).

17.4 GLUTAMINE AND OXIDATIVE STRESS

The glutathione (GSH) system is one of the major mechanisms protecting against oxidative stress in the cells. Glutamate, an amino acid constitutive of GSH, is one of the metabolites of glutamine metabolism. GSH content is decreased in surgical patients in skeletal muscle (Luo et al. 1996) or in the intestinal mucosa during inflammatory disease (Miralles-Barrachina et al. 1999). Glutamine maintained or restored splanchnic GSH production (Cao et al. 1998), as well as tissue concentrations of GSH in catabolic (Hong et al. 1992) or undernourished animals (Belmonte et al. 2007). Glutamine also prevented GSH depletion in Peyer's patches (Manhart et al. 2001) and reduced oxidative stress (Cruzat et al. 2014) in endotoxemic mice.

In surgical patients, glutamine supplementation maintained muscle and plasma GSH concentrations to the preoperative level (Flaring et al. 2003) and improved GSH levels in patients with non-pancreatic complicated surgery (Estivariz et al. 2008). In enterally fed trauma patients, intravenous glutamine supplementation improved plasma GSH levels (Eroglu 2009).

17.5   GLUTAMINE AND IMMUNE FUNCTION

In endotoxemic mice, glutamine maintained B and T lymphocyte population in Peyer's patches by preventing GSH reduction (Manhart et al. 2001). A single administration of glutamine was also able to enhance lymphocyte population both in intestinal (Lee et al. 2012; Tung et al. 2013) and lung (Hou et al. 2013; Hu et al. 2014) tissues by limiting T cell apoptosis.

In critical illness, alterations of immune function have been reported. In monocytes from trauma patients, glutamine parenteral supplementation restored HLA-DR expression that plays a critical role in the induction of the cellular immune response (Boelens et al. 2002). During acute pancreatitis, intravenous glutamine supplementation increased lymphocyte count (de Beaux et al. 1998). Thus, glutamine may improve cellular immune response in critical illness. Concerning innate immune response, experimental data revealed that glutamine may affect toll-like receptor activation, in particular, TLR4 (Mbodji et al. 2011; Ren et al. 2014). However, in trauma patients receiving glutamine, TLR4 and TLR2 on circulating monocytes remained not modified (Perez-Barcena et al. 2010).

17.6   GLUTAMINE AND HEAT SHOCK PROTEINS

Experimental data on cell culture extensively reported that glutamine has protective effect on cells by inducing the production of heat shock proteins (HSPs), which protect cells against toxic agents or pathologic insults (Wischmeyer 2002, 2007). Indeed, glutamine enhanced HSP expression in human peripheral blood mononuclear cells (Wischmeyer et al. 2003) in intestinal epithelial cell lines (Chow and Zhang 1998; Wischmeyer et al. 1997) and in several organs in rats (Wischmeyer et al. 2001). In endotoxemic rats, beneficial effects of intravenous glutamine on inflammatory, apoptotic, and antioxidant responses were related to HSP32 induction (Uehara et al. 2005).

In healthy volunteers, glutamine enhanced HSP32 expression in the intestinal mucosa (Coeffier et al. 2002). In critically ill patients receiving intravenous glutamine, plasma HSP70 concentration was increased (Ziegler et al. 2005) and a correlation between higher plasma HSP70 and better clinical outcomes was observed, suggesting that beneficial effects of glutamine may be related to HSP induction.

17.7   GLUTAMINE AND GLUCOSE HOMEOSTASIS

In critically ill patients, glycemic control is an important issue (Falciglia et al. 2009; Preiser et al. 2002) and the use of intensive insulin therapy with tight glycemic control has been extensively debated in the past few years (Marik and Preiser 2010; Treggiari et al. 2008; van den Berghe et al. 2001). In the French multicenter, randomized, controlled study evaluating the effects of intravenous glutamine, reduced hyperglycemia episodes and insulin needs have been observed in critically ill patients (Dechelotte et al. 2006). This reduction of insulin resistance by glutamine has been confirmed by others (Grau et al. 2011; Grintescu et al. 2015). Studies in healthy controls indicate that enteral infusion of glutamine increased the insulin level (Bouteloup et al. 2000; Coeffier et al. 2003). Recent data indicated that glutamine may affect incretin production (Joshi et al. 2013). Supplementation with glutamine of obese mice resulted in persistent reductions in both plasma glucose and insulin levels (Opara et al. 1996). In dogs, glutamine infusion markedly increased whole-body glucose utilization, mainly muscular and hepatic, and also increased whole-body glucose production to some extent (Borel et al. 1998). In addition, parenteral Ala-Gln administration attenuated insulin resistance and improved glucose utilization in multiple-trauma patients (Bakalar et al. 2006). Thus, glutamine may have potential benefits during clinical situations associated with insulin resistance.

17.8   CONCLUSION AND PERSPECTIVES

In conclusion, several clinical studies performed in parenterally fed critically ill and surgical patients indicate that provision of supplemental intravenous glutamine reduces the rate of infectious

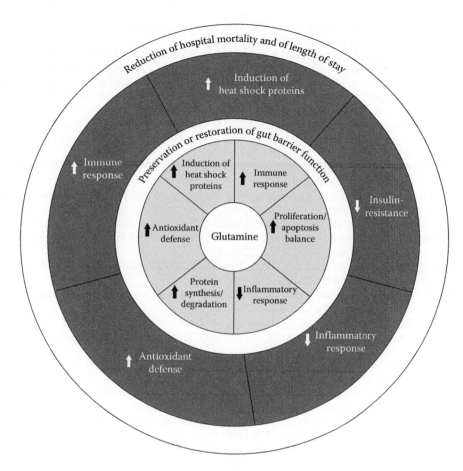

FIGURE 17.2 Putative action mechanisms of glutamine.

complications and length of hospital stay. These beneficial effects may be explained by several mechanisms (Figure 17.2), including the modulation of inflammatory, immune, and oxidative responses as well as the induction of HSPs and the regulation of glucose homeostasis by glutamine.

REFERENCES

Andrews, P. J., A. Avenell, D. W. Noble et al. 2011. Randomised trial of glutamine, selenium, or both, to supplement parenteral nutrition for critically ill patients. *BMJ* 342:d1542.

Aosasa, S., D. Wells-Byrum, J. W. Alexander, and C. K. Ogle. 2003. Influence of glutamine-supplemented Caco-2 cells on cytokine production of mononuclear cells. *JPEN J Parenter Enteral Nutr* 27(5):333–9.

Bakalar, B., F. Duska, J. Pachl et al. 2006. Parenterally administered dipeptide alanyl-glutamine prevents worsening of insulin sensitivity in multiple-trauma patients. *Crit Care Med* 34(2):381–6.

Belmonte, L., M. Coeffier, F. Le Pessot et al. 2007. Effects of glutamine supplementation on gut barrier, glutathione content and acute phase response in malnourished rats during inflammatory shock. *World J Gastroenterol* 13(20):2833–40.

Bertrand, J., A. Goichon, P. Chan et al. 2014. Enteral glutamine infusion modulates ubiquitination of heat shock proteins, Grp-75 and Apg-2, in the human duodenal mucosa. *Amino Acids* 46:1059–67.

Beutheu, S., I. Ghouzali, L. Galas, P. Dechelotte, and M. Coeffier. 2013. Glutamine and arginine improve permeability and tight junction protein expression in methotrexate-treated Caco-2 cells *Clin Nutr* 32(5):863–9.

Beutheu, S., W. Ouelaa, C. Guerin et al. 2014. Glutamine supplementation, but not combined glutamine and arginine supplementation, improves gut barrier function during chemotherapy-induced intestinal mucositis in rats. *Clin Nutr* 33:694–701.

Boelens, P. G., A. P. Houdijk, J. C. Fonk et al. 2002. Glutamine-enriched enteral nutrition increases HLA-DR expression on monocytes of trauma patients. *J Nutr* 132(9):2580–6.

Borel, M. J., P. E. Williams, K. Jabbour, D. Levenhagen, E. Kaizer, and P. J. Flakoll. 1998. Parenteral glutamine infusion alters insulin-mediated glucose metabolism. *JPEN J Parenter Enteral Nutr* 22(5):280–5.

Boukhettala, N., S. Claeyssens, M. Bensifi et al. 2012. Effects of essential amino acids or glutamine deprivation on intestinal permeability and protein synthesis in HCT-8 cells: Involvement of GCN2 and mTOR pathways. *Amino Acids* 42:375–83.

Bouteloup, C., S. Claeyssens, C. Maillot, A. Lavoinne, E. Lerebours, and P. Dechelotte. 2000. Effects of enteral glutamine on gut mucosal protein synthesis in healthy humans receiving glucocorticoids. *Am J Physiol Gastrointest Liver Physiol* 278(5):G677–81.

Cao, Y., Z. Feng, A. Hoos, and V. S. Klimberg. 1998. Glutamine enhances gut glutathione production. *JPEN J Parenter Enteral Nutr* 22(4):224–7.

Chow, A. and R. Zhang. 1998. Glutamine reduces heat shock-induced cell death in rat intestinal epithelial cells. *J Nutr* 128(8):1296–301.

Coeffier, M., S. Claeyssens, B. Hecketsweiler, A. Lavoinne, P. Ducrotte, and P. Dechelotte. 2003. Enteral glutamine stimulates protein synthesis and decreases ubiquitin mRNA level in human gut mucosa. *Am J Physiol Gastrointest Liver Physiol* 285(2):G266–73.

Coeffier, M., F. Le Pessot, A. Leplingard et al. 2002. Acute enteral glutamine infusion enhances heme oxygenase-1 expression in human duodenal mucosa. *J Nutr* 132(9):2570–3.

Coeffier, M., R. Marion, P. Ducrotte, and P. Dechelotte. 2003. Modulating effect of glutamine on IL-1beta-induced cytokine production by human gut. *Clin Nutr* 22(4):407–13.

Coeffier, M., R. Marion, A. Leplingard, E. Lerebours, P. Ducrotte, and P. Dechelotte. 2002. Glutamine decreases interleukin-8 and interleukin-6 but not nitric oxide and prostaglandins e(2) production by human gut *in vitro*. *Cytokine* 18(2):92–7.

Coeffier, M., O. Miralles-Barrachina, F. Le Pessot et al. 2001. Influence of glutamine on cytokine production by human gut *in vitro*. *Cytokine* 13(3):148–54.

Conejero, R., A. Bonet, T. Grau et al. 2002. Effect of a glutamine-enriched enteral diet on intestinal permeability and infectious morbidity at 28 days in critically ill patients with systemic inflammatory response syndrome: A randomized, single-blind, prospective, multicenter study. *Nutrition* 18(9):716–21.

Cruzat, V. F., A. Bittencourt, S. P. Scomazzon, J. S. Leite, P. I. de Bittencourt, Jr., and J. Tirapegui. 2014. Oral free and dipeptide forms of glutamine supplementation attenuate oxidative stress and inflammation induced by endotoxemia. *Nutrition* 30(5):602–11.

De-Souza, D. A. and L. J. Greene. 2005. Intestinal permeability and systemic infections in critically ill patients: Effect of glutamine. *Crit Care Med* 33(5):1125–35.

de Beaux, A. C., M. G. O'Riordain, J. A. Ross, L. Jodozi, D. C. Carter, and K. C. Fearon. 1998. Glutamine-supplemented total parenteral nutrition reduces blood mononuclear cell interleukin-8 release in severe acute pancreatitis. *Nutrition* 14(3):261–5.

Dechelotte, P., M. Hasselmann, L. Cynober et al. 2006. L-alanyl-L-glutamine dipeptide-supplemented total parenteral nutrition reduces infectious complications and glucose intolerance in critically ill patients: The French controlled, randomized, double-blind, multicenter study. *Crit Care Med* 34(3):598–604.

Eroglu, A. 2009. The effect of intravenous alanyl-glutamine supplementation on plasma glutathione levels in intensive care unit trauma patients receiving enteral nutrition: The results of a randomized controlled trial. *Anesth Analg* 109 (2):502–5.

Estivariz, C. F., D. P. Griffith, M. Luo et al. 2008. Efficacy of parenteral nutrition supplemented with glutamine dipeptide to decrease hospital infections in critically ill surgical patients. *JPEN J Parenter Enteral Nutr* 32(4):389–402.

Evans, M. E., D. P. Jones, and T. R. Ziegler. 2003. Glutamine prevents cytokine-induced apoptosis in human colonic epithelial cells. *J Nutr* 133(10):3065–71.

Falciglia, M., R. W. Freyberg, P. L. Almenoff, D. A. D'Alessio, and M. L. Render. 2009. Hyperglycemia-related mortality in critically ill patients varies with admission diagnosis. *Crit Care Med* 37(12):3001–9.

Flaring, U. B., O. E. Rooyackers, J. Wernerman, and F. Hammarqvist. 2003. Glutamine attenuates post-traumatic glutathione depletion in human muscle. *Clin Sci (Lond)* 104(3):275–82.

Fuentes-Orozco, C., G. Cervantes-Guevara, I. Mucino-Hernandez et al. 2008. L-alanyl-L-glutamine-supplemented parenteral nutrition decreases infectious morbidity rate in patients with severe acute pancreatitis. *JPEN J Parenter Enteral Nutr* 32(4):403–11.

Fukatsu, K., K. A. Kudsk, B. L. Zarzaur, Y. Wu, M. K. Hanna, and R. C. DeWitt. 2001. TPN decreases IL-4 and IL-10 mRNA expression in lipopolysaccharide stimulated intestinal lamina propria cells but glutamine supplementation preserves the expression. *Shock* 15(4):318–22.

Garrel, D., J. Patenaude, B. Nedelec et al. 2003. Decreased mortality and infectious morbidity in adult burn patients given enteral glutamine supplements: A prospective, controlled, randomized clinical trial. *Crit Care Med* 31(10):2444–9.

Goeters, C., A. Wenn, N. Mertes et al. 2002. Parenteral L-alanyl-L-glutamine improves 6-month outcome in critically ill patients. *Crit Care Med* 30(9):2032–7.

Grau, T., A. Bonet, E. Minambres et al. 2011. The effect of L-alanyl-L-glutamine dipeptide supplemented total parenteral nutrition on infectious morbidity and insulin sensitivity in critically ill patients. *Crit Care Med* 39(6):1263–8.

Griffiths, R. D., K. D. Allen, F. J. Andrews, and C. Jones. 2002. Infection, multiple organ failure, and survival in the intensive care unit: Influence of glutamine-supplemented parenteral nutrition on acquired infection. *Nutrition* 18(7–8):546–52.

Griffiths, R. D., C. Jones, and T. E. Palmer. 1997. Six-month outcome of critically ill patients given glutamine-supplemented parenteral nutrition. *Nutrition* 13(4):295–302.

Grintescu, I. M., I. Luca Vasiliu, I. Cucereanu Badica et al. 2015. The influence of parenteral glutamine supplementation on glucose homeostasis in critically ill polytrauma patients-A randomized-controlled clinical study. *Clin Nutr* 34(3):377–82.

Hall, J. C., G. Dobb, J. Hall, R. de Sousa, L. Brennan, and R. McCauley. 2003. A prospective randomized trial of enteral glutamine in critical illness. *Intensive Care Med* 29(10):1710–6.

Heyland, D. K. and R. Dhaliwal. 2013. Role of glutamine supplementation in critical illness given the results of the REDOXS study. *JPEN J Parenter Enteral Nutr* 37(4):442–3.

Heyland, D., J. Muscedere, P. E. Wischmeyer et al. 2013. A randomized trial of glutamine and antioxidants in critically ill patients. *N Engl J Med* 368(16):1489–97.

Higashiguchi, T., Y. Noguchi, T. Meyer, J. E. Fischer, and P. O. Hasselgren. 1995. Protein synthesis in isolated enterocytes from septic or endotoxaemic rats: Regulation by glutamine. *Clin Sci (Lond)* 89(3):311–9.

Hong, R. W., J. D. Rounds, W. S. Helton, M. K. Robinson, and D. W. Wilmore. 1992. Glutamine preserves liver glutathione after lethal hepatic injury. *Ann Surg* 215(2):114–9.

Hou, Y. C., M. H. Pai, J. J. Liu, and S. L. Yeh. 2013. Alanyl-glutamine resolves lipopolysaccharide-induced lung injury in mice by modulating the polarization of regulatory T cells and T helper 17 cells. *J Nutr Biochem* 24(9):1555–63.

Houdijk, A. P., E. R. Rijnsburger, J. Jansen et al. 1998. Randomised trial of glutamine-enriched enteral nutrition on infectious morbidity in patients with multiple trauma. *Lancet* 352(9130):772–6.

Hu, Y. M., C. L. Yeh, M. H. Pai, W. Y. Lee, and S. L. Yeh. 2014. Glutamine administration modulates lung gammadelta T lymphocyte expression in mice with polymicrobial sepsis. *Shock* 41(2):115–22.

Huang, Y., N. Li, K. Liboni, and J. Neu. 2003. Glutamine decreases lipopolysaccharide-induced IL-8 production in Caco-2 cells through a non-NF-kappaB p50 mechanism. *Cytokine* 22(3–4):77–83.

Hubert-Buron, A., J. Leblond, A. Jacquot, P. Ducrotte, P. Dechelotte, and M. Coeffier. 2006. Glutamine pre-treatment reduces IL-8 production in human intestinal epithelial cells by limiting IkappaBalpha ubiquitination. *J Nutr* 136(6):1461–5.

Hulsewe, K. W., B. A. van Acker, W. Hameeteman et al. 2004. Does glutamine-enriched parenteral nutrition really affect intestinal morphology and gut permeability? *Clin Nutr* 23(5):1217–25.

Joshi, S., I. R. Tough, and H. M. Cox. 2013. Endogenous PYY and GLP-1 mediate l-glutamine responses in intestinal mucosa. *Br J Pharmacol* 170(5):1092–101.

Kreymann, K. G., M. M. Berger, N. E. Deutz et al. 2006. ESPEN Guidelines on Enteral Nutrition: Intensive care. *Clin Nutr* 25(2):210–23.

Kudsk, K. A., Y. Wu, K. Fukatsu et al. 2000. Glutamine-enriched total parenteral nutrition maintains intestinal interleukin-4 and mucosal immunoglobulin A levels. *JPEN J Parenter Enteral Nutr* 24(5):270–4; discussion 274–5.

Le Bacquer, O., C. Laboisse, and D. Darmaun. 2003. Glutamine preserves protein synthesis and paracellular permeability in Caco-2 cells submitted to "luminal fasting". *Am J Physiol Gastrointest Liver Physiol* 285(1):G128–36.

Lee, W. Y., Y. M. Hu, T. L. Ko, S. L. Yeh, and C. L. Yeh. 2012. Glutamine modulates sepsis-induced changes to intestinal intraepithelial gammadelta T lymphocyte expression in mice. *Shock* 38(3):288–93.

Li, N., P. Lewis, D. Samuelson, K. Liboni, and J. Neu. 2004. Glutamine regulates Caco-2 cell tight junction proteins. *Am J Physiol Gastrointest Liver Physiol* 287(3):G726–33.

Liboni, K. C., N. Li, P. O. Scumpia, and J. Neu. 2005. Glutamine modulates LPS-induced IL-8 production through IkappaB/NF-kappaB in human fetal and adult intestinal epithelium. *J Nutr* 135(2):245–51.

Luo, J. L., F. Hammarqvist, K. Andersson, and J. Wernerman. 1996. Skeletal muscle glutathione after surgical trauma. *Ann Surg* 223(4):420–7.

Manhart, N., K. Vierlinger, A. Spittler, H. Bergmeister, T. Sautner, and E. Roth. 2001. Oral feeding with glutamine prevents lymphocyte and glutathione depletion of Peyer's patches in endotoxemic mice. *Ann Surg* 234(1):92–7.

Marik, P. E. and J. C. Preiser. 2010. Toward understanding tight glycemic control in the ICU: A systematic review and metaanalysis. *Chest* 137(3):544–51.

Marion, R., M. M. Coeffier, G. Gargala, P. Ducrotte, and P. P. Dechelotte. 2004. Glutamine and CXC chemokines IL-8, Mig, IP-10 and I-TAC in human intestinal epithelial cells. *Clin Nutr* 23(4):579–85.

Mbodji, K., S. Torre, V. Haas, P. Dechelotte, and R. Marion-Letellier. 2011. Alanyl-glutamine restores maternal deprivation-induced TLR4 levels in a rat neonatal model. *Clin Nutr* 30(5):672–7.

Miralles-Barrachina, O., G. Savoye, L. Belmonte-Zalar et al. 1999. Low levels of glutathione in endoscopic biopsies of patients with Crohn's colitis: The role of malnutrition. *Clin Nutr* 18(5):313–7.

Ockenga, J., K. Borchert, K. Rifai, M. P. Manns, and S. C. Bischoff. 2002. Effect of glutamine-enriched total parenteral nutrition in patients with acute pancreatitis. *Clin Nutr* 21(5):409–16.

Opara, E. C., A. Petro, A. Tevrizian, M. N. Feinglos, and R. S. Surwit. 1996. L-glutamine supplementation of a high fat diet reduces body weight and attenuates hyperglycemia and hyperinsulinemia in C57BL/6J mice. *J Nutr* 126(1):273–9.

Peng, X., H. Yan, Z. You, P. Wang, and S. Wang. 2004. Effects of enteral supplementation with glutamine granules on intestinal mucosal barrier function in severe burned patients. *Burns* 30(2):135–9.

Perez-Barcena, J., C. Crespi, V. Regueiro et al. 2010. Lack of effect of glutamine administration to boost the innate immune system response in trauma patients in the intensive care unit. *Crit Care* 14(6):R233.

Planas, M., S. Schwartz, M. A. Arbos, and M. Farriol. 1993. Plasma glutamine levels in septic patients. *JPEN J Parenter Enteral Nutr* 17(3):299–300.

Preiser, J. C., P. Devos, and G. Van den Berghe. 2002. Tight control of glycaemia in critically ill patients. *Curr Opin Clin Nutr Metab Care* 5(5):533–7.

Ren, W., J. Duan, J. Yin et al. 2014. Dietary L-glutamine supplementation modulates microbial community and activates innate immunity in the mouse intestine. *Amino Acids* 46(10):2403–13.

Rhoads, J. M., R. A. Argenzio, W. Chen et al. 1997. L-glutamine stimulates intestinal cell proliferation and activates mitogen-activated protein kinases. *Am J Physiol* 272(5 Pt 1):G943–53.

Sakiyama, T., M. W. Musch, M. J. Ropeleski, H. Tsubouchi, and E. B. Chang. 2009. Glutamine increases autophagy under Basal and stressed conditions in intestinal epithelial cells. *Gastroenterology* 136(3):924–32.

Seth, A., S. Basuroy, P. Sheth, and R. K. Rao. 2004. L-Glutamine ameliorates acetaldehyde-induced increase in paracellular permeability in Caco-2 cell monolayer. *Am J Physiol Gastrointest Liver Physiol* 287(3):G510–7.

Singer, P., M. M. Berger, G. Van den Berghe et al. 2009. ESPEN Guidelines on Parenteral Nutrition: Intensive care. *Clin Nutr* 28(4):387–400.

Singleton, K. D., V. E. Beckey, and P. E. Wischmeyer. 2005. Glutamine prevents activation of NF-kappaB and stress kinase pathways, attenuates inflammatory cytokine release, and prevents acute respiratory distress syndrome (ARDS) following sepsis. *Shock* 24(6):583–9.

Singleton, K. D. and P. E. Wischmeyer. 2008. Glutamine attenuates inflammation and NF-kappaB activation via Cullin-1 deneddylation. *Biochem Biophys Res Commun* 373(3):445–9.

Souba, W. W. 1997. Nutritional support. *N Engl J Med* 336(1):41–8.

Tjader, I., O. Rooyackers, A. M. Forsberg, R. F. Vesali, P. J. Garlick, and J. Wernerman. 2004. Effects on skeletal muscle of intravenous glutamine supplementation to ICU patients. *Intensive Care Med* 30(2):266–75.

Treggiari, M. M., V. Karir, N. D. Yanez, N. S. Weiss, S. Daniel, and S. A. Deem. 2008. Intensive insulin therapy and mortality in critically ill patients. *Crit Care* 12(1):R29.

Tung, J. N., W. Y. Lee, M. H. Pai, W. J. Chen, C. L. Yeh, and S. L. Yeh. 2013. Glutamine modulates CD8alphaalpha(+) TCRalphabeta(+) intestinal intraepithelial lymphocyte expression in mice with polymicrobial sepsis. *Nutrition* 29(6):911–7.

Uehara, K., T. Takahashi, H. Fujii et al. 2005. The lower intestinal tract-specific induction of heme oxygenase-1 by glutamine protects against endotoxemic intestinal injury. *Crit Care Med* 33(2):381–90.

van den Berghe, G., P. Wouters, F. Weekers et al. 2001. Intensive insulin therapy in the critically ill patients. *N Engl J Med* 345(19):1359–67.

van der Hulst, R. R., B. K. van Kreel, M. F. von Meyenfeldt et al. 1993. Glutamine and the preservation of gut integrity. *Lancet* 341(8857):1363–5.

Vermeulen, M. A., J. de Jong, M. J. Vaessen, P. A. van Leeuwen, and A. P. Houdijk. 2011. Glutamate reduces experimental intestinal hyperpermeability and facilitates glutamine support of gut integrity. *World J Gastroenterol* 17(12):1569–73.

Vincent, J. L., D. J. Bihari, P. M. Suter et al. 1995. The prevalence of nosocomial infection in intensive care units in Europe. Results of the European Prevalence of Infection in Intensive Care (EPIC) Study. EPIC International Advisory Committee. *JAMA* 274(8):639–44.

Wang, B., G. Wu, Z. Zhou et al. 2015. Glutamine and intestinal barrier function. *Amino Acids* 47(10):243–54.

Wischmeyer, P. E. 2002. Glutamine and heat shock protein expression. *Nutrition* 18(3):225–8.

Wischmeyer, P. E. 2007. Glutamine: Mode of action in critical illness. *Crit Care Med* 35(9 Suppl):S541–4.

Wischmeyer, P. E., R. Dhaliwal, M. McCall, T. R. Ziegler, and D. K. Heyland. 2014. Parenteral glutamine supplementation in critical illness: A systematic review. *Crit Care* 18(2):R76.

Wischmeyer, P. E., M. Kahana, R. Wolfson, H. Ren, M. M. Musch, and E. B. Chang. 2001. Glutamine induces heat shock protein and protects against endotoxin shock in the rat. *J Appl Physiol* 90(6):2403–10.

Wischmeyer, P. E., M. W. Musch, M. B. Madonna, R. Thisted, and E. B. Chang. 1997. Glutamine protects intestinal epithelial cells: Role of inducible HSP70. *Am J Physiol* 272(4 Pt 1):G879–84.

Wischmeyer, P. E., J. Riehm, K. D. Singleton et al. 2003. Glutamine attenuates tumor necrosis factor-alpha release and enhances heat shock protein 72 in human peripheral blood mononuclear cells. *Nutrition* 19(1):1–6.

Xu, C. L., R. Sun, X. J. Qiao, C. C. Xu, X. Y. Shang, and W. N. Niu. 2014. Protective effect of glutamine on intestinal injury and bacterial community in rats exposed to hypobaric hypoxia environment. *World J Gastroenterol* 20(16):4662–74.

Zhou, Y. P., Z. M. Jiang, Y. H. Sun, X. R. Wang, E. L. Ma, and D. Wilmore. 2003. The effect of supplemental enteral glutamine on plasma levels, gut function, and outcome in severe burns: A randomized, double-blind, controlled clinical trial. *JPEN J Parenter Enteral Nutr* 27(4):241–5.

Ziegler, T. R., L. G. Ogden, K. D. Singleton et al. 2005. Parenteral glutamine increases serum heat shock protein 70 in critically ill patients. *Intensive Care Med* 31(8):1079–86.

18 Glutamine Supplementation in Critical Illness
Focus on Renal Injury

Giacomo Garibotto, Alice Bonanni, Giacomo Deferrari, and Daniela Verzola

CONTENTS

18.1 INTRODUCTION

Glutamine, the most abundant amino acid in body fluids, is synthesized *de novo* predominantly in skeletal muscle where it accounts for more than 50% of the free amino acid pool (Bergstrom 1974; Darmaun 1992; Ahlma et al. 1994). In normal healthy conditions, glutamine circulates in plasma at ~0.6 mM/L and accounts for ~25% of circulating free amino acids. The clinical interest of glutamine derives from its different, important physiological roles. The role of glutamine as a substrate for protein synthesis is well recognized (Young 2001). Besides that, glutamine is a central metabolite for amino acid transamination through α-ketoglutarate and glutamic acid. By replenishing Krebs cycle intermediates in proliferating tissues, glutamine serves as a major intermediate in energy metabolism and as anaplerotic substrate (Darmaun and Dechelotte 1991; Soeters 2012). Moreover, glutamine is used as a substrate in the synthesis of peptide and nonpeptide molecules (including glutathione, neurotransmitters, and nucleotide bases) (Young 2001). In addition to its structural role, glutamine has been termed a "competence factor," and by that it stimulates the intestinal fluid electrolyte absorption, intestinal cell proliferation, and the mitogenic response to growth factors by mechanisms that are not still completely understood (Eagle 1959; Young 2001; Soeters 2012).

Glutamine may also contribute to the preservation of tissue metabolic function by maintenance of ATP levels, and may also diminish *inducible NO synthase* (iNOS) expression and enhance GSH levels after stress (Soeters 2012). Finally, glutamine plays a homeostatic role as a regulator of systemic acid–base balance and in the detoxification of ammonia and is one of the osmolytes regulating cells homeostasis in hyper- and hypo-osmolar states (Haussinger 1994).

Glutamine, together with alanine, constitutes the most important nitrogen carrier in body fluids. Most cells and tissues, mainly skeletal muscle, produce glutamine (Eagle 1959; Darmaun 1986). In healthy humans, the daily endogenous glutamine production (about 50–80 g/day or 0.7–1.1 g/kg for a 70-kg individual), exceeds that of all other amino acids (Darmaun 1986). The key enzymes of glutamine metabolism have a different tissue distribution: while glutaminase is mainly present in the liver and kidney, glutamine synthetase is mainly present in skeletal muscle (Krebs 1935), indicating a specific role of individual organs in the fate of this amino acid. In the basal, postabsorptive state, endogenous production (appearance rate) of glutamine can be either derived by *de novo* synthesis via glutamine synthetase or released via the breakdown of proteins. Both during the postabsorptive and protein-fed states, most of the *de novo* glutamine produced is exported from muscle to the splanchnic area (Gelfand et al. 1986; Deferrari et al. 1994) to be used in enterocytes, hepatocytes, immune cells, and kidney cells, mainly proximal tubule cells. In addition, excess glutamine is catabolized to glutamate and urea in selected liver zones (Haussinger 1994; Brosnan 2009).

This chapter summarizes the major findings on glutamine metabolism in kidney injury, including acute kidney injury (AKI) and chronic kidney disease (CKD), that are very common in critically ill patients treated in intensive care units (ICUs). We shall focus on the possible beneficial effects and risks of glutamine supplementation in this subgroup of critically ill patients, an issue that, in fact, has not been addressed in humans up to now. The soundness of glutamine supplementation in critical illness itself is well detailed in Chapter 13 (concerning the neonates) and Chapters 14 through 17 (concerning the adult and aged humans), where the reader will find a lot of data and different points of views among the authors.

18.2   GLUTAMINE AS A NITROGEN SHUTTLE AND ITS ROLE DURING METABOLIC ACIDOSIS

The interorgan nitrogen transport function in humans is unique to glutamine (Elia and Livesey 1983). One of glutamine's major roles is to act as a "nitrogen shuttle," which helps the body to be protected from high levels of ammonia. Thus, glutamine can act as a buffer, accepting excess ammonia (from glutamate to glutamine in muscle) and releasing it when needed, to form ammonia in the kidney and urea in the liver. In muscle, glutamine synthetase utilizes ammonia to produce glutamine in the cytosol, whereas in the kidney, glutaminase and glutamate dehydrogenase produce ammonia in the mitochondria from glutamine and glutamate, respectively (Adeva et al. 2012; Mitch et al. 2015). Ammonia and bicarbonate are used in the liver mitochondria to yield carbamoylphosphate, and thus initiating the urea cycle, the major mechanism of ammonia removal in humans. Well-balanced mechanisms are able to maintain stable glutamine pools. An example of the checks and balances that keep stable glutamine levels is shown by glutamine metabolism during metabolic acidosis. In normal acid–base homeostasis, the kidney supplies ammonia to the body pools (Garibotto et al. 2004; Mitch et al. 2015). However, during chronic metabolic acidosis, the kidney is the major organ in clearing ammonia from the body via generation of ammonia from glutamine and preferential ammonia excretion in the urine (Deferrari et al. 1994). Such a process permits the elimination of excess H^+ from the body. In addition, the accelerated ammonia formation inhibits lysosomal protein degradation in tubule cells, an effect responsible for tubular hypertrophy and progression of chronic renal disease (Garibotto et al. 2004). Therefore, the response of body tissues to chronic metabolic acidosis is a coordinated one that includes both an increase in muscle proteolysis (Tizianello et al. 1978; Bailey et al. 1996) and glutamine release from muscle, as well as an increased glutamine uptake (which is used for ammoniagenesis) and suppression of protein degradation in the kidney. The final effects of acidosis are atrophy (in muscle) and hypertrophy (in the kidney). Theoretically, these changes in glutamine metabolism are able to maintain stable glutamine levels and supply to the kidney. However, reduced glutamine levels have been observed in subjects with acute metabolic acidosis, suggesting that reduced availability of this amino acid may hinder the body response to this condition (Tizianello et al. 1982; Deferrari et al. 1994).

18.3 GLUTAMINE: AN ESSENTIAL FACTOR FOR NATIVE KIDNEY CELLS

Besides the role of glutamine on ammoniagenesis, studies now indicate that this amino acid, either directly or indirectly by the formation of glutamate, can exert different effects on native kidney cells. Glutamine removed by the arterial blood is a major substrate for glutamate formation in the kidney. Recent studies have shown that L-glutamate, besides playing an essential role in the central nervous systems as an excitatory neurotransmitter, also acts in several peripheral tissues, including the kidney. *N-Methyl*-D-aspartate (NMDA) and Group 1 *metabotropic glutamate receptors* (mGluRs) are expressed in the renal cortex and medulla, and appear to play a role in the regulation of renal blood flow, glomerular filtration, proximal tubule reabsorption, and urine concentration within medullary collecting ducts (Dryer 2015). Activation of NMDA receptors induces Ca (2+) influx and oxidative stress, which can lead to glomerulosclerosis (Dryer 2015). Group 1 mGluRs are expressed mainly in podocytes. Mice in which these receptors are knocked out gradually develop albuminuria and glomerulosclerosis. L-Glu receptors may be useful targets for drug therapy, and many selective orally active compounds are studied as potential drug targets for various kidney diseases (Dryer 2015). Of note, a special role of glutamine is evident in podocytes. As a matter of fact, the availability of glutamine may protect the podocyte cytoskeleton by increasing intracellular pH and reducing cytosolic cathepsin L protease activity (Altintas et al. 2014). In addition, podocyte glutamine supplementation has been shown to reduce proteinuria in LPS-treated mice whereas acidification increases glomerular injury (Altintas 2014). The protection of podocyte's survival in humans is of major importance, since these cells, of neural origin, are finally differentiated in adults and cannot be replaced after a loss. In accordance with the aforementioned findings, glutamine supplementation in rats with streptozotocin (STZ)-induced diabetes decreased renal nitrotyrosine level and thioredoxin-interacting protein mRNA expression (Tsai et al. 2012) suggesting that glutamine supplementation attenuates renal oxidative damage in type 1 diabetes. However, other studies (Alba-Loureiro et al. 2010) have shown an increase in proinflammatory interleukins (IL)-1beta and IL-6 after glutamine supplementation in renal cortex of rats with STZ-induced diabetes. These issues need to be approached in humans, since a current hypothesis is that podocyte apoptotic cell loss and inflammation underlie diabetic kidney disease progression (Verzola et al. 2014).

18.4 SEPTIC AND NONSEPTIC ACUTE KIDNEY INJURY: A TARGET FOR GLUTAMINE SUPPLEMENTATION?

Acute kidney injury (AKI) includes a highly heterogeneous group of conditions with widely varying comorbidity and outcomes. Nutritional treatment in these patients typically aims at accelerating kidney recovery and decreasing mortality. Since inflammation and oxidative stress play important roles in the development of AKI, the interventions against AKI have mainly been focused on anti-inflammatory and/or antioxidative approaches. However, currently, there are no proven interventions that can prevent AKI. Moreover, optimal nutritional requirements and nutrient intake composition for patients with AKI remain a partially unresolved issue.

It is curious that, even if uncomplicated nonseptic AKI as an isolated disease is common, there is no study dealing with its effects on glutamine and protein metabolism in humans and our current knowledge comes from studies performed in animals with experimental acute uremia. Early *in vitro* and *in vivo* studies in rats have shown that in AKI, the rate of ureagenesis is accelerated (Persike 1949; Sellers 1957), and is blocked only partially when animals are fed with glucose (Lacy 1969). Frohlich et al. (1974) observed that increased ureagenesis was associated with increased glucose production in the liver of acutely uremic rats. Initially, studies suggested that the degradation of endogenous liver proteins and/or amino acid could provide the substrates for both urea and glucose production. However, Bondy et al. (1949) found that the hepatic increase in urea synthesis in rats with acute uremia was partially prevented by adrenalectomy, suggesting that glucocorticoids are responsible for the increased net catabolism in uremia.

The fact that specific changes in muscle protein metabolism take place in rats with acute uremia has been shown in early studies. Clark and Mitch (1983) observed an increased release of amino acids from the isolated perfused hindquarter of rats with acute uremia. To study whether abnormal protein and carbohydrate metabolism are linked in acute uremia, the effects of insulin on net muscle protein degradation and glucose uptake were measured in the perfused hindquarters of paired acutely uremic and sham-operated rats. At an early stage of uremia, glucose uptake was significantly depressed and muscle protein degradation increased; moreover, rates of protein degradation were only partially responsive to the insulin's antiproteolytic effect. This indicates the occurrence of early concurrent alterations in protein and glucose metabolism. However, after 48 h of acute uremia, net protein breakdown increased further because protein synthesis was also depressed (Clark and Mitch 1983). Flugel-Link et al. (1983) observed that muscle protein synthesis was not altered, but protein degradation was greater in the hindquarters of acute uremic versus sham rats. These results indicated the occurrence of two different alterations, which can cause catabolism in acute uremia: an increase in protein degradation (which appears to be the consequence of altered glucose metabolism and is stimulated by glucocorticoids) and a decrease in protein synthesis.

Price et al. (1998) provided several lines of evidence suggesting that an ATP and ubiquitin-dependent proteolytic pathway is responsible for an increase in muscle protein degradation in AKI. In addition, these authors also observed that the activity of branched-chain ketoacid dehydrogenase (which is the rate-limiting enzyme for branched-chain amino acid oxidation and catabolism) was increased several-fold in skeletal muscle from acutely uremic rats.

There is also clear evidence from experimental studies in animals that acute uremia in muscle depresses amino acid uptake. Arnold and Holliday (1979) observed that both basal and insulin-stimulated uptake of α-aminoisobutyric acid (a nonmetabolizable analog of alanine) were diminished in muscle of acutely uremic rats. The occurrence of such a defect could aggravate net protein catabolism, by decreasing muscle protein synthesis and thereby causing loss of muscle proteins. Of note, Maroni et al. (1990) demonstrated that the insulin-response curve was altered in muscle of acutely uremic rats, with physiologic concentrations of insulin stimulating MeAIB uptake normally, whereas both basal and maximal insulin-stimulated MeAIB uptake were lower in muscles from rats with acute uremia.

All these observations support the conclusion that the activation of ATP-dependent ubiquitin-proteasome proteolytic pathway and changes in amino acid transport and catabolism contribute to the accelerated loss of muscle observed in acutely uremic rats. Metabolic acidosis can also contribute to accelerate the catabolic processes, since it occurs commonly in patients with AKI not only because the elimination of H^+ is diminished, but also because there is an increase in net protein breakdown, with an increased production of H^+.

The picture is even more complex when AKI is a complication of sepsis (Plank et al. 1988; Puthucheary et al. 2013). Development of AKI during sepsis increases morbidity and predicts higher mortality (Lafrance 2010). In addition, septic AKI negatively affects multiple organ functions and is associated with an increased in-hospital length of stay (Uchino et al. 2005). When compared with AKI due to nonseptic causes, septic AKI is characterized by distinct mechanisms and different clinical approaches. Despite current advances in several fields of internal medicine, the diagnostic procedures and appropriate therapeutic interventions in sepsis are still highly questioned. Major obstacles to a progress in our understanding of mechanisms and treatment in sepsis-induced AKI include limited availability of animal models of septic AKI, as well as great clinical variability of patients with this complication. The pathophysiology of septic AKI is complex and multifactorial, including hemodynamic changes, endothelial dysfunction, infiltration of inflammatory cells in the kidney, glomerular thrombosis, and tubular obstruction of tubules with necrotic "debris" (Zarjou and Agarwal 2011). A growing body of evidence suggests that the sepsis-induced immune responses involve the sequential activation of both pro- and anti-inflammatory effectors. It has been shown that sepsis affects several pathways, including *toll-like receptors* (TLRs) (a class of proteins that play an important role in alerting the innate immune system) (Kessel et al. 2008), injury caused by endotoxin, complement cascade, coagulation pathway activation, release of arachidonic acid and nitric oxide, vascular injury, and others that mediate the development and course of sepsis (Zarjou and Agarwal 2011). Such complexity may have been an important contributor to the failure of clinical trials targeting just one of these pathways.

Progressive understanding of the mechanisms causing excessive protein catabolism in AKI, sepsis, and trauma has led to the study of the effects of glutamine to restrict catabolism and protect from kidney damage. Recent research reveals that glutamine plays a vital role in cell signaling and upregulates heat shock proteins (HSPs), which may protect from cellular injury (Peng et al. 2006, pp. 400–406; Langhans and Hrupka 1999). HSPs are expressed at low levels in the normal kidney, but they are upregulated in the renal medulla when exposed to a variety of types of cell stress, as a mechanism of defense (Smoyer et al. 2000). Glutamine is also an important precursor of glutathione, a vital antioxidant molecule.

However, studies on the effects of glutamine supplementation on acute renal damage from the published literature are limited to the *in vitro* or *ex vivo* settings and in part controversial (Fuller et al. 2007; Kim et al. 2009). It has also been hypothesized that glutamine may be beneficial in preventing AKI, an effect induced by the activation of HSP, and/or antioxidant action. The glutamine-induced maintenance of glutathione levels appears to be separated from a renal sparing effect in animal models (Abraham and Isaac 2011). These results suggest that mechanisms other than oxidative stress may be involved in the renal protective effects of glutamine (Santora and Kozar 2008). Oliveira et al. (2009) observed that in a cecal ligation and puncture rodent model, a single intravenous dose of glutamine attenuated epithelial cell apoptosis in the kidneys. Ya-Mei Hu et al. (2012) showed that a single dose of glutamine administered after the initiation of sepsis downregulates the expressions of high-mobility group box (HMGB)-1-related mediators and decreasing oxidative stress in the kidneys. More recently, Fan et al. (2015) observed that enteral nutrition with parenteral glutamine supplementation diminished the release of inflammatory cytokines and improved survival in septic rats.

Despite the promising nephroprotective effects of glutamine in the early phase of acute renal failure in experimental models, there are very few data in the clinical setting of human disease showing a possible role for glutamine both in the prevention of renal damage and in the renal function recovery after the acute phase (Fiaccadori 2013). However, supplementation of large amounts of glutamine has recently been associated with mortality in ICU patients with renal failure (Heyland et al. 2013), suggesting that glutamine catabolism combines with metabolic alterations in uremia to increase toxicity. Overall, there is a need of studies of glutamine supplementation in patients at high risk or at the early stages of AKI.

18.5 GLUTAMINE DEPLETION IN CRITICAL ILLNESSES: DOES IT MATTER?

In normal conditions, glutamine production from muscle (either from protein breakdown or from *de novo* synthesis) declines continuously from infancy through adulthood, but the relative contributions of proteolysis and *de novo* synthesis remain remarkably constant at ≈13% and ≈87%, respectively (Kuhn et al. 1999). Although skeletal muscle contributes only ≈25%–40% to whole-body protein turnover in humans, ≈70% of overall glutamine production in healthy adults arises from skeletal muscle (Tessari et al. 1996). In critical illnesses, the skeletal muscle response includes a resistance to the antiproteolytic action of insulin, an accelerated proteolysis and enhanced efflux of glutamine and other amino acids from muscle, to provide the splanchnic area with precursors for protein synthesis and energy (Nurjhan et al. 1995). Darmaun et al. (1998) raised systemic cortisol levels to mimic moderate stress conditions and observed that glutamine release from proteolysis increased only slightly (by ≈13%), whereas glutamine *de novo* synthesis increased more markedly (by ≈44%) and accounted for the bulk of the extra glutamine produced. Despite accelerated release from muscle, glutamine deficiency, induced by the increased glutamine requirements of intestinal cells, hepatocytes, and immune cells is thought to occur and has led to the idea that glutamine is a "conditionally essential" amino acid during critical illness (Wernerman 2008). Indeed, studies have shown that in the critically ill, glutamine production is insufficient to cope with increased requirements (Berg et al. 2007). A major question is whether glutamine depletion has any functional significance. Glucose and glutamine are indispensible for most cells *in vitro* culture systems (Yin 2012; Qie 2012). In Hep3B, a tumor cell line originated from hepatocytes, both glutamine and glutamate depletion can trigger gene expression reprogramming. Specifically, glutamine depletion leads to repression of transcription regulators controlling cell functions and cell cycle, ultimately leading to the inhibition of cell growth (Qie 2012). Early studies by Vinnars et al. (1975) showed that intracellular free glutamine of skeletal muscle is markedly reduced after operation, trauma, and inflammatory states. Roth et al. (1982) demonstrated a link between muscle glutamine depletion and survival in septic patients, suggesting that reduced intracellular glutamine may be also a prognostic marker. A major clinical effect of glutamine depletion is likely a decrease in muscle protein synthesis. It is worth noting that early studies have shown a direct correlation between intracellular glutamine concentration and protein synthesis in perfused rat skeletal muscle (MacLennan 1987). In addition, a short-term depletion of plasma glutamine decreases the estimates of whole-body protein synthesis (Darmaun et al. 1998) suggesting that glutamine plays a role in the control of protein metabolism in humans. In turn, loss of muscle mass, with no evident upregulation of glutamine synthesis, likely contributes to insufficient glutamine production in patients with protein-energy wasting.

Low glutamine levels have been associated with poor outcomes during several critical illnesses (Bongers 2007; Streat et al. 1987; Wernerman 2008). Notably, during acute illness, both low plasma and mucosal glutamine concentrations are associated with patient nutritional depletion (Askanazi et al. 1980), suggesting a causative role of glutamine levels on wasting and frailty. Oudemans-van Straaten et al. (2001) showed that glutamine depletion was an independent predictor of mortality in a group of ICU patients when dichotomized at a plasma glutamine concentration of 420 µmol/L. Accordingly, this plasma glutamine level has been used to distinguish glutamine-depleted patients. In a prospective single-center study of consecutive patients admitted to the ICU at Karolinska University Hospital, Huddinge, the admission plasma glutamine concentrations were totally independent of the conventional risk scoring at admittance, and a subnormal concentration was an independent predictor of mortality (Rodas et al. 2012). The mortality risk was mainly confined to the post-ICU period. These data suggest that a plasma concentration of glutamine lower than 420 µmol/L at ICU admission is an independent risk factor for post-ICU mortality.

18.6 CHRONIC KIDNEY DISEASE, WASTING, AND MORTALITY

Chronic kidney disease (CKD) is associated with a wasting syndrome that directly correlates with mortality and morbidity (Yoo 2009). The risk of wasting progressively increases as the glomerular filtration rate (GFR) decreases (Kopple et al. 2000) with a high incidence of this complication in patients who are at the beginning of dialytic treatment (Kopple et al. 2000; Lim 2000). Catabolic factors appear to be distinct for patients at different stages of disease. Several conditions associated with CKD, such as metabolic acidosis, physical inactivity, diabetes, and sepsis, can promote muscle wasting through an increase in protein degradation (Lim 2000; Mitch 2002; Stenvinkel 2004; Mitch and Goldberg 1996). Furthermore, specific defects in amino acid metabolism, resistance to growth hormone and insulin-like growth factor 1, or a very low protein intake can reduce muscle protein synthesis (Thissen et al. 1999). Finally, the hemodialytic procedure per se can stimulate protein breakdown or reduce protein synthesis. All these factors may potentiate the effects of concurrent catabolic illnesses, anorexia, and physical inactivity often found in uremic patients.

It is increasingly apparent that uremia per se predisposes to wasting (Mitch 2002; Stenvinkel 2004). Recent advances obtained in experimental uremia have consistently increased our understanding of intracellular pathways producing loss of muscle mass. Acidosis increases protein degradation through an upregulation of the ATP-dependent, ubiquitin-requiring pathway (Du et al. 2004; Lecker 2006). In addition, impaired signaling through the insulin receptor substrate-1

(IRS-1)/phosphoinositide 3-kinase (PI3-kinase)/Akt pathway can predispose to catabolism through the upregulation of atrogin-related proteolytic pathways (Bailey et al. 2006; Workeneh 2010).

It is consistently accepted that in CKD patients, a deficiency in the antioxidant systems combines with an increase in pro-oxidant activity owing to advanced age and comorbidities (Bonanni et al. 2011) and that microinflammation and oxidative stress play a major role on both cardiovascular mortality and wasting. Several visceral proteins and hormones that decrease in blood in response to malnutrition (such as albumin, prealbumin, transferrin, retinol binding protein, and IGF-I) are also negative acute-phase proteins and their liver synthesis is depressed by inflammation. Several investigators have shown that a significant percentage of chronic hemo- and peritoneal dialysis patients have increased levels of proinflammatory cytokines (IL-1, IL-6, and TNF alpha) suggesting that a systemic inflammatory response is common in dialysis-treated patients (Bonanni 2011 for review). Moreover, cross-sectional studies suggest that inflammation is responsible for serologic and anthropometric evidence of malnutrition. Elevated CRP is strongly associated with cardiovascular mortality, so that the association between inflammation and atherosclerosis is particularly strong in dialysis patients. Although precise mechanisms that contribute to the high prevalence of inflammation in CKD are unknown, reactive oxygen species (ROS) have been proposed as a potential contributor. On the one hand, oxidative stress is able to activate transcriptor factors, such as NF-kB, which regulate inflammatory mediator gene expression. On the other hand, chronic inflammation may cause increased oxidative stress, thus creating a vicious circle in the determination of cardiovascular risk in CKD patients (Bonanni 2011; Zhang et al. 2013).

Current evidence indicates that metabolism of glutamine, together with that of branched-chain amino acids (BCAA), is altered in patients with moderate- to advanced-stage chronic renal disease (Broyer et al. 1980; Divino Filho et al. 1997; Bonanni 2011) and could contribute to wasting. Postabsorptive glutamine blood levels have been reported to be normal (Garibotto et al. 1993) or high in patients with CKD, and their increase in blood after amino acid or protein ingestion is inappropriately high (Deferrari et al. 1988; Garibotto et al. 1993). Early studies have shown that in the postabsorptive state, the removal of glutamine by splanchnic organs is blunted in patients with chronic renal failure (Tizianello et al. 1980a,b), probably because of defective removal of glutamine by the intestine (Tizianello et al. 1980a,b).

Recently, alterations in gut microbiota composition and intestinal barrier have been shown to be associated with inflammation and oxidative stress in CKD patients (Vaziri 2012). Of note, a current hypothesis is that the disruption of tight junctions and diffusion of bacterial toxins may play a major role in the pathogenesis of uremic inflammation and toxicity because of colonic epithelial barrier dysfunction endotoxemia. In light of the physiological role of glutamine to maintain the gastrointestinal mucosal homeostasis and preserve the epithelial barrier function (Reeds 2001), one could speculate that defective handling of glutamine by the intestine could affect mucosal integrity and promote endotoxemia. However, the effect of glutamine on endotoxemia and inflammation has never been tested in patients with CKD.

The alterations of amino acid and protein metabolism in patients with CKD may overlap with those induced by dialysis. The effects of dialysis on nutrition are variable. On the one hand, the "amount" of dialysis delivered appears to be an important factor that affects dietary intake and nutritional status of ESRD patients (Schoenfeld et al. 1983). On the other hand, specific dialysis-related factors contribute to increase protein requirements (Kopple et al. 1973; Ikizler et al. 1994; Gutierrez et al. 1990; Lofberg et al. 2000). A hemodialysis session may impair protein metabolism in different ways: (a) because of the associated losses of substrates, and (b) because of the promotion of net protein catabolism by the process itself. About 6–12 g of amino acids are lost in the dialysate per hemodialysis session (Kopple 1973; Ikizler et al. 1994; Gutierrez 1990; Lofberg et al. 2000). It is noteworthy that the amount of amino acids removed during one hemodialysis session is similar or greater than the amino acid content in extracellular fluids (about 5–6 g, for a 70-kg man). However, plasma amino acid levels decline only by 20%–50% after a hemodialysis session (Gutierrez 1990; Lofberg et al. 2000). Therefore, some other organ, such as skeletal muscle or the splanchnic bed, should counterbalance this amino acid loss with an increased efflux. The available data suggest that hemodialysis induces an accelerated efflux of amino acids from peripheral tissues and significant alterations in protein turnover and glutamine release from muscle without significant changes in glutamine synthesis. Therefore, although muscle protein breakdown during hemodialysis provides amino acid substrate for splanchnic protein synthesis, it could lead to progressive muscle wasting with time. Intradialytic replacement of amino acids could increase the substrate availability for protein synthesis, but the utilization of the amino acids may be limited by altered amino acid transport kinetics (Ray et al. 2005).

For ICU patients with multiple organ failure, including acute renal failure, continuous renal replacement therapy (CRRT) is an alternative to intermittent hemodialysis. CRRT carries the risk of high loss of glutamine into the ultrafiltrate/dialysate, particularly when exogenous intravenous glutamine supplementation is given. Berg et al. (2007) investigated glutamine kinetics during CRRT in 12 anuric patients with multiple organ failure with and without intravenous glutamine supplementation. Glutamine losses into the filtration fluids were similar during glutamine infusion and control days (on the average 3.6 and 3.5 g/24 h, respectively). Net glutamine balance across the leg was also similar on treatment and control days. Interestingly, glutamine loss was more related to the filtrated volume than to plasma concentration. Therefore, glutamine loss in patients on CRRT is accelerated by higher filtration volumes and suggests a greater need for exogenous glutamine than in patients without renal failure.

18.7   GLUTAMINE SUPPLEMENTATION IN CRITICALLY ILL PATIENTS

In the REDOXS study, Heyland et al. (2012) tested the hypothesis that patients with multiorgan failure would have greater depletion of glutamine and antioxidants and would benefit the most from a higher dose of these nutrients (Novak et al. 2002). In this large trial, 1223 patients admitted to an ICU with clinical evidence of severe organ dysfunction (i.e., 93% in shock state, 33% with renal failure) were randomized to one of the four treatments: (1) glutamine; (2) antioxidant therapy; (3) glutamine and antioxidant therapy; and (4) placebo. Glutamine was provided by both enteral and parenteral routes. Surprisingly, this study showed that high-dose glutamine (0.78 g/kg/day) starting within the first 24 h of ICU admission, with or without nutrition support, was associated with an absolute increase in mortality (+6.5%) at 6 months. There are several factors that may account for the discrepancy between the results of the REDOXS study and previous findings. The majority of patients treated were in shock and received the highest dose of glutamine prescribed for critically ill patients (i.e., 30 g/day more than the maximal dose used in other studies). In addition, although the percentage was not statistically significant, AKI was more prevalent in the group receiving glutamine (34.7% in controls vs. 38.9% in antioxidant + glutamine group, respectively, $p > 0.05$).

The recent Canadian Guidelines (Dhaliwal et al. 2014) downgraded the previous indications (Singer et al. 2009) for parenteral glutamine from "strongly recommended" to "should be considered," with the caution that glutamine should not to be used in critically ill patients with shock and multiorgan failure. Although there were no new randomized controlled trials of enteral glutamine supplementation, the committee also agreed to add a strong caution for the use of enteral glutamine in all critically ill patients with shock and multiorgan failure in light of the results from the REDOXS study. Interestingly, a post hoc subgroup analysis of the REDOXS trial (Heyland et al. 2015) showed that both glutamine and antioxidants appeared most harmful in patients with baseline renal dysfunction. It is well known that glutamine itself is known to exacerbate defects in ammonia metabolism and ureagenesis. In addition, blood urea levels are a proxy for small-molecule toxicity in uremia and are associated with negative outcome in dialyzed CKD patients (Owen 1993). Overall, one could speculate that ICU patients with AKI are prone to develop increased ureagenesis and toxicity when glutamine is given in extra amounts. The enteral or parenteral route administration could also lead to different toxic effects. In a more recent meta-analysis confined to studies with parenteral glutamine supplementation, Wischmeyer et al. (2014) observed that glutamine supplementation was associated with a trend toward a reduction of overall mortality and a significant reduction in hospital mortality. In addition, parenteral glutamine was associated with a strong trend toward a reduction in infectious complications and significant reduction in hospital stay. The authors suggested that the discrepancy in studies on glutamine supplementation in critically ill patients may derive from intravenous versus parenteral nutrition or a combination of enteral and parenteral nutrition. However, the reasons why different routes of administration of glutamine might lead to protective or toxic effects in renal patients are not explained.

18.8 POSSIBLE TOXIC EFFECTS RELATED TO GLUTAMINE SUPPLEMENTATION IN ICU PATIENTS WITH AKI

On theoretical grounds, chronic glutamine supplementation could be associated with adverse events. These include increase in ureagenesis, alterations in amino acid transport and tissue distribution, decreased body synthesis of glutamine in response to supplements, altered kidney ammonia production, and increase in tumor growth (Holecek 2013; Soeters and Grecu 2012). These possible effects have not been clearly elucidated in clinical trials in humans. Also, it is unknown whether a harmful dose-response exists for glutamine supplementation and it would be of primary importance to understand the effects of glutamine supplementation according to different status/disease and in terms of glutamine deficiency. As a matter of fact, critical illnesses are not always associated with low glutamine levels. In the REDOXS study, only 30% of patients presented with a glutamine <420 μmol/L, and supranormal (>930 μmol) levels were observed in 15% of them. Notably, also higher glutamine levels were associated with mortality. This was also seen in a recent study examining baseline glutamine levels in critically ill patients, which also showed a U-shaped curve, with both glutamine plasma concentration <400 or >930 μmol/L being related to 6-month mortality (Rodas et al. 2012).

While low glutamine levels are explained by accelerated use in different organs or reduced muscle mass, it is possible that high plasma glutamine levels are the effect of an increase in muscle protein breakdown. Kao et al. (2013) recently observed that endogenous leucine flux, an index of whole-body protein breakdown, was greater in patients with sepsis than in controls, and that glutamine accounted for as much as 50% of amino acids released from the accelerated whole-body protein breakdown. In addition, they observed a significant correlation between endogenous leucine flux and glutamine rate of entry into the plasma, indicating that glutamine entry into the plasma in sepsis is closely related to its release from proteolysis. Accordingly, patients with high glutamine levels probably include very catabolic patients with higher proteolytic rates.

The issue that large amounts of glutamine administered as peptide may impair synthesis of endogenous glutamine and enhance glutamate and ammonia production was addressed by Mori et al. (2014), who measured glutamine endogenous rates of appearance of glutamine in ICU patients following glutamine supplementation. It is worth noting that during alanyl-glutamine supplementation, the higher levels of glutamine attained were not followed by a decrease of endogenous glutamine rates of appearance, indicating that the production of glutamine is not controlled by the circulating glutamine levels.

18.9 CONCLUSIONS

In conclusion, there are several unmet needs in the treatment of AKI and CKD. Current standards of care therapies do not arrest or reverse kidney injury. In addition, they do not reduce the mortality associated with kidney dysfunction. Newer therapies targeting multiple molecular pathways involved in renal and systemic inflammation, and oxidative stress, including glutamine supplementation, have shown promise in animal models. Subsequently, glutamine supplementation has been investigated in clinical human trials with mixed results. Even if recent research has added new understanding on the metabolic effects of glutamine supplementation in AKI, many issues still need to be addressed. The relationships among glutamine's effects on oxidation, HSP activation, and clinical outcomes have not been adequately studied. In addition, future studies should address the optimal dosage, and administration route, of glutamine in AKI, as well as the possible indications and hazards associated with its supplementation. The understanding of the effects of glutamine supplementation on preservation of renal function, protein metabolism, and toxicity in AKI will be an important advance for the future.

REFERENCES

Abraham, P. and B. Isaac. 2011. The effects of oral glutamine on cyclophosphamide-induced nephrotoxicity in rats. *Hum Exp Toxicol* 30:616–623.

Adeva, M., G. Souto, N. Blanco, and C. Donapetry. 2012 Ammonium metabolism in humans. *Metabolism* 61:1495–1511.

Ahlma, K., C.E. Leijonmark, O. Ljungqvist et al. 1994. Short-term starvation alters the free amino acid content of the human intestinal mucosa. *Clinical Science* 86:653–662.

Alba-Loureiro, T.C., R.F. Ribeiro, T.M. Zorn et al. 2010. Effects of glutamine supplementation on kidney of diabetic rat. *Amino Acids* 38:1021–1030.

Altintas, M.M., K. Moriwaki, C. Wei et al. 2014. Reduction of proteinuria through podocyte alkalinization. *J Biol Chem* 289:17454–17467.

Arnold, W.C. and M.A. Holliday. 1979. Tissue resistance to insulin stimulation of amino acid uptake in acutely uremic rats. *Kidney Int* 16:124–130.

Askanazi, J., Y.A. Carpentier, C.B. Michelsen et al. 1980. Muscle and plasma amino acids following injury. Influence of intercurrent infection. *Ann Surg* 192:78–85.

Bailey, J.L., S.R. Price, B. Zheng et al. 2006. Chronic kidney disease causes defects in signaling through the insulin receptor substrate/phosphatidylinositol 3-kinase/Akt pathway: Implications for muscle atrophy. *J Am Soc Nephrol* 17:1388–1394.

Bailey, J.L., X. Wang, B.K. England et al. 1996. The acidosis of chronic renal failure activates muscle proteolysis in rats by augmenting transcription of genes encoding proteins of the ATP-dependent ubiquitin proteasome pathway. *J Clin Invest* 15:1447–1453.

Berg, A., A. Norberg, C.R. Martling et al. 2007. Glutamine kinetics during intravenous glutamine supplementation in ICU patients on continuous renal replacement therapy. *Intensive Care Med* 33:660–666.

Bergstrom, J., P. Furst, L. Noree et al. 1974. Intracellular free amino acid concentration in human skeletal muscle. *J Appl Physiol* 36:693–697.

Bonanni, A., I. Mannucci, D. Verzola et al. 2011. Protein-energy wasting and mortality in chronic kidney disease. *Int J Environ Res Public Health* 8:1631–1654.

Bondy, P., F. Engel, and B. Farrar. 1949. The metabolism of amino acids and protein in the adrenalectomized-nephrectomized rat. *Endocrinology* 44:476–482.

Brosnan, M.E. and J.T. Brosnan. 2009. Hepatic glutamate metabolism: A tale of 2 hepatocytes. *Am J Clin Nutr* 90:857S–861S.

Broyer, M., G. Jean, A.M. Dartois, and C. Kleinknecht. 1980. Plasma and muscle free amino acids in children at the early stages of renal failure. *Am J Clin Nutr* 133:1396–401.

Clark, A.S. and W.E. Mitch. 1983. Muscle protein turnover and glucose uptake in acutely uremic rats. Effects of insulin and the duration of renal insufficiency. *J Clin Invest* 72:836–845.

Darmaun, D. 1992. *In vivo* exploration of glutamine metabolism in man. *Diabet Metab* 18:117–121.

Darmaun, D. and P. Dechelotte. 1991. Role of leucine as a precursor of glutamine alpha-amino nitrogen *in vivo* in humans. *Am J Clin Nutr* 260:326–329.

Darmaun, D., D.F. Matthews, and D.M. Bier. 1986. Glutamine and glutamate kinetics in humans. *Am J Physiol* 251:E117–126.

Darmaun, D., S. Welch, A. Rini et al. 1998. Phenylbutyrate-induced glutamine depletion in humans: Effect on leucine metabolism. *Am J Physiol Endocrinol Metab* 274:E801–E807.

Deferrari, G., G. Garibotto, C. Robaudo et al. 1988. Splanchnic exchange of amino acids after amino acid ingestion in patients with chronic renal insufficiency. *Am J Clin Nutr* 48:72–83.

Deferrari, G., G. Garibotto, C. Robaudo et al. 1994. Renal ammoniagenesis and interorgan flow of glutamine in chronic metabolic acidosis. *Contrib Nephrol* 110:144–149.

Dhaliwal, R., R. Cahill, M. Lemieux, and D.K. Heyland. 2014. The Canadian critical care nutrition guidelines in 2013: An update on current recommendations and implementation strategies. *Nutr Clin Pract* 29:29–43.

Divino Filho, J.C., P. Bàràny, P. Stehle et al. 1997. Free amino-acid levels simultaneously collected in plasma, muscle, and erythrocytes of uraemic patients. *Nephrol Dial Transplant* 12:2339–2348.

Dryer, S.E. 2015. Glutamate receptors in the kidney. *Nephrol Dial Transplant* 30:1630–1638.

Du, J., X. Wang, C.L. Meireles et al. 2004. Activation of caspase-3 is an initial step triggering muscle proteolysis in catabolic conditions. *J Clin Invest* 113:115–123.

Eagle, H. 1959. Amino acid metabolism in mammalian cell cultures. *Science* 130:432–437.

Elia, M. and G. Livesey. 1983. Effects of ingested steak and infused leucine on forelimb metabolism in man and the fate of the carbon skeletons and amino groups of branched-chain amino acids. *Clin Sci* 64:517–526.

Fan, J., L. Wu, G. Li et al. 2015. Effects of enteral nutrition with parenteral glutamine supplementation on the immunological function in septic rats. *Br J Nutr* 113:1712–1722.

Fiaccadori, E., G. Regolisti, and U. Maggiore. 2013. Specialized nutritional support interventions in critically ill patients on renal replacement therapy. *Curr Opin Clin Nutr Metab Care* Mar;16(2):217–24.

Flugel-Link, R.M., I.B. Salusky, M.R. Jones et al. 1983. Protein and amino acid metabolism in posterior hemicorpus of acutely uremic rats. *Am J Physiol* 244:E615–E623.

Frohlich, J., J. Scholmreich, G. Hoppe-Seyler et al. 1974. The effect of acute uremia on gluconeogenesis in isolated perfused rat livers. *Eur J Clin Invest* 4:453–459.

Fuller, T.F., F. Rose, K.D. Singleton et al. 2007. Glutamine donor pretreatment in rat kidney transplants with severe preservation reperfusion injury. *J Surg Res* 140:77–83.

Garibotto, G., G. Deferrari, C. Robaudo et al. 1993. Effects of a protein meal on blood amino acid profile in patients with chronic renal failure. *Nephron* 64:216–225.

Garibotto, G., A. Sofia, C. Robaudo et al. 2004. Kidney protein dynamics and ammoniagenesis in humans with chronic metabolic acidosis. *J Am Soc Nephrol* 15:1606–1615.

Gelfand, R.A., M.G. Glickman, R. Jacob et al. 1986. Removal of infused amino acids by splanchnic and leg tissues in humans. *Am J Physiol* 250:E407–E413.

Gutierrez, A., A. Alvestrand, J. Wahren et al. 1990. Effect of *in vivo* contact between blood and dialysis membranes on protein catabolism in humans. *Kidney Int* 38:487–494.

Haussinger, D., F. Lang, and W. Gerok. 1994. Regulation of cell function by the cellular hydration state. *Am J Physiol* 267:E343–E355.

Heyland, D., J. Muscedere, P.E. Wischmeyer et al. 2013. A randomized trial of glutamine and antioxidants in critically ill patients. *N Engl J Med* 368:1489–1497.

Heyland, D.K., G. Elke, D. Cook et al. 2015. Glutamine and antioxidants in the critically ill patient: A post hoc analysis of a large-scale randomized trial. *JPEN J Parenter Enteral Nutr* 39:401–409.

Holecek, M. 2013. Side effects of long-term glutamine supplementation. *JPEN J Parenter Enteral Nutr* 37:607–616.

Kopple, J.D., M.E. Swendseid, J.H. Shinaberger et al. 1973. The free and bound amino acids removed by hemodialysis. *Trans Am Soc Artif Int Org* 19:309–313.

Ikizler, T.A., P.J. Flakoll, R. Parker et al. 1994. Amino acid and albumin losses during hemodialysis. *Kidney Int* 46:830–837.

Kao, C.L., J. Hsu, V. Bandi, and F. Jahoor. 2013. Alterations in glutamine metabolism and its conversion to citrulline in sepsis. *Am J Physiol Endocrinol Metab* 304:E1359–E1364.

Kessel, A., E. Toubi, E. Pavlotzky et al. 2008. Treatment with glutamine is associated with downregulation of toll-like receptor 4 and myeloid differentiation factor 88 expression and decrease in intestinal mucosal injury caused by lipopolysaccharide endotoxemia in a rat. *Clin Exp Immunol* 151:341–347.

Kim, Y.S., M.H. Jung, M.Y. Choi et al. 2009. Glutamine attenuates tubular cell apoptosis in acute kidney injury via inhibition of the c-Jun N-terminal kinase phosphorylation. *Crit Care Med* 37:2033–2044.

Kopple, J.D., T. Greene, W.C. Chumlea et al. 2000. Relationship between nutritional status and the glomerular filtration rate: Results from the MDRD study. *Kidney Int* 57:1688–1703.

Kopple, J.D., M.E. Swendseid, J.H. Shinaberger et al. 1973. The free and bound amino acids removed by hemodialysis. *Trans Am Soc Artif Int Org* 19:309–313.

Krebs, H.A. 1935. Metabolism of amino-acids. IV. The synthesis of glutamine from glutamate and ammonia and the enzymic hydrolysis of glutamine in animal tissues. *Biochem J* 29:1951–1969.

Kuhn, K.S., K. Schuhmann, P. Stehle et al. 1999. Determination of glutamine in muscle protein facilitates accurate assessment of proteolysis and *de novo* synthesis-derived endogenous glutamine production. *Am J Clin Nutr* 70:484–489.

Lacy, W.W. 1969. Effects of acute uremia on amino acid uptake and urea production by perfused rat liver. *Am J Physiol* 216:1300–1305.

Lafrance, J.P. and D.R. Miller. 2010. Acute kidney injury associates with increased long-term mortality. *J Am Soc Nephrol* 21:345–352.

Langhans, W. and B. Hrupka. 1999. Interleukins and tumor necrosis factor as inhibitors of food intake. *Neuropeptides* 33:415–424.

Lecker, S.H., A.L. Goldberg, and W.E. Mitch. 2006. Protein degradation by the ubiquitin-proteasome pathway in normal and disease states. *J Am Soc Nephrol* 17:1807–1819.

Lim, V.S. and J.D. Kopple. 2000. Protein metabolism in patients with chronic renal failure: Role of uraemia and dialysis. *Kidney Int* 58:1–10.

Lofberg, E., P. Essen, M. McNurlan et al. 2000. Effect of hemodialysis on protein synthesis. *Clin Nephrol* 54:284–294.

MacLennan, P.A., R.A. Brown, and M.J. Rennie. 1987. A positive relationship between protein synthetic rate and intracellular glutamine concentration in perfused rat skeletal muscle. *FEBS Lett* 215:187–191.

Maroni, B.J., R.W. Haesemeyer, M.H. Kutner et al. 1990. Kinetics of system A amino acid uptake by muscle: Effects of insulin and acute uremia. *Am J Physiol* 258:F1304–F1310.

Mitch, W.E. 2002. Malnutrition: A frequent misdiagnosis for hemodialysis patients. *J Clin Invest* 110:437–439.

Mitch, W.E. and A.L. Goldberg. 1996. Mechanisms of muscle wasting: The role of ubiquitin-proteasome system. *N Engl J Med* 335:1897–1905.

Mitch, W.E., J.M. Sands, and I.D. Weiner. 2015. Urea and ammonia metabolism and the control of renal nitrogen excretion. *Clin J Am Soc Nephrol* 10:1444–1458.

Mori, M., O. Rooyackers, M. Smedberg et al. 2014. Endogenous glutamine production in critically ill patients: The effect of exogenous glutamine supplementation. *Crit Care* 18:2;R72.

Novak, F., D.K. Heyland, A. Avenell et al. 2002. Glutamine supplementation in serious illness: A systematic review of the evidence. *Crit Care Med* 30:2022–2029.

Nurjhan, N., A. Bucci, G. Perriello et al. 1995. Glutamine: A major gluconeogenic precursor and vehicle for inter-organ carbon transport in man. *J Clin Invest* 95:272–277.

Oliveira, G.P., M.B. Oliveira, R.S. Santos et al. 2009. Intravenous glutamine decreases lung and distal organ injury in an experimental model of abdominal sepsis. *Crit Care* 13:R74.

Oudemans-van Straaten, H.M., R.J. Bosman, M. Treskes et al. 2001. Plasma glutamine depletion and patient outcome in acute ICU admissions. *Intensive Care Med* 27:84–90.

Owen, W.F., N.L. Lew, Y. Liu et al. 1993. The urea reduction ratio and serum albumin concentration as predictors of mortality in patients undergoing hemodialysis. *N Engl J Med* 329:1001–1006.

Peng, Z.Y., C.R. Hamiel, A. Banerjee et al. 2006. Glutamine attenuation of cell death and inducible nitric oxide synthase expression following inflammatory cytokine-induced injury is dependent on heat shock factor-1 expression. *JPEN J Parenter Enteral Nutr* 30:400–406.

Persike, E.C. and T. Addis. 1949. Increased rate of urea formation following removal of renal tissue. *Am J Physiol* 158:149–156.

Plank, L.D., A.B. Connolly, and G.L. Hill. 1988. Sequential changes in metabolic response in severely septic patients during the first 23 days after the onset of peritonitis. *Ann Surg* 208:143–149.

Price, S.R., D. Reaich, A. Marinovic et al. 1998. Mechanisms contributing to muscle-wasting in acute uremia: Activation of amino acid catabolism. *J Am Soc Nephrol* 9:439–443.

Puthucheary, Z.A., J. Rawal, M. McPhail et al. 2013. Acute skeletal muscle wasting in critical illness. *JAMA* 310:1591–1600.

Ray, D.S.C., T. Welbourne, E.A. Dominic et al. 2005. Glutamine kinetics and protein turnover in end stage renal disease. *Am J Physiol Endocrinol Metab* 288:E377–E346.

Reeds, P.J. and D.G. Burrin. 2001. Glutamine and the bowel. *J Nutr* 131:2505S–2508S.

Rodas, P.C., O. Rooyackers, C. Hebert et al. 2012. Glutamine and glutathione at ICU admission in relation to outcome. *Clin Sci* 122:591–597.

Roth, E., J. Furnovies, F. Muhlbacer et al. 1982. Metabolic disorders in severe abdominal sepsis: Glutamine deficiency in skeletal muscle. *Clinical Nutr* 1:25–41.

Santora, R. and R.A. Kozar. 2008. Molecular mechanisms of pharmaconutrients. *J Surg Res* 161:288–294.

Schoenfeld, P.Y., R.R. Henrt, N.M. Laird et al. 1983. Assessment of nutritional status of the national cooperative dialysis study population. *Kidney Int* 23:80–88.

Sellers, A., L. Katz, and J. Marmorsten. 1957. Effect of bilateral nephrectomy on urea formation in rat liver slices. *Am J Physiol* 191:345–349.

Shuo Qie, Dongming Liang, Chengqian Yin et al. 2012. Glutamine depletion and glucose depletion trigger growth inhibition via distinctive gene expression reprogramming. *Cell Cycle* 11:3679–3690.

Singer, P., M.M. Berger, G. Van den Berghe et al. 2009. ESPEN guidelines on parenteral nutrition: Intensive care. *Clin Nutr* 28:387–400.

Smoyer, W.E., R. Ransom, R.C. Harris, M.J. Welsh, G. Lutsch, and R. Benndorf. 2000. Ischemic acute renal failure induces differential expression of small heat shock proteins. *J Am Soc Nephrol* 11:211–221.

Soeters, P.B. and I. Grecu. 2012. Have we enough glutamine and how does it works? A clinician's view. *Annu Nutr Metab* 60:17–26.

Souba, W.W. 1997. Nutritional support. *N Engl J Med* 336:41–48.

Stenvinkel, P., O. Heimburger, and B. Lindholm. 2004. Wasting, but not malnutrition, predicts cardiovascular mortality in end-stage renal disease. *Nephrol Dial Transpl* 19:2181–2183.

Streat, S.J., A.H. Beddoe, and G.L. Hill. 1987. Aggressive nutritional support does not prevent protein loss despite fat gain in septic intensive care patients. *Journal of Trauma* 27:262–264.

Tessari, P., G. Garibotto, S. Inchiostro et al. 1996. Kidney, splanchnic, and leg protein turnover in humans. Insight from leucine and phenylalanine kinetics. *J Clin Invest* 98:1481–1492.

Thissen, J.P., L.E. Underwood, and J.M. Ketelslegers. 1999. Regulation of insulin-like growth factor-I in starvation and injury. *Nutr Rev* 57:167–176.

Tizianello, A., G. De Ferrari, and G. Garibotto. 1978. Effects of chronic renal insufficiency and metabolic acidosis on glutamine metabolism in man. *Clin Sci Mol Med* 55:391–397.

Tizianello, A., G. De Ferrari, G. Garibotto, G.M. Ghiggeri, C. Robaudo, G. Motta, and M. Nahum. 1980a. Ammonia and amino acid metabolism by the portal-vein-drained viscera in chronic renal insufficiency. *Proc Eur Dial Transplant Assoc* 17:695–699.

Tizianello, A., G. Deferrari, G. Garibotto, and C. Robaudo. 1980b. Amino acid metabolism and the liver in renal failure. *Am J Clin Nut* 33:1354–1362.

Tizianello, A., G. Deferrari, G. Garibotto et al. 1982. Renal ammoniagenesis in an early stage of metabolic acidosis in man. *J Clin Invest* 69:240–250.

Tsai, P.H., J.J. Liu, C.L. Yeh et al. 2012. Effects of glutamine supplementation on oxidative stress-related gene expression and antioxidant properties in rats with streptozotocin-induced type 2 diabetes. *Br J Nutr* 107:1112–1118.

Uchino, S., J.A. Kellum, R. Bellomo et al. 2005. Acute renal failure in critically ill patients: A multinational, multicenter study. *JAMA* 294:813–818.

Vaziri, N.D. 2012. CKD impairs barrier function and alters microbial flora of the intestine: A major link to inflammation and uremic toxicity. *Curr Opin Nephrol Hypertens* 21:587–592.

Verzola, D., L. Cappuccino, E. D'Amato et al. 2014. Enhanced glomerular Toll-like receptor 4 expression and signaling in patients with type 2 diabetic nephropathy and microalbuminuria. *Kidney Int* 86:1229–1243.

Vinnars, E., J. Bergstrom, and P. Furst. 1975. Influence of post-operative state on the intracellular free amino acids in human skeletal tissue. *Ann Surg* 182:665–671.

Zarjou, A. and A. Agarwal. 2011. Sepsis and acute kidney injury. *J Am Soc Nephrol* 22, 999–1006.

Wernerman, J. 2008. Clinical use of glutamine supplementation. *J Nutr* 138:2040S–2044S.

Wischmeyer, P.E., R. Dhaliwal, M. McCall et al. 2014. Parenteral glutamine supplementation in critical illness: A systematic review. *Crit Care* 18:R76–R84.

Workeneh, B.T. and W.E. Mitch. 2010. Review of muscle wasting associated with chronic kidney disease. *Am J Clin Nutr* 91:1128S–1132S.

Ya-Mei Hu, Man-Hui Pai, Chiu-Li Yeh, Yu-Chen Hou, and Sung-Ling Yeh. 2012. Glutamine administration ameliorates sepsis-induced kidney injury by downregulating the high-mobility group box protein-1-mediated pathway in mice. *Am J Physiol–Renal* 302:F150–F158.

Yin, C., S. Qie, and N. Sang. 2012. Carbon source metabolism and its regulation in cancer cells. *Crit Rev Eukaryot Gene Expr* 22:17–35.

Yoo, K.H., C.P. Kovesdy, and K. Kalantar Zadeh. 2009. Why is protein energy wasting associated with mortality in chronic kidney disease? *Semin Nephrol* 29:3–14.

Young, V.R. and A.M. Ajami. 2001. Glutamine: The emperor or his clothes? *J Nutr* 131(9S):2449S–2459S.

Zhang, L., J. Pan, Y. Dong et al. 2013. Stat3 activation links C/EBPdelta to myostatin pathway to stimulate loss of muscle mass. *Cell Metabolism* 18:368–379.

Section VIII

Glutamine and the Catabolic State:
Role of Glutamine in Cancer

19 Glutamine Transport and Metabolism in Cancer

Barrie P. Bode

CONTENTS

19.1 GLUTAMINE METABOLISM: INTRODUCTION

The amino acid glutamine has garnered considerable attention over the last three decades due to its prolific roles in metabolism and associated pleiotropic cellular effects. Classified as a "nonessential" amino acid in most textbooks, glutamine is now widely recognized as a "conditionally essential" amino acid under physiological conditions where its consumption outpaces the body's ability to resynthesize it. The complex cell- and context-specific metabolism of glutamine coupled with its designation as conditionally essential has led to its study as a potential adjuvant in patient therapy, as a regulatory nutrient in cellular function, and as a potential metabolic target in cancer therapy and imaging. As such, the focus on glutamine in clinical applications has created a paradox where its uptake and metabolism in critically ill patients is promoted but, conversely, targeted for inhibition in cancer therapy. In Part I of this section (Glutamine and the Catabolic State), glutamine's role as an adjuvant ("nutritional pharmacology") in critical illness is addressed, and in Part II, prospects are provided for exploiting its deranged physiology and biochemistry in cancer for therapeutic and diagnostic purposes.

Here, we discuss glutamine biochemistry, metabolism, and transport as well as the molecular underpinnings of increased glutamine consumption in rapidly proliferating cells. Current foci and frontiers for research on glutamine transport and metabolism are covered, informed by historical foundations, and driven by rapidly emerging results from recent studies. Further advances in this field are likely to yield benefits to patients in the diagnosis, treatment, and management of cancer in the twenty-first century.

19.2 GLUTAMINE BIOCHEMISTRY; ENZYMES AND DISPOSITION

Glutamine is the amino acid of highest circulating concentration in the blood (600 μM:1,000 μM), reflecting its prolific and pleiotropic roles in human metabolism and physiology (Souba 1992). The metabolic disposition of glutamine is complex and cell type specific. In general terms, upon its transport into the cell, initial glutamine metabolism falls into one of three categories:

1. It is directly incorporated into proteins via the action of glutaminyl-tRNA synthetase.
2. It is hydrolyzed by glutaminase (GLS) to glutamate and ammonia.
3. Its amide nitrogen is transferred to specific chemical substrates in biosynthetic reactions by glutamine amidotransferases (GATases).

All the three of these broad pathways are depicted in Figure 19.1 and are enhanced in rapidly proliferating cells, which collectively contribute to the observed increase in glutamine consumption associated with growth (DeBerardinis and Cheng 2010; Wang et al. 2010; Goswami et al. 2015). Examples of GATases are asparagine synthetase, carbamoyl phosphate synthetase (CPS-II), the initial rate-limiting enzyme in *de novo* pyrimidine biosynthesis, phosphoribosyl pyrophosphate amidotransferase (PPAT)—the initial committing enzyme in *de novo* purine biosynthesis, and glutamine:fructose-6-phosphate amidotransferase (GFAT), the initial rate-limiting enzyme in hexosamine biosynthesis (Mouilleron and Golinelli-Pimpaneau 2007). Importantly, both glutaminase

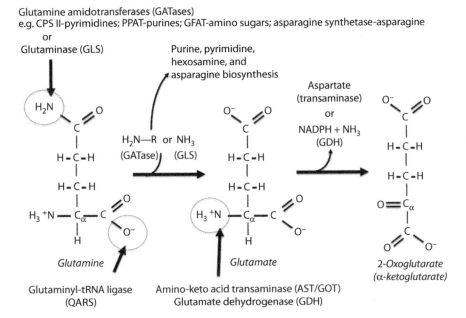

FIGURE 19.1 Metabolism of glutamine to 2-oxoglutarate. The initial metabolism of glutamine can involve its direct incorporation into proteins via glutaminyl-tRNA ligase, or its conversion to glutamate by hydrolysis of its amido nitrogen by glutaminase or by transfer of its amido nitrogen to a receptor substrate via a glutamine amidotransferase (GATase). Examples of GATases are asparagine synthetase, carbamoyl phosphate synthetase (CPS-II), the initial rate-limiting enzyme in *de novo* pyrimidine biosynthesis, phosphoribosyl pyrophosphate amidotransferase (PPAT)—the initial committing enzyme in *de novo* purine biosynthesis, and glutamine:fructose-6-phosphate amidotransferase (GFAT)—the initial rate-limiting enzyme in hexosamine biosynthesis. Glutamate is further metabolized to 2-oxoglutarate by the action of glutamate dehydrogenase (GDH) or by a transamination reaction, such as aspartate amino transferase, each of which removes the alpha amino group forming the keto acid. The 2-oxoglutarate formed engages in the tricarboxylic acid (TCA) cycle, aiding in anaplerosis and helps to drive oxidative metabolism in the mitochondria.

and amidotransferase reactions yield glutamate as a product, which is the first step in the intermediary metabolism of glutamine-derived carbons. Glutamate can likewise undergo a number of enzymatically catalyzed biochemical reactions such as direct charging to a tRNA for protein synthesis, and coupling to cysteine via the enzyme gamma-glutamylcysteine synthetase (glutamate-cysteine ligase [GCL]), the first and rate-limiting step in glutathione (GSH) biosynthesis (Liu et al. 2014). Much of the glutamine-derived glutamate is further metabolized to α-ketoglutarate (2-oxoglutarate) by mitochondrial glutamate dehydrogenase (GDH), or by transaminases such as glutamic-oxaloacetic transaminase ([GOT]; also known as aspartate aminotransferase [AST]). Once formed, 2-oxoglutarate enters the citric acid cycle (also known as the Krebs cycle or tricarboxylic acid [TCA] cycle) and contributes to anaplerosis and oxidative ATP generation. Glutamine-derived 2-oxoglutarate may also be subjected to reductive carboxylation via isocitrate dehydrogenase 1 or 2 (IDH1/2), effectively reversing the first two steps of the citric acid cycle, where it subsequently contributes carbons to fatty acid and membrane biosynthesis via the ATP citrate lyase pathway (Filipp et al. 2012).

Likewise, glutamine is resynthesized in cells via the enzyme glutamine synthetase (gene symbol *GLUL* for *glu*tamate-ammonia *l*igase), which uses the energy of ATP to ligate ammonia to the gamma carboxyl group of glutamate, essentially reversing the glutaminase reaction. The expression and function of glutamine synthetase in human cells is precisely why glutamine has been categorized as a "nonessential" amino acid in textbooks. Glutamine synthetase appears to function as an octamer in eukaryotic (human) cells (Eisenberg et al. 2000; Boksha et al. 2002; Llorca et al. 2006) and its expression is often enhanced in specific cell types within a tissue, where it serves in part to participate in glutamine–glutamate metabolic cycling. Thus, glutamine is consumed and resynthesized within tissues by different cell types, and its overall metabolic disposition both by mode and magnitude is influenced by the prevailing physiological demands of the body (Souba 1992).

19.2.1 GLUTAMINE CYCLES

Glutamine is the major interorgan carbon and nitrogen shuttle and serves with glucose and fatty acids as a primary energy source for specific cells and tissues. Given its myriad roles in human physiology and metabolism, several glutamine cycles function within and between tissues. The mechanisms of glutamine metabolic cycles are depicted in Figure 19.2. These cycles will be mentioned here only briefly for context, as tumors typically function as disruptive "glutamine sinks" when they form within tissues. Two tissue glutamine cycles that have been well characterized function within the liver and the brain (Haussinger and Schliess 2007; Butterworth 2014). In the liver, glutamine entering the tissue via the portal or hepatic arterial circulation is transported into most of the hepatocytes lining the hepatic acinus and consumed by a variety of metabolic pathways. To balance this consumption, a small population of hepatocytes (3%–5%) surrounding the central venous outflow expresses high levels of glutamine synthetase, and regenerates glutamine for export into the venous circulation. By virtue of this intrahepatic metabolic compartmentation, under most conditions, there is net glutamine balance across the liver. This intrahepatic glutamine cycle was elucidated by Dieter Häussinger and colleagues in the 1980s (Haussinger 1983) and the flux through hepatic glutamine-consuming pathways is regulated significantly by its transport across the plasma membrane (Haussinger et al. 1985). As glutamine synthetase in the perivenous hepatocytes incorporates ammonia and glutamate to form glutamine, it is also considered an "ammonia scavenger" system, designed to capture ammonia that escapes detoxification via the urea cycle in the periportal hepatocytes (Haussinger and Gerok 1984).

Another well-characterized glutamine cycle operates in the brain, and in particular in glutamatergic neurons and associated astrocytes. Based on classical work in biochemistry in the 1960s and 1970s, this intercellular neural glutamine–glutamate cycle was likewise elucidated in the mid-1980s when astrocytes were found to manufacture and export glutamine from glutamate via glutamine synthetase (Waniewski and Martin 1986). In general, glutamate, the major excitatory neurotransmitter in the central nervous system, is released into the synaptic cleft by glutamatergic neurons,

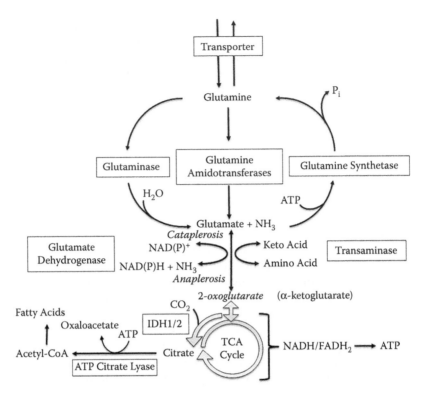

FIGURE 19.2 Glutamine–glutamate cycles. Glutamine is broken down by glutaminase or glutamine amidotransferases to glutamate. Glutamate is subsequently metabolized by glutamate dehydrogenase (GDH) or transaminases to 2-oxoglutarate (α-ketoglutarate) in the mitochondria, where it enters the TCA cycle, and can either contribute to oxidative metabolism, NADH/FADH2 production, and ATP generation (via oxidative phosphorylation), or via reductive carboxylation through isocitrate dehydrogenase (IDH1/2) contribute to the regeneration of citrate for acetyl-CoA production and fatty acid (membrane) biosynthesis via ATP citrate lyase. Likewise, glutamine is regenerated by glutamine synthetase via the ATP-dependent condensation of glutamate with ammonia. Alternatively, glutamate can be exported from the cell through specific transporters and travel to adjacent cells where it is taken up and reconverted to glutamine by glutamine synthetase via the ATP-dependent condensation of ammonia. Glutamine synthesized by the glutamine synthetase pathway is often exported from the cell via specific transporters as part of tissue glutamine cycles.

then rapidly cleared by surrounding astrocytes, which are endowed with prodigious levels of glutamate transporters (Excitatory Amino Acid Transporters or EAATs) (Kanai et al. 2013). Similar to perivenous hepatocytes, astrocytes express significant levels of glutamine synthetase, and utilize transported glutamate to manufacture glutamine from ammonia and ATP. Newly synthesized glutamine is exported from the astrocyte where it is taken up by adjacent neurons and hydrolyzed by glutaminase back to glutamate, which is packaged into synaptic vesicles. This cycle, while not stoichiometric (McKenna 2007), largely drives the glutamine–glutamate cycle in the brain and has been recognized as such since the late 1980s (Torgner and Kvamme 1990). Integration of these two glutamine cycles occurs in liver failure (from chronic or acute conditions), when increasing plasma ammonia levels secondary to loss of hepatic urea cycle leads to neurotoxicity, a state termed "hepatic encephalopathy." The underlying causes of ammonia toxicity to the brain are likely multifaceted and remain the subject of much scientific research and debate (Parekh and Balart 2015). The liver and brain intercellular glutamine cycles are the most prolific and well studied, and are used here as examples of how tissues rely on them for normal physiological function. However, other glutamine cycles occur within different tissues, and their role in physiological function continues to emerge from ongoing research. For example, a glutamine–GABA–glutamate cycle functions in the endocrine pancreas and plays a role in the secretion of insulin and glucagon (Jenstad and Chaudhry 2013).

Intertissue glutamine cycles also function in the body and will be mentioned only briefly here as they are covered more in-depth in other chapters of this book. During critical illness and catabolic states, skeletal muscle releases net amounts of glutamine into the circulation, where other organs and tissues such as liver and immune cells transport and metabolize it at enhanced rates (Souba 1992; Fischer et al. 1995; Marelli-Berg et al. 2012). Muscle represents the largest repository of glutamine in the body, and early observations in the 1980s regarding its transport and relationship to muscle protein synthesis (Rennie et al. 1986) have led to numerous studies regarding nutritional pharmacology with glutamine, its derivatives, and precursors (Wernerman 2011). During physiologic stress, induction of glutamine synthetase in tissues such as the lung and skeletal muscle are believed to contribute to mobilization and export of glutamine into the circulation (Abcouwer et al. 1995). Renal glutaminolysis and ammoniagenesis, which involves increased glutamine uptake and glutaminase activity, is deployed in response to acidosis as a mechanism for systemic pH regulation (Weiner and Verlander 2013). Cogent to this chapter, cancer leads to loss of muscle glutamine content, which is ostensibly mobilized to support either the tumor or immune cells (Parry-Billings et al. 1991; Pisters and Pearlstone 1993; Newsholme and Calder 1997; Yoshida et al. 2001).

The point and relevance of inter- and intratissue glutamine cycles in the context of cancer is that tumors disrupt these programmed physiological systems, and must by definition also develop glutamine cycles within their diverse cellular populations to support growth. Just as the glutamine cycles allow tissues to function normally, glutamine cycles must also evolve and operate between stromal and tumor cells in a symbiotic commensal arrangement. Elucidation of how these glutamine economies evolve within tumors, and how those arrangements are distinct from the normal tissue in which they arise is poorly understood, and is one of the key emerging frontiers in finding the metabolic "Achilles' heel" of cancer that may lead to more targeted and specific therapies (Icard et al. 2014).

19.3   CELL PROLIFERATION, THE WARBURG EFFECT, AND GLUTAMINE METABOLISM

The central role of glutamine in cellular proliferation was established in the 1950s by Harry Eagle, who showed that glutamine is required at concentrations above all other amino acids to sustain the growth and proliferation of cultured cells (Eagle et al. 1956); indeed, every scientist who does cell culture knows that growth medium must be supplemented with glutamine at supraphysiological concentrations of 2–4 mM in order to support optimal growth conditions. *In vivo*, the physiological role of glutamine in driving cell growth and regeneration is reflected by its consumption and use as a primary metabolic fuel in proliferative tissues such as activated immune cells and gut epithelia (Windmueller and Spaeth 1978; Newsholme 2001; Macintyre and Rathmell 2013).

Cell proliferation likewise obviously plays a central role in tumorigenesis; thus, alteration of glutamine metabolism in cancer has garnered progressively increased attention over the last decade. These contemporary efforts reprise of some of the seminal works performed in the twentieth century but are now guided and informed by data from the human genome project and technological advances in molecular biology, imaging, proteomics, and metabolomics. A search of PubMed confirms this perception: the number of articles published on "glutamine metabolism" and cancer from 2004 to 2008 was 18. The subsequent 5-year period from 2009 to 2013 yielded 88 published articles. In 2014 alone, 39 articles on this topic were published, and in 10 months into 2015, 44 articles have appeared on this topic. The graph shown in Figure 19.3 displays this trend. Increased interest in glutamine metabolism parallels the resurrected interest of the cancer research community in targeting metabolic alterations in carcinogenesis as potential therapies (Jang et al. 2013). Leading this vanguard was the rediscovery of the "Warburg effect"—enhanced rates of glycolytic metabolism even in the face of normal oxygen tensions, named after Otto Warburg, the Nobel

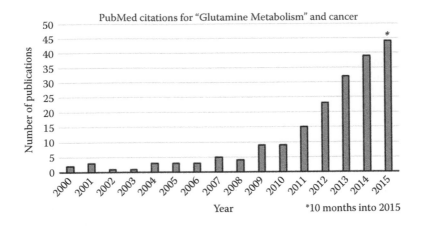

PubMed citations for "Glutamine Metabolism" and cancer

*10 months into 2015

FIGURE 19.3   Growing research interest in cancer glutamine metabolism. The number of publications focusing on glutamine metabolism in cancer as indexed by PubMed. Note the annual increase in publications since 2010. The first 10 years of the twenty-first century yielded 34 publications; the ensuing five years (2010–2014) yielded 118, with 65 in 2015. The entire twentieth century produced 64 papers on this topic (within the limits of search error), many of which laid the foundation for current research in this resurrected field.

Prize-winning biochemist who first made this observation in cancerous versus normal tissues (Hsu and Sabatini 2008). Both glucose and glutamine metabolism are altered and enhanced as part of the Warburg effect (Vander Heiden et al. 2009) through familiar oncogenic signaling pathways such as Myc and E2F/Rb (Dang 2012; Reynolds et al. 2014) that increase glutaminase and glutamine transporter expression (Dang 2010). Indeed, the core principles and mechanisms that are deployed to achieve rapid cellular proliferation in normal physiological functions such as lymphocyte activation (Macintyre and Rathmell 2013) appear to be coopted and sustained in cancer (Diaz-Ruiz et al. 2011; Agathocleous and Harris 2013).

Glutamine has widely been considered to be predominantly metabolized as a primary oxidative fuel for ATP generation via the TCA cycle such as in enterocytes as shown by the seminal work of Herbert Windmueller (Windmueller and Spaeth 1978) and in activated immune cells (Le et al. 2012). However, a long hypothesized and recently demonstrated role for glutamine in lipid biosynthesis has gained recognition, and is prominent particularly under conditions of hypoxia or the Warburg effect. This pathway involves the reductive carboxylation of glutamine-derived 2-oxoglutarate (α-ketoglutarate) by IDH1 (Metallo et al. 2012). A PubMed search reveals that this pathway was first described in cancer cells in 1995, (Holleran et al. 1995) and then for over a decade nothing more was published. From 2007 to 2015, a flourish of 23 papers were published on this pathway from a number of groups, demonstrating that a substantial disposition of glutamine-derived carbons into lipids occurs in cancer cells via the reductive carboxylation of 2-oxoglutarate by IDH1, essentially reversing the first two steps of the TCA cycle, reforming citrate, which is subsequently converted to oxaloacetate and acetyl-CoA by ATP citrate lyase. While the reductive carboxylation of glutamine-derived 2-oxoglutarate provides building blocks (acetyl-CoA and NADPH) for membrane biosynthesis, mutations in IDH1 likewise lead to the production of 2-hydroxyglutarate, a novel metabolite that exerts several oncogenic effects on cells (Yen et al. 2010). The mutations in IDH1 are druggable, and might offer therapeutic opportunities for cancer (Li et al. 2015). IDH1/2 thus serves as a nexus for glutamine-related metabolic therapy in cancer.

19.3.1   TUMOR GLUTAMINE CYCLES AND METABOLISM

Tumors have been characterized as "glutamine sinks" as their consumption of this amino acid is typically excessive relative to normal tissue (Hirayama et al. 1987; DeBerardinis et al. 2007). However, much of what we know about tumor glutamine metabolism is based on whole tissue measurements (the black box) or work in isolated cell lines *in vitro*, with little insight into the complex interaction between tumor cell types and the microenvironments that collectively yield the "glutamine sink." Over the last 5 years, studies have begun to emerge focusing on the development of intratumoral glutamine and other metabolic economies between cancerous and stromal cells in the tumor microenvironment particularly in breast cancer (Choi et al. 2013; Kim et al. 2013a,b; Lisanti et al. 2013; Mao et al. 2013; Icard et al. 2014; Martinez-Outschoorn et al. 2014; Morandi and Chiarugi 2014; Otto et al. 2015). Data to date suggest that epithelial carcinoma cells consume glutamine via oxidative metabolism and build mitochondrial biomass while producing reactive oxygen species (ROS), simultaneously inducing a glycolytic and autophagic phenotype in stromal cells (cancer-associated fibroblasts, or CAFs), which in turn supply the cancer cells with metabolic fuels such as lactate and ketones produced as by-products of the Warburg effect (Ko et al. 2011; Martinez-Outschoorn et al. 2014). This relationship between stromal and cancer cells has been designated as "metabolic asymmetry" and "reverse Warburg effect," where recruited and conscripted CAFs supply the carcinoma cells with glycolytic products such as lactate as well as autophagy-generated glutamine and fatty acids. Cancer cells utilize these fuels via oxidative metabolism (Martinez-Outschoorn et al. 2014). Solid tumors are heterogeneous with multiple cell types and dynamic microenvironments with variable oxygen tensions, which in turn impact metabolic profiles in carcinoma cells (Guillaumond et al. 2014). How these variables affect this emerging model of the "reverse Warburg effect" remain to be determined.

In addition to enhanced glutamine transport, which is discussed in the next section of the chapter, "glutamine addiction" by tumors involves enhanced myc-dependent expression and activation of mitochondrial glutaminase (Wise et al. 2008). Humans express four isoforms of glutaminase, encoded by two separate genes: kidney-type glutaminase (KGA) encoded by *GLS1* and liver-type glutaminase (LGA) encoded by *GLS2*, each of which is alternatively spliced (Lukey et al. 2013). Of the glutaminase isoforms, the shorter version of kidney-type (phosphate-activated) glutaminase (*GLS1*), termed "glutaminase C (GAC)" and identified in 1999 (Elgadi et al. 1999), appears to be most active and important in cancer glutamine metabolism (Cassago et al. 2012). GAC is activated by inorganic phosphate, which is enhanced under hypoxic conditions, and oligomerizes into functional tetramers that further assemble into helical fibers—a mode of allosteric activation that is amenable to druggable inhibition (Ferreira et al. 2013). GAC clearly plays a central role in glutamine consumption, and is induced in cancer cells as part of the "reverse Warburg effect" in stromal-carcinoma interactions (Ko et al. 2011).

Glutamine synthetase (GLUL) plays a role in glutamine cycles, but its role in tumor biology is unclear at the mechanistic level, especially in the context of the carcinoma-stromal metabolic asymmetry and the Warburg effect. Glutamine synthetase is associated with activating β-catenin mutations in several cancers, but its specific role in tumor initiation and progression has not yet been established (Rajagopalan and DeBerardinis 2011). For example, it has garnered interest as a diagnostic and prognostic marker for hepatocellular carcinoma (HCC) (Dal Bello et al. 2010; Lo and Ng 2011), but whether tumoral glutamine synthetase contributes to glutamine efflux as part of stromal-carcinoma metabolic cycling or simply provides the glutamine necessary for purine, pyrimidine, or amino sugar biosynthetic reactions remains to be established. GLUL expression is negatively regulated by feedback from its product, glutamine, and conversely stimulated by glutamine deficit (Labow et al. 2001). Such regulation infers the intracellular metabolic disposition of GLUL-generated glutamine rather than export, especially in the context of the cell autonomous environment of cell culture, under which most of those regulatory studies were performed.

In this regard, a metabolic pathway dependent on enhanced glutamine and glucose supply (Wellen et al. 2010) and upregulated in cancer is the hexosamine biosynthetic pathway involving the glutamine-fructose-6-phosphate amidotransferase (GFAT) (Vasconcelos-Dos-Santos et al. 2015). One hexosamine derivative, *N*-acetylglucosamine (GlcNAc) through its protein-ligating enzyme, *O*-GlcNAc transferase (OGT) is implicated in driving aberrant protein glycosylation characteristic of tumor progression particularly in prostate and pancreatic cancer (Ma and Vosseller 2014). For example, the transcription factor NF-kB, which is linked to inflammatory and oncogenic signaling, is O-GlcNAc modified in pancreatic cancer cells (Ma et al. 2013). In sum, enhanced glutamine-dependent metabolic pathways contribute to the "nitrogen trap" or "glutamine sink" phenotypes of tumors (DeBerardinis et al. 2007). Rather than participation in stromal-carcinoma glutamine cycles, enhanced glutamine synthetase expression may supply glutamine for use in biosynthetic pathways in the face of nutrient austerity in some tumors.

These studies are significant because they begin to address how glutamine economies are established within tumors (Martinez-Outschoorn et al. 2014). More work clearly remains to be performed in this area, including the roles of other cell types (immune cells, endothelial cells, etc.) in tumor glutamine cycles, but such available information helps to establish the initial framework for this research frontier in cancer metabolism.

19.4 GLUTAMINE TRANSPORT

Before glutamine can be metabolized, it must first be transported across the plasma membrane into cells, and conversely, exported from cells as part of local or systemic metabolic cycles. To date, several transporters have been identified in human cells that can mediate the uni- or bidirectional movement of glutamine across the plasma membrane (Bode 2001; Pochini et al. 2014). The properties of these glutamine transporters and the implication of some of them in supporting the growth of tumors and are described in this section.

19.4.1 SOLUTE CARRIER FAMILIES AND GLUTAMINE TRANSPORTERS

As the human genome sequencing project was completed at the beginning of the twenty-first century, information on the genes that encode for solute transporters came into greater focus, and facilitated the cloning and characterization of specific transporters. Most of this work occurred in the 1990s and continued into the 2000s. Elucidation of the properties and characteristics of "orphan" transporters (those for which no known function has yet been established) remains an ongoing research pursuit, and is guided by the homology to known transporters as a first step in the process. Confronted with a deluge of data and disparate transporter nomenclature, in the early 2000s, a consortium of scientists established a systematic nomenclature for the transporters, which is organized by a gene family curated and updated in the *Solute Carrier Tables* (SLC) database (http://slc.bioparadigms.org/) (Hediger et al. 2004, 2013). Given the important role that solute transporters play in metabolism, physiology, and pharmacology, a recent call was published to expend greater effort and resources on transporter research (Cesar-Razquin et al. 2015) similar to past efforts on kinases and drug-metabolizing enzymes.

Among the solute carriers are amino acid transporters, and among those are transporters that mediate glutamine movement across membranes. A focused review on the genes and physiological properties of glutamine transporters was published in 2001 (Bode 2001), and has since been updated (Pochini et al. 2014). Currently, 17 glutamine transporters distributed over four different transporter gene families have been characterized, and are depicted in Figure 19.4. Glutamine transporters are integral membrane proteins encoded by specific genes, and each exhibits distinct physiological properties. A brief explanation of the nomenclature used to describe them is warranted here.

The genes on specific chromosomes that encode for human glutamine transporters are italicized and begin with "SLC" for solute carrier, followed by a gene family number, an "A" (for *a*mino acid transporter) and another number for the transporter within that family. For example, *SLC1A5* represents the gene (and cognate mRNA) that encodes for the glutamine transporter ASCT2 (discussed later), and indicates that it is in the SLC1 gene family, and is the fifth member of the SLC1 amino acid transporter family designated or described (Kanai et al. 2013). The names of the glutamine transporter proteins are less rooted in formal genetic rubrics and are typically acronyms reflective

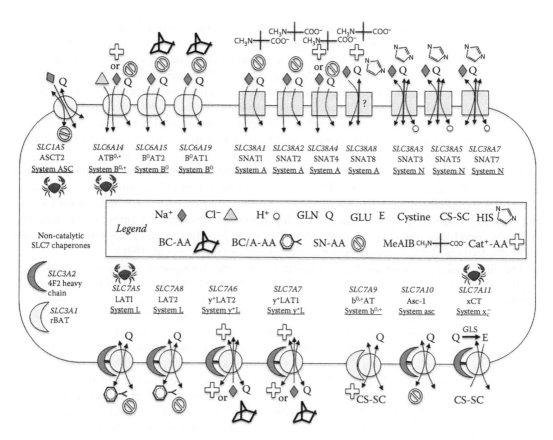

FIGURE 19.4 Solute carrier (SLC) transporters involved in glutamine transport. Transporter genes (italics), proteins, and the corresponding physiological transport activity ("systems") they mediate (underline) as well as their substrates and transport mechanism are illustrated. BC-AA = branched-chain amino acid; BC/A-AA = branched-chain/aromatic amino acid; SN-AA = small neutral amino acid; Cat + -AA = cationic amino acid; MeAIB = alpha-(methylamino)-isobutyric acid. SLC7A11 (xCT), while not a glutamine transporter, uses glutaminase (GLS)-derived glutamate to drive the uptake of cystine into the cell to support glutathione (GSH) biosynthesis. The crab icon indicates transporters implicated in cancer biology.

of their functional characteristics or family. ASCT2, for example, is named for its transport of *ala*nine, *s*erine, and *c*ysteine as characteristic substrates, and was the second of two such transporters present in the SLC1 gene family. Transporter proteins are designated by uppercase letters. Prior to the advent of the molecular cloning and identification of amino transporters, their activities were described as "systems" based on functional characteristics such as ion dependence, substrate preferences, sensitivity to small molecular inhibitors or pH, and kinetic profiles (Christensen et al. 1994). ASCT2 is named not only for three of its primary substrates, but also because it exhibits "System ASC" activity, which was historically described as the sodium-dependent transport of small neutral amino acids (like alanine, serine, and cysteine), insensitive to inhibition by the amino acid analog alpha-(methylamino)-isobutyric acid (MeAIB) (Kilberg et al. 1979). Thus, *SLC1A5* encodes for the ASCT2 protein, which exhibits System ASC activity. Such nomenclature is used to describe other glutamine transporters, which designates their genes and mRNA (molecular biology), protein (cell biology and biochemistry), and activity (physiology), respectively.

Four amino acid transporter families have members that transport glutamine. The SLC1 family, also known as the "excitatory amino acid transporter" family, has one transporter, ASCT2, which transports glutamine and plays a particularly prolific role in cancer biology, as discussed later. ASCT1 transports small neutral amino acids like ASCT2, but does not transport the amides (glutamine and asparagine) (Kanai et al. 2013; Scalise et al. 2014). ASCT2 is a sodium-dependent neutral amino acid exchanger that was originally designated as ATB^0 in 1996 (Kekuda et al. 1996). Its homology to other SLC1 family members (the anionic sodium-dependent glutamate transporters) including ASCT1 led to its subsequent designation as ASCT2 since 2004. The SLC1 family has also since been renamed as the *high-affinity glutamate and neutral amino acid transporter family* due to the low K$_m$'s (high affinity) of constituent transporters for their substrate amino acids.

The SLC6 family or "sodium- and chloride-dependent neurotransmitter transporter family" (Rudnick et al. 2014) harbors three members that are demonstrated to be capable of mediating glutamine uptake. Among these transporters is ATB$^{0,+}$, encoded by the *SLC6A14* gene, which mediates the uptake of glutamine, other neutral amino acids (the "0" designation), and cationic amino acids (the " + " designation). Like ASCT2, ATB$^{0,+}$ has been implicated in driving growth in specific cancers (Karunakaran et al. 2011; Babu et al. 2015). The other two members, BOAT1 (SLC6A19) and BOAT2 (SLC6A15), mediate the sodium-dependent uptake of neutral amino acids, including glutamine, and likely represent the true System B^0 activity for which ASCT2 was originally named ATB^0 due to their highly similar functional characteristics (Kekuda et al. 1996).

The SLC7 family, designated as "cationic amino acid transporter/glycoprotein-associated family" (Fotiadis et al. 2013), and formerly "CATs and HATs" (Verrey et al. 2004) (for *c*ationic *a*mino acid *t*ransporters/*h*eterodimeric *a*mino acid *t*ransporters), is a large and diverse transporter family whose membership mediates the transport of the entire spectrum of amino acids: small neutral, large branched-chain/aromatic, cationic, and anionic. Among the 14 members, six are capable of mediating the bidirectional movement of glutamine across the plasma membrane by exchange mechanisms. All six of these SLC7 transporters are in the "HAT" (heterodimeric amino acid transporter) subfamily as they are covalently linked to members of the SLC3 non-transporter carrier chaperone proteins (Fotiadis et al. 2013). Based on their activities and kinetic asymmetries, three of the SLC7 family members (LAT1 [SLC7A5], LAT2 [SLC7A8], and b$^{0,+}$AT [SLC7A9]) are more inclined to mediate glutamine efflux, two likely mediate net glutamine uptake (y + LAT1 (SLC7A7), y + LAT2 (SLC7A6)), and one facilitates relatively unbiased glutamine exchange (asc-1 [SLC7A10]) (Fotiadis et al. 2013). Another SLC7 family transporter that is not a glutamine transporter but warrants mention is xCT (SLC7A11), as it mediates the exchange of intracellular glutamine-derived glutamate (via glutaminase or amidotransferase activity) for extracellular cystine, used in GSH biosynthesis (Bannai and Ishii 1988). The xCT transporter has received considerable attention for its implicated role in cancer biology over the last few years (Bhutia et al. 2015).

The most prolific glutamine transporter family is the SLC38, or "SNAT" family (for *System N* and *System A Transporters*) (Broer 2014). This family of sodium-dependent glutamine transporters has 11 family members, seven of which have been characterized. The System N transporters (SNAT3 [SLC38A3], SNAT5 [SLC38A5], and SNAT7 [SLC38A7]) and System A transporters (SNAT1 [SLC38A1], SNAT2 [SLC38A2], SNAT4 [SLC38A4], and SNAT8 [SLC38A8]) are distinguished by two primary features: System A transporters accept the nonmetabolizable N-methylated amino acid analog MeAIB as a substrate, whereas System N transporters do not; also, System N transporters can mediate the bidirectional transport of glutamine through a sodium–proton exchange mechanism, whereas System A transporters mediate only the inward transport of their substrate amino acids, and are thus concentrative. The System N transporters are more glutamine-selective than the System A transporters, as they primarily mediate glutamine and histidine transport (Kilberg et al. 1980), with secondary preference for a limited panel small neutral amino acids such as asparagine, alanine, and serine (Broer 2014).

In summary, to date, 17 glutamine transporters have been identified that mediate the movement of this prolific amino acid across the plasma membrane of cells. These transporters act in concert to collectively support our physiology and metabolism in a cell-specific manner. During the cancerous transformation of cells and tissues, a subset of these transporters appears to be consistently selected to drive the tumor growth and progression.

19.4.2 Glutamine Transporters Implicated in Cancer

To date, four amino acid transporters have been found to be consistently or variably induced in human cancers: SLC1A5 (ASCT2), SLC7A5 (LAT1), SLC7A11 (xCT), and SLC6A14 (ATB$^{0,+}$) (Bhutia et al. 2015). Of these transporters, ASCT2 is most intimately linked to glutamine uptake, LAT1 to essential amino acid (EAA) import (and glutamine export), xCT to cystine uptake for GSH biosynthesis, and ATB$^{0,+}$ to the concentrative uptake of cationic and neutral amino acids. Evidence regarding the alleged role of each in cancer biology is briefly presented here.

A System ASC-like amino acid transporter was first shown to mediate the markedly enhanced glutamine transport rates in human liver cancer cells relative to System N-mediated uptake in normal human hepatocytes (Bode et al. 1995). This transporter was later identified as ASCT2 (Bode et al. 2002), which also mediates most glutamine uptake in human prostate (Wang et al. 2015), breast (Collins et al. 1998; Jeon et al. 2015), lung (Hassanein et al. 2016), and colon (Huang et al. 2014) cancer cells, among others. Likewise, targeting ASCT2 as a therapy has been successful in human cell lines and some animal models for HCC (Fuchs et al. 2004, 2007), lung cancer (Hassanein et al. 2013, 2016), prostate cancer (Wang et al. 2015), breast cancer (Chen et al. 2015; Jeon et al. 2015; van Geldermalsen et al. 2016), melanoma (Wang et al. 2014), and colon cancer (Huang et al. 2014). In 2005, a bioinformatics-based study indicated that ASCT2 was consistently upregulated in a broad spectrum of human cancers in conjunction with LAT1 (Fuchs and Bode 2005). LAT1 is a transporter that is responsible for the uptake of essential branched-chain and aromatic amino acids through an exchange mechanism, as well as several drugs like melphalan (Yanagida et al. 2001) were previously linked to cell activation and transformation and referred to as "CD98 light chain" (Mannion et al. 1998; Storey et al. 2005). Significantly, another paper appeared in 2005 that corroborated the inferred relationship between LAT1 and ASCT2, when crosslinking and proteomics analyses demonstrated that these transporters were physically associated along with monocarboxylate transporters (MCTs) and CD147 in the plasma membrane of cancer cells (Xu and Hemler 2005). This complex was designated the "metabolic activation-related complex." Subsequently, over the ensuing decade, several studies have examined ASCT2 and LAT1 as cohorts through immunohistochemistry for their prognostic and diagnostic value in several primary human cancers, most recently esophageal and lung cancer (Yen et al. 2010; Nikkuni et al. 2015). Most of these studies have concluded that elevated expression of both transporters, alone or in combination with other markers in patient tumors, are associated with poorer clinical outcomes.

A teleological hypothesis for the observed ASCT2 and LAT1 relationship was formulated whereby the two amino acid transporters cooperate through their exchange mechanisms to stimulate mammalian target-of-rapamycin (mTOR) growth signaling (Fuchs and Bode 2005). The mTOR kinase complex integrates multiple signaling pathways to regulate and drive cap-dependent translation in the cell, and is stimulated by amino acids, particularly EAAs such as leucine (Efeyan et al. 2012). Likewise, mTOR has been the focus of intense investigation for its role in cancer biology and, by extension, a target for oncology patients through novel rapamycin analogs (mTOR kinase inhibitors) (Meng and Zheng 2015). The hypothesized link between ASCT2/LAT1 and mTOR stimulation involves a "tertiary active transport mechanism," whereby the sodium-dependent uptake of amino acids through ASCT2 (secondary active transport) supplies intracellular substrates for LAT1-mediated exchange, which in turn imports EAAs that stimulate mTOR complex 1 (mTORC1) signaling. The hypothesis was based on earlier work proposing such a relationship between sodium-dependent transporters and facilitative exchangers in maintaining intracellular amino acid pools (Broer 2002; Verrey 2003). An initial test of this hypothesis indeed demonstrated that targeted silencing of ASCT2 expression in human liver cancer cells reduced mTORC1 signaling, which preceded programmed cell death (Fuchs et al. 2007). A subsequent study examined the entire relationship and showed that ASCT2-supplied glutamine drove LAT1 exchange and mTORC1 signaling in cancer cells through this tertiary active transport arrangement (Nicklin et al. 2009). Whether this

ASCT2/LAT1/mTORC1 axis operates *in vivo* and is amenable to targeted therapy is the subject of ongoing research.

In addition to ASCT2 and LAT1, $ATB^{0,+}$ encoded by the *SLC6A14* gene transports glutamine and has recently been implicated in a number of human cancers, including colon (Gupta et al. 2005) and breast (Karunakaran et al. 2011; Babu et al. 2015). Significantly, $ATB^{0,+}$ is upregulated in breast cancer cells when co-incubated with fibroblasts; conversely, LAT1 is downregulated in breast carcinoma cells and instead enhanced in the fibroblasts (Ko et al. 2011). This finding plays into the notion that LAT1 mediates net glutamine efflux, and concentrative transporters like $ATB^{0,+}$ mediate net glutamine uptake. Unlike ASCT2, $ATB^{0,+}$ is a concentrative (not exchange-driven) transporter capable of driving glutamine as well as cationic amino acid accumulation in the cell. ASCT2 likewise drives net glutamine delivery to cancer cells, but relies on a "glutamine sink" in the form of rapid glutamine metabolism to do so, as it is an exchanger capable of mediating glutamine efflux as well. The relative contribution of each of these transporters to cancer biology is an area of active investigation.

Finally, xCT (SLC7A11) has recently received considerable attention for its hypothesized role in cancer biology. xCT mediates the uptake of cystine in exchange for intracellular glutamate to support GSH biosynthesis, and thus plays a particularly pivotal role in the cellular response to ROS and oxidative stress (Ishii and Mann 2014). As cells metabolize glutamine and other oxidizable substrates via the TCA cycle, ROS are a natural by-product and place a strain on the intracellular reduced GSH pools. At first glance, enhanced glutamine transport and oxidative metabolism increases intracellular ROS, but proportionally provides more glutamine-derived glutamate to drive cystine uptake through xCT to sustain GSH biosynthesis. Thus, xCT under these conditions plays a notable rate-limiting step in the impact of ROS on the cell, and therefore represents a potential target for cancer therapy. Indeed, many of glutamine's antiapoptotic effects may be tied to its role in maintaining intracellular GSH levels (Fuchs and Bode 2006). Recent observations are particularly relevant in this regard: The tumor suppressor p53, whose role in cancer biology is well documented, inhibits glycolysis (Warburg effect) through the induction of protein TIGAR (*TP53-I*nduced *G*lycolysis and *A*poptosis *R*egulator) (Bensaad et al. 2006), but also suppresses the expression of *SLC7A11* (xCT) (Jiang et al. 2015). TIGAR likewise prevents ROS-mediated and p53-induced apoptosis (Bensaad et al. 2009). One hypothesized way it achieves this goal is by directing glucose to the pentose-phosphate shunt, which generates NADPH necessary to sustain reduced GSH pools and neutralize ROS damage (Green and Chipuk 2006). TIGAR likewise is induced in breast carcinoma cells by coincubation with fibroblasts along with mitochondrial biogenesis, glutamine transport, and metabolism (Martinez-Outschoorn et al. 2011). Inhibition of xCT under these conditions might lead to carcinoma-selective death, which is the framework for ongoing studies into transport targeting xCT in cancer (Dai et al. 2014). In sum, xCT is tied to glutamine through glutamate and oxidative metabolism and has gained increasing attention in the redox-focused formulation of potential cancer therapies (Ishii and Mann 2014).

19.5 TARGETING GLUTAMINE TRANSPORT AND METABOLISM IN CANCER IMAGING AND THERAPY

The quest for improved cancer therapies and detection based on glutamine's role in cancer biology has been an ongoing translational research pursuit for several years. As with many other facets of cancer research, glutamine transport and metabolism in cancerous cells share significantly overlapping mechanisms with normal cellular populations that rely on proliferation for their function, such as the deployment of ASCT2, upregulation of glutaminase, and mTOR activation (Marelli-Berg et al. 2012; Nakaya et al. 2014; Macintyre and Rathmell 2013). In spite of these challenges, researchers press on in their goals to leverage differences between normal and cancerous growth mechanisms in the development of therapies and imaging agents based on the magnitude or mechanism of glutamine transport and metabolism. Here, we discuss recent developments in glutamine-based therapy and imaging.

19.5.1 GLUTAMINE-TARGETED IMAGING AND CANCER DIAGNOSTICS

Fluorodeoxyglucose (FDG) labeled with ^{18}F (^{18}FDG), developed in the 1970s (Alavi and Reivich 2002), has been used in positron emission tomography (PET) imaging for the detection of metabolically active tumors since the 1990s based on the Warburg effect, but with variable success and several limitations. Thus, the development of diagnostic substrates for enhanced cancer detection remains an active area of research (Kumar et al. 2008). The coordinately enhanced consumption of glutamine by rapidly proliferating cells in the Warburg effect has led to the exploration of ^{13}C-labeled glutamine to image cancers such as HCC and prostate using hyperpolarized nuclear magnetic resonance spectroscopy (MRS) (Gallagher et al. 2008; Qu et al. 2011a,b; Wilson and Kurhanewicz 2014). The editor of this book, Dominique Meynial-Denis, addresses glutamine as a new therapeutic target in cancer, with a focus on hyperpolarized MRS, in the next chapter. With regard to the development of glutamine-based imaging agents for both PET and hyperpolarized MRS in tumor diagnostics, the group led by Hank Kung at the University of Pennsylvania (where FDG-based PET imaging was first conceived and implemented [Alavi and Reivich 2002]) has been particularly active (Lieberman et al. 2011; Qu et al. 2011a,b; Ploessl et al. 2012; Qu et al. 2012; Wu et al. 2014), as has the lab of Kevin Brindle at the University of Cambridge (Witney and Brindle 2010).

FDG-based PET imaging has been successful for the detection of many actively growing cancers because it involves the transport (by GLUT1) and phosphorylation (by hexokinase) of a glucose analog that is nonmetabolizable (deoxyglucose), which subsequently accumulates within cells to yield an image. Among the challenges for the development of glutamine-based imaging molecules is the similar requirement to match robust and specific transport to nonmetabolizable substrates, such that their residence time and accumulation within the tumor is sufficient for imaging purposes. Given the rapid metabolism of glutamine within cells, an imperative exists to develop such synthetic substrates. Most synthetic ASCT2 substrates, to date, have been based on a derivatized aromatic ring linked to either glutamine's amide nitrogen (such as the gamma-glutamyl transferase substrate gamma-glutamyl para-nitroanilide) (Esslinger et al. 2005; Schulte et al. 2015), serine's hydroxyl group or cysteine's sulfur group (benzylserine or benzylcysteine derivatives, respectively) (Grewer and Grabsch 2004; Albers et al. 2012). Recent work using computer modeling generated five new activators and two inhibitors for ASCT2 (Colas et al. 2015). While many of these synthetic ligands modulate ASCT2's activity, whether they are actively transported and accumulated by ASCT2 or simply bind to the protein remains to be determined and they have not been applied to PET imaging to date. However, one synthetic substrate of trans-1-amino-3-^{18}F-fluorocyclobutanecarboxylic acid (anti-^{18}F-FACBC) is transported predominantly by ASCT2 in prostate carcinoma and glioma cells (Okudaira et al. 2011, 2013; Ono et al. 2013, 2015) and has been tested in preclinical (animal) models, in healthy volunteers (Schuster et al. 2014) and some initial prostate cancer patient cohorts with promising results (Brunocilla et al. 2014; Kairemo and Rasulova 2014; Ren et al. 2016). Incremental progress continues in this area of nonmetabolizable glutamine transporter substrates, and will certainly be both informed and driven by basic research studies in transporter biology.

In addition to nonmetabolizable ASCT2 substrates, glutamine that is directly fluorinated at the 4-position (4-^{18}F-(2S,4R)-fluoroglutamine) has been developed and tested as a PET imaging agent, both in preclinical lung cancer models (Hassanein et al. 2016) and recently in glioma patients, where it has yielded promising results for improved PET imaging versus ^{18}FDG (Venneti et al. 2015). Its PET imaging utility surprisingly occurs in the face of its active metabolism, and superior to its ^{18}F-(2S,4R)-fluoroglutamate derivative in cells based partly on its incorporation into intracellular macromolecules (Cooper et al. 2012; Ploessl et al. 2012; Kairemo and Rasulova 2014). Both radiolabeled analogs for glutamine and glutamate are transported largely by two transporters implicated in cancer biology—ASCT2 and xCT, respectively (Ploessl et al. 2012; Venneti et al. 2015). Continued testing and improvement in this area should lead to superior cancer-specific imaging agents with increased diagnostic value relative to the current FDG-based modalities.

19.5.2 GLUTAMINE-TARGETED THERAPIES

Glutamine transport and metabolism serve a multitude of essential roles in human physiology, so the targeting glutamine per se for cancer therapy has been difficult with regard to specificity. For example, early work with glutamine analogs including acivicin, L-diazo-norleucine (L-DON), and azaserine resulted in significant toxicity, including neurotoxicity, to patients (Ahluwalia et al. 1990). There have, however, been two recent primary advancements in glutamine-associated cancer therapies: glutaminase inhibitors and isocitrate dehydrogenase (IDH) inhibitors, both of which may be linked in some cancers (Emadi et al. 2014).

As discussed earlier in the chapter, the shorter version of kidney-type (phosphate-activated) glutaminase (GLS1) (Elgadi et al. 1999), termed "glutaminase C" appears to be most active and

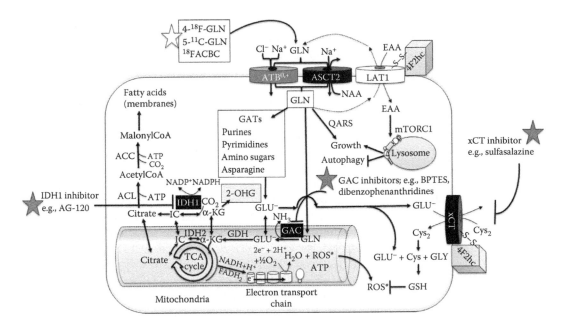

FIGURE 19.5 Cancer glutamine addiction and targets for glutamine-related cancer detection and therapies. As part of the Warburg effect, the myc transcription factor family drives the expression of transporters (ASCT2) and enzymes (glutaminase C [GAC]) that contribute to "glutamine addiction" for cancer growth. Once imported, glutamine contributes substantially to the biosynthesis of nucleic acids and hexosamines via glutamine amidotransferase (GATases) enzymes; to translation via charging to tRNA (glutamine-tRNA synthetase [QARS]); to growth via the tertiary transport mechanism (dashed arrow lines) via LAT1 for essential amino acid (EAA) import that stimulates mTOR complex 1 (mTORC1) signaling; to the anaplerotic production of α-ketoglutarate via GAC and glutamate dehydrogenase (GDH) for oxidation in the TCA cycle and ATP production or the production of citrate (reverse TCA) via reductive carboxylation mediated by isocitrate dehydrogenase (IDH). Mutant IDH1 or IDH2 can likewise form the "oncometabolite" 2-hydroxyglutarate (2-OHG), which exerts proto-oncogenic effects on cells. Citrate formed via glutamine-derived α-ketoglutarate is acted on by ATP-citrate lyase to form acetyl-CoA for fatty acid biosynthesis; thus, a significant level of glutamine-derived carbons can be found in the membranes of cancer cells. Glutamate produced by glutaminolysis or GAT reactions is also utilized to drive the uptake of cystine into the cell (via xCT) and to produce glutathione (GSH) by conjugation to cysteine in a feed-forward system. High levels of GAC activity can lead to increased oxidative metabolism and the production of reactive oxygen species (ROS*), but the commensurate increase in cellular glutamate levels drives higher exchange-mediate cystine import to produce more GSH to offset the ROS production. Thus, inhibition of xCT under these conditions would render the cancer cells susceptible to ROS-mediated stress and death. The components of this "glutamine addiction pathway" that are currently being targeted for the development of imaging agents and therapies are indicated in black with white text. Stars indicate imaging (white) or therapeutic (dark) tools under development.

important in cancer glutamine metabolism. Two classes of GAC inhibitors have been developed that have shown initial promise. A class of GAC allosteric inhibitors, dibenzophenanthridines (Katt et al. 2012), inhibit cancer cell growth without affecting their normal cellular counterparts by preventing the tetrameric association of GAC monomeric subunits for enzyme activation (Ferreira et al. 2013; Stalnecker et al. 2015). Another class of glutaminase inhibitors—bis-2-(5-phenylacetamido-1,2,4-thiadiazol-2-yl)ethyl sulfide (BPTES)—were developed in 2007 and selectively inhibit the kidney isoform but not the liver isoform of glutaminase (Robinson et al. 2007). Inhibition of GAC with BPTES preferentially slows the growth of glioma (Seltzer et al. 2010) and myeloid leukemia cells (Emadi et al. 2014) with IDH1 mutations. This link is based on the glutaminase-dependent production of glutamate for α-ketoglutarate, the substrate for IDH1 or IDH2. This connection is reinforced by the requirement for GDH in "glutamine addiction" of cancer cells (Yang et al. 2009). Likewise, mutant IDH molecular inhibitors are currently being clinically tested for a variety of malignancies (Parker and Metallo 2015) to prevent the production of the oncogenic metabolite 2-hydroxyglutarate. The clinical efficacy of all of these glutamine metabolism-targeted cancer therapies remains to be determined in large randomized clinical trials.

19.6 CONCLUSIONS AND FUTURE DIRECTIONS

The last decade (2005–2015) has been characterized by a dramatic increase in the number of biomedical research studies focused on glutamine transport and metabolism in cancer. The prolific metabolic role that this "conditionally essential" amino acid plays in the body is paralleled by its equally essential role in cancer biology, including myc-driven "glutamine addiction" as a corollary to the Warburg effect. The search for the metabolic "Achilles' heel" of cancer is squarely dependent on the discovery of distinctions between normal and deranged mechanisms of glutamine transport and metabolism. In this regard, thus far, a small cohort of transporters (ASCT2, ATB$^{0,+}$, LAT1, and xCT) and enzymes (GAC and IDH1/2) have emerged as the most promising targets for the development of cancer detection tools and therapies (Figure 19.5). This is a field that is likely to grow for years, where bioinformatics, bench science, animal models, and clinical application merge to yield effective tools targeting deranged glutamine biology in the ongoing crusade against cancer.

REFERENCES

Abcouwer, S. F., B. P. Bode, and W. W. Souba. 1995. Glucocorticoids regulate rat glutamine synthetase expression in a tissue-specific manner. *J Surg Res* 59(1):59–65, doi: 10.1006/jsre.1995.1132.

Agathocleous, M. and W. A. Harris. 2013. Metabolism in physiological cell proliferation and differentiation. *Trends Cell Biol* 23(10):484–92, doi: 10.1016/j.tcb.2013.05.004.

Ahluwalia, G. S., J. L. Grem, Z. Hao, and D. A. Cooney. 1990. Metabolism and action of amino acid analog anti-cancer agents. *Pharmacol Ther* 46(2):243–71.

Alavi, A. and M. Reivich. 2002. Guest editorial: The conception of FDG-PET imaging. *Semin Nucl Med* 32(1):2–5, doi: 10.1053/snuc.2002.29269.

Albers, T., W. Marsiglia, T. Thomas, A. Gameiro, and C. Grewer. 2012. Defining substrate and blocker activity of alanine-serine-cysteine transporter 2 (ASCT2) Ligands with Novel Serine Analogs. *Mol Pharmacol* 81(3):356–65, doi: 10.1124/mol.111.075648.

Babu, E., Y. D. Bhutia, S. Ramachandran, J. P. Gnanaprakasam, P. D. Prasad, M. Thangaraju, and V. Ganapathy. 2015. Deletion of the amino acid transporter Slc6a14 suppresses tumour growth in spontaneous mouse models of breast cancer. *Biochem J* 469(1):17–23, doi: 10.1042/bj20150437.

Bannai, S. and T. Ishii. 1988. A novel function of glutamine in cell culture: Utilization of glutamine for the uptake of cystine in human fibroblasts. *J Cell Physiol* 137(2):360–6, doi: 10.1002/jcp.1041370221.

Bensaad, K., E. C. Cheung, and K. H. Vousden. 2009. Modulation of intracellular ROS levels by TIGAR controls autophagy. *EMBO J* 28(19):3015–26, doi: 10.1038/emboj.2009.242.

Bensaad, K., A. Tsuruta, M. A. Selak, M. N. Vidal, K. Nakano, R. Bartrons, E. Gottlieb, and K. H. Vousden. 2006. TIGAR, a p53-inducible regulator of glycolysis and apoptosis. *Cell* 126(1):107–20, doi: 10.1016/j. cell.2006.05.036.

Bhutia, Y. D., E. Babu, S. Ramachandran, and V. Ganapathy. 2015. Amino Acid transporters in cancer and their relevance to "glutamine addiction": Novel targets for the design of a new class of anticancer drugs. *Cancer Res* 75(9):1782–8, doi: 10.1158/0008-5472.can-14-3745.

Bode, B. P. 2001. Recent molecular advances in mammalian glutamine transport. *J Nutr* 131(9 Suppl):2475S–85S; discussion 2486S–7S.

Bode, B. P., B. C. Fuchs, B. P. Hurley, J. L. Conroy, J. E. Suetterlin, K. K. Tanabe, D. B. Rhoads, S. F. Abcouwer, and W. W. Souba. 2002. Molecular and functional analysis of glutamine uptake in human hepatoma and liver-derived cells. *Am J Physiol Gastrointest Liver Physiol* 283(5):G1062–73, doi: 10.1152/ajpgi.00031.2002.

Bode, B. P., D. L. Kaminski, W. W. Souba, and A. P. Li. 1995. Glutamine transport in isolated human hepatocytes and transformed liver cells. *Hepatology* 21(2):511–5.

Boksha, I. S., H. J. Schonfeld, H. Langen, F. Muller, E. B. Tereshkina, and GSh Burbaeva. 2002. Glutamine synthetase isolated from human brain: Octameric structure and homology of partial primary structure with human liver glutamine synthetase. *Biochemistry (Mosc)* 67(9):1012–20.

Broer, S. 2002. Adaptation of plasma membrane amino acid transport mechanisms to physiological demands. *Pflugers Arch* 444(4):457–66, doi: 10.1007/s00424-002-0840-y.

Broer, S. 2014. The SLC38 family of sodium-amino acid co-transporters. *Pflugers Arch* 466(1):155–72, doi: 10.1007/s00424-013-1393-y.

Brunocilla, E., R. Schiavina, C. Nanni et al. 2014. First case of 18F-FACBC PET/CT-guided salvage radiotherapy for local relapse after radical prostatectomy with negative 11C-Choline PET/CT and multiparametric MRI: New imaging techniques may improve patient selection. *Arch Ital Urol Androl* 86(3):239–40, doi: 10.4081/aiua.2014.3.239.

Butterworth, R. F. 2014. Pathophysiology of brain dysfunction in hyperammonemic syndromes: The many faces of glutamine. *Mol Genet Metab* 113(1–2):113–7, doi: 10.1016/j.ymgme.2014.06.003.

Cassago, A., A. P. Ferreira, I. M. Ferreira, C. Fornezari, E. R. Gomes, K. S. Greene, H. M. Pereira, R. C. Garratt, S. M. Dias, and A. L. Ambrosio. 2012. Mitochondrial localization and structure-based phosphate activation mechanism of Glutaminase C with implications for cancer metabolism. *Proc Natl Acad Sci U S A* 109(4):1092–7, doi: 10.1073/pnas.1112495109.

Cesar-Razquin, A., B. Snijder, T. Frappier-Brinton et al. 2015. A call for systematic research on solute carriers. *Cell* 162(3):478–87, doi: 10.1016/j.cell.2015.07.022.

Chen, Z., Y. Wang, C. Warden, and S. Chen. 2015. Cross-talk between ER and HER2 regulates c-MYC-mediated glutamine metabolism in aromatase inhibitor resistant breast cancer cells. *J Steroid Biochem Mol Biol* 149:118–27, doi: 10.1016/j.jsbmb.2015.02.004.

Choi, J., H. Kim do, W. H. Jung, and J. S. Koo. 2013. Metabolic interaction between cancer cells and stromal cells according to breast cancer molecular subtype. *Breast Cancer Res* 15(5):R78, doi: 10.1186/bcr3472.

Christensen, H. N., L. M. Albritton, D. K. Kakuda, and C. L. MacLeod. 1994. Gene-product designations for amino acid transporters. *J Exp Biol* 196:51–7.

Colas, C., C. Grewer, N. J. Otte, A. Gameiro, T. Albers, K. Singh, H. Shere, M. Bonomi, J. Holst, and A. Schlessinger. 2015. Ligand Discovery for the Alanine-Serine-Cysteine Transporter (ASCT2, SLC1A5) from Homology Modeling and Virtual Screening. *PLoS Comput Biol* 11(10):e1004477, doi: 10.1371/journal.pcbi.1004477.

Collins, C. L., M. Wasa, W. W. Souba, and S. F. Abcouwer. 1998. Determinants of glutamine dependence and utilization by normal and tumor-derived breast cell lines. *J Cell Physiol* 176(1):166–78, doi: 10.1002/(sici)1097–4652(199807)176:1 < 166::aid-jcp18 > 3.0.co;2-5.

Cooper, A. J., B. F. Krasnikov, J. T. Pinto, H. F. Kung, J. Li, and K. Ploessl. 2012. Comparative enzymology of (2S,4R)4-fluoroglutamine and (2S,4R)4-fluoroglutamate. *Comp Biochem Physiol B Biochem Mol Biol* 163(1):108–20, doi: 10.1016/j.cbpb.2012.05.010.

Dai, L., Y. Cao, Y. Chen, C. Parsons, and Z. Qin. 2014. Targeting xCT, a cystine-glutamate transporter induces apoptosis and tumor regression for KSHV/HIV-associated lymphoma. *J Hematol Oncol* 7:30, doi: 10.1186/1756-8722-7-30.

Dal Bello, B., L. Rosa, N. Campanini, C. Tinelli, F. Torello Viera, G. D'Ambrosio, S. Rossi, and E. M. Silini. 2010. Glutamine synthetase immunostaining correlates with pathologic features of hepatocellular carcinoma and better survival after radiofrequency thermal ablation. *Clin Cancer Res* 16(7):2157–66, doi: 10.1158/1078-0432.ccr-09-1978.

Dang, C. V. 2010. Rethinking the Warburg effect with Myc micromanaging glutamine metabolism. *Cancer Res* 70(3):859–62, doi: 10.1158/0008-5472.CAN-09-3556.

Dang, C. V. 2012. MYC on the path to cancer. *Cell* 149(1):22–35, doi: 10.1016/j.cell.2012.03.003.

DeBerardinis, R. J. and T. Cheng. 2010. Q's next: The diverse functions of glutamine in metabolism, cell biology and cancer. *Oncogene* 29(3):313–24, doi: 10.1038/onc.2009.358.

DeBerardinis, R. J., A. Mancuso, E. Daikhin, I. Nissim, M. Yudkoff, S. Wehrli, and C. B. Thompson. 2007. Beyond aerobic glycolysis: Transformed cells can engage in glutamine metabolism that exceeds the requirement for protein and nucleotide synthesis. *Proc Natl Acad Sci U S A* 104(49):19345–50, doi: 10.1073/pnas.0709747104.

Diaz-Ruiz, R., M. Rigoulet, and A. Devin. 2011. The Warburg and Crabtree effects: On the origin of cancer cell energy metabolism and of yeast glucose repression. *Biochim Biophys Acta* 1807(6):568–76, doi: 10.1016/j.bbabio.2010.08.010.

Eagle, H., V. I. Oyama, M. Levy, C. L. Horton, and R. Fleischman. 1956. The growth response of mammalian cells in tissue culture to L-glutamine and L-glutamic acid. *J Biol Chem* 218(2):607–16.

Efeyan, A., R. Zoncu, and D. M. Sabatini. 2012. Amino acids and mTORC1: From lysosomes to disease. *Trends Mol Med* 18(9):524–33, doi: 10.1016/j.molmed.2012.05.007.

Eisenberg, D., H. S. Gill, G. M. Pfluegl, and S. H. Rotstein. 2000. Structure-function relationships of glutamine synthetases. *Biochim Biophys Acta* 1477(1–2):122–45.

Elgadi, K. M., R. A. Meguid, M. Qian, W. W. Souba, and S. F. Abcouwer. 1999. Cloning and analysis of unique human glutaminase isoforms generated by tissue-specific alternative splicing. *Physiol Genom* 1(2):51–62.

Emadi, A., S. A. Jun, T. Tsukamoto, A. T. Fathi, M. D. Minden, and C. V. Dang. 2014. Inhibition of glutaminase selectively suppresses the growth of primary acute myeloid leukemia cells with IDH mutations. *Exp Hematol* 42(4):247–51, doi: 10.1016/j.exphem.2013.12.001.

Esslinger, C. S., K. A. Cybulski, and J. F. Rhoderick. 2005. Ngamma-aryl glutamine analogues as probes of the ASCT2 neutral amino acid transporter binding site. *Bioorg Med Chem* 13(4):1111–8, doi: 10.1016/j.bmc.2004.11.028.

Ferreira, A. P., A. Cassago, A. Goncalves Kde et al. 2013. Active glutaminase C self-assembles into a supratetrameric oligomer that can be disrupted by an allosteric inhibitor. *J Biol Chem* 288(39):28009–20, doi: 10.1074/jbc.M113.501346.

Filipp, F. V., D. A. Scott, Z. A. Ronai, A. L. Osterman, and J. W. Smith. 2012. Reverse TCA cycle flux through isocitrate dehydrogenases 1 and 2 is required for lipogenesis in hypoxic melanoma cells. *Pigment Cell Melanoma Res* 25(3):375–83, doi: 10.1111/j.1755-148X.2012.00989.x.

Fischer, C. P., B. P. Bode, S. F. Abcouwer, G. C. Lukaszewicz, and W. W. Souba. 1995. Hepatic uptake of glutamine and other amino acids during infection and inflammation. *Shock* 3(5):315–22.

Fotiadis, D., Y. Kanai, and M. Palacin. 2013. The SLC3 and SLC7 families of amino acid transporters. *Mol Aspects Med* 34(2–3):139–58, doi: 10.1016/j.mam.2012.10.007.

Fuchs, B. C. and B. P. Bode. 2005. Amino acid transporters ASCT2 and LAT1 in cancer: Partners in crime? *Semin Cancer Biol* 15(4):254–66, doi: 10.1016/j.semcancer.2005.04.005.

Fuchs, B. C. and B. P. Bode. 2006. Stressing out over survival: Glutamine as an apoptotic modulator. *J Surg Res* 131(1):26–40, doi: 10.1016/j.jss.2005.07.013.

Fuchs, B. C., R. E. Finger, M. C. Onan, and B. P. Bode. 2007. ASCT2 silencing regulates mammalian target-of-rapamycin growth and survival signaling in human hepatoma cells. *Am J Physiol Cell Physiol* 293(1):C55–63, doi: 10.1152/ajpcell.00330.2006.

Fuchs, B. C., J. C. Perez, J. E. Suetterlin, S. B. Chaudhry, and B. P. Bode. 2004. Inducible antisense RNA targeting amino acid transporter ATB0/ASCT2 elicits apoptosis in human hepatoma cells. *Am J Physiol Gastrointest Liver Physiol* 286(3):G467–78.

Gallagher, F. A., M. I. Kettunen, S. E. Day, M. Lerche, and K. M. Brindle. 2008. 13C MR spectroscopy measurements of glutaminase activity in human hepatocellular carcinoma cells using hyperpolarized 13C-labeled glutamine. *Magn Reson Med* 60(2):253–7, doi: 10.1002/mrm.21650.

Goswami, M. T., G. Chen, B. V. Chakravarthi et al. 2015. Role and regulation of coordinately expressed *de novo* purine biosynthetic enzymes PPAT and PAICS in lung cancer. *Oncotarget* 6(27):23445–61.

Green, D. R. and J. E. Chipuk. 2006. p53 and metabolism: Inside the TIGAR. *Cell* 126(1):30–2, doi: 10.1016/j.cell.2006.06.032.

Grewer, C. and E. Grabsch. 2004. New inhibitors for the neutral amino acid transporter ASCT2 reveal its Na + -dependent anion leak. *J Physiol* 557(Pt 3):747–59, doi: 10.1113/jphysiol.2004.062521.

Guillaumond, F., J. L. Iovanna, and S. Vasseur. 2014. Pancreatic tumor cell metabolism: Focus on glycolysis and its connected metabolic pathways. *Arch Biochem Biophys* 545:69–73, doi: 10.1016/j.abb.2013.12.019.

Gupta, N., S. Miyauchi, R. G. Martindale, A. V. Herdman, R. Podolsky, K. Miyake, S. Mager, P. D. Prasad, M. E. Ganapathy, and V. Ganapathy. 2005. Upregulation of the amino acid transporter ATB0,+ (SLC6A14) in colorectal cancer and metastasis in humans. *Biochim Biophys Acta* 1741(1–2):215–23, doi: 10.1016/j.bbadis.2005.04.002.

Hassanein, M., M. R. Hight, J. R. Buck, M. N. Tantawy, M. L. Nickels, M. D. Hoeksema, B. K. Harris, K. Boyd, P. P. Massion, and H. C. Manning. 2016. Preclinical evaluation of 4-[F] fluoroglutamine PET to assess ASCT2 expression in lung cancer. *Mol Imaging Biol* 18(1):18–23, doi: 10.1007/s11307-015-0862-4.

Hassanein, M., M. D. Hoeksema, M. Shiota, J. Qian, B. K. Harris, H. Chen, J. E. Clark, W. E. Alborn, R. Eisenberg, and P. P. Massion. 2013. SLC1A5 mediates glutamine transport required for lung cancer cell growth and survival. *Clin Cancer Res* 19(3):560–70, doi: 10.1158/1078-0432.ccr-12-2334.

Hassanein, M., J. Qian, M. D. Hoeksema et al. 2015. Targeting SLC1a5-mediated glutamine dependence in non-small cell lung cancer. *Int J Cancer* 137(7):1587–97, doi: 10.1002/ijc.29535.

Haussinger, D. 1983. Hepatocyte heterogeneity in glutamine and ammonia metabolism and the role of an intercellular glutamine cycle during ureogenesis in perfused rat liver. *Eur J Biochem* 133(2):269–75.

Haussinger, D. and W. Gerok. 1984. Hepatocyte heterogeneity in ammonia metabolism: Impairment of glutamine synthesis in CCl4 induced liver cell necrosis with no effect on urea synthesis. *Chem Biol Interact* 48(2):191–4.

Haussinger, D. and F. Schliess. 2007. Glutamine metabolism and signaling in the liver. *Front Biosci* 12:371–91.

Haussinger, D., S. Soboll, A. J. Meijer, W. Gerok, J. M. Tager, and H. Sies. 1985. Role of plasma membrane transport in hepatic glutamine metabolism. *Eur J Biochem* 152(3):597–603.

Hediger, M. A., B. Clemencon, R. E. Burrier, and E. A. Bruford. 2013. The ABCs of membrane transporters in health and disease (SLC series): Introduction. *Mol Aspects Med* 34(2–3):95–107, doi: 10.1016/j.mam.2012.12.009.

Hediger, M. A., M. F. Romero, J. B. Peng, A. Rolfs, H. Takanaga, and E. A. Bruford. 2004. The ABCs of solute carriers: Physiological, pathological and therapeutic implications of human membrane transport proteinsIntroduction. *Pflugers Arch* 447(5):465–8, doi: 10.1007/s00424-003-1192-y.

Hirayama, C., K. Suyama, Y. Horie, K. Tanimoto, and S. Kato. 1987. Plasma amino acid patterns in hepatocellular carcinoma. *Biochem Med Metab Biol* 38(2):127–33.

Holleran, A. L., D. A. Briscoe, G. Fiskum, and J. K. Kelleher. 1995. Glutamine metabolism in AS-30D hepatoma cells. Evidence for its conversion into lipids via reductive carboxylation. *Mol Cell Biochem* 152(2):95–101.

Hsu, Peggy P., and David M. Sabatini. 2008. Cancer cell metabolism: Warburg and beyond. *Cell* 134(5):703–7. doi: http://dx.doi.org/10.1016/j.cell.2008.08.021

Huang, F., Y. Zhao, J. Zhao, S. Wu, Y. Jiang, H. Ma, and T. Zhang. 2014. Upregulated SLC1A5 promotes cell growth and survival in colorectal cancer. *Int J Clin Exp Pathol* 7(9):6006–14.

Icard, P., P. Kafara, J. M. Steyaert, L. Schwartz, and H. Lincet. 2014. The metabolic cooperation between cells in solid cancer tumors. *Biochim Biophys Acta* 1846(1):216–25, doi: 10.1016/j.bbcan.2014.06.002.

Ishii, T. and G. E. Mann. 2014. Redox status in mammalian cells and stem cells during culture *in vitro*: Critical roles of Nrf2 and cystine transporter activity in the maintenance of redox balance. *Redox Biol* 2:786–94, doi: 10.1016/j.redox.2014.04.008.

Jang, M., S. S. Kim, and J. Lee. 2013. Cancer cell metabolism: Implications for therapeutic targets. *Exp Mol Med* 45:e45, doi: 10.1038/emm.2013.85.

Jenstad, M. and F. A. Chaudhry. 2013. The Amino Acid Transporters of the Glutamate/GABA-Glutamine Cycle and Their Impact on Insulin and Glucagon Secretion. *Front Endocrinol (Lausanne)* 4:199, doi: 10.3389/fendo.2013.00199.

Jeon, Y. J., S. Khelifa, B. Ratnikov et al. 2015. Regulation of glutamine carrier proteins by RNF5 determines breast cancer response to ER stress-inducing chemotherapies. *Cancer Cell* 27(3):354–69, doi: 10.1016/j.ccell.2015.02.006.

Jiang, L., N. Kon, T. Li, S. J. Wang, T. Su, H. Hibshoosh, R. Baer, and W. Gu. 2015. Ferroptosis as a p53-mediated activity during tumour suppression. *Nature* 520(7545):57–62, doi: 10.1038/nature14344.

Kairemo, K. and N. Rasulova. 2014. Preliminary clinical experience of trans-1-amino-3-(18)F-fluorocyclobutane carboxylic acid (anti-(18)F-FACBC) PET/CT imaging in prostate cancer patients. 2014:305182, doi: 10.1155/2014/305182.

Kanai, Y., B. Clemencon, A. Simonin, M. Leuenberger, M. Lochner, M. Weisstanner, and M. A. Hediger. 2013. The SLC1 high-affinity glutamate and neutral amino acid transporter family. *Mol Aspects Med* 34(2–3):108–20, doi: 10.1016/j.mam.2013.01.001.

Karunakaran, S., S. Ramachandran, V. Coothankandaswamy et al. 2011. SLC6A14 (ATB0,+) protein, a highly concentrative and broad specific amino acid transporter, is a novel and effective drug target for treatment of estrogen receptor-positive breast cancer. *J Biol Chem* 286(36):31830–8, doi: 10.1074/jbc.M111.229518.

Katt, W. P., S. Ramachandran, J. W. Erickson, and R. A. Cerione. 2012. Dibenzophenanthridines as inhibitors of glutaminase C and cancer cell proliferation. *Mol Cancer Ther* 11(6):1269–78, doi: 10.1158/1535-7163. mct-11-0942.

Kekuda, R., P. D. Prasad, Y. J. Fei, V. Torres-Zamorano, S. Sinha, T. L. Yang-Feng, F. H. Leibach, and V. Ganapathy. 1996. Cloning of the sodium-dependent, broad-scope, neutral amino acid transporter Bo from a human placental choriocarcinoma cell line. *J Biol Chem* 271(31):18657–61.

Kilberg, M. S., H. N. Christensen, and M. E. Handlogten. 1979. Cysteine as a system-specific substrate for transport system ASC in rat hepatocytes. *Biochem Biophys Res Commun* 88(2):744–51.

Kilberg, M. S., M. E. Handlogten, and H. N. Christensen. 1980. Characteristics of an amino acid transport system in rat liver for glutamine, asparagine, histidine, and closely related analogs. *J Biol Chem* 255(9):4011–9.

Kim, S., W. H. Jung, and J. S. Koo. 2013a. The expression of glutamine-metabolism-related proteins in breast phyllodes tumors. *Tumour Biol* 34(5):2683–9, doi: 10.1007/s13277-013-0819-7.

Kim, S., H. Kim do, W. H. Jung, and J. S. Koo. 2013b. Expression of glutamine metabolism-related proteins according to molecular subtype of breast cancer. *Endocr Relat Cancer* 20(3):339–48, doi: 10.1530/ERC-12-0398.

Ko, Y. H., Z. Lin, N. Flomenberg, R. G. Pestell, A. Howell, F. Sotgia, M. P. Lisanti, and U. E. Martinez-Outschoorn. 2011. Glutamine fuels a vicious cycle of autophagy in the tumor stroma and oxidative mitochondrial metabolism in epithelial cancer cells: Implications for preventing chemotherapy resistance. *Cancer Biol Ther* 12(12):1085–97, doi: 10.4161/cbt.12.12.18671.

Kumar, R., H. Dhanpathi, S. Basu, D. Rubello, S. Fanti, and A. Alavi. 2008. Oncologic PET tracers beyond [(18)F]FDG and the novel quantitative approaches in PET imaging. *Q J Nucl Med Mol Imaging* 52(1):50–65.

Labow, B. I., W. W. Souba, and S. F. Abcouwer. 2001. Mechanisms governing the expression of the enzymes of glutamine metabolism—glutaminase and glutamine synthetase. *J Nutr* 131(9 Suppl):2467S–74S; discussion 2486S–7S.

Le, A., A. N. Lane, M. Hamaker et al. 2012. Glucose-independent glutamine metabolism via TCA cycling for proliferation and survival in B cells. *Cell Metab* 15(1):110–21, doi: 10.1016/j.cmet.2011.12.009.

Li, L., A. C. Paz, B. A. Wilky, B. Johnson, K. Galoian, A. Rosenberg, G. Hu, G. Tinoco, O. Bodamer, and J. C. Trent. 2015. Treatment with a small molecule mutant IDH1 inhibitor suppresses tumorigenic activity and decreases production of the oncometabolite 2-Hydroxyglutarate in human chondrosarcoma cells. *PLoS One* 10(9):e0133813, doi: 10.1371/journal.pone.0133813.

Lieberman, B. P., K. Ploessl, L. Wang, W. Qu, Z. Zha, D. R. Wise, L. A. Chodosh, G. Belka, C. B. Thompson, and H. F. Kung. 2011. PET imaging of glutaminolysis in tumors by 18F-(2S,4R)4-fluoroglutamine. *J Nucl Med* 52(12):1947–55, doi: 10.2967/jnumed.111.093815.

Lisanti, M. P., U. E. Martinez-Outschoorn, and F. Sotgia. 2013. Oncogenes induce the cancer-associated fibroblast phenotype: Metabolic symbiosis and "fibroblast addiction" are new therapeutic targets for drug discovery. *Cell Cycle* 12(17):2723–32, doi: 10.4161/cc.25695.

Liu, Y., A. S. Hyde, M. A. Simpson, and J. J. Barycki. 2014. Emerging regulatory paradigms in glutathione metabolism. *Adv Cancer Res* 122:69–101, doi: 10.1016/b978-0-12-420117-0.00002-5.

Llorca, O., M. Betti, J. M. Gonzalez, A. Valencia, A. J. Marquez, and J. M. Valpuesta. 2006. The three-dimensional structure of an eukaryotic glutamine synthetase: Functional implications of its oligomeric structure. *J Struct Biol* 156(3):469–79, doi: 10.1016/j.jsb.2006.06.003.

Lo, R. C. and I. O. Ng. 2011. Hepatocellular tumors: Immunohistochemical analyses for classification and prognostication. *Chin J Cancer Res* 23(4):245–53, doi: 10.1007/s11670-011-0245-6.

Lukey, M. J., K. F. Wilson, and R. A. Cerione. 2013. Therapeutic strategies impacting cancer cell glutamine metabolism. *Future Med Chem* 5(14):1685–700, doi: 10.4155/fmc.13.130.

Ma, Z., D. J. Vocadlo, and K. Vosseller. 2013. Hyper-O-GlcNAcylation is anti-apoptotic and maintains constitutive NF-kappaB activity in pancreatic cancer cells. *J Biol Chem* 288(21):15121–30, doi: 10.1074/jbc.M113.470047.

Ma, Z. and K. Vosseller. 2014. Cancer metabolism and elevated O-GlcNAc in oncogenic signaling. *J Biol Chem* 289(50):34457–65, doi: 10.1074/jbc.R114.577718.

Macintyre, A. N. and J. C. Rathmell. 2013. Activated lymphocytes as a metabolic model for carcinogenesis. *Cancer Metab* 1(1):5, doi: 10.1186/2049-3002-1-5.

Mannion, B. A., T. V. Kolesnikova, S. H. Lin, S. Wang, N. L. Thompson, and M. E. Hemler. 1998. The light chain of CD98 is identified as E16/TA1 protein. *J Biol Chem* 273(50):33127–9.

Mao, Y., E. T. Keller, D. H. Garfield, K. Shen, and J. Wang. 2013. Stromal cells in tumor microenvironment and breast cancer. *Cancer Metastasis Rev* 32(1–2):303–15, doi: 10.1007/s10555-012-9415-3.

Marelli-Berg, F. M., H. Fu, and C. Mauro. 2012. Molecular mechanisms of metabolic reprogramming in proliferating cells: Implications for T-cell-mediated immunity. *Immunology* 136(4):363–9, doi: 10.1111/j.1365-2567.2012.03583.x.

Martinez-Outschoorn, U. E., M. P. Lisanti, and F. Sotgia. 2014. Catabolic cancer-associated fibroblasts transfer energy and biomass to anabolic cancer cells, fueling tumor growth. *Semin Cancer Biol* 25:47–60, doi: 10.1016/j.semcancer.2014.01.005.

Martinez-Outschoorn, U. E., S. Pavlides, A. Howell, R. G. Pestell, H. B. Tanowitz, F. Sotgia, and M. P. Lisanti. 2011. Stromal-epithelial metabolic coupling in cancer: Integrating autophagy and metabolism in the tumor microenvironment. *Int J Biochem Cell Biol* 43(7):1045–51, doi: 10.1016/j.biocel.2011.01.023.

Martinez-Outschoorn, U., F. Sotgia, and M. P. Lisanti. 2014. Tumor microenvironment and metabolic synergy in breast cancers: Critical importance of mitochondrial fuels and function. *Semin Oncol* 41(2):195–216, doi: 10.1053/j.seminoncol.2014.03.002.

McKenna, M. C. 2007. The glutamate-glutamine cycle is not stoichiometric: Fates of glutamate in brain. *J Neurosci Res* 85(15):3347–58, doi: 10.1002/jnr.21444.

Meng, L. H. and X. S. Zheng. 2015. Toward rapamycin analog (rapalog)-based precision cancer therapy. *Acta Pharmacol Sin* 36(10):1163–9, doi: 10.1038/aps.2015.68.

Metallo, C. M., P. A. Gameiro, E. L. Bell et al. 2012. Reductive glutamine metabolism by IDH1 mediates lipogenesis under hypoxia. *Nature* 481(7381):380–4, doi: 10.1038/nature10602.

Morandi, A. and P. Chiarugi. 2014. Metabolic implication of tumor:stroma crosstalk in breast cancer. *J Mol Med (Berl)* 92(2):117–26, doi: 10.1007/s00109-014-1124-7.

Mouilleron, S. and B. Golinelli-Pimpaneau. 2007. Conformational changes in ammonia-channeling glutamine amidotransferases. *Curr Opin Struct Biol* 17(6):653–64, doi: 10.1016/j.sbi.2007.09.003.

Nakaya, M., Y. Xiao, X. Zhou, J. H. Chang, M. Chang, X. Cheng, M. Blonska, X. Lin, and S. C. Sun. 2014. Inflammatory T cell responses rely on amino acid transporter ASCT2 facilitation of glutamine uptake and mTORC1 kinase activation. *Immunity* 40(5):692–705, doi: 10.1016/j.immuni.2014.04.007.

Newsholme, E. A. and P. C. Calder. 1997. The proposed role of glutamine in some cells of the immune system and speculative consequences for the whole animal. *Nutrition* 13(7–8):728–30.

Newsholme, P. 2001. Why is L-glutamine metabolism important to cells of the immune system in health, postinjury, surgery or infection? *J Nutr* 131(9 Suppl):2515S–22S; discussion 2523S–4S.

Nicklin, P., P. Bergman, B. Zhang et al. 2009. Bidirectional transport of amino acids regulates mTOR and autophagy. *Cell* 136(3):521–34, doi: 10.1016/j.cell.2008.11.044.

Nikkuni, O., K. Kaira, M. Toyoda et al. 2015. Expression of amino acid transporters (LAT1 and ASCT2) in patients with stage III/IV laryngeal squamous cell carcinoma. *Pathol Oncol Res* 21(4):1175–81, doi: 10.1007/s12253-015-9954-3.

Okudaira, H., T. Nakanishi, S. Oka, M. Kobayashi, H. Tamagami, D. M. Schuster, M. M. Goodman, Y. Shirakami, I. Tamai, and K. Kawai. 2013. Kinetic analyses of trans-1-amino-3-[18F]fluorocyclobutanecarboxylic acid transport in Xenopus laevis oocytes expressing human ASCT2 and SNAT2. *Nucl Med Biol* 40(5):670–5, doi: 10.1016/j.nucmedbio.2013.03.009.

Okudaira, H., N. Shikano, R. Nishii et al. 2011. Putative transport mechanism and intracellular fate of trans-1-amino-3-18F-fluorocyclobutanecarboxylic acid in human prostate cancer. *J Nucl Med* 52(5):822–9, doi: 10.2967/jnumed.110.086074.

Ono, M., S. Oka, H. Okudaira, T. Nakanishi, A. Mizokami, M. Kobayashi, D. M. Schuster, M. M. Goodman, Y. Shirakami, and K. Kawai. 2015. [(14)C]Fluciclovine (alias anti-[(14)C]FACBC) uptake and ASCT2 expression in castration-resistant prostate cancer cells. *Nucl Med Biol* 42(11):887–92, doi: 10.1016/j.nucmedbio.2015.07.005.

Ono, M., S. Oka, H. Okudaira, D. M. Schuster, M. M. Goodman, K. Kawai, and Y. Shirakami. 2013. Comparative evaluation of transport mechanisms of trans-1-amino-3-[(1)(8)F]fluorocyclobutanecarboxylic acid and L-[methyl-(1)(1)C]methionine in human glioma cell lines. *Brain Res* 1535:24–37, doi: 10.1016/j.brainres.2013.08.037.

Otto, A. M., J. Hintermair, and C. Janzon. 2015. NADH-Linked metabolic plasticity of MCF-7 breast cancer cells surviving in a nutrient-deprived microenvironment. *J Cell Biochem* 116(5):822–35, doi: 10.1002/jcb.25038.

Parekh, P. J. and L. A. Balart. 2015. Ammonia and its role in the pathogenesis of hepatic encephalopathy. *Clin Liver Dis* 19(3):529–37, doi: 10.1016/j.cld.2015.05.002.

Parker, S. J. and C. M. Metallo. 2015. Metabolic consequences of oncogenic IDH mutations. *Pharmacol Ther* 152:54–62, doi: 10.1016/j.pharmthera.2015.05.003.

Parry-Billings, M., B. Leighton, G. D. Dimitriadis, R. Curi, J. Bond, S. Bevan, A. Colquhoun, and E. A. Newsholme. 1991. The effect of tumour bearing on skeletal muscle glutamine metabolism. *Int J Biochem* 23(9):933–7.

Pisters, P. W. and D. B. Pearlstone. 1993. Protein and amino acid metabolism in cancer cachexia: Investigative techniques and therapeutic interventions. *Crit Rev Clin Lab Sci* 30(3):223–72, doi: 10.3109/10408369309084669.

Ploessl, K., L. Wang, B. P. Lieberman, W. Qu, and H. F. Kung. 2012. Comparative evaluation of 18F-labeled glutamic acid and glutamine as tumor metabolic imaging agents. *J Nucl Med* 53(10):1616–24. doi: 10.2967/jnumed.111.101279.

Pochini, L., M. Scalise, M. Galluccio, and C. Indiveri. 2014. Membrane transporters for the special amino acid glutamine: Structure/function relationships and relevance to human health. *Front Chem* 2:61. doi: 10.3389/fchem.2014.00061.

Qu, W., S. Oya, B. P. Lieberman, K. Ploessl, L. Wang, D. R. Wise, C. R. Divgi, L. A. Chodosh, C. B. Thompson, and H. F. Kung. 2012. Preparation and characterization of L-[5-11C]-glutamine for metabolic imaging of tumors. *J Nucl Med* 53(1):98–105, doi: 10.2967/jnumed.111.093831.

Qu, W., Z. Zha, B. P. Lieberman, A. Mancuso, M. Stetz, R. Rizzi, K. Ploessl, D. Wise, C. Thompson, and H. F. Kung. 2011a. Facile synthesis [5-(13)C-4-(2)H(2)]-L-glutamine for hyperpolarized MRS imaging of cancer cell metabolism. *Acad Radiol* 18(8):932–9, doi: 10.1016/j.acra.2011.05.002.

Qu, W., Z. Zha, K. Ploessl, B. P. Lieberman, L. Zhu, D. R. Wise, C. B. Thompson, and H. F. Kung. 2011b. Synthesis of optically pure 4-fluoro-glutamines as potential metabolic imaging agents for tumors. *J Am Chem Soc* 133(4):1122–33, doi: 10.1021/ja109203d.

Rajagopalan, K. N. and R. J. DeBerardinis. 2011. Role of glutamine in cancer: Therapeutic and imaging implications. *J Nucl Med* 52(7):1005–8, doi: 10.2967/jnumed.110.084244.

Ren, J., L. Yuan, G. Wen, and J. Yang. 2016. The value of anti-1-amino-3-18F-fluorocyclobutane-1-carboxylic acid PET/CT in the diagnosis of recurrent prostate carcinoma: A meta-analysis. *Acta Radiol* 57(4): 487–93, doi: 10.1177/0284185115581541.

Rennie, M. J., H. S. Hundal, P. Babij, P. MacLennan, P. M. Taylor, P. W. Watt, M. M. Jepson, and D. J. Millward. 1986. Characteristics of a glutamine carrier in skeletal muscle have important consequences for nitrogen loss in injury, infection, and chronic disease. *Lancet* 2(8514):1008–12.

Reynolds, M. R., A. N. Lane, B. Robertson, S. Kemp, Y. Liu, B. G. Hill, D. C. Dean, and B. F. Clem. 2014. Control of glutamine metabolism by the tumor suppressor Rb. *Oncogene* 33(5):556–66, doi: 10.1038/onc.2012.635.

Robinson, M. M., S. J. McBryant, T. Tsukamoto, C. Rojas, D. V. Ferraris, S. K. Hamilton, J. C. Hansen, and N. P. Curthoys. 2007. Novel mechanism of inhibition of rat kidney-type glutaminase by bis-2-(5-phenylacetamido-1,2,4-thiadiazol-2-yl)ethyl sulfide (BPTES). *Biochem J* 406 (3):407–14, doi: 10.1042/bj20070039.

Rudnick, G., R. Kramer, R. D. Blakely, D. L. Murphy, and F. Verrey. 2014. The SLC6 transporters: Perspectives on structure, functions, regulation, and models for transporter dysfunction. *Pflugers Arch* 466(1):25–42, doi: 10.1007/s00424-013-1410-1.

Scalise, M., L. Pochini, S. Panni, P. Pingitore, K. Hedfalk, and C. Indiveri. 2014. Transport mechanism and regulatory properties of the human amino acid transporter ASCT2 (SLC1A5). *Amino Acids* 46(11):2463–75, doi: 10.1007/s00726-014-1808-x.

Schulte, M. L., E. S. Dawson, S. A. Saleh, M. L. Cuthbertson, and H. C. Manning. 2015. 2-Substituted Ngamma-glutamylanilides as novel probes of ASCT2 with improved potency. *Bioorg Med Chem Lett* 25(1):113–6, doi: 10.1016/j.bmcl.2014.10.098.

Schuster, D. M., C. Nanni, S. Fanti et al. 2014. Anti-1-amino-3-18F-fluorocyclobutane-1-carboxylic acid: Physiologic uptake patterns, incidental findings, and variants that may simulate disease. *J Nucl Med* 55(12):1986–92, doi: 10.2967/jnumed.114.143628.

Seltzer, M. J., B. D. Bennett, A. D. Joshi et al. 2010. Inhibition of glutaminase preferentially slows growth of glioma cells with mutant IDH1. *Cancer Res* 70(22):8981–7, doi: 10.1158/0008-5472.can-10-1666.

Souba, W. W. 1992. *Glutamine: Physiology, Biochemistry and Nutrition in Critical Illness, Medical Intelligence Unit.* Austin, TX: R.G. Landes Co.

Stalnecker, C. A., S. M. Ulrich, Y. Li, S. Ramachandran, M. K. McBrayer, R. J. DeBerardinis, R. A. Cerione, and J. W. Erickson. 2015. Mechanism by which a recently discovered allosteric inhibitor blocks glutamine metabolism in transformed cells. *Proc Natl Acad Sci U S A* 112(2):394–9, doi: 10.1073/pnas.1414056112.

Storey, B. T., C. Fugere, A. Lesieur-Brooks, C. Vaslet, and N. L. Thompson. 2005. Adenoviral modulation of the tumor-associated system L amino acid transporter, LAT1, alters amino acid transport, cell growth and 4F2/CD98 expressionwith cell-type specific effects in cultured hepatic cells. *Int J Cancer* 117(3):387–97, doi: 10.1002/ijc.21169.

Torgner, I. and E. Kvamme. 1990. Synthesis of transmitter glutamate and the glial-neuron interrelationship. *Mol Chem Neuropathol* 12(1):11–7.

van Geldermalsen, M., Q. Wang, R. Nagarajah et al. 2016. ASCT2/SLC1A5 controls glutamine uptake and tumour growth in triple-negative basal-like breast cancer. *Oncogene* 35(24):3201–8, doi: 10.1038/onc.2015.381.

Vander Heiden, M. G., L. C. Cantley, and C. B. Thompson. 2009. Understanding the Warburg effect: The metabolic requirements of cell proliferation. *Science* 324(5930):1029–33, doi: 10.1126/science.1160809.

Vasconcelos-Dos-Santos, A., I. A. Oliveira, M. C. Lucena, N. R. Mantuano, S. A. Whelan, W. B. Dias, and A. R. Todeschini. 2015. Biosynthetic machinery involved in aberrant glycosylation: Promising targets for developing of drugs against cancer. *Front Oncol* 5:138, doi: 10.3389/fonc.2015.00138.

Venneti, S., M. P. Dunphy, H. Zhang et al. 2015. Glutamine-based PET imaging facilitates enhanced metabolic evaluation of gliomas *in vivo. Sci Transl Med* 7(274):274ra17, doi: 10.1126/scitranslmed.aaa1009.

Verrey, F. 2003. System L: Heteromeric exchangers of large, neutral amino acids involved in directional transport. *Pflugers Arch* 445(5):529–33, doi: 10.1007/s00424-002-0973-z.

Verrey, F., E. I. Closs, C. A. Wagner, M. Palacin, H. Endou, and Y. Kanai. 2004. CATs and HATs: The SLC7 family of amino acid transporters. *Pflugers Arch* 447(5):532–42, doi: 10.1007/s00424-003-1086-z.

Wang, J. B., J. W. Erickson, R. Fuji et al. 2010. Targeting mitochondrial glutaminase activity inhibits oncogenic transformation. *Cancer Cell* 18(3):207–19, doi: 10.1016/j.ccr.2010.08.009.

Wang, Q., K. A. Beaumont, N. J. Otte et al. 2014. Targeting glutamine transport to suppress melanoma cell growth. *Int J Cancer* 135(5):1060–71, doi: 10.1002/ijc.28749.

Wang, Q., R. A. Hardie, A. J. Hoy et al. 2015. Targeting ASCT2-mediated glutamine uptake blocks prostate cancer growth and tumour development. *J Pathol* 236(3):278–89, doi: 10.1002/path.4518.

Waniewski, R. A. and D. L. Martin. 1986. Exogenous glutamate is metabolized to glutamine and exported by rat primary astrocyte cultures. *J Neurochem* 47(1):304–13.

Weiner, I. D. and J. W. Verlander. 2013. Renal ammonia metabolism and transport. *Compr Physiol* 3(1):201–20, doi: 10.1002/cphy.c120010.

Wellen, K. E., C. Lu, A. Mancuso, J. M. Lemons, M. Ryczko, J. W. Dennis, J. D. Rabinowitz, H. A. Coller, and C. B. Thompson. 2010. The hexosamine biosynthetic pathway couples growth factor-induced glutamine uptake to glucose metabolism. *Genes Dev* 24(24):2784–99, doi: 10.1101/gad.1985910.

Wernerman, J. 2011. Glutamine supplementation. *Ann Intensive Care* 1(1):25.

Wilson, D. M. and J. Kurhanewicz. 2014. Hyperpolarized 13C MR for molecular imaging of prostate cancer. *J Nucl Med* 55(10):1567–72, doi: 10.2967/jnumed.114.141705.

Windmueller, H. G. and A. E. Spaeth. 1978. Identification of ketone bodies and glutamine as the major respiratory fuels *in vivo* for postabsorptive rat small intestine. *J Biol Chem* 253(1):69–76.

Wise, D. R., R. J. DeBerardinis, A. Mancuso et al. 2008. Myc regulates a transcriptional program that stimulates mitochondrial glutaminolysis and leads to glutamine addiction. *Proc Natl Acad Sci U S A* 105(48):18782–7, doi: 10.1073/pnas.0810199105.

Witney, T. H. and K. M. Brindle. 2010. Imaging tumour cell metabolism using hyperpolarized 13C magnetic resonance spectroscopy. *Biochem Soc Trans* 38(5):1220–4, doi: 10.1042/BST0381220.

Wu, Z., Z. Zha, G. Li, B. P. Lieberman, S. R. Choi, K. Ploessl, and H. F. Kung. 2014. [(18)F](2S,4S)-4-(3-Fluoropropyl) glutamine as a tumor imaging agent. *Mol Pharm* 11(11):3852–66, doi: 10.1021/mp500236y.

Xu, D. and M. E. Hemler. 2005. Metabolic activation-related CD147-CD98 complex. *Mol Cell Proteomics* 4(8):1061–71, doi: 10.1074/mcp.M400207-MCP200.

Yanagida, O., Y. Kanai, A. Chairoungdua et al. 2001. Human L-type amino acid transporter 1 (LAT1): Characterization of function and expression in tumor cell lines. *Biochim Biophys Acta* 1514(2):291–302.

Yang, C., J. Sudderth, T. Dang, R. M. Bachoo, J. G. McDonald, and R. J. DeBerardinis. 2009. Glioblastoma cells require glutamate dehydrogenase to survive impairments of glucose metabolism or Akt signaling. *Cancer Res* 69(20):7986–93, doi: 10.1158/0008-5472.can-09-2266.

Yen, K. E., M. A. Bittinger, S. M. Su, and V. R. Fantin. 2010. Cancer-associated IDH mutations: Biomarker and therapeutic opportunities. *Oncogene* 29(49):6409–17, doi: 10.1038/onc.2010.444.

Yoshida, S., A. Kaibara, N. Ishibashi, and K. Shirouzu. 2001. Glutamine supplementation in cancer patients. *Nutrition* 17(9):766–8.

20 Glutamine as a New Therapeutic Target in Cancer
Use of Hyperpolarized Magnetic Resonance Spectroscopy

Dominique Meynial-Denis and Jean-Pierre Renou

CONTENTS

20.1 HYPERPOLARIZATION

20.1.1 RULES

Nuclear magnetic resonance (NMR) is a noninvasive and nondestructive technique, which is inherently low sensitive. Magnetic resonance imaging (MRI) is widely used in clinical applications because its low sensitivity is compensated for by the high concentration of water in the human body. Although the ^{1}H NMR image can be acquired easily and quickly, the method cannot be used for metabolism studies. Metabolite concentrations (close to mM) are much lower than water concentration in biological tissues (Ross et al. 2003). ^{13}C is the only isotope of carbon observable in metabolic studies. For example, despite the low natural abundance of ^{13}C (1.1%) and its gyromagnetic ratio, ^{13}C spectroscopy has uncovered hitherto unknown brain disorders *in vivo* and is an inexpensive method of diagnosis in neonates, children, adults, and elderly patients (Ross et al. 2003). Hyperpolarized MRI is a powerful technique that allows real-time monitoring of metabolites at concentration levels not accessible by standard MRI techniques. Hyperpolarization has extended the ability to detect and quantify cellular metabolism *in vivo*. Different methods can enhance the polarization of nuclear spins. One of these, Dynamic Nuclear Polarization (DNP), involves transfer of polarization from an electron spin to a nuclear spin in the solid state (Abragam and Goldman 1978). A small aliquot of metabolites is polarized and paramagnetic radicals are mixed and rapidly frozen. In glass phase, the mixture is placed in the hyperpolarizer magnet. The electronic spins in the radicals are in the low-energy state and aligned with the main magnetic field. This polarization is transferred to the nuclear spins by microwave irradiation close to the electronic Larmor frequency. The frozen hyperpolarized material is then quickly melted and dissolved in a preheated and pressurized (~1000 kPa) buffered aqueous solution. The dissolved material is collected at room temperature for its injection (Leftin et al. 2014).

Enhanced polarization, which is due mainly to the solid effect and the thermal mixing mechanism, produces a drastic 10,000-fold gain of ^{13}C detection (Ardenkjaer-Larsen et al. 2003). Although the DNP methodology is very versatile, it can be applied to a wide range of molecules labeled with ^{13}C or any other nucleus such as ^{15}N (Nonaka et al. 2013). A method for simultaneous polarization of four ^{13}C labeled substrates ([1-^{13}C] pyruvate, ^{13}C sodium bicarbonate, [1,4-^{13}C] fumarate, and ^{13}C urea) was recently developed; so, a single intravenous bolus of these metabolites provided multiple metabolic and physiological measurements in a single *in vivo* experiment (Wilson et al. 2010). A polarizer equipped with a magnet having a large homogeneous volume is able to polarize four samples in parallel (Ardenkjaer-Larsen et al. 2011; Hu et al. 2013). Improvements have also been made in the dissolution process for studies involving compounds with limited solubility (Bowen and Ardenkjaer-Larsen 2014).

20.1.2 SAFETY

The hyperpolarized agents prepared via DNP are injected into cell suspensions or the whole body of animals or humans. For clinical applications, a sterile fluid path was developed to maintain all products involved in the DNP process in a sterile environment (Ardenkjaer-Larsen et al. 2011). Most of the radicals can be filtered out before injection (Nelson et al. 2013). However, the filtering step is time consuming and slows down the protocol, thereby leading to reduced sensitivity. Eichhorn et al. developed a variant of dissolution DNP of frozen neat pyruvic acid (Eichhorn et al. 2013), without the explicit addition of persistent radicals by ultraviolet irradiation.

20.1.3 ACQUISITION

A principal limitation of the technique is the very short lifetime of the hyperpolarization. The loss of hyperpolarization is determined by the longitudinal relaxation time (T_1) (Rowland et al. 2010). Protonated carbons have a short T_1 owing to the dipole–dipole relaxation mechanism. The use of deuterated molecules in deuterated water extends the lifetime of polarization (Allouche-Arnon et al. 2011; Barb et al. 2011, 2013). Other techniques using long-lived singlet states can extend the hyperpolarized lifetime and therefore the potential imaging window (Warren et al. 2009; Pileio et al. 2010; Mishkovsky et al. 2012; Feng et al. 2013). These transfer pulse sequences, which enhance the signal of short-T_1 nuclear spins, have to be simple in order to be implemented on clinical spectrometers and compatible with surface coils.

Specific pulse sequences have been developed to accelerate acquisitions, and thus to improve sensitivity (signal to noise ratio) (Josan et al. 2011; Tropp et al. 2011; von Morze et al. 2011). Selective excitation of the limited frequency band has been proposed as a means to overcome the large frequency range (160 ppm for ^{13}C) to be covered (Josan et al. 2014; Larson et al. 2010, 2011). A recent study showed that it was possible to obtain two-dimensional images *in vivo* simultaneously for several compounds within 100 ms by single-shot spatiotemporal encoding (Schmidt et al. 2014). Different strategies have been developed to reduce the acquisition time. Parallel imaging associated with partial Fourier acquisition provided a 3.75 factor acceleration (Ohliger et al. 2013) of the same order of magnitude as that found with reconstruction based on compressed sensing (Hu et al. 2010). These developments open up possible applications in a clinical setting.

20.1.4 MODELING

The observed rate of hyperpolarized substances depends on the rate of delivery to the tumor, transport into the cell, and enzymatic activity. Quantification of metabolic conversion by kinetic modeling has been developed for the analysis of pyruvate to lactate exchange (Lupo et al. 2010; Zierhut et al. 2010; Harrison et al. 2012; Kazan et al. 2013).

20.2 HYPERPOLARIZATION AND ONCOLOGY

A major challenge in cancer biology is to monitor and understand cancer metabolism *in vivo* with the aim of improving diagnosis and possibly therapy. Metabolic properties in cancer cells differ from those in normal tissue. The energy needed for cellular processes arises from aerobic glycolysis in cancer cells (glucose is actively consumed by these cells leading to the formation of lactate) while in normal cells it arises primarily from oxidative phosphorylation (Vander Heiden et al. 2009). This phenomenon, known as "the Warburg effect," is illustrated in the case of glutamine in this chapter (Section 20.3.1). For this, mitochondrial *glutaminase*, which is a hallmark of tumor metabolism, is studied with the isotopes ^{13}C and ^{2}D.

A major issue involving hyperpolarized Magnetic Resonance Spectroscopy (MRS) is the relatively short duration of polarization. This means that, to study metabolism, the substrate must be rapidly transported through the bloodstream to the tissue of interest, be rapidly taken up by the cell, and be rapidly metabolized. Information on the metabolism of substances that are quickly metabolized can be obtained by detection of hyperpolarized products that are imaged (Kurhanewicz et al. 2011). The section below describes the potential of the different substrates that have been successfully hyperpolarized and how they can improve imaging cellular metabolism in cancer in both preclinical and clinical models.

20.2.1 HYPERPOLARIZED ^{13}C PYRUVATE

[1-^{13}C] pyruvate is the most widely investigated hyperpolarized molecular probe (Day et al. 2007). It has excellent physical properties: a relatively long T_1 relaxation time, ease of high polarization, and fast polarization build-up. The pyruvate molecule plays a key role in cellular metabolism owing to its very rapid transport across the cell membrane and consequently, pyruvate has been widely used to detect metabolic changes. The high solubility of this molecule in water is an important factor because it means that the concentration of the hyperpolarized pyruvate is still relatively high after dissolution. Pyruvate, the end product of glycolysis, can be reduced to lactate in the reaction catalyzed by the enzyme *lactate dehydrogenase (LDH)*. Alternatively, pyruvate undergoes transamination with glutamate to form alanine, in the reaction catalyzed by *alanine transaminase (ALT)*. A third reaction involves the irreversible decarboxylation of [1-^{13}C] pyruvate to hyperpolarized ^{13}C-labeled carbon dioxide in the reaction catalyzed by the mitochondrial enzyme, *pyruvate dehydrogenase (PDH)*. The reactions catalyzed by LDH and ALT are altered in cancer. Indeed, an increase in aerobic glycolysis is a fundamental property of cancer cells. The transformation of injected pyruvate into alanine and lactate can be noninvasively imaged and used to map the metabolic differences between normal and cancerous tissue within a biologically relevant time frame (seconds) (Golman et al. 2006). It has been shown that in precancerous tissue, pyruvate is converted to alanine before the morphological and histological change induced by the cancer (Hu et al. 2011). Hyperpolarized [1-^{3}C] pyruvate has shown promising results in patients with prostate cancer (Nelson et al. 2013). In addition, raised hyperpolarized lactate and total hyperpolarized carbon (lactate + pyruvate + alanine) are used to characterize the various histological grades of prostate cancer (Albers et al. 2008). One of the challenges in cancer biology was to use hyperpolarized [1-^{13}C] pyruvate as a method to monitor therapy response (Day et al. 2007). This molecule has been used to follow glycolysis during tumor formation (increase in lactate formation) and regression (inhibition of lactate formation as tumors begin to regress). Hyperpolarized [1-3C] pyruvate has also been used to detect treatment response in a glioma tumor model: after radiotherapy of the whole brain (15 Gy), the ratio of hyperpolarized [1-3C] lactate compared to the maximum pyruvate signal in blood vessels in tumor was drastically decreased (34%) (Day et al. 2011). ^{13}C isotopomer analysis combined with hyperpolarized ^{13}C spectroscopy allows quantitative flux measurements in living tumors (Yang et al. 2014). In the rat brain *in vivo*, injection of [2-^{13}C] pyruvate leads only to the detection of [2-^{13}C] lactate, whereas [1-^{13}C] pyruvate is able to detect both [1-^{13}C] lactate and ^{13}C bicarbonate. A metabolic model was used to fit the hyperpolarized ^{13}C time courses obtained during infusion of [1-^{13}C] pyruvate and to determine the values of rates of both PDH and LDH. The rapid determination of these values (approximately 1 min of data acquisition) opens up new avenues for the study of brain metabolism (Marjanska et al. 2010).

20.2.2   HYPERPOLARIZED ^{13}C BICARBONATE

Injection of hyperpolarized ^{13}C bicarbonate is one of the NMR techniques for imaging pH (Gallagher et al. 2011). This method, which exploits pH-dependent chemical shift, results in the rapid production of hyperpolarized ^{13}CO$_2$ in the reaction catalyzed by *carbonic anhydrase*. As this reaction is close to equilibrium in the body and is pH dependent, the ratio of the ^{13}C signal intensities from H^{13}CO$_3^-$ and ^{13}CO$_2$ measured by MRS can be used to calculate tissue pH *in vivo* by the Henderson–Hasselbalch equation:

$$pH = pK_a + \log_{10}\left(\frac{[HCO_3^-]}{[CO_2]}\right)$$

This technique was used in a mouse tumor model, which showed that the average interstitial pH in the tumor was significantly lower than in the surrounding tissue.

Recent initiatives in molecular biology have provided unique opportunities to characterize the tumor environment and to understand its impact on the growth of tumors, the metastatic dissemination of cancer, and response to treatment (Gillies et al. 2002). Thus, pH imaging *in vivo* could be a helpful early biomarker for the detection and therapeutic follow-up of cancers.

20.2.3   HYPERPOLARIZED ^{13}C GLUCOSE

Glucose imaging could also be useful in the diagnosis and characterization of cancer *in vivo*. Hyperpolarized [U-^{2}H,U-^{13}C] glucose has been studied in living breast cancer cell cultures and ^{13}C lactate (labeled in C1 and C3) detected (Harris et al. 2013). Hyperpolarized glucose images were obtained in the live rat with deuterated glucose (Allouche-Arnon et al. 2013). The deuteration of protonated carbons of glucose drastically increases T_1. In a recent study, glycolysis was monitored in mouse lymphoma and lung tumors (Rodrigues et al. 2014). ^{13}C lactate was detected only in the tumors (and not in the surrounding normal tissue) and it was markedly decreased at 24 h after treatment with a chemotherapeutic drug. These observations could lead to a new approach to following tumor treatment response.

20.2.4   HYPERPOLARIZED ^{13}C CHOLINE

Aberrant choline phospholipid metabolism of malignant cells often results in increased concentration of phosphocholine (Glunde et al. 2009; Kurhanewicz et al. 2011). ^{1}H and ^{31}P MRS have shown elevated levels of this metabolite in many different forms of tumor compared with those of normal tissue (Podo 1999). A recent study was made of the hyperpolarized choline molecular probe for monitoring acetylcholine synthesis (Allouche-Arnon et al. 2011). The feasibility of such an *in vivo* study was performed on healthy rats with [1,1,2,2-^{2}H, 1-^{13}C] choline (Friesen-Waldner et al. 2014). However, the main drawback with choline arises from the short T_1 values for the carbons. Because choline has a quaternary nitrogen, ^{15}N-labeled choline is a potential agent that can be hyperpolarized. Its long T_1 (~4 min) would make it suitable for imaging in live animal studies (Cudalbu et al. 2010). Although the ^{15}N resonances of choline and phosphocholine are very close (0.2 ppm) and would hamper an *in vivo* study, DNP is able to address this problem (Gabellieri et al. 2008; Sarkar et al. 2009).

20.2.5 HYPERPOLARIZED ^{13}C FUMARATE

The hyperpolarized [1,4-^{13}C] fumarate is transformed into [1,4-^{13}C] malate that can be accumulated by a block of the tricarboxylic cycle during cell death. Indeed, in necrotizing cells, the plasma membrane permeability barrier is damaged (Neves and Brindle 2014), and fumarate enters the cell rapidly and is converted into malate in the hydration reaction catalyzed by the abundant enzyme *fumarase*. This transformation is potentially a sensitive marker of tumor cell death *in vivo* and could be clinically used to detect the early response of tumors to treatment. It has been used in different tumor types (Gallagher et al. 2009; Bohndiek et al. 2010; Witney et al. 2010; Clatworthy et al. 2012; Mignion et al. 2014).

20.3 INTEREST OF HYPERPOLARIZED GLUTAMINE IN THE DETECTION OF CANCER

20.3.1 WHY GLUTAMINE METABOLISM IS INTERESTING IN IMAGING TUMOR CELLS?

Cancer cells have a different metabolic profile to that of normal cells. The Warburg effect (increased aerobic glycolysis) and glutaminolysis (increased mitochondrial activity from glutamine catabolism) are well-known hallmarks of cancer and are accompanied by increased production of lactate, hyperpolarized mitochondrial membrane, and reactive oxygen species. Moreover, it has been recently shown how glutamine transporters ASCT2 (System ASC, a Na$^+$-coupled transporter for alanine, serine, cysteine, and glutamine, which activates mammalian target of rapamycin (mTOR) signaling and is both a target for the oncogene c-MYc and a driving growth for cancer cells), ATB$^{0,+}$ (amino acid transporter with neutral, denoted by "0," and cationic, denoted by " + ," amino acids as substrates), LAT1 and LAT4 (System L, Na$^+$-independent transporters 1 and 4, which have affinity for large neutral amino acids) and xCT (System x, Na$^+$-independent obligatory exchanger and means that cysteine entry into cells is coupled mandatorily to glutamate efflux) and enzymes, *glutaminase C* and *isocitrate dehydrogenase (IDH)*, have emerged as the most promising targets for the development of cancer detection tools and therapies (Bhutia et al. 2015). Indeed, mutations in a subset of metabolic enzymes such as *glutaminase* and IDH result in perturbations of intermediary metabolism (Dang et al. 2009; Parsons et al. 2008). In brief, ASCT2 is most intimately linked to glutamine uptake, LAT1 to essential amino acid import (and glutamine export), xCT to cystine uptake for glutathione biosynthesis, which reduces oxidative damage and protects the cancer cells from apoptosis, and ATB$^{0,+}$ to the concentrative uptake of cationic and neutral amino acids, as reported by Barrie Bode in Chapter 19.

Consequently, glutamine plays a central role in tumor metabolism. Accordingly, glutaminolysis is considered as a hallmark of tumor cell metabolism. The oxidation of the carbon backbone of glutamine, which occurs in mitochondria, requires conversion of glutamine to 2-oxoglutarate via glutamate. Tumor cells have large intracellular pools of glutamate and to maintain these pools, glutamine is converted to glutamate by the enzyme *glutaminase*. This mitochondrial enzyme is overexpressed in many tumor tissues. *Glutaminase* expression correlates with tumor growth rates and therefore the assessment of its activity is essential to characterize the metabolic phenotype of growing tumors.

Measurements of the conversion of hyperpolarized [5-^{13}C] glutamine into glutamate have been used to detect intramitochondrial *glutaminase* activity in intact hepatoma cells (Gallagher et al. 2008; Witney and Brindle 2010; Cabella et al. 2013). However, it seems better to use deuterated

TABLE 20.1

DNP-Polarized Glutamine and PET Tracers with Imaging Potential in Cancer Metabolism

Molecule	DNP or PET	Biological Mechanism Responsible for Signal	Comments	References
[5-^{13}C] Glutamine	DNP	Based on changes in *glutaminase* activity in hepatocellular cancer: the signal of [5-^{13}C] glutamate is higher in cancerous tissue owing to its higher rate of transport rather than to its higher expression of *glutaminase*	The correlation between glutaminolysis and tumor cell proliferation and survival suggests that it is possible to monitor response to chemotherapy with the [5-^{13}C] glutamine marker	Cabella et al. (2013)
^{18}F-Labeled glutamine	PET	Glutamine transporter ASCT2, which is a key mediator of glutamine uptake by many tumor cells	Radiolabeled amino acids and their transporters are used as oncologic imaging agents	Huang and McConathy (2013)
[5-^{11}C] Glutamine	PET	The upregulation of the oncogene myc can regulate glutamine uptake and its metabolism through glutaminolysis to provide the cancer cell with a replacement energy source	[5-^{11}C] glutamine might be useful for probing *in vivo* tumor metabolism in glutaminolytic tumors, which are not detected by ^{18}F-FDG-PET	Qu et al. (2012)
^{18}F-Fluorodeoxyglucose (^{18}F-FDG) and glutamine-based PET	PET	Target glutamine provides a useful window into tumor biology that would complement ^{18}F-FDG-PET	Target glutamine is used in cancer cells as a complement to glucose	Rajagopalan and DeBerardinis (2011)
^{18}F-(2*S*,4*R*)4-Fluoroglutamine	PET	Selective uptake and trap of ^{18}F-(2*S*,4*R*)4-fluoroglutamine by tumor cells	An alternative metabolic tracer for tumors, ^{18}F-(2*S*,4*R*)4-fluoroglutamine, was developed as a PET tracer for mapping glutaminolytic tumors	Lieberman et al. (2011); Chopra (2012)
[5-(13)C-4-(2)H(2)]-L-Glutamine	DNP	Hyperpolarized glutamine is converted into glutamate within seconds in cancerous cells or tissues	First report of specifically deuterated [5-(13)C-4-(2)H(2)]-L-glutamine in conjunction with hyperpolarized MRS for studying glutaminolysis in proliferating tumor cells	Qu et al. (2011)
[5-^{13}C] Glutamine	DNP	*Glutaminase* activity may be a useful surrogate marker for the proliferative state of cancer cells and loss of activity and indication of positive response to cytostatic therapies	Nuclear spin hyperpolarization increases MRI sensitivity by ~10,000-fold	Gallagher et al. (2008); Witney and Brindle (2010)

[5-^{13}C] glutamine to image tumor *glutaminase* activity (Qu et al. 2011; Kennedy et al. 2012). It is difficult to follow *glutaminase* activity and thus there is increased proliferation from glutamine conversion to glutamate following treatment and the cells become necrotic, as observed with fumarate (Kurhanewicz et al. 2011; Neves and Brindle 2014). In necrotic cells, in which the permeability barrier of the plasma membrane is compromised, glutamine enters the cell rapidly and is converted into glutamate catalyzed by the abundant enzyme *glutaminase*. In contrast, in viable cells, the transport rate of glutamine into the mitochondria is too slow to allow the observation of labeled glutamine within the lifetime of the polarization. However, if this permeability barrier is removed, as it is in necrotic cells, then glutamine conversion to glutamate can be observed.

20.3.2 Use of Hyperpolarized ^{13}C Glutamine in Comparison with Positron Emission Tomography Tracers in the Detection of *In Vivo* Cancer

DNP can be an alternative to ^{18}fludeoxyglucose-positron emission tomography (FDG-PET) for imaging tumor treatment response in the clinic via the flux between pyruvate and lactate (Witney et al. 2009). Other authors have reviewed the following: (1) the potential of hyperpolarized MRS for studying the cross talk between oncogenic cell signaling and for probing diagnostic biomarkers of therapeutic response in cancer (Dafni and Ronen 2010) and (2) the direct information provided by hyperpolarized ^{13}C MRI, which may allow direct molecular imaging of tissues and cells (Rodrigues et al. 2009). The benefits of DNP-polarized glutamine and PET tracers are shown in Table 20.1: glutaminolysis and tumor cell proliferation/survival were followed by DNP with carbon 13 or deuterated glutamine (Gallagher et al. 2008; Witney and Brindle 2010; Qu et al. 2011; Cabella et al. 2013), an alternative metabolic tracer for tumors, ^{18}F-fluoroglutamine was developed as a PET tracer for mapping glutaminolytic tumors (Chopra 2004; Lieberman et al. 2011; Rajagopalan and DeBerardinis 2011; Qu et al. 2012; Huang and McConathy 2013). In conclusion, although PET is already established as a clinical tool (Bading and Shields 2008), hyperpolarized ^{13}C glutamine and its DNP should be adopted as a routine clinical imaging tool (Gallagher et al. 2011).

20.4 SUMMARY AND CONCLUSIONS

Imaging glutamine metabolism is a major challenge in cancer biology to monitor and understand cancer metabolism *in vivo* with the aim of improving diagnosis and, perhaps, therapy. Glutamine is a marker of tumor growth and division and can be safely administered to humans in a clinical setting. In particular, strong correlations have been reported between oncogene expression and the activity of the enzyme *glutaminase*. This mitochondrial enzyme, which is responsible for the deamidation of glutamine to form glutamate, is overexpressed in many tumor tissues. The changes in *glutaminase* activity allow tumor progression to be followed. Thus, with hyperpolarized [5-^{13}C] glutamine (improvement in sensitivity of ^{13}C MRS by a factor of 10,000 via DNP preparation), it may be possible to use this conditionally essential amino acid to assess the effect of tumor treatment with cytostatic drugs.

REFERENCES

Abragam, A. and M. Goldman. 1978. Principles of dynamic nuclear-polarization. *Rep Prog Phys* 41:395–467.

Albers, M. J., R. Bok, A. P. Chen et al. 2008. Hyperpolarized 13C lactate, pyruvate, and alanine: Noninvasive biomarkers for prostate cancer detection and grading. *Cancer Res* 68(20):8607–15.

Allouche-Arnon, H., A. Gamliel, C. M. Barzilay et al. 2011. A hyperpolarized choline molecular probe for monitoring acetylcholine synthesis. *Contrast Media Mol Imaging* 6(3):139–47.

Allouche-Arnon, H., M. H. Lerche, M. Karlsson, R. E. Lenkinski, and R. Katz-Brull. 2011. Deuteration of a molecular probe for DNP hyperpolarization—a new approach and validation for choline chloride. *Contrast Media Mol Imaging* 6(6):499–506.

Allouche-Arnon, H., T. Wade, L. F. Waldner et al. 2013. *In vivo* magnetic resonance imaging of glucose—Initial experience. *Contrast Media Mol Imaging* 8(1):72–82.

Ardenkjaer-Larsen, J. H., B. Fridlund, A. Gram et al. 2003. Increase in signal-to-noise ratio of >10,000 times in liquid-state NMR. *Proc Natl Acad Sci USA* 100(18):10158–63.

Ardenkjaer-Larsen, J. H., A. M. Leach, N. Clarke, J. Urbahn, D. Anderson, and T. W. Skloss. 2011. Dynamic nuclear polarization polarizer for sterile use intent. *NMR Biomed* 24(8):927–32.

Bading, J. R. and A. F. Shields. 2008. Imaging of cell proliferation: Status and prospects. *J Nucl Med* 49 Suppl 2:64S–80S.

Barb, A. W., S. K. Hekmatyar, J. N. Glushka, and J. H. Prestegard. 2011. Exchange facilitated indirect detection of hyperpolarized 15ND2-amido-glutamine. *J Magn Reson* 212(2):304–10.

Barb, A. W., S. K. Hekmatyar, J. N. Glushka, and J. H. Prestegard. 2013. Probing alanine transaminase catalysis with hyperpolarized 13CD3-pyruvate. *J Magn Reson* 228:59–65.

Bhutia, Y. D., E. Babu, S. Ramachandran, and V. Ganapathy. 2015. Amino Acid transporters in cancer and their relevance to "glutamine addiction": Novel targets for the design of a new class of anticancer drugs. *Cancer Res* 75(9):1782–8.

Bohndiek, S. E., M. I. Kettunen, D. E. Hu et al. 2010. Detection of tumor response to a vascular disrupting agent by hyperpolarized 13C magnetic resonance spectroscopy. *Mol Cancer Ther* 9(12):3278–88.

Bowen, S. and J. H. Ardenkjaer-Larsen. 2014. Enhanced performance large volume dissolution-DNP. *J Magn Reson* 240:90–4.

Cabella, C., M. Karlsson, C. Canape et al. 2013. *In vivo* and *in vitro* liver cancer metabolism observed with hyperpolarized [5-(13)C]glutamine. *J Magn Reson* 232:45–52.

Chopra, A. 2004. 18F-(2S,4R)4-fluoroglutamine. In *Molecular Imaging and Contrast Agent Database (MICAD)*. Bethesda, MD.

Clatworthy, M. R., M. I. Kettunen, D. E. Hu et al. 2012. Magnetic resonance imaging with hyperpolarized [1,4-(13)C2]fumarate allows detection of early renal acute tubular necrosis. *Proc Natl Acad Sci USA* 109(33):13374–9.

Cudalbu, C., A. Comment, F. Kurdzesau et al. 2010. Feasibility of *in vivo* 15N MRS detection of hyperpolarized 15N labeled choline in rats. *Phys Chem Chem Phys* 12(22):5818–23.

Dafni, H. and S. M. Ronen. 2010. Dynamic nuclear polarization in metabolic imaging of metastasis: Common sense, hypersense and compressed sensing. *Cancer Biomark* 7(4):189–99.

Dang, L., D. W. White, S. Gross et al. 2009. Cancer-associated IDH1 mutations produce 2-hydroxyglutarate. *Nature* 462(7274):739–44.

Day, S. E., M. I. Kettunen, M. K. Cherukuri et al. 2011. Detecting response of rat C6 glioma tumors to radiotherapy using hyperpolarized [1–13C]pyruvate and 13C magnetic resonance spectroscopic imaging. *Magn Reson Med* 65(2):557–63.

Day, S. E., M. I. Kettunen, F. A. Gallagher et al. 2007. Detecting tumor response to treatment using hyperpolarized 13C magnetic resonance imaging and spectroscopy. *Nat Med* 13(11):1382–7.

Eichhorn, T. R., Y. Takado, N. Salameh et al. 2013. Hyperpolarization without persistent radicals for *in vivo* real-time metabolic imaging. *Proc Natl Acad Sci U S A* 110(45):18064–9.

Feng, Y., T. Theis, X. Liang, Q. Wang, P. Zhou, and W. S. Warren. 2013. Storage of hydrogen spin polarization in long-lived 13C2 singlet order and implications for hyperpolarized magnetic resonance imaging. *J Am Chem Soc* 135(26):9632–5.

Friesen-Waldner, L. J., T. P. Wade, K. Thind et al. 2014. Hyperpolarized choline as an MR imaging molecular probe: Feasibility of *in vivo* imaging in a rat model. *J Magn Reson Imaging* 41(4):917–23.

Gabellieri, C., S. Reynolds, A. Lavie, G. S. Payne, M. O. Leach, and T. R. Eykyn. 2008. Therapeutic target metabolism observed using hyperpolarized 15N choline. *J Am Chem Soc* 130(14):4598–9.

Gallagher, F. A., S. E. Bohndiek, M. I. Kettunen, D. Y. Lewis, D. Soloviev, and K. M. Brindle. 2011. Hyperpolarized 13C MRI and PET: *In vivo* tumor biochemistry. *J Nucl Med* 52(9):1333–6.

Gallagher, F. A., M. I. Kettunen, and K. M. Brindle. 2011. Imaging pH with hyperpolarized 13C. *NMR Biomed* 24(8):1006–15.

Gallagher, F. A., M. I. Kettunen, S. E. Day, M. Lerche, and K. M. Brindle. 2008. 13C MR spectroscopy measurements of glutaminase activity in human hepatocellular carcinoma cells using hyperpolarized 13C-labeled glutamine. *Magnetic Resonance in Medicine* 60(2):253–257.

Gallagher, F. A., M. I. Kettunen, D. E. Hu et al. 2009. Production of hyperpolarized [1,4–13C2]malate from [1,4–13C2]fumarate is a marker of cell necrosis and treatment response in tumors. *Proc Natl Acad Sci U S A* 106(47):19801–6.

Gillies, R. J., N. Raghunand, G. S. Karczmar, and Z. M. Bhujwalla. 2002. MRI of the tumor microenvironment. *J Magn Reson Imaging* 16(4):430–50.

Glunde, K., M. A. Jacobs, A. P. Pathak, D. Artemov, and Z. M. Bhujwalla. 2009. Molecular and functional imaging of breast cancer. *NMR Biomed* 22(1):92–103.

Golman, K., R. I. Zandt, M. Lerche, R. Pehrson, and J. H. Ardenkjaer-Larsen. 2006. Metabolic imaging by hyperpolarized 13C magnetic resonance imaging for *in vivo* tumor diagnosis. *Cancer Res* 66(22):10855–60.

Harris, T., H. Degani, and L. Frydman. 2013. Hyperpolarized 13C NMR studies of glucose metabolism in living breast cancer cell cultures. *NMR Biomed* 26(12):1831–43.

Harrison, C., C. Yang, A. Jindal et al. 2012. Comparison of kinetic models for analysis of pyruvate-to-lactate exchange by hyperpolarized 13 C NMR. *NMR Biomed* 25(11):1286–94.

Hu, S., A. Balakrishnan, R. A. Bok et al. 2011. 13C-pyruvate imaging reveals alterations in glycolysis that precede c-Myc-induced tumor formation and regression. *Cell Metab* 14(1):131–42.

Hu, S., P. E. Larson, M. Vancriekinge et al. 2013. Rapid sequential injections of hyperpolarized [1-(1)(3)C] pyruvate *in vivo* using a sub-kelvin, multi-sample DNP polarizer. *Magn Reson Imaging* 31(4):490–6.

Hu, S., M. Lustig, A. Balakrishnan et al. 2010. 3D compressed sensing for highly accelerated hyperpolarized (13)C MRSI with *in vivo* applications to transgenic mouse models of cancer. *Magn Reson Med* 63(2):312–21.

Huang, C. and J. McConathy. 2013. Radiolabeled amino acids for oncologic imaging. *J Nucl Med* 54(7):1007–10.

Josan, S., R. Hurd, J. M. Park et al. 2014. Dynamic metabolic imaging of hyperpolarized [2-(13) C]pyruvate using spiral chemical shift imaging with alternating spectral band excitation. *Magn Reson Med* 71(6):2051–8.

Josan, S., Y. F. Yen, R. Hurd, A. Pfefferbaum, D. Spielman, and D. Mayer. 2011. Application of double spin echo spiral chemical shift imaging to rapid metabolic mapping of hyperpolarized [1-(1)(3)C]-pyruvate. *J Magn Reson* 209(2):332–6.

Kazan, S. M., S. Reynolds, A. Kennerley et al. 2013. Kinetic modeling of hyperpolarized (13)C pyruvate metabolism in tumors using a measured arterial input function. *Magn Reson Med* 70(4):943–53.

Kennedy, B. W., M. I. Kettunen, D. E. Hu, and K. M. Brindle. 2012. Probing lactate dehydrogenase activity in tumors by measuring hydrogen/deuterium exchange in hyperpolarized l-[1-(13)C,U-(2)H]lactate. *J Am Chem Soc* 134(10):4969–77.

Kurhanewicz, J., D. B. Vigneron, K. Brindle et al. 2011. Analysis of cancer metabolism by imaging hyperpolarized nuclei: Prospects for translation to clinical research. *Neoplasia* 13(2):81–97.

Larson, P. E., R. Bok, A. B. Kerr et al. 2010. Investigation of tumor hyperpolarized [1–13C]-pyruvate dynamics using time-resolved multiband RF excitation echo-planar MRSI. *Magn Reson Med* 63(3):582–91.

Larson, P. E., S. Hu, M. Lustig et al. 2011. Fast dynamic 3D MR spectroscopic imaging with compressed sensing and multiband excitation pulses for hyperpolarized 13C studies. *Magn Reson Med* 65(3):610–9.

Leftin, A., T. Roussel, and L. Frydman. 2014. Hyperpolarized functional magnetic resonance of murine skeletal muscle enabled by multiple tracer-paradigm synchronizations. *PLoS One* 9(4):e96399.

Lieberman, B. P., K. Ploessl, L. Wang et al. 2011. PET imaging of glutaminolysis in tumors by 18F-(2S,4R)4-fluoroglutamine. *J Nucl Med* 52(12):1947–55.

Lupo, J. M., A. P. Chen, M. L. Zierhut et al. 2010. Analysis of hyperpolarized dynamic 13C lactate imaging in a transgenic mouse model of prostate cancer. *Magn Reson Imaging* 28(2):153–62.

Marjanska, M., I. Iltis, A. A. Shestov et al. 2010. *In vivo* 13C spectroscopy in the rat brain using hyperpolarized [1-(13)C]pyruvate and [2-(13)C]pyruvate. *J Magn Reson* 206(2):210–8.

Mignion, L., P. Dutta, G. V. Martinez, P. Foroutan, R. J. Gillies, and B. F. Jordan. 2014. Monitoring chemotherapeutic response by hyperpolarized 13C-fumarate MRS and diffusion MRI. *Cancer Res* 74(3):686–94.

Mishkovsky, M., T. Cheng, A. Comment, and R. Gruetter. 2012. Localized *in vivo* hyperpolarization transfer sequences. *Magn Reson Med* 68(2):349–52.

Nelson, S. J., J. Kurhanewicz, D. B. Vigneron et al. 2013. Metabolic imaging of patients with prostate cancer using hyperpolarized [1-(1)(3)C]pyruvate. *Sci Transl Med* 5(198):198ra108.

Neves, A. A. and K. M. Brindle. 2014. Imaging cell death. *J Nucl Med* 55(1):1–4.

Nonaka, H., R. Hata, T. Doura et al. 2013. A platform for designing hyperpolarized magnetic resonance chemical probes. *Nat Commun* 4:2411.

Ohliger, M. A., P. E. Larson, R. A. Bok et al. 2013. Combined parallel and partial fourier MR reconstruction for accelerated 8-channel hyperpolarized carbon-13 *in vivo* magnetic resonance Spectroscopic imaging (MRSI). *J Magn Reson Imaging* 38(3):701–13.

Parsons, D. W., S. Jones, X. Zhang et al. 2008. An integrated genomic analysis of human glioblastoma multiforme. *Science* 321(5897):1807–12.

Pileio, G., M. Carravetta, and M. H. Levitt. 2010. Storage of nuclear magnetization as long-lived singlet order in low magnetic field. *Proc Natl Acad Sci U S A* 107(40):17135–9.

Podo, F. 1999. Tumour phospholipid metabolism. *NMR Biomed* 12(7):413–39.

Qu, W., S. Oya, B. P. Lieberman et al. 2012. Preparation and characterization of L-[5–11C]-glutamine for metabolic imaging of tumors. *J Nucl Med* 53(1):98–105.

Qu, W., Z. Zha, B. P. Lieberman et al. 2011. Facile synthesis [5-(13)C-4-(2)H(2)]-L-glutamine for hyperpolarized MRS imaging of cancer cell metabolism. *Acad Radiol* 18(8):932–9.

Rajagopalan, K. N. and R. J. DeBerardinis. 2011. Role of glutamine in cancer: Therapeutic and imaging implications. *J Nucl Med* 52(7):1005–8.

Rodrigues, T. B., C. P. Fonseca, M. M. Castro, S. Cerdan, and C. F. Geraldes. 2009. 13C NMR tracers in neurochemistry: Implications for molecular imaging. *Q J Nucl Med Mol Imaging* 53(6):631–45.

Rodrigues, T. B., E. M. Serrao, B. W. Kennedy, D. E. Hu, M. I. Kettunen, and K. M. Brindle. 2014. Magnetic resonance imaging of tumor glycolysis using hyperpolarized 13C-labeled glucose. *Nat Med* 20(1):93–7.

Ross, B., A. Lin, K. Harris, P. Bhattacharya, and B. Schweinsburg. 2003. Clinical experience with 13C MRS *in vivo*. *NMR Biomed* 16(6–7):358–69.

Rowland, I. J., E. T. Peterson, J. W. Gordon, and S. B. Fain. 2010. Hyperpolarized 13carbon MR. *Curr Pharm Biotechnol* 11(6):709–19.

Sarkar, R., A. Comment, P. R. Vasos et al. 2009. Proton NMR of (15)N-choline metabolites enhanced by dynamic nuclear polarization. *J Am Chem Soc* 131(44):16014–5.

Schmidt, R., C. Laustsen, J. N. Dumez et al. 2014. *In vivo* single-shot 13C spectroscopic imaging of hyperpolarized metabolites by spatiotemporal encoding. *J Magn Reson* 240:8–15.

Tropp, J., J. M. Lupo, A. Chen et al. 2011. Multi-channel metabolic imaging, with SENSE reconstruction, of hyperpolarized [1-(13)C] pyruvate in a live rat at 3.0 tesla on a clinical MR scanner. *J Magn Reson* 208(1):171–7.

Vander Heiden, M. G., L. C. Cantley, and C. B. Thompson. 2009. Understanding the Warburg effect: The metabolic requirements of cell proliferation. *Science* 324(5930):1029–33.

von Morze, C., G. Reed, P. Shin et al. 2011. Multi-band frequency encoding method for metabolic imaging with hyperpolarized [1-(13)C]pyruvate. *J Magn Reson* 211(2):109–13.

Warren, W. S., E. Jenista, R. T. Branca, and X. Chen. 2009. Increasing hyperpolarized spin lifetimes through true singlet eigen states. *Science* 323(5922):1711–4.

Wilson, D. M., K. R. Keshari, P. E. Larson et al. 2010. Multi-compound polarization by DNP allows simultaneous assessment of multiple enzymatic activities *in vivo*. *J Magn Reson* 205(1):141–7.

Witney, T. H. and K. M. Brindle. 2010. Imaging tumour cell metabolism using hyperpolarized 13C magnetic resonance spectroscopy. *Biochem Soc Trans* 38(5):1220–4.

Witney, T. H., M. I. Kettunen, S. E. Day et al. 2009. A comparison between radiolabeled fluorodeoxyglucose uptake and hyperpolarized (13)C-labeled pyruvate utilization as methods for detecting tumor response to treatment. *Neoplasia* 11(6):574–82, 1 p following 582.

Witney, T. H., M. I. Kettunen, D. E. Hu et al. 2010. Detecting treatment response in a model of human breast adenocarcinoma using hyperpolarised [1–13C]pyruvate and [1,4–13C2]fumarate. *Br J Cancer* 103(9):1400–6.

Yang, C., C. Harrison, E. S. Jin et al. 2014. Simultaneous steady-state and dynamic 13C NMR can differentiate alternative routes of pyruvate metabolism in living cancer cells. *J Biol Chem* 289(9):6212–24.

Zierhut, M. L., Y. F. Yen, A. P. Chen et al. 2010. Kinetic modeling of hyperpolarized 13C1-pyruvate metabolism in normal rats and TRAMP mice. *J Magn Reson* 202(1):85–92.

Section IX

Glutamine, Immunity, and Exercise

21 Glutamine and the Immune System

Luise V. Marino and Philip C. Calder

CONTENTS

21.1 INTRODUCTION

Glutamine is a very important amino acid in supporting the immune response, and it is thought that one of the contributors to impaired immunity in catabolic stress states is a diminished supply of glutamine. The aim of this chapter is to review the metabolism of glutamine by cells of the immune system; the role(s) of glutamine in supporting specific immune cell functions; the evidence from animal models and human clinical trials around glutamine, immunity, infection, and inflammation; and the mechanisms of action of glutamine within the immune system, with an emphasis on the role of heat shock proteins. Prior to discussing glutamine, the chapter describes in brief the immune system and its function in health and disease. The effects of glutamine on the immune system in the context of exercise are covered in Chapters 22 and 23.

21.2   IMMUNE SYSTEM

21.2.1   Overview

The role of the immune system is to protect the host from infectious agents that exist in the environment, such as bacteria, viruses, fungi, and parasites, from other noxious environmental insults, and from tumor cells. The immune system is complex and involves many different cell types that are distributed in many locations throughout the body and travel between those locations in the lymph and the bloodstream. In some locations in the body, immune cells are organized into discrete lymphoid organs, classified as primary lymphoid organs where immune cells arise and mature (bone marrow and thymus) and secondary lymphoid organs (e.g., lymph nodes, spleen, gut-associated lymphoid tissue) where mature immune cells interact and respond to antigens. The immune system has two broad functional divisions called the innate (or natural) immune system and the acquired (or specific or adaptive) immune system.

21.2.2   Innate Immunity

Components of the innate immune system include physical barriers, soluble factors in the bloodstream and in secretions like saliva and tears, and phagocytic cells that include granulocytes (neutrophils, basophils, eosinophils), monocytes, and macrophages. Innate immunity has no memory and so is not affected by prior exposure to an organism or other immune trigger. The soluble factors of innate immunity include complement proteins. Phagocytic cells recognize certain common structures on bacteria and other microorganisms via surface receptors called pattern recognition receptors; the structures they recognize are called pathogen-associated molecular patterns. Binding of the organism to one of these receptors triggers phagocytosis (engulfing) and subsequent destruction of the pathogenic microorganism by toxic chemicals, such as superoxide radicals and hydrogen peroxide. Natural killer cells also possess surface receptors and destroy their target cells by the release of cytotoxic proteins. In this way, innate immunity provides a first line of defense against invading pathogens. However, an immune response often requires the coordinated actions of both innate and acquired immunity.

21.2.3   Acquired Immunity

In contrast to innate immunity, which is not very specific, acquired immunity involves the specific recognition of molecules (termed antigens) derived from an invading pathogen and which distinguishes it as being foreign to the host. Acquired immunity is also involved in ensuring tolerance to sources of nonthreatening antigens such as nonpathogenic bacteria, food, and the host's own tissues. The main cells involved in acquired immunity are the lymphocytes, which are classified into T and B lymphocytes (also called T cells and B cells). B lymphocytes undergo development and maturation in the bone marrow before being released into the circulation, while T lymphocytes mature in the thymus. From the bloodstream, lymphocytes can enter secondary lymphoid organs, like the spleen and lymph nodes. Immune responses occur largely in these lymphoid organs, which are highly organized to favor the interactions between cells and antigens that are required for an effective immune response.

The acquired immune response is highly specific and becomes effective over several days after its initial activation. It also persists for some time after the removal of the initiating antigen. This persistence gives rise to immunological memory, which is also a characteristic feature of acquired immunity. Memory is the basis for a stronger, more effective immune response to re-exposure to an antigen (i.e., reinfection with the same pathogen) and is the rationale for vaccination. Eventually, the immune system will re-establish homeostasis using self-regulatory mechanisms.

B-lymphocytes produce antibodies (soluble antigen-specific immunoglobulins). This form of immune protection is called humoral immunity. Antibodies bind to the surface of microorganisms bearing the antigen the antibody was raised against and this promotes the recognition and phago-cytosis of the organism by phagocytic cells. The organisms being dealt with by humoral immunity are extracellular until they are phagocytosed. However, some pathogens, particularly viruses, but also certain bacteria, infect individuals by entering cells. These pathogens will escape humoral immunity and are instead dealt with by cell-mediated immunity, which is conferred by T lympho-cytes. T lymphocytes express antigen-specific T-cell receptors on their surface. They are only able to recognize antigens that are presented to them on another cell surface (the cell presenting the antigen to the T lymphocyte is termed an antigen presenting cell or APC). Activation of the T-cell receptor results in proliferation of the T-cell and secretion of the cytokine interleukin (IL)-2, which promotes proliferation and differentiation. This process greatly increases the number of antigen-specific T lymphocytes. There are three principal types of T lymphocytes; cytotoxic T cells, helper T cells, and regulatory T cells. Cytotoxic T lymphocytes carry the surface protein marker CD8 and kill infected cells and tumor cells by secretion of cytotoxic enzymes, which cause lysis of the target cell. Helper T lymphocytes carry the surface protein marker CD4 and eliminate pathogens by stim-ulating the phagocytic activity of macrophages and the proliferation of, and antibody secretion by, B lymphocytes. Helper T lymphocytes have traditionally been subdivided into two broad categories according to the pattern of cytokines they produce. Th1 cells produce IL-2 and interferon (IFN)-γ, which activate macrophages, natural killer cells, and cytotoxic T-lymphocytes. Antigens derived from bacteria, viruses, and fungi tend to induce a Th1 dominant response. Th2 cells produce IL-4, which stimulates immunoglobulin (Ig)E production, and IL-5, an eosinophil-activating factor. Th2 cells are responsible for the defense against helminthic parasites, which is due to IgE-mediated activation of mast cells and basophils. Other categories of helper T cells, including Th17 cells, have been described. Regulatory T cells produce IL-10 and transforming growth factor-β and suppress the activities of B cells and other T cells preventing inappropriate activation.

21.2.4 GUT-ASSOCIATED IMMUNE SYSTEM

Mucosal surfaces have a strong immune component because they are a site of interaction with the environment. The immune system of the gut (sometimes termed the gut-associated immune system or gut-associated lymphoid tissue) is extensive and is believed to contain up to 70% of the immune cells in the human body. This makes sense because it is the site of continuous exposure to patho-genic and nonpathogenic microorganisms from within the gut lumen and to food-borne antigens. The gut-associated immune system includes the physical barrier of the intestine, as well as compo-nents of the innate and acquired immune systems. The physical barrier includes acid in the stomach, mucus, and tightly connected epithelial cells, which collectively prevent the entry of pathogens. The cells of the gut-associated immune system are organized into specialized structures, termed Peyer's patches, which are located directly beneath the epithelium in the lamina propria. This also contains so-called M cells, which sample small particles from the gut lumen; these particles can be derived from food or from microorganisms. The gut-associated immune system has a vital role in ensur-ing host defense against pathogens within the gastrointestinal lumen and in generating tolerogenic responses to harmless microorganisms and to food components.

21.3 GLUTAMINE METABOLISM BY CELLS OF THE IMMUNE SYSTEM

Thirty years ago it was identified that lymphoid organs, including the spleen, thymus, lymph nodes, Peyer's patches and bone marrow, isolated lymphocytes, and isolated macrophages, exhibit a high activity of glutaminase (Ardawi and Newsholme, 1982; Newsholme et al., 1986; Ardawi, 1988a; Keast and Newsholme, 1990), the enzyme responsible for the conversion of glutamine to glutamate. Later, neutrophils were also shown to also have a high glutaminase activity (Curi et al., 1997). Furthermore, glutaminase activity of the rat popliteal lymph node was increased in response to an immunologic challenge (Ardawi and Newsholme, 1982). In accordance with the high glutaminase activity, glutamine is utilized at a high rate by cultured lymphocytes (Ardawi and Newsholme, 1983; Brand, 1985; Ardawi, 1988a; Brand et al., 1989; O'Rourke and Rider, 1989; Wu et al., 1991), macrophages (Newsholme et al., 1987; Newsholme and Newsholme, 1989; Spolarics et al., 1991), and neutrophils (Curi et al., 1997; Pithon-Curi et al., 2002, 2004). Table 21.1 compares the rates of glutamine and glucose utilization by cultured rodent immune cells and describes the principal metabolic products seen *in vitro*. Mitogens and antigens trigger T-lymphocyte activation and lead to production of cytokines and to proliferation. Immune stimulation has been demonstrated to induce expression of genes encoding glutamine transporters in some cell types (Wang et al., 2011) and to enhance the rates of glutamine transport into T lymphocytes (Carr et al., 2010), glutaminase activity (Brand, 1985), and glutamine utilization (Ardawi and Newsholme, 1983; Brand, 1985; Ardawi, 1988a; Brand et al., 1989; O'Rourke and Rider, 1989; Wu et al., 1992). More recent work has demonstrated that activation of certain kinases in T cells (e.g., some extracellular signal regulated kinases (ERKs)/mitogen-activated protein kinases (MAPKs)) leads to increased glutamine uptake and metabolism (Carr et al., 2010), showing a direct link between the molecular events of T-cell activation and increased glutamine metabolism. Activation of macrophages *in vivo* or *in vitro* increases glutamine utilization (Murphy and Newsholme, 1998). In culture, the major products of glutamine metabolism by immune cells are glutamate, aspartate, lactate, and ammonia, although alanine and pyruvate are also produced and as much as 25% of glutamine used is completely oxidized (Ardawi and Newsholme, 1983; Brand, 1985; Newsholme et al., 1987; Ardawi, 1988a; Brand et al., 1989; Newsholme and Newsholme, 1989; O'Rourke and Rider, 1989). Figure 21.1 describes the metabolism of glutamine into these products.

Newsholme (1987) estimated that the rate of oxygen consumption by murine macrophages in culture (~500 nmol/h per mg cell protein) is similar to that of sheep heart (~700 nmol/h per mg protein) and rat liver (~500 nmol/h per mg protein). Furthermore, it was calculated that the rate of adenosine triphosphate (ATP) generation by macrophages *in vitro* in the presence of high concentrations of both glucose and glutamine was about 1000 nmol/h per mg cell protein. It was estimated that glucose contributed 62% of cellular energy requirement and glutamine 38%. Other researchers calculated that glutamine can contribute up to 35% of the energy requirement of immune cells in culture (Spolarics et al., 1991). These calculations do not consider any contribution from fatty acid oxidation and so are likely to be an overestimate. Nevertheless, it seems likely that glutamine makes a considerable contribution to the energy needs of cells of the immune system.

TABLE 21.1

Rates of Utilization of Glucose or Glutamine and of Production of Various Metabolites by Isolated Rat Lymphocytes, Mouse Macrophages, and Rat Neutrophils

Cell Type	Substrate	Rate of Utilization		Rate of Production		
		Glutamine	Glucose	Lactate	Glutamate	Aspartate
Lymphocyte	Glutamine	223	–	9	132	59
	Glucose	–	42	91	–	–
Macrophage	Glutamine	186	–	33	137	25
	Glucose	–	355	632	–	–
Neutrophil	Glutamine	770	–	320	250	68
	Glucose	–	460	550	–	–

Source: Data are from Ardawi, M.S. and E.A. Newsholme. 1983. *Biochem. J.* 212: 835–842 (lymphocytes); Newsholme, P., S. Gordon, and E.A. Newsholme. 1987. *Biochem. J.* 242: 631–636 (macrophages); and Curi, T.C et al. *Am. J. Physiol.* 273: C1124–C1129 (neutrophils).

Note: Units are nmol/h per mg cell protein.

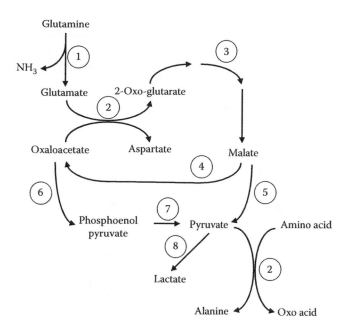

FIGURE 21.1 Glutamine metabolism. Enzymes are numbered as follows: 1, glutaminase; 2, transaminase; 3, part of the citric acid cycle; 4, malate dehydrogenase; 5, malic enzyme; 6, phosphoenolpyruvate carboxykinase; 7, pyruvate kinase; 8, lactate dehydrogenase.

The high rate of glutamine utilization by neutrophils, macrophages, and lymphocytes and its increase when these cells are immunologically challenged suggest that provision of sufficient glutamine might be important to support the function of these cells and therefore the ability of the host to mount an effective immune response.

21.4 GLUTAMINE AND THE FUNCTION OF CELLS OF THE IMMUNE SYSTEM

21.4.1 T Lymphocytes

T lymphocytes proliferate poorly in culture medium that lacks glutamine (Ardawi and Newsholme, 1983; Szondy and Newsholme, 1989; Chuang et al., 1990; Griffiths and Keast, 1990; Parry-Billings et al., 1990a; Hörig et al., 1993; Yaqoob and Calder, 1997; Chang et al., 1999a,b) and enzymatic destruction of glutamine in culture medium prevents T-lymphocyte proliferation (Hirsch, 1970; Simberkoff and Thomas, 1970). As shown in Figure 21.2 the human blood T-lymphocyte proliferative response to stimulation *in vitro* increases with increasing glutamine concentration and is maximal at the normal physiological concentration. Other amino acids including glutamate, aspartate, and arginine cannot substitute for glutamine to support T-lymphocyte proliferation *in vitro* (Ardawi and Newsholme, 1983; Calder, 1995a). However, hydrolyzable dipeptides that contain glutamine, such as alanyl-glutamine or glycyl-glutamine can replace glutamine in cell culture (Brand et al., 1989; Kweon et al., 1991; Köhler et al., 2000).

As part of the T-cell proliferative process IL-2 is produced and IL-2 receptor expression is increased. Th1-type lymphocytes produce IFN-γ, which is important in antibacterial and antiviral immunity. IL-2 production by mitogen stimulated rat, mouse, and human T lymphocytes in culture was enhanced with increased glutamine availability (Calder and Newsholme, 1992; Rohde et al., 1996; Yaqoob and Calder, 1997, 1998; Chang et al., 1999b). Furthermore, increased glutamine availability was linked with higher IL-2 receptor expression on mitogen-stimulated lymphocytes from rats (Yaqoob and Calder, 1997) and humans (Hörig et al., 1993). Production of IFN-γ by human

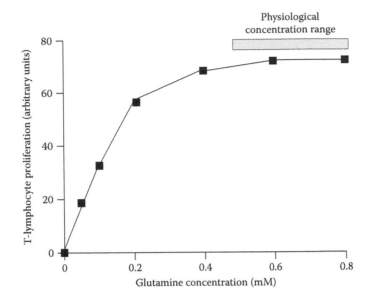

FIGURE 21.2 Human blood lymphocyte proliferation *in vitro* as a function of the concentration of gluta-mine in the culture medium. Unpublished data.

blood lymphocytes in culture increased with increasing glutamine availability (Hörig et al., 1993; Heberer et al., 1996; Rohde et al., 1996; Yaqoob and Calder, 1998; Chang et al., 1999b). Thus, increased glutamine availability in the medium of cultured lymphocytes appears to favor a Th1-type response, which is associated with defense against bacteria, viruses, and fungi.

Increasing the amount of glutamine in the diet of laboratory rodents also seems to increase T-lymphocyte function. For example, Kew et al. (1999) reported that feeding mice a diet containing about 2.5 times the normal amount of glutamine increased the number of CD4[+] cells in the spleen, increased spleen T-lymphocyte proliferation and IL-2 production, and increased the number of lymphocytes bearing the IL-2 receptor.

21.4.2 B LYMPHOCYTES

There are limited studies of glutamine and B-lymphocyte function. It was demonstrated that differentiation of B lymphocytes into antibody producing cells *in vitro* is dependent upon glutamine and increases over the physiological range of glutamine concentration (Crawford and Cohen, 1985).

21.4.3 MONOCYTES AND MACROPHAGES

Spittler et al. (1995, 1997) demonstrated that the expression of various molecules involved in phago-cytosis and in antigen presentation on the surface of human blood monocytes is influenced by the concentration of glutamine in which the cells are cultured. This was linked with increased func-tion, including increased phagocytosis and antigen presentation, with increasing glutamine avail-ability (Spittler et al., 1995, 1997). Other studies have demonstrated that glutamine availability influences phagocytosis by cultured murine macrophages (Parry-Billings et al., 1990a; Wallace and Keast, 1992). Glutamine also influences production of cytokines by monocytes and macrophages. For example, Wallace and Keast (1992) demonstrated that glutamine increased the IL-1 response to murine macrophages to bacterial lipopolysaccharide (LPS). Similarly, rat macrophages showed increased production of tumor necrosis factor (TNF)-α with increasing glutamine availability (Murphy and Newsholme, 1999). Glutamine addition to the culture medium of rat macrophages increased LPS-stimulated IL-1 and IL-6 gene expression and secreted protein (Yassad et al., 2000). Glutamine also increased LPS-stimulated IL-8 production by cultured human blood monocytes (Murphy and Newsholme, 1999).

Wells et al. (1999) reported that feeding mice a diet containing about 2.5 times the normal amount of glutamine increased the production of TNF-α, IL-1β, and IL-6 by LPS-stimulated macrophages.

21.4.4 NEUTROPHILS

Glutamine availability supported reactive oxygen species production by neutrophils (Pithon-Curi et al., 2002). Neutrophils from the blood of patients with burns or postsurgery show impaired anti-microbial activities including decreased reactive oxygen species production, phagocytosis, and bactericidal activity. Addition of glutamine to cultures of such cells restored function (Ogle et al., 1994; Furukawa et al., 1997, 2000a,b). Garcia et al. (1999) showed that glutamine prevented the stress hormone-induced inhibition of neutrophil superoxide production.

21.4.5 GUT-ASSOCIATED IMMUNE SYSTEM

Rats fed a glutamine-deficient diet for 7 days showed decreased mucosal wet weight and a decreased number of intraepithelial lymphocytes (Horvath et al., 1996). Intravenous glutamine increased the concentration of secretory IgA in the intestinal lumen of mice and increased intestine IL-4 and IL-10 concentrations (Kudsk et al., 2000). Oral glutamine maintained gut-associated lymphoid tissue and secretory IgA concentrations in mice (Alverdy, 1990).

21.5 PLASMA AND MUSCLE GLUTAMINE IN CATABOLIC STATES

Skeletal muscle is the major site of glutamine biosynthesis and an early response to stress is an increase in glutamine export from skeletal muscle. This could potentially lead to a lower skeletal muscle glutamine concentration, but is partly offset by increased protein breakdown, and enhanced *de novo* glutamine synthesis from other amino acids. Skeletal muscle glutamine synthetase is upregulated by glucocorticoids (Max et al., 1988) and by TNF-α (Chakrabarti, 1998). Furthermore, glucocorticoids increase glutamine efflux from muscle (Muhlbacher et al., 1984; Parry-Billings et al., 1990b). Thus, it appears that physiological stress induces processes to maintain or even enhance the supply of glutamine from skeletal muscle to the rest of the body. Nevertheless, glucocorticoid treatment decreases both skeletal muscle and plasma glutamine concentrations (Muhlbacher et al., 1984; Parry-Billings et al., 1990b), suggesting that the demand for glutamine can exceed the supply.

A number of animal studies report that skeletal muscle and plasma glutamine concentrations are decreased during catabolic stress situations such as sepsis, cancer cachexia, and following burns or major surgery; some studies in this area are summarized in Table 21.2. As shown in Table 21.3, several studies in humans also show lower concentrations of skeletal muscle and plasma glutamine in a number of patient groups than in healthy controls. Plasma glutamine concentration might be up to 50% lower in these conditions than seen in controls (Table 21.3). It is possible that plasma glutamine concentrations may fall below those necessary to support optimal immune function and this may contribute to increased susceptibility to infection, more severe infections, progression of sepsis, and poor patient outcome. In accordance with this, one study reported that a plasma glutamine concentration of <0.42 mM at admission to the intensive care unit (ICU) was associated with higher severity of illness and greater mortality than a concentration >0.42 mM (Oudemans-van Straaten et al., 2001). It is interesting to note that this concentration is almost precisely that at which T-lymphocyte proliferative responses *in vitro* become suboptimal (Figure 21.2). Skeletal muscle glutamine concentration may be decreased to less than 50% of that seen in controls (Table 21.3). This suggests that skeletal muscle supply of glutamine is exceeded by the demand of the liver, kidney, intestine, and immune system. Consequently, it has been suggested that glutamine should be considered to be

TABLE 21.2
Plasma and Skeletal Muscle Glutamine Concentrations Reported in Various Animal Models

Species	Model	Plasma Glutamine		Skeletal Muscle Glutamine		Reference
		Control	Experimental	Control	Experimental	
Rat	Injury	–	–	9.9	5.9	Albina et al. (1987)
Rat	Sepsis	1.1	0.8	3.8	1.5	Parry-Billings et al. (1989)
Rat	Cancer cachexia	1.0	0.8	5.1	2.3	Parry-Billings et al. (1991)
Rat	Burn	0.7	0.5	4.1	2.7	Ardawi (1988b)
Dog	Burn	0.7	0.5	7.6	6.0	Stinnett et al. (1982)
Pig	Surgery	0.3	0.2	–	–	Deutz et al. (1992)

Note: Units are mM.

TABLE 21.3
Plasma and Skeletal Muscle Glutamine Concentrations Seen in Humans in Different Catabolic States

	Plasma Glutamine		Skeletal Muscle Glutamine		Reference
	Controls	Patients	Controls	Patients	
Trauma/burn	0.60	0.70	20.0	10.0	Furst et al. (1979)
Injury	0.78	0.51	20.5	9.1	Askanazi et al. (1980)
Sepsis	0.53	0.37	19.3	6.7	Roth et al. (1982)
Sepsis	0.78	0.62	20.5	9.5	Askanazi et al. (1980)
Sepsis	0.38	0.30	22.0	4.0	Milewski et al. (1982)
Burn	0.62	0.30	–	–	Parry-Billings et al. (1990a)
Burn	0.83	0.50	–	–	Stinnett et al. (1982)
Surgery	0.65	0.48	–	–	Parry-Billings et al. (1992)
Surgery	0.46	0.36	–	–	Lund et al. (1986)
Surgery	0.69	0.59	18.8	9.5	Askanazi et al. (1978)
Surgery	0.60	0.70	20.0	10.0	Askanazi et al. (1980)
Surgery	0.62	0.48	–	–	Powell et al. (1994)

Note: Units are mM.

conditionally essential in catabolic states (Lacey and Wilmore, 1990; Wilmore and Shabert, 1998). Thus, there has been much interest in investigating the effect of adding exogenous glutamine in models of infection or catabolic stress and in patients with relevant conditions.

21.6 EFFECT OF EXOGENOUS GLUTAMINE ON IMMUNE FUNCTION AND SURVIVAL IN ANIMAL MODELS OF INFECTION AND INFLAMMATION

If glutamine is important in supporting an optimal immune response, then provision of exogenous glutamine may be important at times of muscle and plasma glutamine depletion, especially where there is a risk or presence of infection. A number of studies in mice and rats have investigated the

TABLE 21.4

Effect of Exogenous Glutamine on Survival in Animal Models of Infection

Species	Mode of Infection	How Extra Glutamine Was Provided	% Mortality Control	% Mortality Experimental	Reference
Rat	Cecal ligation and puncture	Intravenous	75	25	Ardawi (1991)
Rat	Intraperitoneal *Escherichia coli*	Intravenous	45	8	Inoue et al. (1993)
Rat	Intraperitoneal *E. coli*	Intravenous	66	14	Naka et al. (1996)
Rat	Intratracheal *Pseudomonas*	Intravenous	75	30	DeWitt et al. (1999)
Mouse	Intravenous *Staphylococcus aureus*	Oral	80	60, 30[a]	Suzuki et al. (1993)
Mouse	Intravenous *S. aureus*	Oral	80	40	Adjei et al. (1994)

[a] Two different doses of glutamine were used.

effect of additional dietary glutamine or intravenous (parenteral) glutamine on response to infection; some of these studies are summarized in Table 21.4. They consistently show markedly improved survival when glutamine is provided orally or intravenously in amounts much greater than those that are present in the standard laboratory rodent diet. Unfortunately, most of these studies have not reported immune function measures and so the link between glutamine-enhanced improvement in immune function and in handling pathogens cannot be established precisely. However, the studies do show that in these models glutamine decreased muscle breakdown, diminished the decline in muscle glutamine and improved nitrogen balance (Ardawi, 1991), increased plasma glutamine concentration (Inoue et al., 1993), and improved intestinal integrity and function (Inoue et al., 1993; Naka et al., 1996).

Although studies listed in Table 21.4 did not assess immune function, other similar studies have done so. For example, Yoo et al. (1997) reported that proliferation of blood lymphocytes from *E. coli* infected piglets was higher if the animals received a glutamine-enriched diet compared with a diet without glutamine. Shewchuk et al. (1997) reported that proliferation of spleen lymphocytes from tumor bearing rats was higher if the animals received a glutamine-enriched diet compared with a standard diet. Parenteral glutamine increased phagocytosis by lung macrophages from tumor bearing rats (Kweon et al., 1991) and proliferation of blood lymphocytes from septic rats (Yoshida et al., 1992).

In a mouse hyperoxia model, glutamine provided as a dipeptide with arginine and in combination with omega-3 fatty acids attenuated intestinal inflammation (Li et al., 2012) and lung injury and inflammation, including effects on myeloperoxidase and inflammatory cytokines (e.g., IL-6) and chemokines (Ma et al., 2012).

Studies have also investigated the effect of exogenous glutamine on the gut-associated lymphoid system in infected animals. Intravenous glutamine prevented the influenza virus infection associated loss of Peyer patches lymphocytes and intestinal integrity in mice (Li et al., 1997, 1998). Oral glutamine increased total cellularity of Peyer's patches in LPS-treated mice (Manhart et al., 2000), an effect mainly due to T cells.

21.7 GLUTAMINE, IMMUNITY, AND INFECTION IN HOSPITALIZED PATIENTS

Glutamine has been used in patients in various catabolic states to help maintain nitrogen balance, muscle mass, and gut integrity, rather than to support the immune system. However, an intervention that prevents, or reverses, the decline in glutamine concentration might have a beneficial influence on the immune system. Quite a number of studies have investigated the effect of exogenously supplied glutamine on immunity and infection in catabolic stress states in various patient groups. In these studies glutamine has been provided intravenously or enterally. Patients who received intravenous glutamine postsurgery showed higher ex vivo T-lymphocyte proliferation (O'Riordain et al., 1994), higher blood lymphocyte numbers (Morlion et al., 1998), better expression of molecules involved in antigen presentation on the surface of monocytes (Spittler et al., 2001), and had a shorter stay in hospital (Morlion et al., 1998). Intravenous administration of glutamine reduced infection rate (12% of patients vs. 42% in the control group) and length of hospital stay (average of 29 days vs. 36 days) in patients who had received bone marrow transplantation (Ziegler et al., 1992). Glutamine administration also resulted in higher numbers of lymphocytes, T lymphocytes, and CD4+ lymphocytes, but not B lymphocytes or natural killer cells, in the bloodstream (Ziegler et al., 1998). A glutamine-enriched feeding formula decreased sepsis rate in very low birth weight babies (11% vs. 31% in the control group) (Neu et al., 1997). Griffiths et al. (1997) reported that ICU patients who received intravenous glutamine had less "late" mortality than seen in a control group (43% vs. 67%) and this was related to a different pattern of infections in the two groups (Griffiths et al., 2002). Jensen et al. (1996) earlier reported that enteral glutamine increased the ratio of CD4+ to CD8+ cells in ICU patients. Trauma patients who received enteral glutamine had less risk of pneumonia (17% vs. 45% in the control group), bacteremia (7% vs. 42%), and severe sepsis (4% vs. 26%) (Houdijk et al., 1998). Boelens et al. (2002, 2004) reported that enteral glutamine increased Human leukocyte antigen–antigen D related (HLA-DR) expression on monocytes and IFN-γ production by T cells from trauma patients. Enteral glutamine decreased infection rate, and mortality, in adult burn patients (Garrel et al., 2003). In contrast to these positive studies, more recently Andrews et al. (2011) saw no effect of intravenous glutamine on infections, antibiotic use or mortality in ICU patients.

Studies of glutamine and clinical outcomes have been subject to several meta-analyses. Wang et al. (2010) identified that intravenous glutamine (used in hydrolysable dipeptide form) resulted in fewer infections and shorter hospital stay in gastrointestinal surgery patients. More recently, Bollhalder et al. (2013) identified that intravenous glutamine resulted in fewer infections and shorter hospital length of stay, with larger effects seen in surgical than critically ill patients. Earlier, Novak et al. (2002) conducted a meta-analysis of intravenous and enteral glutamine use in surgical and critically ill patients. They identified that glutamine use resulted in fewer infections and shorter hospital stay and that these benefits were associated with providing intravenous glutamine and using glutamine at a dose greater than 0.2 g/kg/day and were more likely seen in surgical patients.

Based upon positive trials and meta-analyses, the American Society of Parenteral and Enteral Nutrition and the European Society for Clinical Nutrition and Metabolism both recommend that 0.3–0.5 g/kg of glutamine is added to parenteral nutrition for critically ill adults (Singer et al., 2009; McClave et al., 2009), a dose that has been shown to restore glutamine levels in critical illness (Tjader et al., 2004; Berg et al., 2005). However, recent work has questioned the efficacy of providing additional glutamine to septic adults, as administration of glutamine (0.8 g/kg/day) by both intravenous and enteral routes led to increased mortality compared to those who did not receive supplementation (Heyland et al., 2013). Other work has shown that critically ill septic patients who have either very low (<0.42 mM; Oudemans-van Straaten et al., 2001) or very high (>0.93 mM; Rodas et al., 2012) plasma glutamine concentrations are at risk of increased mortality, although it has been argued that very high glutamine levels could be more a marker of organ failure and severe shock rather than a cause of harm per se (Wischmeyer, 2015). Nevertheless, it is possible that providing too much glutamine could drive plasma concentrations too high and this may not be beneficial. In this context, the effects of hyperlevel glutamine on immune responses and inflammation during sepsis are unknown. In in vitro models, high levels of glutamine (5 mM) resulted in respiratory uncoupling and energy wasting within mitochondria and were associated with cell death (Krajcova et al., 2015). It is important to note that Wischmeyer (2015) suggests that while septic patients should not receive additional glutamine, certain patient populations may benefit from glutamine supplementation, for example, adults with burns, malignancies, trauma, or those requiring parenteral nutrition.

21.8   MECHANISMS OF GLUTAMINE ACTION

21.8.1   METABOLIC ROLES OF GLUTAMINE

Glutamine makes a significant contribution to energy generation in cells of the immune system (see Section 21.3). However, oxidation of glutamine is only partial and immune cells can use other substrates to generate energy (Calder, 1995b; Maciolek et al., 2014). Thus, it seems unlikely that the importance of glutamine to the immune system is related solely to its role as an energy yielding substrate.

Glutamine acts as a substrate for biosynthesis of purines and pyrimidines that are building blocks for RNA and DNA and so necessary for protein synthesis and cell division. However, the rate of synthesis of nucleotides in T-lymphocytes is low relative to the rate of glutamine utilization (Szondy and Newsholme, 1989), suggesting that, although this may be an important metabolic fate of glutamine, it probably does not provide the sole mechanism of glutamine action in immune cells.

Nicotinamide adenine dinucleotide phosphate (NADPH) is required by enzymes that are responsible for the formation of nitric oxide (inducible nitric oxide synthase) and superoxide (NADPH oxidase), the formation of reduced glutathione, and the *de novo* synthesis of RNA, DNA, and fatty acids. Glutamine metabolism via $NADP^+$-dependent malate dehydrogenase (aka malic enzyme) can generate considerable amounts of NADPH to support these diverse cellular requirements. Glutamine has been shown to enhance superoxide generation by neutrophils and monocytes (Garcia et al., 1999; Saito et al., 1999; Furukawa et al., 2000a,b), suggesting a link between glutamine availability of NADPH oxidase activity.

Glutamine has a number of roles as a biosynthetic precursor. One important role is as a source of glutamate for synthesis of the antioxidant tripeptide glutathione. Glutathione itself promotes T-lymphocyte activity (Dröge et al., 1994; Chang et al., 1999a) but is depleted during infection and trauma. Glutamine has been shown to preserve glutathione levels in rats (Hong et al., 1992; Welbourne et al., 1993; Denno et al., 1996; Cao et al., 1998) and in cultured human immune cells (Chang et al., 1999a). Indeed, Roth et al. (2002) reported a strong link between glutamine concentration, intracellular glutathione content, and lymphocyte proliferation *in vitro*. The effect of oral glutamine on T-cell number in the spleen and Peyer's patches of LPS-treated mice was related to increased glutathione content of those tissues (Manhart et al. 2000). Conversely, use of an inhibitor of glutathione synthesis reduced the number of lymphocytes in Peyer's patches (Manhart et al., 2000). These studies suggest that glutamine promotes glutathione synthesis in T lymphocytes (and elsewhere) and that this is associated with increased lymphocyte number and improved lymphocyte function.

21.8.2   GLUTAMINE AND HEAT SHOCK PROTEINS IN IMMUNITY AND INFLAMMATION

21.8.2.1   Heat Shock Proteins

Heat shock proteins (HSPs) are highly conserved proteins functioning in the unstressed state as intracellular molecular chaperones, maintaining homeostatic function, including protein refolding, movement of proteins across membranes, and gene regulation (Leppa and Sistonen, 1997). Cellular stress affects protein homeostasis resulting in misfolding and clumping of proteins (both self and nonself). The HSP response has evolved with the principal task of restoring protein homeostasis: repairing damage to proteins and re-establishing normal growth conditions (Wu, 1995; Leppa and Sistonen, 1997; Morimoto and Santoro, 1998; Laramie et al., 2008). HSPs are involved in numerous biological processes including the cell cycle, cell proliferation, differentiation, and apoptosis (Milarski and Morimoto, 1986; Hang et al., 1995). Numerous HSPs have been described and subsequently have been classified into six main families: HSP27, HSP40, HSP60, HSP70, HSP90, and HSP110. Of these, the HSP70 family is one of the most well studied and understood (Milarski and Morimoto, 1986; Jerome et al., 1993; Hang et al., 1995; Jaattela, 1999).

HSP70 is constitutively expressed and required at all times for cells to function normally. It is present in various cells including embryo cells, glial cells, dendritic cells (DCs), endothelial cells, monocytes, granulocytes, macrophages, B and T lymphocytes, and vascular smooth muscle cells (Hunter-Lavin et al., 2004). HSP70 comprises 1%–5% of cellular protein and is found in the cytoplasm, nucleus, mitochondria, and endoplasmic reticulum (Morimoto and Santoro, 1998).

HSP70 also occurs in an inducible form (Nam et al., 2007). The heat shock response is rapid, occurring within minutes of stress recognition (Morimoto and Santoro, 1998), resulting in the ubiquitous release of HSP70 (Maugeri et al., 2010). HSP70 is released in response to environmental stress (e.g., heat shock, heavy metals, oxidative stress) and pathological stress (e.g., ischemic and reperfusion injury and inflammatory response) (Laramie et al., 2008). Cytoplasmic HSP70 accumulation is relative to the degree of cellular stress (Morimoto and Santoro, 1998), conferring cytoprotection, in addition to acting as an extracellular chemokine to neighboring cells. Under these circumstances inducible HSP70 can comprise up to 20% of cell protein content (Pockley et al., 2008). HSP70 also acts to increase phagocytosis and uptake of foreign antigens and upregulates costimulatory molecules (de Jong et al., 2009).

Elevated levels of HSP70 remain within the cell for several hours conferring protection from subsequent insults (Balakrishnan and De Maio, 2006). However, ongoing HSP70 expression in an unstressed state has been found to be detrimental to cells and as a result mechanisms have evolved to ensure the timely resolution of the heat shock response (Li et al., 1991; Arispe et al., 2004).

21.8.2.2 Clinical Consequences of Upregulated HSP70 Release

Circulating HSP70 is part of a network of molecules arising from stressed or damaged cells, which stimulate immune activation (Matzinger, 1998, 2002; Gallucci and Matzinger, 2001; Vega et al., 2008), maintenance of cell homeostasis, and cellular protection (Henderson and Pockley, 2010), preventing apoptosis and death (Ribeiro et al., 1994, 1995, 1996; Villar et al., 1994; de Maio, 1999). Increased HSP70 expression has been shown to occur in trauma (Pittet et al., 2002), head injury (da Rocha et al., 2005), infection (Kimura et al., 2004), lung injury (Ganter et al., 2006), critical illness (Ziegler et al., 2005), and septic shock (Delogu et al., 1997; Wheeler et al., 2005). Experimental burns in rats and severe burns in adult humans have shown that upregulation of HSP70 expression (Meyer et al., 2000; Ogura et al., 2002) protects against organ damage, leading to increased survival (Ribeiro et al., 1995; Bruemmer-Smith et al., 2001). In humans, HSP70 expression occurs within minutes of the stress/insult with detectable levels in the plasma within the first few hours postinsult (Delogu et al., 1997; Pittet et al., 2002; Wheeler et al., 2005; Tang et al., 2008), with peaks between day 2 and 6 (Hashiguchi et al., 2001; Hu et al., 2005), although elevated levels are still detected at day 28 (Meyer et al., 2000; Ogura et al., 2002). In adults, HSP70 levels ≥15 ng/mL are associated with increased survival following severe trauma (Pittet et al., 2002). Conversely, high levels of HSP70 are associated with an increased risk of mortality in traumatic brain injury in adults (da Rocha et al., 2005), and severe sepsis in both adults (Gelain et al., 2011) and children (Wheeler et al., 2005). However, these high levels may be more reflective of overwhelming sepsis and pervasive HSP70 release from dying or necrotic cells rather than a cytotoxic effect of HSP70 itself (Wheeler et al., 2005; Gelain et al., 2011), especially since overall enhanced expression of HSP70 in adults (Ziegler et al., 2005; Wheeler et al., 2007) and in experimental animal models of sepsis appears to be protective (Weiss et al., 2000; Bruemmer-Smith et al., 2001; Rozhkova et al., 2010). Wheeler et al. (2005) describe high levels of HSP70 on hospital admission in children with septic shock and in other work in critically ill children with meningococcal disease, HSP70 levels decline over time as the sepsis resolves (Marino et al., 2014).

21.8.2.3 The Effect of HSP70 on the Inflammatory and Immune Response

HSP70 has a range of immunoregulatory and inflammatory functions and is capable of promoting either a pro- or anti-inflammatory response dependent on its location (within or external to the cell), the receptor sites it binds to (e.g., toll-like receptor [TLR] 2 or 4), and the type of T-cells stimulated, which ultimately influences the mix of cytokines released (Pockley et al., 2008). Under normal circumstances HSP70 is detectable in plasma of healthy individuals (who have no evidence of inflammation), suggesting that during times of homeostasis HSP70 does not promote an inflammatory response and its immunoregulatory/inflammatory functions are tightly controlled (Pockley et al., 2008). During times of stress, HSP70 is able to interact with APCs performing two distinct functions. The first is to present HSP:protein complexes, which are taken up by APC for processing, activating acquired immunity. The second function relates to HSP70 being able to stimulate the innate immune response and the secretion of cytokines and chemokines, such as TNF-α, IL-10, IL-6, IL-1β (amongst others), by macrophages and DCs (Binder et al., 2004; Quintana and Cohen, 2005). As the stress response resolves, HSP70 acts to dampen the inflammatory and immunoregulatory response, restoring homeostasis (Binder et al., 2004; van Eden et al., 2012). HSP70 therefore appears to play an important role in the modulation of both immune and inflammatory responses.

21.8.2.4 Glutamine and the Upregulation of HSP70

The benefits of glutamine in critical illness are believed to be due in part to the increased release of HSP70. Glutamine supplementation *in vitro* upregulates HSP70 release by lung macrophages and epithelial cells (Singleton et al., 2005a,b), protecting against sepsis-related injury (Singleton et al., 2005a,b). The efficacy of glutamine appears to be HSP70 dependent, since the benefit of glutamine during murine sepsis was not seen in HSP70 knockout mice (Singleton and Wischmeyer, 2007). In experimentally induced respiratory distress syndrome, glutamine supplementation has been shown to improve ATP levels reversing lactate accumulation and restoring HSP70 levels (Ziegler et al., 2005; Wischmeyer, 2006, 2009). HSP70 deficiency in a rat model of sepsis leads to a decline in lung tissue metabolism, lung injury, and organ failure (Singleton et al., 2005a,b).

Glutamine depletion appears to affect HSP70 production downstream of transcriptional and translational sites. This affects HSP70 mRNA stability, which in glutamine depleted cells significantly reduces their half-life (Eliasen et al., 2006). Glutamine has also been shown to exert an effect on HSP70 production relative to the upstream influence of glutamine on HSP70 gene expression (Morrison et al., 2006).

Hamiel et al. (2009) hypothesized that the effect of glutamine on HSP70 upregulation is dependent on the hexosamine biosynthetic molecular pathway (Figure 21.3). Glutamine is metabolized via this pathway, which appears to be part of an early cellular protective response to stress and glutamine is a key substrate required for optimal activity of the pathway. It appears that glutamine enhances hexosamine biosynthetic activity ultimately leading to increased HSP70 levels within the cell (Gong and Jing, 2011). It is thought that glutamine deficiency leads to a loss of activity of this pathway and so a reduction in HSP70 levels (Hamiel et al., 2009).

21.9 SUMMARY AND CONCLUSIONS

Glutamine is used at a high rate by cells of the immune system but not all of the glutamine used is fully oxidized. Glutamine is converted to a number of metabolites involved in signaling, biosynthesis, immune cell turnover and function, and cell and tissue protection and preservation (Figure 21.4). Enhanced synthesis of HSP70 seems to be an important mechanism by which glutamine exerts its effects on some aspects of immune function. Glutamine utilization is increased when immune cells are activated and this increases the demand for an optimal supply of glutamine. Glutamine at normal physiological concentrations seems to be necessary to support optimal function of T cells, B cells, monocytes, macrophages, neutrophils, and the gut-associated lymphoid tissue. The effects of glutamine on T-cell functions have been studied in detail. Here it is described that activation increases glutamine transport and metabolism and that an optimal glutamine supply supports proliferation, surface receptor expression, and Th1 cytokine production. These findings suggest that providing exogenous glutamine would improve host defense against bacteria and viruses in situations where the endogenous supply was limited. A number of studies in rats and mice support this idea. In

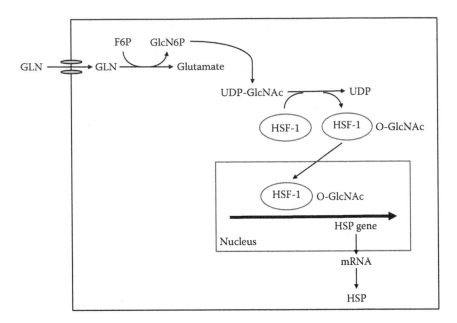

FIGURE 21.3 Proposed mechanism for glutamine-mediated upregulation of HSP70 synthesis. Glutamine (GLN) is metabolized via the hexosamine biosynthetic pathway to UDP-*N*-acetylglucosamine (UDP-GlcNAc). This covalently modifies the heat shock transcription factor (HSF)-1, which translocates to the nucleus and binds to the HSP promoter region. Other abbreviations: F6P, fructose 6-phosphate; GlcN6P, glucosamine 6-phosphate; OGlcNAc, O-linked GlcNAc; NUDP, uridine diphosphate.

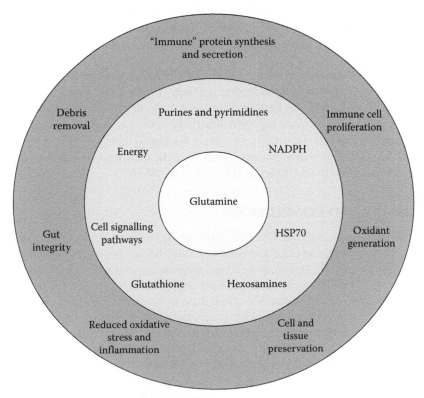

FIGURE 21.4 Influence of glutamine on immune function and related activities highlighting the key underlying mechanisms involved.

humans major surgery, injury, trauma, critical illness, and sepsis all result in lowered glutamine availability seen as lower than normal concentrations of glutamine in skeletal muscle, the site of its synthesis, and in blood plasma, suggesting that demand for glutamine may be exceeding supply. It is possible that lowered glutamine availability is in part responsible for the impaired immune function and the increased susceptibility to infections seen in those patient groups. Provision of glutamine either intravenously or enterally to such patients is associated with improvements in immune function, where this has been examined, and in improved clinical outcome, including fewer infections. A recent study in critically ill patients where a very high amount of glutamine was given by both enteral and intravenous routes did not find a benefit and even identified some harm. This suggests that more needs to be known about the dose-dependent effects of glutamine on target cell function (e.g., the immune response) and on clinical outcomes. However, glutamine is safe and effective in most patient groups in whom its use is indicated by lowered plasma concentration.

REFERENCES

Adjei, A.A., Y. Matsumoto, T. Oku, Y. Hiroi and S. Yamamoto. 1994. Dietary arginine and glutamine combination improves survival in septic mice. *Nutr. Res.* 14: 1591–1599.

Albina, J.E., W. Henry, P.A. King, J. Shearer, B. Mastrofrancesco, L. Goldstein and M.D. Caldwell. 1987. Glutamine metabolism in rat skeletal muscle wounded with lambda-carrageenan. *Am. J. Physiol.* 252: E49–E56.

Alverdy, J.C. 1990. Effects of glutamine-supplemented diets on immunology of the gut. *J. Parenter. Enteral Nutr.* 14(4 Suppl): 109S–113S.

Andrews, P.J., A. Avenell, D.W. Noble, M.K. Campbell, B.L. Croal, W.G. Simpson, L.D. Vale, C.G. Battison, D.J. Jenkinson, J.A. Cook JÁ and the Scottish Intensive care Glutamine or selenium Evaluative Trial Trials Group. 2011. Randomised trial of glutamine, selenium, or both, to supplement parenteral nutrition for critically ill patients. *Brit. Med. J.* 342: d1542.

Ardawi, M.S. 1988a. Glutamine and glucose metabolism in human peripheral lymphocytes. *Metabolism* 37: 99–103.

Ardawi, M.S. 1988b. Skeletal muscle glutamine production in thermally injured rats. *Clin. Sci.* 74: 165–172.

Ardawi, M.S. 1991. Effect of glutamine-enriched total parenteral nutrition on septic rats. *Clin. Sci.* 81: 215–222.

Ardawi, M.S. and E.A. Newsholme. 1982. Maximum activities of some enzymes of glycolysis, the tricarboxylic acid cycle and ketone-body and glutamine utilization pathways in lymphocytes of the rat. *Biochem. J.* 208: 743–748.

Ardawi, M.S. and E.A. Newsholme. 1983. Glutamine metabolism in lymphocytes of the rat. *Biochem. J.* 212: 835–842.

Arispe, N., M. Doh, O. Simakova, B. Kurganov and A. De Maio. 2004. Hsc70 and Hsp70 interact with phosphatidylserine on the surface of PC12 cells resulting in a decrease of viability. *FASEB J.* 18: 1636–1645.

Askanazi, J., Y.A. Carpentier, C.B. Michelsen, D.H. Elwyn, P. Furst, L.R. Kantrowitz, F.E. Gump and J.M. Kinney. 1980. Muscle and plasma amino acids following injury. Influence of intercurrent infection. *Ann. Surg.* 192: 78–85.

Askanazi, J., D.H. Elwyn, J.M. Kinney, F.E. Gump, C.B. Michelsen, F.E. Stinchfield, P. Fürst, E. Vinnars and J. Bergström. 1978. Muscle and plasma amino acids after injury: The role of inactivity. *Ann. Surg.* 188: 797–803.

Balakrishnan, K. and A. De Maio. 2006. Heat shock protein 70 binds its own messenger ribonucleic acid as part of a gene expression self-limiting mechanism. *Cell Stress Chaperones* 11: 44–50.

Berg, A., O. Rooyackers, A. Norberg and J. Wernerman. 2005. Elimination kinetics of L-alanyl-L-glutamine in ICU patients. *Amino Acids* 29: 221–228.

Binder, R.J., R. Vatner and P. Srivastava. 2004. The heat-shock protein receptors: Some answers and more questions. *Tissue Antigen* 64: 442–451.

Boelens, P.G., A.P. Houdijk, J.C. Fonk, R.J. Nijveldt, C.C. Ferwerda, B.M. Von Blomberg-Van Der Flier, L.G. Thijs, H.J. Haarman, J.C. Puyana and P.A. Van Leeuwen PA. 2002. Glutamine-enriched enteral nutrition increases HLA-DR expression on monocytes of trauma patients. *J. Nutr.* 132: 2580–2586.

Boelens, P.G., A.P. Houdijk, J.C. Fonk, J.C. Puyana, H.J. Haarman, M.E. von Blomberg-van der Flier and P.A. van Leeuwen PA. 2004. Glutamine-enriched enteral nutrition increases *in vitro* interferon-gamma production but does not influence the *in vivo* specific antibody response to KLH after severe trauma. A prospective, double blind, randomized clinical study. *Clin. Nutr.* 23: 391–400.

Bollhalder, L., A.M. Pfeil, Y. Tomonaga and M. Schwenkglenks. 2013. A systematic literature review and meta-analysis of randomized clinical trials of parenteral glutamine supplementation. *Clin. Nutr.* 32: 213–223.

Brand, K. 1985. Glutamine and glucose metabolism during thymocyte proliferation. Pathways of glutamine and glutamate metabolism. *Biochem. J.* 228: 353–361.

Brand, K., W. Fekl, J. von Hintzenstern, K. Langer, P. Luppa and C. Schoerner. 1989. Metabolism of glutamine in lymphocytes. *Metabolism* 38(Suppl 1): 29–33.

Bruemmer-Smith, S., F. Stuber and S. Schroeder. 2001. Protective functions of intracellular heat-shock protein (HSP) 70-expression in patients with severe sepsis. *Intensive Care Med.* 27: 1835–1841.

Calder, P.C. 1995a. Requirement of both glutamine and arginine by proliferating lymphocytes. *Proc. Nutr. Soc.* 54: 123A.

Calder, P.C. 1995b. Fuel utilisation by cells of the immune system. *Proc. Nutr. Soc.* 54: 65–82.

Calder, P.C. and E.A. Newsholme. 1992. Glutamine promotes interleukin-2 production by concanavalin A-stimulated lymphocytes. *Proc. Nutr. Soc.* 51: 105A.

Cao, Y., Z. Feng, A. Hoos and V.S. Klimberg. 1998. Glutamine enhances gut glutathione production. *J. Parenter. Enteral Nutr.* 22: 224–227.

Carr, E.L., A. Kelman, G.S. Wu, R. Gopaul, E. Senkevitch, A. Aghvanyan, A.M. Turay and K.A. Frauwirth. 2010. Glutamine uptake and metabolism are coordinately regulated by ERK/MAPK during T lymphocyte activation. *J. Immunol.* 185: 1037–1044.

Chakrabarti, R.1998. Transcriptional regulation of the rat glutamine synthetase gene by tumor necrosis factor-alpha. *Eur. J. Biochem.* 254: 70–74.

Chang, W.K., K.D. Yang and M.F. Shaio. 1999a. Lymphocyte proliferation modulated by glutamine: Involved in the endogenous redox reaction. *Clin. Exp. Immunol.* 117: 482–488.

Chang, W.K., K.D. Yang and M.F. Shaio. 1999b. Effect of glutamine on Th1 and Th2 cytokine responses of human peripheral blood mononuclear cells. *Clin. Immunol.* 93: 294–301.

Chuang, J.C., C.L. Yu and S.R. Wang. 1990. Modulation of human lymphocyte proliferation by amino acids. *Clin. Exp. Immunol.* 81: 173–176.

Crawford, J. and H.J. Cohen. 1985. The essential role of L-glutamine in lymphocyte differentiation *in vitro*. *J. Cell Physiol.* 124: 275–282.

Curi, T.C., M.P. De Melo, R.B. De Azevedo, T.M. Zorn and R. Curi. 1997. Glutamine utilization by rat neutrophils: Presence of phosphate-dependent glutaminase. *Am. J. Physiol.* 273: C1124–C1129.

da Rocha, A.B., C. Zanoni, G.R. de Freitas, C. Andre, S. Himelfarb, R.F. Schneider, I. Grivicich et al. 2005. Serum Hsp70 as an early predictor of fatal outcome after severe traumatic brain injury in males. *J. Neurotrauma* 22: 966–977.

de Jong, P.R., A.W. Schadenberg, N.L. Jansen and B.J. Prakken. 2009. Hsp70 and cardiac surgery: Molecular chaperone and inflammatory regulator with compartmentalized effects. *Cell Stress Chaperones* 14: 117–131.

Delogu, G., L. Lo Bosco, M. Marandola, G. Famularo, L. Lenti, F. Ippoliti and L. Signore. 1997. Heat shock protein (HSP70) expression in septic patients. *J. Crit. Care.* 12: 188–192.

de Maio, A. 1999. Heat shock proteins: Facts, thoughts, and dreams. *Shock* 11: 1–12.

Denno, R., J.D. Rounds, R. Faris, L.B. Holejko and D.W. Wilmore. 1996. Glutamine-enriched total parenteral nutrition enhances plasma glutathione in the resting state. *J. Surg. Res.* 61: 35–38.

Deutz, N.E., P.L. Reijven, G. Athanasas and P.B. Soeters. 1992. Post-operative changes in hepatic, intestinal, splenic and muscle fluxes of amino acids and ammonia in pigs. *Clin. Sci.* 83: 607–614.

DeWitt, R.C., Y. Wu, K.B. Renegar and K.A. Kudsk. 1999. Glutamine-enriched total parenteral nutrition preserves respiratory immunity and improves survival to a Pseudomonas Pneumonia. *J. Surg. Res.* 84: 13–18.

Dröge, W., S. Mihm, M. Bockstette and S. Roth. 1994. Effect of reactive oxygen intermediates and antioxidants on proliferation and function of T lymphocytes. *Meth. Enzymol.* 234: 135–151.

Eliasen, M.M., M. Brabec, C. Gerner, J. Pollheimer, H. Auer, M. Zellner, G. Weingartmann, F. Garo, E. Roth and R. Oehler. 2006 Reduced stress tolerance of glutamine-deprived human monocytic cells is associated with selective down-regulation of Hsp70 by decreased mRNA stability. *J. Mol. Med.* 84: 147–58.

Furst, P., J. Bergstrom, L. Chao, J. Larsson, S-O. Liljedahl, M. Neuhauser, B. Schildt and E. Vinnars. 1979. Influence of amino acid supply on nitrogen and amino acid metabolism in severe trauma. *Acta Chir. Scand.* 494 (Suppl. 1): 136–138.

Furukawa, S., H. Saito, K. Fukatsu, Y. Hashiguchi, T. Inaba, M.T. Lin, T. Inoue, I. Han, T. Matsuda and T. Muto. 1997. Glutamine-enhanced bacterial killing by neutrophils from postoperative patients. *Nutrition* 13: 863–869.

Furukawa, S., H. Saito, T. Inoue, T. Matsuda, K. Fukatsu, I. Han, S. Ikeda and A. Hidemura. 2000a. Supplemental glutamine augments phagocytosis and reactive oxygen intermediate production by neutrophils and monocytes from postoperative patients *in vitro*. *Nutrition* 16: 323–329.

Furukawa, S., H. Saito, T. Matsuda, T. Inoue, K. Fukatsu, I. Han, S. Ikeda, A. Hidemura and T. Muto. 2000b. Relative effects of glucose and glutamine on reactive oxygen intermediate production by neutrophils. *Shock* 13: 274–278.

Gallucci, S. and P. Matzinger. 2001. Danger signals: SOS to the immune system. *Curr. Opin. Immunol.* 13: 114–119.

Ganter, M.T., L.B. Ware, M. Howard, J. Roux, B. Gartland, M.A. Matthay, M. Fleshner, F. Pittet. 2006. Extracellular heat shock protein 72 is a marker of the stress protein response in acute lung injury. *Am. J. Physiol.* 291: L354–L361.

Garcia, C., T.C. Pithon-Curi, M. de Lourdes Firmano, M. Pires de Melo, P. Newsholme and R. Curi. 1999. Effects of adrenaline on glucose and glutamine metabolism and superoxide production by rat neutrophils. *Clin. Sci.* 96: 549–555.

Garrel, D., J. Patenaude, B. Nedelec, L. Samson, J. Dorais, J. Champoux, M. D'Elia and J. Bernier. 2003. Decreased mortality and infectious morbidity in adult burn patients given enteral glutamine supplements: A prospective, controlled, randomized clinical trial. *Crit. Care Med.* 31: 2444–2449.

Gelain, D.P., M.A. de Bittencourt Pasquali, C Comim, M.S. Grunwald, C. Ritter, C.D. Tomasi, S.C. Alves, J. Quevedo, F. Dal-Pizzol and J.C. Moreira. 2011. Serum heat shock protein 70 levels, oxidant status, and mortality in sepsis. *Shock* 35: 466–470.

Gong, J. and L. Jing. 2011. Glutamine induces heat shock protein 70 expression via O-GlcNAc modification and subsequent increased expression and transcriptional activity of heat shock factor-1. *Minerva Anesthesiol.* 77: 488–495.

Griffiths, M. and D. Keast. 1990. The effect of glutamine on murine splenic leukocyte responses to T and B cell mitogens. *Immunol. Cell Biol.* 68: 405–408.

Griffiths, R.D., K.D. Allen, F.J. Andrews and C. Jones. 2002. Infection, multiple organ failure, and survival in the intensive care unit: Influence of glutamine-supplemented parenteral nutrition on acquired infection. *Nutrition* 18: 546–552.

Griffiths, R.D., C. Jones and T.E. Palmer. 1997. Six-month outcome of critically ill patients given glutamine-supplemented parenteral nutrition. *Nutrition* 13: 295–302.

Hamiel, C.R., S. Pinto, A. Hau and P.E. Wischmeyer. 2009. Glutamine enhances heat shock protein 70 expression via increased hexosamine biosynthetic pathway activity. *Am. J. Physiol.* 297: C1509–C1519.

Hang, H., L. He and M.H. Fox. 1995. Cell cycle variation of Hsp70 levels in HeLa cells at 37 degrees C and after a heat shock. *J. Cell Physiol.* 165: 367–375.

Hashiguchi, N., H. Ogura, H. Tanaka, T. Koh, M. Aoki, T. Shiozaki, T. Matsuoka, T. Shimazu and H. Sugimoto. 2001. Enhanced expression of heat shock proteins in leukocytes from trauma patients. *J. Trauma* 50: 102–107.

Heberer, M., R. Babst, A. Juretic, T. Gross, H. Hörig, F. Harder and G.C. Spagnoli. 1996. Role of glutamine in the immune response in critical illness. *Nutrition* 12: S71–S72.

Henderson, B. and A.G. Pockley. 2010. Molecular chaperones and protein-folding catalysts as intercellular signaling regulators in immunity and inflammation. *J. Leukoc. Biol.* 88: 445–462.

Heyland, D., J. Muscedere, P.E. Wischmeyer, D. Cook, G. Jones, M. Albert, G. Elke, M.M. Berger, A.G. Day, Canadian Critical Care Trials Group. 2013. A randomized trial of glutamine and antioxidants in critically ill patients. *N. Engl. J. Med.* 368: 1489–1497.

Hirsch, E.M. 1970. L-glutaminase: Suppression of lymphocyte blastogenic responses *in vitro*. *Science* 172: 736–738.

Hong, R.W., J.D. Rounds, W.S. Helton, M.K. Robinson and D.W. Wilmore. 1992. Glutamine preserves liver glutathione after lethal hepatic injury. *Ann. Surg.* 215: 114–119.

Hörig, H., G.C. Spagnoli, L. Filgueira, R. Babst, H. Gallati, F. Harder, A. Juretic and H. Heberer. 1993. Exogenous glutamine requirement is confined to late events of T cell activation. *J. Cell Biochem.* 53: 343–351.

Horvath, K., M. Jami, I.D. Hill, J.C. Papadimitriou, L.S. Magder and S. Chanasongcram. 1996. Isocaloric glutamine-free diet and the morphology and function of rat small intestine. *J. Parenter. Enteral Nutr.* 20: 128–134.

Houdijk, A.P., E.R. Rijnsburger, J. Jansen, R.I. Wesdorp, J.K. Weiss, M.A. McCamish, T. Teerlink et al. 1998. Randomised trial of glutamine-enriched enteral nutrition on infectious morbidity in patients with multiple trauma. *Lancet* 352: 772–776.

Hu, D., Y. Qu, F.Q. Chen and B. Luo. 2005. Expression of heat shock protein 72 in leukocytes from patients with acute trauma and its relationship with survival. *Zhongguo Wei Zhong Bing Ji Jiu Yi Xue* 17: 299–301.

Hunter-Lavin, C., E.L. Davies, M.M. Bacelar, M.J. Marshall, S.M. Andrew and J.H. Williams. 2004. Hsp70 release from peripheral blood mononuclear cells. *Biochem. Biophys. Res. Commun.* 324: 511–517.

Inoue, Y., J.P. Grant and P.J. Snyder. 1993. Effect of glutamine-supplemented intravenous nutrition on survival after Escherichia coli-induced peritonitis. *J. Parenter. Enteral Nutr.* 17: 41–46.

Jaattela, M. 1999. Heat shock proteins as cellular lifeguards. *Ann. Med.* 31: 261–271.

Jensen, G.L., R.H. Miller, D.G. Talabiska, J. Fish and L. Gianferante. 1996. A double-blind, prospective, randomized study of glutamine-enriched compared with standard peptide-based feeding in critically ill patients. *Am. J. Clin. Nutr.* 64: 615–621.

Jerome, V., C. Vourc'h, E.E. Baulieu and M.G. Catelli. 1993. Cell cycle regulation of the chicken hsp90 alpha expression. *Exp. Cell Res.* 205: 44–51.

Keast, D. and E.A. Newsholme. 1990. Effect of mitogens on the maximum activities of hexokinase, lactate dehydrogenase, citrate synthase and glutaminase in rat mesenteric lymph node lymphocytes and splenocytes during the early period of culture. *Int. J. Biochem.* 22: 133–136.

Kew, S., S.M. Wells, P. Yaqoob, F.A. Wallace, E.A. Miles and P.C. Calder. 1999. Dietary glutamine enhances murine T-lymphocyte responsiveness. *J. Nutr.* 129: 1524–1531.

Kimura, F., H. Itoh, S. Ambiru, H. Shimizu, A. Togawa, H. Yoshidome, M. Ohtsuka et al. 2004. Circulating heat-shock protein 70 is associated with postoperative infection and organ dysfunction after liver resection. *Am. J. Surg.* 187: 777–784.

Köhler, H., H. Hartig-Knecht, J. Rüggeberg, R. Adam and H. Schroten. 2000. Lymphocyte proliferation is possible with low concentrations of glycyl-glutamine. *Eur. J. Nutr.* 39: 103–105.

Krajcova, A., J. Ziak, K. Jiroutkova, J. Patkova, M. Elkalaf, V. Dzupa, J. Trnka and F. Duska. 2015. Normalizing glutamine concentration causes mitochondrial uncoupling in an *in vitro* model of human skeletal muscle. *J. Parenter. Enteral Nutr.* 39: 180–189.

Kudsk, K.A., Y. Wu, K. Fukatsu, B.L. Zarzaur, C.D. Johnson, R. Wang and M.K. Hanna. 2000. Glutamine-enriched total parenteral nutrition maintains intestinal interleukin-4 and mucosal immunoglobulin A levels. *J. Parenter. Enteral Nutr.* 24: 270–274.

Kweon, M.N., S. Moriguchi, K. Mukai and Y. Kishino. 1991. Effect of alanylglutamine-enriched infusion on tumor growth and cellular immune function in rats. *Amino Acids* 1: 7–16.

Lacey, J.M. and D.W. Wilmore. 1990. Is glutamine a conditionally essential amino acid? *Nutr. Rev.* 48: 297–309.

Laramie, J.M., T.P. Chung, B. Brownstein, G.D. Stormo and J.T. Cobb. 2008. Transcriptional profiles of human epithelial cells in response to heat: Computational evidence for novel heat shock proteins. *Shock* 29: 623–630.

Leppa, S. and L. Sistonen. 1997. Heat shock response—pathophysiological implications. *Ann. Med.* 29: 73–78.

Li, G.C., G. Li, Y.K. Liu, J.Y. Mak, L.L. Chen and W.M. Lee. 1991. Thermal response of rat fibroblasts stably transfected with the human 70-kDa heat shock protein-encoding gene. *Proc. Natl. Acad. Sci. USA* 88: 1681–1685.

Li, J., B.K. King, P.G. Janu, K.B. Renegar and K.A. Kudsk KA. 1998. Glycyl-L-glutamine-enriched total parenteral nutrition maintains small intestine gut-associated lymphoid tissue and upper respiratory tract immunity. *J. Parenter. Enteral Nutr.* 22: 31–36.

Li, J., K.A. Kudsk, P. Janu and K.B. Renegar. 1997. Effect of glutamine-enriched total parenteral nutrition on small intestinal gut-associated lymphoid tissue and upper respiratory tract immunity. *Surgery* 121: 542–549.

Li, N., L. Ma, X. Liu, L. Shaw, S. Li Calzi, M.B. Grant and J. Neu. 2012. Arginyl-glutamine dipeptide or docosahexaenoic acid attenuates hyperoxia-induced small intestinal injury in neonatal mice. *J. Pediatr. Gastroenterol. Nutr.* 54: 499–504.

Lund, J., H. Stjernström, E. Vinnars, L. Jorfeldt, U. Bergholm and L. Wiklund. 1986. The influence of abdominal surgery on the splanchnic exchange of amino acids. *Acta Chir. Scand.* 152: 191–197.

Ma, L., N. Li, X. Liu, L. Shaw, s. Li Calzi, M.B. Grant and J. Neu. 2012. Arginyl-glutamine dipeptide or docosahexaenoic acid attenuate hyperoxia-induced lung injury in neonatal mice. *Nutrition* 28: 1186–1191.

Maciolek, J.A., J.A. Pasternak and H.L. Wilson. 2014. Metabolism of activated T lymphocytes. *Curr. Opin. Immunol.* 27: 60–74.

Manhart, N., K. Vierlinger, R. Akomeah, H. Bergmeister, A. Spittler and E. Roth. 2000. Influence of enteral diets supplemented with key nutrients on lymphocyte subpopulations in Peyer's patches of endotoxin-boostered mice. *Clin. Nutr.* 19: 265–269.

Marino, L.V., N. Pathan, R. Meyer, V. Wright and P. Habibi. 2014. Glutamine depletion and heat shock protein 70 (HSP70) in children with meningococcal disease. *Clin. Nutr.* 33: 915–921.

Matzinger, P. 1998. An innate sense of danger. *Semin. Immunol.* 10: 399–415.

Matzinger, P. 2002. The danger model: A renewed sense of self. *Science* 296: 301–305.

Maugeri, N., J. Radhakrishnan and J.C. Knight. 2010. Genetic determinants of HSP70 gene expression following heat shock. *Hum. Mol. Genet.* 19: 4939–4947.

Max, S.R., J. Mill, K. Mearow, M. Konagaya, Y. Konagaya, J.W. Thomas, C. Banner and L. Vitković, 1988. Dexamethasone regulates glutamine synthetase expression in rat skeletal muscles. *Am. J. Physiol.* 255: E397–E402.

McClave, S.A., R.G. Martindale, V.W. Vanek, M. McCarthy, P. Roberts, B. Taylor, J.B. Ochoa, L. Napolitano, G. Cresci, A.S.P.E.N. Board of Directors, American College of Critical Care Medicine, Society of Critical Care Medicine. 2009. Guidelines for the provision and assessment of nutrition support therapy in the adult critically ill patient: Society of Critical Care Medicine (SCCM) and American Society for Parenteral and Enteral Nutrition (A.S.P.E.N.). *J. Parenter. Enteral Nutr.* 33: 277–316.

Meyer, T.N., A.L. da Silva, E.C. Vieira and A.C. Alves. 2000. Heat shock response reduces mortality after severe experimental burns. *Burns* 26: 233–238.

Milarski, K.L. and R.I. Morimoto. 1986. Expression of human HSP70 during the synthetic phase of the cell cycle. *Proc. Natl. Acad. Sci. USA* 83: 9517–9521.

Milewski, P.J., C.J. Threlfall, D.F. Heath, I.B. Holbrook, K. Wilford and M.H. Irving. 1982. Intracellular free amino acids in undernourished patients with or without sepsis. *Clin. Sci.* 62: 83–91.

Morimoto, R.I. and M.G. Santoro. 1998. Stress-inducible responses and heat shock proteins: New pharmacologic targets for cytoprotection. *Nat. Biotechnol.* 16: 833–838.

Morlion, B.J., P. Stehle, P. Wachtler, H.P. Siedhoff, M. Köller, W. König, P. Fürst and C. Puchstein. 1998. Total parenteral nutrition with glutamine dipeptide after major abdominal surgery: A randomized, double-blind, controlled study. *Ann. Surg.* 227: 302–308.

Morrison, A.L., M. Dinges, K.D. Singleton, K. Odoms, H.R. Wong and P.E. Wischmeyer. 2006. Glutamine's protection against cellular injury is dependent on heat shock factor-1. *Am. J. Physiol.* 290: C1625–C1632.

Muhlbacher, F., C.R. Kapadia, M.F. Colpoys, R.J. Smith and D.W. Wilmore. 1984. Effects of glucocorticoids on glutamine metabolism in skeletal muscle. *Am. J. Physiol.* 247: E75–E83.

Murphy, C. and P. Newsholme. 1998. Importance of glutamine metabolism in murine macrophages and human monocytes to L-arginine biosynthesis and rates of nitrite or urea production. *Clin. Sci.* 95: 397–407.

Murphy, C. and E.A. Newsholme. 1999. Macrophage-mediated lysis of a beta-cell line, tumour necrosis factor-alpha release from bacillus Calmette-Guérin (BCG)-activated murine macrophages and interleukin-8 release from human monocytes are dependent on extracellular glutamine concentration and glutamine metabolism. *Clin. Sci.* 96: 89–97.

Naka, S., H. Saito, Y. Hashiguchi, M.T. Lin, S. Furukawa, T. Inaba, R. Fukushima, N. Wada and T. Muto. 1996. Alanyl-glutamine-supplemented total parenteral nutrition improves survival and protein metabolism in rat protracted bacterial peritonitis model. *J. Parenter. Enteral Nutr.* 20: 417–423.

Nam, S.Y., N. Kim, J.S. Kim, S.H. Lim, H.C. Jung and I.S. Song, 2007. Heat shock protein gene 70–2 polymorphism is differentially associated with the clinical phenotypes of ulcerative colitis and Crohn's disease. *J. Gastroenterol. Hepatol.* 22: 1032–1038.

Neu, J., J.C. Roig, W.H. Meetze, M. Veerman, C. Carter, C. Millsaps, D. Bowling, M.J. Dallas, J. Sleasman, T. Knight and N. Auestad. 1997. Enteral glutamine supplementation for very low birth weight infants decreases morbidity. *J. Pediatr.* 131: 691–699.

Newsholme, P. 1987. Studies on metabolism in macrophages. PhD thesis, University of Oxford.

Newsholme, P., R. Curi, S. Gordon and E.A. Newsholme. 1986. Metabolism of glucose, glutamine, long-chain fatty acids and ketone bodies by murine macrophages. *Biochem. J.* 239: 121–125.

Newsholme, P., S. Gordon and E.A. Newsholme. 1987. Rates of utilization and fates of glucose, glutamine, pyruvate, fatty acids and ketone bodies by mouse macrophages. *Biochem. J.* 242: 631–636.

Newsholme, P. and E.A. Newsholme. 1989. Rates of utilization of glucose, glutamine and oleate and formation of end-products by mouse peritoneal macrophages in culture. *Biochem. J.* 261: 211–218.

Novak, F., D.K. Heyland, A. Avenell, J.W. Drover and X. Su. 2002. Glutamine supplementation in serious illness: A systematic review of the evidence. *Crit. Care Med.* 30: 2022–2029.

Ogle, C.K., J.D. Ogle, J.X. Mao, J. Simon, J.G. Noel, B.G. Li and J.W. Alexander. 1994. Effect of glutamine on phagocytosis and bacterial killing by normal and pediatric burn patient neutrophils. *J. Parenter. Enteral Nutr.* 18: 128–133.

Ogura, H., N. Hashiguchi, H. Tanaka, T. Koh, M. Noborio, Y. Nakamori, M. Nishino, Y. Kuwagata, T. Shimazu and H.Y. Sugimoto. 2002. Long-term enhanced expression of heat shock proteins and decelerated apoptosis in polymorphonuclear leukocytes from major burn patients. *J. Burn Care Rehabil.* 23: 103–109.

O'Riordain, M.G., K.C. Fearon, J.A. Ross, P. Rogers, J.S. Falconer, D.C. Bartolo, O.J. Garden and D.C. Carter. 1994. Glutamine-supplemented total parenteral nutrition enhances T-lymphocyte response in surgical patients undergoing colorectal resection. *Ann. Surg.* 220: 212–221.

O'Rourke, A.M. and C.C. Rider. 1989. Glucose, glutamine and ketone body utilisation by resting and concanavalin A activated rat splenic lymphocytes. *Biochim. Biophys. Acta* 1010: 342–345.

Oudemans-van Straaten, H., R.J. Bosman, M. Treskes, H.J. van der Spoel and D.F. Zandstra. 2001. Plasma glutamine depletion and patient outcome in acute ICU admissions. *Intensive Care Med.* 27: 84–90.

Parry-Billings, M., R.J. Baigrie, P.M. Lamont, P.J. Morris and E.A. Newsholme. 1992. Effects of major and minor surgery on plasma glutamine and cytokine levels. *Arch. Surg.* 127: 1237–1240.

Parry-Billings, M., J. Evans, P.C. Calder and E.A. Newsholme. 1990a. Does glutamine contribute to immunosuppression after major burns? *Lancet* 336: 523–525.

Parry-Billings, M., B. Leighton, G.D. Dimitriadis, J. Bond and E.A. Newsholme. 1990b. Effects of physiological and pathological levels of glucocorticoids on skeletal muscle glutamine metabolism in the rat. *Biochem. Pharmacol.* 40: 1145–1148.

Parry-Billings, M., B. Leighton, G.D. Dimitriadis, R. Curi, J. Bond, S. Bevan, A. Colquhoun and E.A. Newsholme. 1991. The effect of tumour bearing on skeletal muscle glutamine metabolism. *Int. J. Biochem.* 23: 933–937.

Parry-Billings, M., B. Leighton, G. Dimitriadis, P.R. de Vasconcelos and E.A. Newsholme. 1989. Skeletal muscle glutamine metabolism during sepsis in the rat. *Int. J. Biochem.* 21: 419–423.

Pithon-Curi, T.C., M.P. De Melo and R. Curi, 2004. Glucose and glutamine utilization by rat lymphocytes, monocytes and neutrophils in culture: A comparative study. *Cell Biochem. Funct.* 22: 321–326.

Pithon-Curi, T.C., A.C. Levada, L.R. Lopes, S.Q. Doi and R. Curi. 2002. Glutamine plays a role in superoxide production and the expression of p47phox, p22phox and gp91phox in rat neutrophils. *Clin. Sci.* 103: 403–408.

Pittet, J.F., H. Lee, D. Morabito, M.B. Howard, W.I. Welch and R.C. Mackersie. 2002. Serum levels of Hsp 72 measured early after trauma correlate with survival. *J. Trauma* 52: 611–617.

Pockley, A.G., M. Muthana and S.K. Calderwood. 2008. The dual immunoregulatory roles of stress proteins. *Trends Biochem. Sci.* 33: 71–79.

Powell, H., L.M. Castell, M. Parry-Billings, J.P. Desborough, G.M. Hall and E.A. Newsholme. 1994. Growth hormone suppression and glutamine flux associated with cardiac surgery. *Clin. Physiol.* 14: 569–580.

Quintana, F.J. and I.R. Cohen. 2005. Heat shock proteins as endogenous adjuvants in sterile and septic inflammation. *J. Immunol.* 175: 2777–2782.

Ribeiro, S.P., J. Villar, G.P. Downey, J.D. Edelson and A.S. Slutsky. 1994. Sodium arsenite induces heat shock protein-72 kilodalton expression in the lungs and protects rats against sepsis. *Crit. Care Med.* 22: 922–929.

Ribeiro, S.P., J. Villar, G.P. Downey, J.D. Edelson and A.S. Slutsky. 1996. Effects of the stress response in septic rats and LPS-stimulated alveolar macrophages: Evidence for TNF-alpha posttranslational regulation. *Am. J. Respir. Crit. Care Med.* 154: 1843–1850.

Ribeiro, S.P., J. Villar and A.S. Slutsky. 1995 Induction of the stress response to prevent organ injury. *New Horiz.* 3: 301–311.

Rodas, P.C., O. Rooyackers, C. Hebert, A. Norberg and J. Wernerman. 2012. Glutamine and glutathione at ICU admission in relation to outcome. *Clin. Sci.* 122: 591–597.

Rohde, T., D.A. MacLean and B. Klarlund Pedersen. 1996. Glutamine, lymphocyte proliferation and cytokine production. *Scand. J. Immunol.* 44: 648–650.

Roth, E., J. Funovics, F. Mühlbacher, M. Schemper, W. Mauritz, P. Sporn and A. Fritsch. 1982. Metabolic disorders in severe abdominal sepsis: Glutamine deficiency in skeletal muscle. *Clin. Nutr.* 1: 25–41.

Roth, E., R. Oehler, N. Manhart, R. Exner, B. Wessner, E. Strasser and A. Spittler. 2002. Regulative potential of glutamine—elation to glutathione metabolism. *Nutrition* 18: 217–221.

Rozhkova, E., M. Yurinskaya, O. Zatsepina, D. Garbuz, V. Karpov, S. Surkov, A. Murashev et al. 2010. Exogenous mammalian extracellular HSP70 reduces endotoxin manifestations at the cellular and organism levels. *Ann. N. Y. Acad Sci.* 1197: 94–107.

Saito, H., S. Furukawa and T. Matsuda. 1999. Glutamine as an immunoenhancing nutrient. *J. Parenter. Enteral Nutr.* 23(5 Suppl): S59–S61.

Shewchuk, L.D., V.E. Baracos and C.J. Field. 1997. Dietary L-glutamine supplementation reduces the growth of the Morris Hepatoma 7777 in exercise-trained and sedentary rats. *J. Nutr.* 127: 158–166.

Simberkoff, M.S. and L. Thomas. 1970. Reversal by L-glutamine of the inhibition of lymphocyte mitosis caused by E. coli asparaginase. *Proc. Soc. Exp. Biol. Med.* 133: 642–644.

Singer, P., M.M. Berger, G. Van den Berghe, G. Biolo, P. Calder, A. Forbes, R. Griffiths, G. Kreyman, X. Leverve and C. Pichard. 2009. ESPEN Guidelines on Parenteral Nutrition: Intensive care. *Clin. Nutr.* 28: 387–400.

Singleton, K.D., N. Serkova, A. Banerjee, X. Meng, F. Gamboni-Robertson and P.E. Wischmeyer. 2005b. Glutamine attenuates endotoxin-induced lung metabolic dysfunction: Potential role of enhanced heat shock protein 70. *Nutrition* 21: 214–223.

Singleton, K.D., N. Serkova, V.E. Beckey and P.E. Wischmeyer. 2005a. Glutamine attenuates lung injury and improves survival after sepsis: Role of enhanced heat shock protein expression. *Crit. Care Med.* 33: 1206–1213.

Singleton, K.D. and P.E. Wischmeyer. 2007. Glutamine's protection against sepsis and lung injury is dependent on heat shock protein 70 expression. *Am. J. Physiol.* 292: R1839–R1845.

Spittler, A., S. Holzer, R. Oehler, G. Boltz-Nitulescu and E. Roth. 1997. A glutamine deficiency impairs the function of cultured human monocytes. *Clin. Nutr.* 16: 97–99.

Spittler, A., T. Sautner, A. Gornikiewicz, N. Manhart, R. Oehler, M. Bergmann, R. Függer and E. Roth. 2001. Postoperative glycyl-glutamine infusion reduces immunosuppression: Partial prevention of the surgery induced decrease in HLA-DR expression on monocytes. *Clin. Nutr.* 20: 37–42.

Spittler, A., S. Winkler, P. Götzinger, R. Oehler, M. Willheim, C. Tempfer, G. Weigel, R. Függer, G. Boltz-Nitulescu and E. Roth. 1995. Influence of glutamine on the phenotype and function of human monocytes. *Blood* 86: 1564–1569.

Spolarics, Z., C.H. Lang, G.J. Bagby and J.J. Spitzer. 1991. Glutamine and fatty acid oxidation are the main sources of energy for Kupffer and endothelial cells. *Am. J. Physiol.* 261: G185–G190.

Stinnett, J.D., J.W. Alexander, C. Watanabe, B.G. MacMillan, J.E. Fischer, M.J. Morris, O. Trocki, P., Miskell, L., Edwards and H. James. 1982. Plasma and skeletal muscle amino acids following severe burn injury in patients and experimental animals. *Ann. Surg.* 195: 75–89.

Suzuki, I., Y. Matsumoto, A.A. Adjei, L. Asato, S. Shinjo and S. Yamamoto. 1993. Effect of a glutamine-supplemented diet on response to methicillin-resistant Staphylococcus aureus infection in mice. *J. Nutr. Sci. Vitaminol.* 39: 405–410.

Szondy, Z. and E.A. Newsholme. 1989. The effect of glutamine concentration on the activity of carbamoyl-phosphate synthase II and on the incorporation of [3H]thymidine into DNA in rat mesenteric lymphocytes stimulated by phytohaemagglutinin. *Biochem. J.* 261: 979–983.

Tang, D., R. Kang, L. Cao, G. Zhang, Y. Yu, W. Xiao, H. Wang and X. Xiao. 2008. A pilot study to detect high mobility group box 1 and heat shock protein 72 in cerebrospinal fluid of pediatric patients with meningitis. *Crit. Care Med.* 36: 291–295.

Tjader, I., O. Rooyackers, A.M. Forsberg, R.F. Vesali, P.J. Garlick and J. Wernerman. 2004. Effects on skeletal muscle of intravenous glutamine supplementation to ICU patients. *Intensive Care Med.* 30: 266–275.

van Eden, W., R. Spiering, F. Broere and R. van der Zee. 2012. A case of mistaken identity: HSPs are no DAMPs but DAMPERs. *Cell Stress Chaperones* 17: 281–292.

Vega, V.L., M. Rodriguez-Silva, T. Frey, M. Gehrmann, J.C. Diaz, C. Steinem, G. Multhoff, N. Arispe and A. De Maio. 2008. Hsp70 translocates into the plasma membrane after stress and is released into the extracellular environment in a membrane-associated form that activates macrophages. *J. Immunol.* 180: 4299–4307.

Villar, J., S.P. Ribeiro, J.B. Mullen, M. Kuliszewski, M. Post and A.S. Slutsky. 1994. Induction of the heat shock response reduces mortality rate and organ damage in a sepsis-induced acute lung injury model. *Crit. Care Med.* 22: 914–921.

Wallace, C. and D. Keast. 1992. Glutamine and macrophage function. *Metabolism* 41: 1016–1020.

Wang, W., Y. Li, W. Zhang, F. Zhang and J. Li. 2011. Changes of plasma glutamine concentration and hepatocyte membrane system N transporters expression in early endotoxemia. *J. Surg. Res.* 166: 290–297.

Wang, Y., Z.M. Jiang, M.T. Nolan, H. Jiang, H.R. Han, K. Yu, H.L. Li, B. Jie and X.K. Liang. 2010. The impact of glutamine dipeptide-supplemented parenteral nutrition on outcomes of surgical patients: A meta-analysis of randomized clinical trials. *J. Parenter. Enteral Nutr.* 34: 521–529.

Weiss, Y.G., A. Bouwman, B. Gehan, G. Schears, N. Raj and C.S. Deutschman. 2000. Cecal ligation and double puncture impairs heat shock protein 70 (HSP-70) expression in the lungs of rats. *Shock* 13: 19–23.

Welbourne, T.C., A.B. King and K. Horton. 1993. Enteral glutamine supports hepatic glutathione efflux during inflammation. *J. Nutr. Biochem.* 4: 236–242.

Wells, S.M., S. Kew, P. Yaqoob, F.A. Wallace and P.C. Calder. 1999. Dietary glutamine enhances cytokine production by murine macrophages. *Nutrition* 15: 881–884.

Wheeler, D.S., L.E. Fisher Jr., J.D. Catravas, B.R. Jacobs, J.A. Carcillo and H.R. Wong. 2005. Extracellular hsp70 levels in children with septic shock. *Pediatr. Crit. Care Med.* 6: 308–311.

Wheeler, D.S., P. Lahni, K. Odoms, B.R. Jacobs, J.A. Carcillo, L.A. Doughty and H.R. Wong. 2007. Extracellular heat shock protein 60 (Hsp60) levels in children with septic shock. *Inflamm. Res.* 56: 216–219.

Wilmore, D.W. and J.K. Shabert. 1998. Role of glutamine in immunologic responses. *Nutrition* 14: 618–626.

Wischmeyer, P.E. 2006. Glutamine: The first clinically relevant pharmacological regulator of heat shock protein expression? *Curr. Opin. Clin. Nutr. Metab. Care* 9: 201–206.

Wischmeyer, P.E. 2009. Glutamine in acute lung injury: The experimental model matters. *Am. J. Physiol.* 296: L286–L287.

Wischmeyer, P. 2015. Glutamine supplementation in parenteral nutrition and intensive care unit patients: Are we throwing the baby out with the bathwater? *J. Parenter. Enteral Nutr.* 39: 893–897.

Wu, C. 1995. Heat shock transcription factors: Structure and regulation. *Annu. Rev. Cell. Dev. Biol.* 11: 441–469.

Wu, G., C.J. Field and E.B. Marliss. 1992. Enhanced glutamine and glucose metabolism in cultured rat splenocytes stimulated by phorbol myristate acetate plus ionomycin. *Metabolism* 41: 982–988.

Wu, G.Y., C.J. Field and E.B. Marliss. 1991. Glutamine and glucose metabolism in thymocytes from normal and spontaneously diabetic BB rats. *Biochem. Cell. Biol.* 69: 801–808.

Yaqoob, P. and P.C. Calder. 1997. Glutamine requirement of proliferating T lymphocytes. *Nutrition* 13: 646–651.

Yaqoob, P. and P.C. Calder. 1998. Cytokine production by human peripheral blood mononuclear cells: Differential sensitivity to glutamine availability. *Cytokine* 10: 790–794.

Yassad, A., A. Husson, A. Bion and A. Lavoinne. 2000. Synthesis of interleukin 1beta and interleukin 6 by stimulated rat peritoneal macrophages: Modulation by glutamine. *Cytokine* 12: 1288–1291.

Yoo, S.S., C.J. Field and M.I. McBurney. 1997. Glutamine supplementation maintains intramuscular glutamine concentrations and normalizes lymphocyte function in infected early weaned pigs. *J. Nutr.* 127: 2253–2259.

Yoshida, S., M.J. Leskiw, M.D. Schluter, K.T. Bush, R.G. Nagele, S. Lanza-Jacoby and T.P Stein. 1992. Effect of total parenteral nutrition, systemic sepsis, and glutamine on gut mucosa in rats. *Am. J. Physiol.* 263: E368–E373.

Ziegler, T.R., R.L. Bye, R.L. Persinger, L.S. Young, J.H. Antin and D.W. Wilmore. 1998. Effects of glutamine supplementation on circulating lymphocytes after bone marrow transplantation: A pilot study. *Am. J. Med. Sci.* 315: 4–10.

Ziegler, T.R., L.G. Ogden, K.D. Singleton, M. Luo, C. Fernandez-Estivariz, D.P. Griffith, J.R. Galloway and P.E. Wischmeyer. 2005. Parenteral glutamine increases serum heat shock protein 70 in critically ill patients. *Intensive Care Med.* 31: 1079–1086.

Ziegler, T.R., L.S. Young, K. Benfell, M. Scheltinga, K. Hortos, R. Bye, F.D. Morrow et al. 1992. Clinical and metabolic efficacy of glutamine-supplemented parenteral nutrition after bone marrow transplantation. A randomized, double-blind, controlled study. *Ann. Intern. Med.* 116: 821–828.

22 Glutamine and Exercise and Immune System

Marcelo Macedo Rogero and Ronaldo Vagner Thomatieli dos Santos

CONTENTS

This chapter will focus on the main advances in the study of glutamine, nutrition, and immune response during physical exercise. The chapter is divided into five sections. In the first section, the physiological functions of glutamine and its importance to the immune system are discussed. The second section deals with the effects of exercise on glutamine concentration and availability. The third section explains how nutrition and glutamine can modulate the immune response during acute and chronic exercise. The fourth section discusses the importance of glutamine supplementation for the immune response after exercise, and the final section consists of a brief conclusion about all the topics dealt with.

22.1 GLUTAMINE AND ITS IMPORTANCE FOR THE IMMUNE SYSTEM

Historically, in terms of scientific research about glutamine, it was verified during the 1930s in studies about the metabolism of this amino acid that the tissues of mammals are able to both hydrolyze and synthesize this amino acid. In the 1950s, it was proved that glutamine is important for *in vitro* cells and that glutamine concentration in the bloodstream is more than twice the amount of any other amino acid (Eagle et al. 1955; Hiscock and Pedersen 2002).

Glutamine is a five-carbon amino acid, classified as a neutral amino acid with 146.15 molecular weight and physiological pH. Nutritionally, glutamine is classified as a conditionally indispensable amino acid, since the body can synthesize this amino acid in normal conditions to achieve this metabolic necessity, however, in certain physiological or physiopathological conditions a necessity to ingest this amino acid can occur (Lacey and Wilmore 1990). It is worth noting that glutamine is the highest-concentration free-form amino acid in skeletal muscles and in human plasma, and it is also found in many other tissues in relatively high concentrations. Plasma glutamine concentration after fasting for 12 h is between 500 and 750 µmol/L, depending on the balance of glutamine release and intake by several tissues and body organs (Moskovitz et al. 1994).

Glutamine is involved in the transference of nitrogen among organs, detox of ammonia, and maintenance of the acid–base balance during acidosis, a possible direct regulation of protein synthesis and degradation, and a precursor of nitrogen for nucleotide synthesis. It is necessary for cell growth and differentiation, carbon-chain transportation among organs, and supplying energy to high-proliferation cells, like enterocytes and immune system cells. It acts as a precursor of ureogenesis and hepatic gluconeogenesis and of mediators such as gamma-aminobutyric acid and glutamate; promotes an increase in the intestine permeability and integrity, increases the resistance to infection by increasing phagocytosis function, and provides energy to the fibroblasts, increasing collagen synthesis (Smith 1990; Young and Ajami 2001; Rogero et al. 2004, 2006).

Glutamine synthetase and glutaminase are the two main intracellular enzymes involved in glutamine metabolism. The first is responsible for the reaction that synthesizes glutamine from ammonia and glutamate, in the presence of ATP, whereas the latter is responsible for hydrolysis of glutamine, converting it into glutamate and ammonia. As for intracellular localization, glutamine synthetase is primarily found in the cytosol, whereas glutaminase in its active form presents itself mainly in the mitochondrial interior (Neu et al. 1996; Walsh et al. 1998; Labow et al. 1999).

Skeletal muscles, lungs, liver, brain, and possibly adipose tissue present activity of enzyme glutamine synthetase and represent important organs involved in the synthesis of glutamine. On the other hand, enterocytes, leucocytes, and kidney tubular cells are primarily glutamine consumers, as well as present high activity of glutaminase enzyme. Under certain conditions, such as reduced carbohydrate intake, the liver may become a consumer site of glutamine (Souba 1993; Antonio and Street 1999; Labow and Souba 2000).

The main body organ for the uptake and metabolism of glutamine is the intestine. The necessary glutamine for the intestine is consumed primarily by the small intestine mucosa, which represents the largest amount of cells of fast proliferation in a normal human body. Diversely, the skeletal muscle is quantitatively the most relevant place of storage, synthesis, and release of glutamine. Intramuscular content of glutamine corresponds to 50%–60% of the free amino acid amount in this tissue. Approximately, 80% of the body glutamine is in the skeletal muscle and this concentration is 30 times higher than that found in the plasma (Windmueller and Spaeth 1975; Smith 1990; Souba et al. 1990; Souba 1993; Darmaun et al. 1994).

The free glutamine concentration in the muscle tissue depends on the type of muscle fiber. Therefore, glutamine storage is three times higher in slow twitch muscle fibers (type 1 fibers) than in fast twitch muscle fibers (type 2 fibers), considering that this fact may be a result of high activity of the glutamine synthetase enzyme and of more adenosine triphosphate (ATP) available to synthesize glutamine into type 1 fibers (Rowbottom et al. 1996; Walsh et al. 1998).

Glutamine is a very important nutrient for the immune function. Lymphocytes and macrophages are able to use glucose and glutamine to obtain energy and precursors to obtain biosynthesis of macromolecules. Glucose is converted mainly into lactate (glycolysis), whereas glutamine converts into glutamate and aspartate, suffering partial oxidation to CO_2 through a process called glutaminolysis, which is essential for the effective functioning of these immune system cells. Glycolysis provides ribose-5-phosphate, precursor of RNA and DNA synthesis, and glycerol-3-phosphate to synthesize phospholipids. Glutaminolysis provides glutamine, ammonia, and aspartate, which are used to synthesize purines and pyrimidines, both essential for DNA and RNA formation. It is worth noting that the processes of lymphocyte proliferation, as well as protein synthesis rates, interleukin-2 (IL-2) production, and antibody synthesis of these cells depend on glutamine. In macrophages, proinflammatory cytokine synthesis and secretions such as tumor necrosis factor alpha (TNF-α), IL-1, and IL-6, which are quantitatively relevant cytokines synthesized by macrophages, represent a process that depends on extracellular glutamine concentration (Newsholme et al. 1989; Calder 1995; Rowbottom et al. 1995; Newsholme et al. 1999).

Neutrophils present an increase in consumption related to the process of endocytosis and generation of oxygen reactive species. However, glucose is not the only energetic metabolite used by these cells. Recent studies demonstrate that neutrophils also actively consume glutamine, inasmuch as the quantity of glutamine used by neutrophils, as well as by lymphocytes and macrophages, is similar or even higher when compared to those of glucose (Newsholme et al. 1999).

Lymphocytes show a high activity of phosphate-dependent glutaminase enzyme and, considering that the latter is a mitochondrial enzyme, a possible metabolic way of glutamine in the mitochondria may be given as glutamine → glutamate → oxoglutarate → succinyl-CoA → succinate → fumarate → malate. Part of malate could be converted into oxaloacetate, which could be transaminated with glutamate to produce oxoglutarate and aspartate. The rest of the malate could be transported within cytosol, where it could undergo the following reaction: conversion into oxaloacetate, which could be transaminated with glutamate by the enzyme cytosolic aspartate aminotransferase, or converted into phosphoenolpyruvate through carboxykinase to form pyruvate and, consequently, lactate through pyruvate kinase and lactate dehydrogenase, respectively (Koyama et al. 1998; Rohde et al. 1998a; Rohde et al. 1998b; Curi 2000).

The plasma and tissue glutamine concentrations are reduced in clinical and catabolic situations such as trauma, burns, sepsis, postoperatory, and after exhaustive exercising or intense training. During these circumstances, glutaminemia reduction occurs because the uptake and utilization rates of this amino acid by several tissues are superior to the speed of synthesis and release by skeletal muscles. Furthermore, during catabolic processes, glutamine uptake by the intestine and kidney from bloodstream is increased. These situations are associated with an increase in susceptibility to infections, which is suggested to be partially related to a decrease in the glutamine supply for immune competent cells, such as lymphocytes (Smith 1990; Rowbottom et al. 1995). Moreover, several studies have demonstrated that the restoration of plasma glutamine concentration results in partial attenuate of inflammation. The mechanism of anti-inflammatory effects of glutamine is not well described; however, it has been suggested that regulation can be mediated by the Th1/Th2 (Yeh et al. 2005) balance in the expression of proinflammatory and anti-inflammatory cytokines (Chu et al. 2012), by decreasing the leakage of endotoxin, and by inhibiting cPLA2 phosphorylation in allergy (Kim et al. 2006; Ko et al. 2008). For more information about glutamine and the immune system, see Chapter 21.

22.2 GLUTAMINE AND EXERCISE

Intense and prolonged exercises are followed by alterations in plasma concentration of some amino acids, including, mainly, glutamine and branched chain amino acids (Hood and Terjung 1990, 1994). Studies with humans show that exercise is initially followed by an accelerated release of glutamine from skeletal muscles and a subsequent increase of glutaminemia. Accordingly, Babij et al. (1983) observed an increase of plasma glutamine concentration from 575 μmol/L at rest to 734 μmol/L during exercise at 100% VO_{2max} (maximum rate of oxygen consumption), whereas Eriksson et al. (1985) reported an increase in the beginning of the exercise from 538 μmol/L to 666 μmol/L after 45 min of exercise in ergometer cycle at 80% VO_{2max}. These results are sustained by Katz et al. (1986) who verified an increase of plasma glutamine concentration from 555 to 699 μmol/L after 4 min of exercise in ergometer cycle at 100% VO_{2max}. According to Hood and Terjung (1990), such an increase of plasma glutamine concentration is related to an increase of intramuscular synthesis of ammonia during the exercise, which, associated with glutamate in the reactions catalyzed by enzyme glutamine synthetase, form glutamine. The increase of intramuscular ammonia concentration during high-intensity and short-duration exercises is resultant of deamination of adenosine monophosphate (AMP) into inosine monophosphate (IMP) (Walsh et al. 1998). Moreover, a possible occurrence of hemoconcentration could also be, partially, responsible for an increase of glutaminemia (Sewell et al. 1994).

Nevertheless, a subsequent reduction in plasma glutamine concentration has been observed whenever the exercise is performed for more than 1 h. According to Parry-Billings et al. (1992), after a marathon, glutaminemia was reduced from 600 to 500 μmol/L among the athletes studied. Rennie et al. (1981) observed a reduction of plasma glutamine concentration from 557 μmol/L at rest to 470 μmol/L immediately after 225 min of cycling at 50% VO_{2max}. In this very study, a decline of plasma glutamine concentration to 391 μmol/L 2 h after finishing the exercise was also observed. In another study, Robson et al. (1998) studied 18 healthy men who cycled for 3 h at 55% VO_{2max}, and a decrease of 23% of plasma glutamine concentration 1 h after the exercise from 580 μmol/L (pre-exercise) to 447 μmol/L (1 h postexercise) was verified. However, when these individuals were submitted to an exhaustive test (cycling), performed at an intensity corresponding 80% VO_{2max}, with an average time of effort tolerance of 38 min, no alteration was observed at plasma glutamine concentration between pre-exercise values and the postexercise recovery period. Furthermore, Lehmann et al. (1995) verified that athletes, who took part in the ultra-*triathlon*, presented a reduction in plasma glutamine concentration from 468 μmol/L to 318 μmol/L 30 min after finishing the competition.

One of the possible reasons associated with above-mentioned results refers to the glutamine release capacity of skeletal muscle during intense and prolonged exercise.

Muscle glutamine production is controlled by glutamine synthetase, which catalyzes the synthesis of glutamine from glutamate and ammonia (Wagenmakers 1998). The control of the glutamine synthetase activity is undertaken by various substances such as cortisol (Gebhardt et al. 1998; Kimura et al. 2001), alanine, and glutamine (Meister 1985). In addition (Table 22.1), glutamine synthetase activity may also be influenced by blood pH (Conjard et al. 2003).

Both the plasma concentration of hormones and amino acids are strongly influenced by exercise and training, raising the suspicion that strenuous physical training can change the ability of glutamine synthesis and thus interfere with the regulation of its plasma concentration. One of the few studies that have proposed to observe the effects of exercise on the activity of the enzyme glutamine synthetase reported decreased activity of this enzyme in plantaris muscle (a muscle composed of type II muscle fibers) after the training period, and decreasing the expression of glutamine synthetase mRNA (Falduto et al. 1989). This finding was subsequently confirmed by Falduto et al. (1992), who observed that the action of exercise, reducing the increase in glutamine synthetase after treatment with glucocorticoids, is restricted to muscle fibers recruited for training. Posteriorly, it

TABLE 22.1
Effect of Exercise on Glutamine Concentration

Authors	Model	Exercise	Change in Glutamine Concentration	Glutamine Concentration (μmol/L)
Babij et al. (1983)	Human	10 min at each of three workloads (25%, 50%, and 75% VO_{2max}) and completed the exercise by working at VO_{2max} to exhaustion	↑ 27%	575–734
Christophe et al. (1971)	Rats	Moderate exercise	↓ 25%	
Dohm et al. (1981)	Rats	To exhaustion	↓ 19%	
Santos et al. (2009)	Rats	Exhaustive training, 6 weeks	↓ 16% (plasma) No change (skeletal muscle)	
Santos et al. (2007)	Rats	Exhaustive training, 6 weeks	↓ 15%	
Eriksson et al. (1985)	Human	45 min at 80% VO_{2max}	↑ 24%	538–666
Graham and Maclean (1998)	Rats	To exhaustion	≅ ↓17%	
Katz et al. (1986)	Human	4 min at 100% VO_{2max}	↑ 26%	555–699
Keast et al. (1995)	Human	Interval training sessions twice daily for 10 days, followed by a 6-day recovery period	↓ 55%	
Lehmann et al. (1995)	Human	Ultra-triathlon	↓ 32%	
Mackinnon and Hooper (1996)	Human	Overtrained vs. control athletes	No change	
Parry-Billings et al. (1992)	Human	Marathon	↓ 17%	600–500
Rennie et al. (1981)	Human	225 min at 50% VO_{2max}	↓ 30%	557–391
Robson et al. (1998)	Human	180 min at 50% VO_{2max} 80% VO_{2max} to exhaustion	↓ 23% No change	580–447 No change
Rowbottom et al. (1995)	Human	Overtrained athletes	↓ 30%	468–318
Walsh et al. (1998)	Human	20 × 1 min at 100% VO_{2max} separated by 2 min at 30% VO_{2max}	↓ 13%	

was observed that moderate training in rats partially reversed the increase in glutamine synthetase mRNA expression increased by malnutrition (Cunha et al. 2003).

Accordingly, results of *in vitro* studies using skeletal muscles of rats indicated that a prolonged and intense exercise provokes reduction of glutamine release from the muscles used as well as promotes reduction of plasma glutamine concentration (Walsh et al. 1998). Dohm et al. (1981) verified, in relation to muscle amino acid concentration, that rats that run on treadmills until exhaustion during a variable time of 1–3 h presented a reduction only of glutamine (19%) and glutamate (39%) after the exercise. In another study, performed by Graham and Maclean (1998), rats running until exhaustion or swimming for 2 h also presented reduction of intramuscular concentrations from 19% to 15% respectively. Rennie et al. (1981) observed a reduction of glutamine 34% of muscle glutamine concentration in humans immediately after a 225-min exercise (50% of VO_{2max}). In another study (Christophe et al. 1971), rats submitted to swimming with an overload of 6% of their bodyweight and aiming to impose an intense exercise presenting a reduction of 25% of glutamine in the gastrocnemius muscle.

Skeletal muscle has an extremely important role, not only to be the main site producer, but also for controlling the glutamine flow into the bloodstream through a membrane transport system, which is designed to guarantee the contribution glutamine to other tissues (Parry-Billings et al. 1991; Ahmed et al. 1993; Castell and Newsholme 1998).

This transport is accomplished by transporter similar to the one previously described in the liver named N transport system, however, with some differences that led to the designation, in skeletal muscle, Nm (Wagenmakers 1998). The Nm transport system regulates both the input and output of glutamine in muscle tissue, being responsible for up to 40 times difference between plasma and muscle glutamine concentrations (Rennie et al. 1998; Wagenmakers 1998). This transport system is dependent on Na^+ intracellular concentration and is regulated by plasma concentrations of glucocorticoids, insulin, and glutamine, as well as the blood pH (Rennie et al. 1998; Wagenmakers 1998). Accordingly, there must be doubts about which mechanism may lead to the reduction of plasma and muscle glutamine concentrations during and after a prolonged physical exercise. Among these possible mechanisms, it is noted that during prolonged physical exercise an increase of cortisol concentration occurs, which stimulates both muscle glutamine efflux and glutamine uptake from the liver. Therefore, in the presence of glutamine in the liver, associated with storage reduction of hepatic glycogen and an increase of cortisol concentration promote an increased stimulation of hepatic gluconeogenesis from glutamine (Dohm et al. 1981; Bishop et al. 1999).

Another mechanism implied in reducing glutaminemia during prolonged physical exercise refers to an increase of blood lactate concentration, which alters blood pH (metabolic acidosis) and, consequently, results in higher uptake of glutamine by the kidneys. Kidney elimination of H^+ ion involves supply of glutamine ammonia. Glutamine ammonia escapes from kidney tubular cells through a process of passive diffusion and joins H^+ protons to form ammonium ions (NH_4^+). The loss of hydrogen ions helps to maintain the acid–base balance (Walsh et al. 1998; Smith and Norris 2000). Moreover, according to Mackinnon and Hooper (1996), an increase of glutamine uptake from immune system cells, mainly when activated, can collaborate to reduce plasma glutamine concentration induced by physical exercise.

As a conclusion, an increase of plasma glutamine concentration during and immediately after high-intensity and short-duration exercise can be explained by the occurrence of hemoconcentration and increase of ammoniagenesis from deamination of AMP into inosine monophosphate (IMP) (Figure 22.1). On the other hand, during a recovery period after an intense and prolonged exercise, the reduction of plasma glutamine concentration is related mainly to an increase in the uptake of this amino acid by other tissues (liver, kidney, leucocytes), which surpasses the release rate of glutamine by the skeletal muscles stimulated by cortisol; alternatively to reduction of synthesis/alteration of kinetic transportation of this amino acid, resulting in a reduction of muscle glutamine efflux (Walsh et al. 1998).

Aside from the acute effects over glutamine metabolism, training is observed to provoke a relative increase of glutamine concentration in athletes at rest, when compared to clinically normal

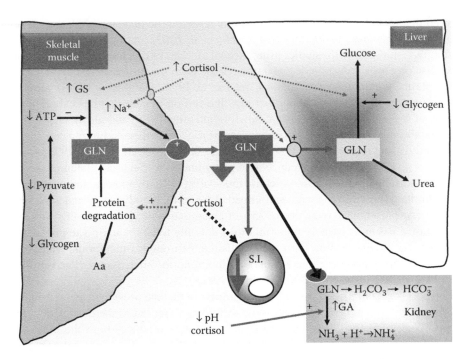

FIGURE 22.1 **(See color insert.)** Alteration in the kinetics of transport of glutamine (GLN) in muscle tissue, resulting in decreased release of GLN during and after exercise.

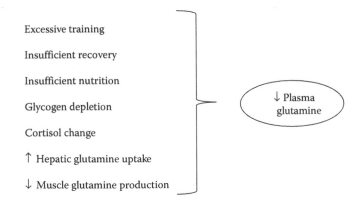

FIGURE 22.2 Conditions associated to glutamine decrease after exercise.

values or to those of nonathletes. However, plasma glutamine concentration can be significantly reduced during intense training periods or in athletes with overtraining syndrome (Keast et al. 1995; Lehmann et al. 1995; Rowbottom et al. 1995, Mackinnon and Hooper 1996), see later for more details in this chapter (Figure 22.2).

22.3   GLUTAMINE, DIET, AND EXERCISE IN THE POSTEXERCISE IMMUNOMODULATION

The plasma and tissue glutamine concentrations can be affected by acute exercise or training; diet can also alter these concentrations according to the proportion or quantity of each macronutrient previously offered to perform physical exercise.

Zanker et al. (1997) studied the effect of an exhaustive exercise associated with diet manipulation over plasma glutamine concentrations. Initially, individuals were submitted to a protocol (exercise and diet) aiming to deplete the storage of body glycogen. Participants were submitted to two tests, both involved 14 h of fasting and a 60-min running at 75% VO_{2max}. The first group remained fasting, whereas the other one ingested a meal rich in carbohydrates (CHO) (80% CHO, 10% protein, and 10% lipids) 3 h before exercising. Plasma glutamine concentration was not altered by the exercise in the fasting group; however, the fed group presented a significant increase of plasma concentration of glutamine as a response to the exercise. Although glycogen concentration has not been determined, authors suggest that there was an increase of glycogen availability after consuming a meal rich in carbohydrates and this stimulated the synthesis and release of glutamine by skeletal muscles.

Gleeson et al. (1998) verified that the consumption of a low-carb diet (7%) administered for 3 days prior to an ergometer cycle exercise (60 min at 70% VO_{2max}) was associated with a lower glutamine concentration at rest in relation to the group with normal CHO ingestion. Individuals submitted to low-carb diets demonstrated a significant reduction of plasma glutamine concentration at 150 min postexercise in relation to the group with a normal diet. Among the possible causes of these results cited by the authors are (i) occurrence of metabolic acidosis at rest in individuals submitted to low-carb diets, which promotes an increase in kidney glutamine uptake to maintain acid–base equilibrium and at the same time the plasma glutamine concentration is reduced; (ii) utilization of glutamine as a gluconeogenic precursor in the liver in situations of low-carb ingestion; (iii) small release of glutamine by muscle tissue during exercise because of a reduced concentration of glycogen (Table 22.2).

Many athletes are incentivized to and convinced that an increase of protein in the diet promotes a better performance. However, an excess of protein in diet can be as harmful to glutamine metabolism, as is a lack of protein. Greenhaff et al. (1988) demonstrated that a diet with high concentrations of protein (24%) and extremely low in CHO (3%), consumed during 4 days, resulted in the reduction of approximately 25% of plasma and muscle glutamine concentrations. Blanchard et al. (2001) investigated if diet manipulation (45% CHO or 70% CHO) and high-intensity exercise during 3 consecutive days exerted influence on plasma and muscle glutamine concentrations. The 70%-CHO group presented a plasma glutamine concentration significantly higher than the 45%-CHO group during three consecutive days of high-intensity exercises, whereas muscle glutamine concentrations presented no significant alterations in both groups. Both Greenhaff et al. (1988) and Blanchard et al. (2001) suggested that low-carb diets and simultaneous increase of protein ingestion result in metabolic acidosis, which lead to an increase of kidney uptake of glutamine to maintain the acid–base equilibrium and subsequent reduction of plasma glutamine concentration.

Kingsbury et al. (1998) verified the relation between plasma glutamine concentration, chronic fatigue, and protein intake in elite athletes in three situations, namely, during a period of intense training, prior to the Olympic Games of 1992; during a period of light training after competition; and after the intake of additional 20–30 g of protein per day in the form of food—for example, meats and cheeses—during a 3-week period. During the time prior to the competition, it was observed that 11 athletes presented infection and fatigue symptoms, simultaneously with the reduction of plasma glutamine concentration (lower than 450 μmol/L). Eight of these athletes continued to present low plasma glutamine concentration during the postcompetition time. With the intake of additional 20–30 g of protein during 3 weeks, an increase of plasma glutamine concentration (53%) and a substantial reduction of plasma glutamate concentration were registered. Six out of 10 athletes who consumed protein supplementation increased the training intensity during the 3 weeks of nutritional intervention.

When the training schedule requires the athlete to undergo several grueling training sessions, without adequate rest, a condition named overreaching can be triggered that is similar to excessive fatigue or overtraining syndrome when it is characterized by chronic severe fatigue with significant worsening of performance (Mackinnon and Hooper 1996; Smith 2003; Carfagno and Hendrix 2014).

TABLE 22.2

Influence of Nutrition on Glutamine Concentration

Authors	Model	Exercise	Diet	Results
Bacurau et al. (2002)	Human	6×20 min in 90% anaerobic threshold	Carbohydrate supplementation (solution at 10% with 95% of glucose polymers and 5% of fructose), 1 g/kg/h	Supplementation avoiding change in GLN
Bassit et al. (2000)	Human	Olympic triathlon	BCAA supplementation (6 g/day; leucine 60%, valine 20%, and isoleucine 20%) was ingested during 30 days before the triathlon competition. A BCAA dose of 3 g was ingested 30 min before the triathlon competition, and 7 days subsequent to the completion of the triathlon	Maintenance in GLN and immune function after supplementation
Bassit et al. (2002)	Human	Olympic tor 30 km run	BCAA supplementation (6 g/day; leucine 60%, valine 20%, and isoleucine 20%) was ingested during 30 days before the triathlon competition. A BCAA dose of 3 g was ingested 30 min before the triathlon competition, and 7 days subsequent to the completion of the triathlon	Maintenance in GLN and Th1/Th2 response
Blanchard et al. (2001)	Human	Two intense exercise through 2 weeks	Diets provided 45% or 70% of the energy as CHO. Four days of inactivity and consumption of a 55% CHO diet separated the two randomized trials	↑ Plasma GLN but not muscle glycogen
Castell et al. (1996)	Human	After intense training	The placebo group received a solution of maltodextrin and the supplemented group, a glutamine solution (5 g in 330 mL of water) immediately after exercise and 2 h after finishing competition or intense training	GLN supplementation ↓ infection
Castell and Newsholme (1997)	Human	Exhaustive exercise	Oral administration of solution with 5 g of glutamine in 330 mL of water immediately after the exercise	The ratio of T-helper/ T-suppressor cells ↑ after GLN supplementation
Gleeson et al. (1998)	Human	60 min at 70% VO_{2max}	High-CHO diet (75 ± 8% CHO) or a low-CHO diet (7 ± 4% CHO)	↓ GLN after 150 min after exercise
Greenhaff et al. (1988)	Human	Rest	Low carbohydrate (3 ± 0%), high fat (73 ± 2%), high protein (24 ± 3%) diet or a high carbohydrate (82 ± 1%), low fat (8 ± 1%) low protein (10 ± 1%) diet	↓ Plasma and muscle GLN
Kingsbury et al. (1998)	Human	Exhaustive training	Intake of additional 20–30 g of protein per day in form of food—for example, meats and cheeses—during a 3-week period	↓ GLN during chronic fatigue and infection
Klassen et al. (2000)	Human	Rest	Acute supplementation with 20 g of L-alanyl-L-glutamine dipeptide	↑ GLN
Krzywkowski et al. (2001a)	Human	2 h at 75% VO_{2max}	Supplementation during and 2 h after the exercise with L-glutamine (17.5 g), protein (68.5 g), or placebo	Neutrocytosis was less pronounced in supplemented group

(Continued)

TABLE 22.2 (*Continued*)
Influence of Nutrition on Glutamine Concentration

Authors	Model	Exercise	Diet	Results
Krzywkowski et al. (2001b)	Human	2 h at 75% VO$_{2max}$	GLN supplementation (500 mL of solution of either 3.5 g of glutamine or 3.5 g of maltodextrin and subsequent four doses of the beverage were ingested at intervals of 45 min)	Maintenance in GLN after supplementation
Rogero et al. (2004)	Rats	Rest	ALA-GLN (1.5 g/kg body weight) or GLN (1 g GLN/kg body weight) supplementation. In the acute study, rats were supplemented after a 14-h fast, whereas in the chronic study animals were supplemented for 21 days	Acute ALA-GLN supplementation promoted a greater increase in glutaminemia, and chronic supplementation increased muscle and liver GLN stores
Rogero et al. (2006)	Rats	Exercise to exhaustion	ALA-GLN (1.5 g/kg body weight) or GLN (1 g GLN/kg body weight) supplementation during the final 21 days of the training protocol	Chronic supplementation with DIP promoted a higher muscle glutamine concentration than chronic supplementation with glutamine immediately after exercise
Rohde et al. (1998a,b)	Human	60, 45, and 30 min at 75% VO$_{2max}$ separated by 2 h of rest	The individuals were supplemented with glutamine (100 mg of glutamine/kg of body mass) 30 min before finishing exercise, immediately after and 2 h after finishing each exercise	Maintenance of glutaminemia above pre-exercise values
Zanker et al. (1997)	Human	2 × 60 min at 70% VO$_{2max}$	Two dietary conditions: after a 14-h fast (fasted) and after ingestion of a high carbohydrate meal (30 kJ/kg: 80% carbohydrate, 10% protein, 10% fat) 3 h before running (fed)	↑ GLN after supplementation

Abbreviations: Branched-chain amino acid (BCAA); dipeptide (DIP); glutamine (GLN).

Several studies have suggested parameters that may be useful in early diagnosis of overtraining. Smith and Norris (2000) indicated that a decrease in glutamine/glutamate ratio measured in the plasma at rest, can be an efficient indicator of overtraining, since the decrease in plasma glutamine can indicate tolerance to exercise, while the increase in glutamate would be an indicator of the intensity of training and efficiency of recovery.

In fact, Parry-Billings et al. (1992) observed a decrease of about 9% of plasma glutamine concentration in athletes suffering from overtraining (Figure 22.3). This decrease was confirmed by another study in which decrease in glutamine during overreaching/overtraining was found (Parry-Billings et al. 1992; Keast et al. 1995; Rowbottom et al. 1995; Halson et al. 2003). More recently, it has been demonstrated that the decrease in plasma glutamine concentration in rats with signs of overtraining is accompanied by a decrease in muscle glutamate concentration and decrease in glutamine synthetase activity (Dos Santos et al. 2009).

Exercise immunology is an active area of research that studies acute and chronic effects of physical exercise over several variables related to immune competence evaluation. The study of physical exercise over the immune system is very important because of the increasing number of reports referring to infectious diseases and reduction of performance in athletes, primarily when they are engaged in exhaustive trainings (Shewchuck et al. 1997).

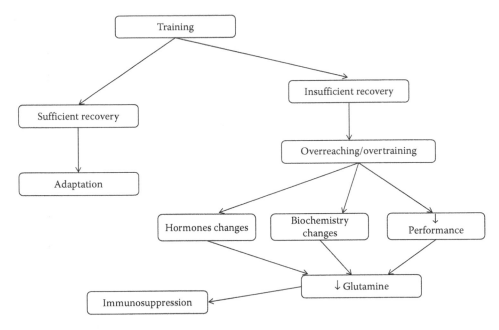

FIGURE 22.3 Overtraining and glutamine.

The effects of exercise on the immune system are influenced by the intensity, duration, and type of exercise, physical condition, environmental conditions, and nutritional status. Athletes involved in intense training programs, particularly endurance events, are more susceptible to infections, mainly of the upper respiratory tract. Diversely, studies suggest that moderate intensity exercises can reduce the risk of upper respiratory tract infections. After an intense and prolonged exercise, a momentary partial suppression of several parameters related to immune competence of athletes is verified, and this period has been called an "open window" for the invasion of microorganisms (Nieman and Pedersen 1999; Woods et al. 1999).

A question in this field that does not present a definitive answer is, How does a moderate exercise precisely act over immune system improving the individual immune function? Laboratory parameters, which can explain clinical benefits, include an increase of phagocytosis, microbicidal activity, and cytotoxic activity of natural killer (NK) cells, associated with an increased expression of adhesion molecule. Furthermore, many alterations that were verified could be, partly, the resultant of changes that occurred in the cell count of peripheral blood (Nieman and Pedersen 1999; Woods et al. 1999).

Among the alterations of the immune function induced by exhaustive exercise are reduction of neutrophil activity, harm to antibody synthesis, reduction of blood and saliva concentration of antibody, activity reduction of cytolytic NK cells, decline of T-lymphocyte circulating number for 3–4 h after exercise, reduction of proliferative capacity of lymphocytes stimulated by mitogens, and substantial alterations of postexercise cytokine concentration, including an increase of about 100 times of the IL-6 concentration together with elevation of anti-inflammatory mediators. These alterations are transitory and most of them return to basal levels within some hours after finishing the exercise (Castell and Newsholme 1998; Pedersen and Toft 2000).

However, there are some alterations in the immune response of athletes that persist for a longer period. Innate immune system seems to respond differently to chronic stress induced by intense exercise, with the activity of NK cell tending to be high, whereas that of neutrophil is reduced. Contrarily, exhaustive training does not affect much the adaptive immune system. Despite these facts, the clinical meaning of such alterations still needs to be elucidated (Pedersen and Toft 2000).

Physical exercise also affects the immune system by means of circulatory alterations (hemody-namic) and release of cortisol and catecholamine. Additionally, modulation in immune-mediated response by exercise can be linked to metabolic factors, such as plasma glutamine concentration (Parry-Billings et al. 1992; Bassit et al. 2000). In relation to glutamine, skeletal muscle is the main tissue involved in synthesizing and releasing this amino acid to bloodstream, and simultaneously this tissue plays an important role in maintaining the process of glutamine utilization by immune system cells. Consequently, skeletal muscle activity can directly affect the immune system (Newsholme 1989).

22.4   GLUTAMINE SUPPLEMENTATION, EXERCISE, AND IMMUNE FUNCTION

Several studies have demonstrated the capacity of acute oral supplementation with glutamine to increase glutaminemia, both in its free form and in dipeptide form. According to Castell and Newsholme (1998), acute oral ingestion of L-glutamine dissolved in water at 0.1 g/kg of body weight or a single dose of 5 g increased plasma glutamine concentration by 100% 30 min after ingestion, considering that glutaminemia returned to its basal levels 2 h after supplementation. Ziegler et al. (1990) verified that acute oral administration of L-glutamine increased plasma glutamine concentration between 30 and 45 min after ingestion, considering that glutaminemia returned close to basal values after 90–120 min of oral ingestion. Klassen et al. (2000) observed that acute supplementation with 20 g of L-alanyl-L-glutamine dipeptide increased the plasma glutamine concentration by 140% in relation to basal concentration 30 min after supplementation, returning to basal value 120 min after ingestion.

Studies with acute oral administration of L-glutamine demonstrate that the dose-dependent increase of plasma glutamine concentration indicates that the main fraction of glutamine administered is supposedly metabolized by enterocytes, although enteral way represents an efficient form of increasing glutamine concentration in peripheral circulation. *In vivo*, approximately 50% of glutamine absorbed in intestine lumen is subsequently metabolized in the intestine and liver (Ziegler et al. 1990; Déchelotte et al. 1991).

Considering the capacity of oral supplementation of glutamine to promote an increase of plasma concentration of this amino acid, even transitorily, several studies aim to investigate the possible role of this amino acid in relation to immune function of individuals engaged in intense and prolonged exercises. Therefore, Castell et al. (1996) verified the effects of oral supplementation of glutamine on infections in athletes. Ultra-marathoners, marathoners, medium-distance runners (participants of 10 km competitions), and rowers composed the group of athletes studied. The placebo group received a solution of maltodextrin and the supplemented group, a glutamine solution (5 g in 330 mL of water) immediately after exercise and 2 h after finishing competition or intense training. The athletes received questionnaires to report infections during 7 days after finishing the competition. In the glutamine supplemented group (n = 72), only 19% reported some kind of infection in that period. Among athletes that received placebo (n = 79), 51% presented some kind of infection in the same period. Although the incidence of infection has increased in both groups, authors concluded that glutamine supplementation during the first 2 h after exercising reduced the occurrence of infections in the week after the event.

In another study, Castell and Newsholme (1997) verified a significant increase in total leucocyte count immediately after the exhaustive exercise, followed by a reduction in lymphocyte count. Oral administration of solution with 5 g of glutamine in 330 mL of water immediately after the exercise resulted in more ratio of lymphocytes T CD4+ : CD8+ in relation to placebo group 1 h after finishing the exercise. Additionally, Hack et al. (1997) observed that a reduction of plasma glutamine concentration presented strong positive correlation with a reduction in the number of T CD4+ cells after 8 weeks of anaerobic training.

Moriguchi et al. (1995) verified the effect of glutamine chronic supplementation added to food on immune response of rats submitted to treadmill exercise. Plasma glutamine concentration was significantly lower in trained control group immediately after the last day of training (20 m/min, 60 min), unlike the supplemented group that maintained glutaminemia compared to control group at rest. Proliferation of lymphocytes and synthesis of IL-2 reduced significantly in the control group at training, whereas these parameters were maintained in the supplemented group immediately after the exercise. Authors concluded that glutamine supplementation prevented a reduction of proliferation response of lymphocytes induced by exercise, due to an increase of uptake and utilization of glutamine by lymphocytes to energy substrate and to biosynthesis of nucleotides.

However, other studies related to glutamine supplementation demonstrated little or no positive effect over immunocompetence of individuals submitted to exhaustive training or intense and prolonged exercise.

Supplementation with four doses of L-glutamine (100 mg/kg of bodyweight) administered at 0, 30, 60, and 90 min after a marathon maintained the plasma concentration of glutamine near preexercise values; however, no effect over proliferative response of lymphocytes, activity of lymphokine-activated "killer" cells, and over exercise-induced alterations on concentration and percentage of some subpopulations of leucocytes was observed (Rohde et al. 1998a,b).

Glutamine supplementation (500 mL of solution of either 3.5 g of glutamine or 3.5 g of maltodextrin and subsequent four doses of the beverage were ingested at intervals of 45 min) effect over the reduction of lymphocyte function induced by exhaustive exercise was also investigated in athletes after ergometer cycle exercise (2 h at 75% VO_{2max}) (Krzywrowski et al. 2001). Glutamine oral supplementation during and 2 h after the exercise prevented the decline of postexercise plasma glutamine concentration; however, it did not affect the activity of NK cells and lymphokine-activated killer cells, the proliferation of T lymphocytes, and catecholamine concentration, growth hormone, insulin, and glucose. Despite these results, it was observed that exercise-induced neutrophil was less pronounced in the group supplemented with glutamine; notwithstanding, it is possible that this result does not have any significant clinical meaning.

Rohde et al. (1998a,b) verified the effect of glutamine supplementation on exercise-induced alterations in the immune system. Eight healthy individuals performed three series of exercises in the ergometer cycle during 60, 45, and 30 min at 75% VO_{2max}, within a 2-h interval. The individuals were supplemented with glutamine (100 mg of glutamine/kg of body mass) 30 min before finishing exercise, immediately after and 2 h after finishing each exercise. Arterial plasma glutamine concentration reduced from 508 ± 35 μM (pre-exercise) to 402 ± 38 μM (2 h after last series of exercises) in the placebo group, whereas this concentration increased above pre-exercise values in L-glutamine supplemented group. Lymphocyte circulating number and lymphocyte proliferation response reduced 2 h after the first and second series, respectively, whereas activity of lymphokine-activated killer cells declined 2 h after finishing the third series. Glutamine supplementation *in vivo* did not influence these alterations in postexercise immune response, despite the maintenance of glutaminemia above pre-exercise values.

Some researchers propose one possible relation between glutaminemia reduction and IgA salivary concentration after intense and prolonged exercise. Krzywkowski et al. (2001a, 2001b) investigated this relation in athletes submitted to a 2-h ergometer cycle exercise (75% VO_{2max}) and supplemented during and 2 h after the exercise with L-glutamine (17.5 g), protein (68.5 g), or placebo. Plasma glutamine concentration reduced by 15% 2 h after finishing the exercise in the placebo group, whereas this reduction was prevented in supplemented groups with glutamine and protein. However, none of the supplements were efficient to prevent reduction of concentration and release of IgA salivary induced by exercise.

Studies prove that neutrophils actively consume glutamine and, consequently, Walsh et al. (2000) investigated the influence of glutamine oral supplementation on degranulation and oxidative burst of neutrophils stimulated after a 2-h exercise (60% VO_{2max}) in trained individuals. Glutamine supplementation was administered during and after finishing the exercise, although none of the parameters of neutrophil function have been altered through this nutritional intervention.

Aside from glutamine supplementation, other nutrients have been used for maintenance of plasma glutamine concentration and immunocompetence of athletes submitted to exhaustive exercises. Accordingly, Bacurau et al. (2002) verified the carbohydrate supplementation effect (solution at 10%

with 95% of glucose polymers and 5% of fructose), 1 g/kg/h, on plasma glutamine concentration and immunocompetence in cyclists who cycled at a speed corresponding to 90% of that obtained at the anaerobic threshold. The athletes cycled for 20 min and rested for 20 min, and this protocol was repeated six times. Exercise induced a reduction in peripheral blood mononuclear cell proliferation as well as in the production of cytokines by cultured cells (IL-1, IL-2, TNF-α, and IFN-γ). All of these changes were prevented by the ingestion of a carbohydrate drink by the athletes, except that in IFN-γ production, which was equally decreased (17%) after the second trial. Also, carbohydrate supplementation resulted in the maintenance of plasma glutamine concentration.

Branched chain amino acids can act as precursors of glutamine synthesis in muscle tissue. These amino acids supply amino groups in transamination reactions, which result in the formation of glutamate that, afterward, at a reaction catalyzed by the enzyme glutamine synthetase, participates in the glutamine synthesis (Gleeson et al. 1998; Wagenmakers 1998). In this context, some studies have evaluated the effectiveness of supplementation of branched chain amino acids to maintain plasma glutamine concentration and modify the immune response to exhaustive endurance exercise.

Concerning the study about the effect of branched chain amino acid supplementation during exhaustive exercise on plasma glutamine concentration, Parry-Billings et al. (1992) evaluated the effect of branched amino acid supplementation (ingestion of four beverages, containing 4 g of branched chain amino acid diluted in 100 mL of each beverage, in a total of 16 g of branched chain amino acids), which was offered to healthy individuals after 10.5, 20.5, 32.5, and 37.5 km throughout a marathon (42.2 km). Branched chain amino acid supplementation promoted an increase of plasma branched chain amino acid concentration, at the same time it maintained plasma glutamine concentration at the end of the marathon. On the other hand, the placebo group had a significant reduction of plasma glutamine concentration (16%) and of branched chain amino acids (18%).

Bassit et al. (2000) evaluated the effect of branched chain amino acid supplementation on immune response and plasma glutamine concentration in triathletes who performed an Olympic triathlon (swim 1.5 km, bike 40 km, and run 10 km). Individuals were distributed in a placebo group or in a group supplemented with branched chain amino acids 30 days prior to triathlon. Branched chain amino acid supplementation (6 g/day; leucine 60%, valine 20%, and isoleucine 20%) was ingested 30 days before the triathlon competition. A branched chain amino acid dose of 3 g was ingested 30 min before the triathlon competition, and 7 days subsequent to the completion of the triathlon. The authors verified that the plasma glutamine concentration after the triathlon was maintained in relation to basal values in the branched chain amino acid supplemented group, whereas there was a significant reduction of plasma glutamine concentration in the placebo group after the triathlon. Regarding immune response, supplemented group presented a higher in vitro IL-1, IL-2, TNF-α, and IFN-γ synthesis from mononuclear cells of peripheral blood at posttriathlon in relation to placebo group. Furthermore, branched chain amino acid supplementation promoted a higher capacity of peripheral blood lymphocyte proliferation when stimulated with mitogens in relation to the placebo group either before or after the triathlon competition. Simultaneously to these effects, this study also demonstrated a reduction of infection symptom rate (34%) reported by athletes supplemented with branched chain amino acids throughout supplementation period—30 days before and the week after the triathlon.

In another study (BASSIT et al. 2002), the effect of branched chain amino acid supplementation on immune response of marathoners submitted to a 30 km run was evaluated. The supplementation protocol was identical to that in the above described study of Bassit et al. (2000). Placebo group marathoners presented a reduction of plasma glutamine concentration of 24% by the end of the competition, whereas the supplementation of branched chain amino acids prevented this reduction. Supplemented group presented higher proliferation response of peripheral blood lymphocytes in relation to placebo group. Cytokine synthesis—IL-1, IL-4, TNF-α, IFN-γ—from mononuclear cells of peripheral blood was reduced after exercising in comparison to pre-exercise values in the placebo group, whereas branched chain amino acid supplementation restored the synthesis of TNF-α and IL-1 and increased the synthesis of IFN-γ and IL-2 and Th1 response.

Accordingly, the maintenance of plasma glutamine concentration through branched chain amino acid supplementation presents beneficial effects over the immunocompetence of athletes; however, studies with glutamine supplementation during and after endurance exercises indicate that this nutritional intervention does not prevent a reduction of immunocompetence induced by exercise. Under these circumstances, it is not clear which mechanism of branched chain amino acid supplementation acts over immunocompetence, that is to say, if it is an effect resultant of maintenance of plasma glutamine concentration, or if it is a direct effect of branched chain amino acids.

22.5 CONCLUSION

The immune system is acutely and, to a lesser extent, chronically influenced by exercising. Epidemiologic and experimental data suggest that moderate exercise increases immune function, whereas during intense training and after a competition an increase of incidence of upper respiratory tract infections occurs in athletes. Studies demonstrated that exercise could induce significant perturbation in both immune system divisions (innate and acquired), including distribution of leucocyte subclasses, peripheral concentration of lymphocyte subclasses, functional activities of effector cells, such as neutrophils and NK cells, and serum concentration of antibody and cytokines. As a result, the studied hypothesis is that during intense and prolonged exercise, the demand over skeletal muscles and other organs for glutamine increases, resulting in a reduction of supply of this amino acid for immune system cells, temporarily affecting its functionality. Therefore, factors that directly or indirectly actuate on synthesis and release of glutamine could influence on immune competence. Additionally, plasma and tissue glutamine concentration significantly reduces after intense and prolonged exercise, which has been suggested as a possible mechanism of immune suppression.

REFERENCES

Ahmed, A., D.L. Maxwell, P.M. Taylor, and M.J. Rennie. 1993. Glutamine transport in human skeletal muscle. *Am J Physiol* 264: E993–E1000.

Antonio, J. and C. Street. 1999. Glutamine: A potentially useful supplement for athletes. *Can J Appl Physiol* 24: 1–14.

Babij, P., S.M. Matthews, and M.J. Rennie. 1983. Changes in blood ammonia, lactate and amino acids in relation to workload during bicycle ergometer exercise in man. *Eur J Appl Physiol* 50: 405–411.

Bacurau, R.F., R.A. Bassit, L. Sawada, F. Navarro, E. Martins Jr., and L.F. Costa Rosa. 2002. Carbohydrate supplementation during exercise and the immune response of cyclists. *Clin Nutr* 21: 423–429.

Bassit, R.A., L.A. Sawada, R.F. Bacurau, F. Navarro, and L.F. Costa Rosa. 2000. The effect of BCAA supplementation upon the immune response of triathletes. *Med Sci Sports Exerc* 32: 1214–1219.

Bassit, R.A., L.A. Sawada, R.F. Bacurau et al. 2002. Branched-chain amino acid supplementation and the immune response of long-distance athletes. *Nutrition* 18: 376–379.

Bishop, N.C., A.K. Blannin, N.P. Walsh, P.J. Robson, and M. Gleeson. 1999. Nutritional aspects of immunosupression in athletes. *Sports Med* 28: 151–176.

Blanchard, M.A., G. Jordan, B. Desbrow, L.T. MacKinnon, and D.G. Jenkins. 2001. The influence of diet and exercise on muscle and plasma glutamine concentrations. *Med Sci Sports Exerc* 33: 69–74.

Calder, P.C. 1995. Fuel utilization by cells of the immune system. *Proc Nutr Soc* 54: 65–82.

Carfagno, D.G. and J.C. Hendrix. 2014. Overtraining syndrome in the athlete: Current clinical practice. *Curr Sports Med Rep* 13: 45–51.

Castell, L.M. and E.A. Newsholme. 1997. The effect of oral glutamine supplementation on athletes after prolonged, exhaustive exercise. *Nutrition* 13: 738–742.

Castell, L.M. and E.A. Newsholme. 1998. Glutamine and the effects of exhaustive exercise upon the immune response. *Can J Physiol Pharmacol* 76: 524–532.

Castell, L.M., J.R. Poortmans, and E.A. Newsholme. 1996. Does glutamine have a role in reducing infections in athletes? *Eur J Appl Physiol Occup Physiol* 73: 488–490.

Christophe, J., J. Winand, R. Kutzner, and M. Hebbelinck. 1971. Amino acid levels in plasma, liver, muscle, and kidney during and after exercise in fasted and fed rats. *Am J Physiol* 221: 453–457.

Chu, C.C., Y.C. Hou, M.H. Pai, C.J. Chao, S.L. Yeh. 2012. Pretreatment with alanyl-glutamine suppresses T-helper-cell-associated cytokine expression and reduces inflammatory responses in mice with acute DSS-induced colitis. *J Nutr Biochem* 23: 1092–1099.

Conjard, A., O. Komaty, H. Delage et al. 2003. Inhibition of glutamine synthetase in the mouse kidney: A novel mechanism of adaptation to metabolic acidosis. *J Biol Chem* 278: 38159–38166.

Cunha, W.D., G. Friedler, M. Vaisberg, M.I. Egami, and L.F. Costa Rosa. 2003. Immunossupression in under-nutrition rats: The effects of glutamine supplementation. *Clin Nutr* 22: 453–457.

Curi, R. 2000. *Glutamina: metabolismo e aplicações clínicas e no esporte*. Rio de Janeiro: Sprint. 264.

Darmaun, D., B. Just, B. Messing et al. 1994. Glutamine metabolism in healthy adult men: Response to enteral and intravenous feeding. *Am J Clin Nutr* 59: 1395–1402.

Déchelotte, P., D. Darmaun, M. Rongier, B. Hecketsweiler, O. Rigal, and J.F. Desjeux. 1991. Absorption and metabolic effects of enterally administered glutamine in humans. *Am J Physiol* 260: G677–G682.

Dohm, G.L., G.R. Beecher, and R.Q. Warren. 1981. Influence of exercise on free amino acid concentrations in rat tissues. *J Appl Physiol* 50: 41–44.

dos Santos, R.V., E.C. Caperuto, M.T. de Mello, M.L. Batista Jr., and L.F. Rosa. 2009. Effect of exercise on glu-tamine synthesis and transport in skeletal muscle from rats. *Clin Exp Pharmacol Physiol* 36: 770–775.

Eagle, H., V.I. Oyama, and M. Levy. 1955. The growth response of mammalian cells in tissue culture to L-glutamine and L-glutamic acid. *J Biol Chem* 18: 607–617.

Eriksson, L.S., S. Broberg, O. Björkman, and J. Wahren. 1985. Ammonia metabolism during exercise in man. *Clin Physiol* 5: 325–336.

Falduto, M.T., R.C. Hickson, and A.P. Young. 1989. Antagonism by glucocorticoids and exercise on expression of glutamine synthetase in skeletal muscle. *Faseb J* 3: 2623–2628.

Falduto, M.T., A.P. Young, and R.C. Hickson. 1992. Exercise inhibits glucocorticoids-induced glutamine syn-thetase expression in red skeletal muscle. *Am J Physiol* 262: C214–C220.

Gebhardt, R., M. Schuler, and D. Schörner. 1998. The spontaneous induction of glutamine synthetase in pig hepatocytes cocultured with RL-ET-14 cells is completely inhibited by trijodothyronine and okadaic acid. *Biochem Biophys Res Commun* 246: 895–898.

Gleeson, M., A.K. Blannin, N.P. Walsh, N.C. Bishop, and A.M. Clark. 1998. Effect of low- and high-carbo-hydrates diets on the plasma glutamine and circulating leukocyte responses to exercise. *Int J Sport Nut* 8: 49–59.

Graham, T.E. and D.A. Maclean. 1998. Ammonia and amino acid metabolism in skeletal muscle: Human, rodent and canine models. *Med Sci Sport Exerc* 30: 34–46.

Greenhaff, P.L., M. Gleeson, and R.J. Maughan. 1988. The effects of diet on muscle pH and metabolism dur-ing high intensity exercise. *Eur J Appl Physiol* 57: 531–539.

Hack, V., C. Weiss, B. Friedmann et al. 1997. Decrease plasma glutamine level and CD4+ T cell number in response to 8 wk of anaerobic training. *Am J Physiol* 272: E788–E795.

Halson, S.L., G.I. Lancaster, A.E. Jeukendrup, and M. Gleeson. 2003. Immunological responses to overreach-ing in cyclists. *Med Sci Sports Exerc* 35: 854–861.

Hiscock, N. and B.K. Pedersen. 2002. Exercise-induced immunodepression-plasma glutamine is not the link. *J Appl Physiol* 93: 813–822.

Hood, D.A. and R.L. Terjung. 1990. Amino acid metabolism during exercise and following endurance train-ing. *Sports Med* 9: 23–35.

Hood, D.A. and R.L. Terjung. 1994. Endurance training alters alanine and glutamine release from muscle during contractions. *FEBS Letters* 340: 287–290.

Katz, A., S. Broberg, K. Sahlin, and J. Wahren. 1986. Muscle ammonia and amino acid metabolism during dynamic exercise in man. *Clin Physiol Funct Imaging* 6: 365–379.

Keast, D., D. Arstein, W. Harper, R.W. Fry, and A.R. Morton. 1995. Depression of plasma glutamine con-centration after exercise stress and its possible influence on the immune system. *Med J Australia* 162: 15–18.

Kim, Y.S., G.Y. Kim, J.H. Kim et al. 2006. Glutamine inhibits lipopolysaccharide-induced cytoplasmic phos-pholipase A2 activation and protects against endotoxin shock in mouse. *Shock* 25: 290–294.

Kimura, K., F. Kanda, S. Okuda, and K. Chihara. 2001. Insulin-like growth factor 1 inhibits glucocorticoid-induced glutamine synthetase activity in cultured L6 rat skeletal muscle. *Neuro Lett* 302: 154–156.

Kingsbury, K.J., L. Kay, and M. Hjelm. 1998. Contrasting plasma free amino acid patterns in elite athletes: Association with fatigue and infection. *British J Sports Med* 32: 25–33.

Klassen, P., M. Mazariegos, N.W. Solomons, and P. Fürst. 2000. The pharmacokinetic responses of humans to 20 g of alanyl-glutamine dipeptide differ with the dosing protocol but not with gastric acidity or in patient with acute dengue fever. *J Nutr* 170: 177–182.

Ko, H.M., N.I. Kang, Y.S. Kim et al. 2008. Glutamine preferentially inhibits T-helper type 2 cell-mediated airway inflammation and late airway hyperresponsiveness through the inhibition of cytosolic phospholipase A(2) activity in a murine asthma model. *Clin Exp Allergy* 38: 357–364.

Koyama, K., M. Kaya, J. Tsujita, and S. Hori. 1998. Effects of decrease plasma glutamine concentrations on peripheral lymphocyte proliferation in rats. *Eur J Appl Physiol* 77: 25–31.

Krzywkowski, K., E.W. Petersen, K. Ostrowski, J.H. Kristensen, J. Boza, B.K. Pedersen. 2001a. Effect of glutamine supplementation on exercise-induced changes in lymphocyte function. *Am J Physiol* 281: C1259–1265.

Krzywkowski, K., E.W. Petersen, K. Ostrowski et al. 2001b. Effect of glutamine supplementation and protein supplementation on exercise-induced decreases in salivary IgA. *J Appl Physiol* 91: 832–838.

Labow, B.I. and W.W. Souba. 2000. Glutamine. *World J Surg* 24: 1503–1513.

Labow, B.I., W.W. Souba, and S.F. Abccouwer. 1999. Glutamine synthetase expression in muscle is regulated by transcriptional and posttranscriptional mechanisms. *Am J Physiol* 276: E1136–E1145.

Lacey, J.M. and D.W. Wilmore. 1990. Is glutamine a conditionally essential amino acid? *Nut Rev* 48: 297–309.

Lehmann M., M. Huonker, F. Dimeo et al. 1995. Serum amino acid concentrations in nine athletes before and after the 1993 Colmar Ultra Triathlon. *Inter J Sports Med* 16: 155–159.

Mackinnon, L.T. and S.L. Hooper. 1996. Plasma glutamine and upper respiratory tract infection during intensified training in swimmers. *Med Sci Sports Exerc* 28: 285–290.

Meister, A. 1985. Glutamine sinthetase from mammalian tissues. *Methods Enzimatic* 113: 185–199.

Moriguchi, S., H. Miwa, and Y. Kishino. 1995. Glutamine supplementation prevents the decrease of mitogen response after a treadmill exercise in rats. *J Nutr Sci Vitaminol* 41: 115–125.

Moskovitz, B., Y. Katz, P. Singer, O. Nativ, and B. Rosenberg. 1994. Glutamine metabolism and utilization: Relevance to major problems in health care. *Pharmacol Res* 30: 61–71.

Neu, J., V. Shenoy, and Chakrabarti 1996. Glutamine nutrition and metabolism: Where do we go from here? *Faseb J* 10: 829–837.

Newsholme, E.A., Newsholme, P., Curi, R., Crabtree, B., and Ardawi, M.S.M. 1989. Glutamine metabolism in different tissues: Its physiological and pathological importance. In: *Perspectives in Clinical Nutrition*. Kinney, J.M. and Borum, P.R. (eds.), Urban, Schwarzenberg, Baltimore, MD, USA.

Newsholme, P., R. Curi, T.C. Pithon Curi, C.J. Murphy, C. Garcia, and M. Pires de Melo. 1999. Glutamine metabolism by lymphocytes, macrophages, and neutrophils: Its importance in health and disease. *J Nut Biochem* 10: 316–324.

Nieman, D.C. and B.K. Pedersen. 1999. Exercise and immune function. *Sports Med* 27: 73–80.

Parry-Billings, M., R. Budgett, Y. Koutedakis et al. 1992. Plasma amino acid concentration in the overtraining syndrome: Possible effects on the immune system. *Med Sci Sport Exerc* 24: 1353–1358.

Parry-Billings, M., B. Leighton, G.D. Dimitriadis et al. 1991. The effect of tumour bearing on skeletal muscle glutamine metabolism. *Int J Biochem* 23: 933–937.

Pedersen, B.K. and A.D. Toft. 2000. Effects of exercise on lymphocytes and cytokines. *Br J Sports Med* 34: 246–251.

Rennie, M.J., R.H. Edwards, S. Krywawych et al. 1981. Effect of exercise on protein turnover in man. *Clin Sci* 61: 627–639.

Rennie, M.J., S.Y. Low, P.M. Taylor, S.E. Khogali, P.C. Yao, and A. Ahmed. 1998. Amino acid transport during muscle contraction and its relevance to exercise. *Adv Exp Medicine Biol* 441: 299–305.

Robson, P.J., A.K. Blannin, N.P. Walsh, L.M. Castell, and M. Gleeson. 1998. Effect of exercise intensity and duration on plasma glutamine responses following exercise and the time course of recovery in physically active men. *J Physiol* 506: 118–119.

Rogero, M.M., J. Tirapegui, R.G. Pedrosa, I.A. Castro, and I.S. Pires. 2004. Plasma and tissue glutamine response to acute and chronic supplementation with L-alanyl-L-glutamine rats. *Nut Res* 24: 261–270.

Rogero, M.M., J. Tirapegui, R.G. Pedrosa, I.A. Castro, and I.S. Pires. 2006. Effect of alanyl-glutamine supplementation on plasma and tissue glutamine concentrations in rats submitted to exhaustive exercise. *Nutrition* 22: 564–571.

Rohde, T., S. Asp, D.A. MacLean, and B.K. Pedersen. 1998a. Competitive sustained exercise in humans, limphokine activated killer cell activity, and glutamine: An intervention study. *Eur J Appl Physiol* 78: 448–453.

Rohde, T., S. Asp, D.A. MacLean, and B.K Pedersen. 1998b. Effect of glutamine supplementation on changes in the immune system induced by repeated exercise. *Med Sci Sports Exerc* 30: 856–862.

Rowbottom, D.G., D. Keast, C. Goodman, and A.R. Morton. 1995. The haematological, biochemical profile of athletes suffering from the overtraining syndrome. *Eur J Appl Physiol* 70: 502–509.

Rowbottom, D.G., D. Keast, and A.R. Morton. 1996. The emerging role of glutamine as an indicator of exercise stress and overtraining. *Sports Med* 21: 80–97.

Santos, R.V., Caperuto, E.C., and Costa Rosa, L.F. 2007. Effects of acute exhaustive physical exercise upon glutamine metabolism of lymphocytes from trained rats. *Life Sci* 80(6): 573–578.

Sewell, D.A., M. Gleeson, and A.K. Blannin. 1994. Hyperammonaemia in relation to high-intensity exercise duration in man. *Eur J Appl Physiol* 69: 350–364.

Shewchuck, L.D., V.E. Baracos, and C.J. Field. 1997. Dietary l-glutamine supplementation reduces the growth of the Morris hepatoma 7777 in exercise-trained and sedentary rats. *J Nut* 127: 158–166.

Smith, D.J. 2003. A framawork for understanding the training process leading to elite performance. *Sports Med* 33: 1103–1126.

Smith, D.J. and S.R. Norris. 2000. Changes in glutamine and glutamate concentrations for tracking training tolerance. *Med Sci Sports Exerc* 32: 684–689.

Smith, R.J. 1990. Glutamine metabolism and its physiologic importance. *J Parenteral Enteral Nut* 14: 40–44.

Souba, W.W. 1993. Intestinal glutamine metabolism and nutrition. *J Nut Biochem* 4: 2–9.

Souba, W.W., K. Herskowitz, R.M. Salloum, M.K. Chen, T.R. Austgen. 1990. *J Parenteral Enteral Nut* 14: 45–50.

Wagenmakers, A.J.M. 1998. Muscle amino acid metabolism at rest and during exercise: Role in human physiology and metabolism. *Exerc Sport Sci Rev* 26: 287–314.

Walsh, N.P., A.K. Blannin, N.C. Bishop, P.J. Robson, and M. Gleeson. 2000. Effect of oral glutamine supplementation on human neutrophils lipopolysaccharide-stimulated degranulation following prolonged exercise. *Int J Sports Nut Exerc Metabol* 10: 39–50.

Walsh, N.P., A.K. Blannin, A.M. Clark, L. Cook, P.J. Robson, and M. Gleeson. 1998. The effects of high-intensity intermittent exercise on the plasma concentrations of glutamine and organics acids. *Eur J Appl Physiol* 77: 434–438.

Walsh, N.P., A.K. Blannin, P.J. Robson, and M. Gleeson. 1998. Glutamine, exercise and immune function: Links and possible mechanisms. *Sports Med* 26: 177–191.

Windmueller, H.G. and A.E. Spaeth. 1975. Intestinal metabolism of glutamine and glutamate from the lumen as compared to glutamine from blood. *Arc Biochem Biophysics* 171: 662–672.

Woods, J.A., J.M. Davis, J.A. Smith, and D.C. Nieman. 1999. Exercise and cellular innate immune function. *Med Sci Sports Exerc* 31: 57–66.

Yeh, C.L., C.S. Hsu, S.L. Yeh, and W.J. Chen. 2005. Dietary glutamine supplementation modulates Th1/Th2 cytokine and interleukin-6 expressions in septic mice. *Cytokine* 31: 329–334.

Young, V.R. and A.M. Ajami. 2001. Glutamine: The emperor or his clothes? *J Nut* 131: 2449–2459.

Zanker, C.L., I.L. Swaine, L.M. Castell, and E.A. Newsholme. 1997. Responses of plasma glutamine, free tryptophan and branched-chain amino acids to prolonged exercise after a regime designed to reduce muscle glycogen. *Eur J Appl Physiol* 75: 543–548.

Ziegler, T.R., K. Benfell, R.J. Smith et al. 1990. Safety and metabolic effects of L-glutamine administration in humans. *J Parenteral Enteral Nut* 14: 137–146.

23 Role of Glutamine in Exercise-Induced Immunodepression in Man

Lindy Castell and Natalie Redgrave

CONTENTS

23.1 ROLE OF GLUTAMINE IN HUMANS

The role of glutamine in many conditions has been described elsewhere in this book. Thus, apart from a brief section on the relevant mechanisms of its action, this chapter will focus upon glutamine in association with exercise in humans.

Glutamine was originally classified as a nonessential amino acid (Rose, 1938). However, since the 1990s there has been increasing evidence that glutamine becomes "conditionally essential" in specific conditions of stress, including strenuous exercise (Lacey and Wilmore, 1990; Newsholme and Castell, 2000).

23.2 EXERCISE-INDUCED ILLNESS IN HUMANS

Compared with the normal sedentary population, endurance athletes can suffer from an abnormally high incidence of relatively minor illnesses, in particular upper respiratory tract infections (URTI), and also from gastrointestinal problems. Although moderate, regular physical activity may improve resistance to infections, an unusually heavy level of physical activity can produce apparent immunodepression in athletes. This is summed up in the description of a J-shaped curve by Nieman (1994).

Approximately 40% of URTI in adults are caused by rhinoviruses, which are characterized by the well-known symptoms of the common cold: nasal congestion, rhinorrhea, pharyngeal irritation, sore throat, and general malaise. The coronaviruses are the second most frequent cause of the common cold, with a slightly longer incubation time but the cold is of shorter duration. The main transmission of both of these is thought to be via aerosol routes. However, they can also be spread very efficiently by hand-to-hand transmission, for example, by playing contact sports or handling contaminated sports equipment. Gwaltney et al. (1978) undertook a simple experiment in which an individual with rhinovirus self-contaminated his hands and then shook hands with 15 individuals: 11 out of 15 recipients of the contaminated handshake were infected with the same rhinovirus. Thus, the athlete's lifestyle and attention to hygiene can be important factors in their susceptibility to infections.

In winter, a 50% increase in the incidence of URTI was observed in military personnel (Casey and Dick, 1990). This may well be attributable to the fact that they were more exposed to the cold virus in environments such as crowded dormitories, gymnasiums, and so on, during the colder months. The present authors observed a high incidence of URTI in rowers who traveled several miles to and from daily training sessions on the river. Within 3 weeks of starting their rigorous winter training sessions, many were suffering from a URTI. This seems likely to be because they traveled to and from training in close confinement with any colleagues incubating an infection.

In addition to the problems associated with cold weather, a higher training mileage, stress of competition, low body mass, oronasal breathing (which impedes cilia activity by drying up bronchial secretions) are also risk factors for increased incidence of URTI. It is likely that stress-induced immunodepression is associated with the risk, or cause of, URTI (Kemeny and Schedlowski, 2007).

The first investigation of the incidence of URTI in endurance athletes was reported by Peters and Bateman (1983) who studied participants 14 days after the Two Oceans Ultra-Marathon. They found that those who completed the race in the fastest time subsequently had the highest incidence of URTI compared with a much lower incidence in those who were the slowest. Nieman et al. (1990) studied participants in the Los Angeles marathon compared with noncompeting athletes: they found that the number of those with no infection before the race who became ill during the week after the race was almost sixfold higher than those who had undergone similar training schedules but who did not participate in the marathon. Several studies on the incidence of URTI in athletes have been reviewed by Weidner (1994).

The term URTI has generally been used to denote URT infections in all the early studies. However, Spence et al. (2007) investigated whether or not the URT symptoms reported in these studies on athletes were actually due to infections. They studied elite and recreational athletes versus sedentary controls for 5 months during training and competition. Swabs were taken to establish whether or not an infectious agent was responsible for an episode of upper respiratory tract illness (URI). In 28 participants, 37 episodes were reported, with risk factors being highest for sedentary controls and elite athletes, demonstrating a pattern similar to Nieman's J-curve. However, of these episodes, only 11% had a pathogenic origin (mostly rhinovirus), despite marked symptoms being present for some time. According to Spence et al. (2007) further work would be needed to uncover the causes of unidentified but symptomatic URI in athletes.

As indicated, the majority of studies published on exercise-induced illness used the term URTI without being aware whether or not an infectious agent was involved. Thus, it is becoming more usual to regard the "I" as referring to "illness," unless appropriate tests have been done to identify the infectious agent. The term "URI" will be used in the rest of this chapter.

However, there is undoubtedly some evidence of exercise-induced immunodepression, which is particularly likely to occur in those who do not allow sufficient recovery time between endurance events. Similarly, immunodepression may occur in those undertaking prolonged, exhaustive exercise in inhospitable environments, for example, military personnel on strenuous training regimens (Castell et al., 2010). In this study on marines undergoing training at altitude in winter, there was an extremely high incidence of illness, for which medication was required, predominantly URI but also gastrointestinal problems.

23.3 MECHANISM OF ACTION OF GLUTAMINE IN THE IMMUNE SYSTEM AND IN EXERCISE-INDUCED IMMUNODEPRESSION

Glutamine is synthesized, stored, and released predominantly by skeletal muscle and, to a lesser extent, by adipocytes, liver, and lung: it is taken up by intestinal cells, such as enterocytes and colonocytes, by the kidney, liver, pancreatic islet cells, and immune cells such as lymphocytes, macrophages, and neutrophils (see also Chapter 21).

Glutamine is required by rapidly dividing cells (Krebs, 1980) and provides nitrogen for the synthesis of purine and pyrimidine nucleotides, enabling synthesis of new DNA and RNA, for mRNA synthesis and DNA repair. Ardawi and Newsholme (1983, 1985) observed a surprisingly high utilization of glutamine by resting, unstimulated human lymphocytes. Subsequent *in vitro* work (Parry-Billings et al., 1992) showed that, despite the presence of all other nutrients, only when glutamine was reduced in the culture medium did a decrease occur in the proliferative ability of human lymphocytes. In addition, the response time to mitogenic stimulation of the lymphocytes was slowed *in vitro*. When it was established that plasma glutamine decreased by approximately 25% after prolonged, exhaustive exercise, it was decided to investigate whether or not this might have ramifications for immune function in athletes.

During physiological stress such as exercise, an increase in the concentration of cortisol in the blood can initiate proteolysis of muscle proteins, transamination of amino acids to glutamate, and the synthesis and increased release of glutamine. About 8–9 g of glutamine per day is released from the entire human musculature (see Elia et al., 1990). Muscle glutamine in humans is ca. 20 mM, which is approximately 60% of the intramuscular pool (Bergstrom et al., 1974). The rate of release across the plasma membrane occurs via a specific transporter. It is controlled by factors such as the hormonal milieu and cytokines. The release of cytokines from cells of the immune system leads to communication with skeletal muscle (Newsholme and Parry-Billings, 1990). It has been demonstrated that the secretion of cytokines or cell surface activation markers is glutamine dependent (Horig et al., 1993; Murphy and Newsholme, 1999).

Glutaminase is the major degradation enzyme of glutamine. The presence of glutaminase in human neutrophils was established in 2004 by Castell et al., who also observed increased oxidative burst in human neutrophils after adding glutamine *in vitro*. Neutrophil function decreases in cyclists undertaking prolonged exercise (Robson et al., 1999) and in cross-country runners immediately after VO_{2max} tests (Castell et al., 1999). The major chemoattractant for neutrophils is the chemokine interleukin-8 (IL-8), and there appears to be a link between its production and the concentration of glutamine. The provision of glutamine as a supplement to athletes has regularly resulted in a decrease in IL-8 production after mitogenic stimulation *in vitro* (Castell, 2003). IL-8 was also observed to be similarly reduced in clinical studies, for example, in patients with acute pancreatitis (De Beaux et al., 1998). It is, therefore, suggested that provision of exogenous glutamine might lead to enhanced function of neutrophils and to a decrease in the requirement for IL-8 secretion to attract more neutrophils to the site of tissue damage.

23.4 GLUTAMINE AND HEAT SHOCK PROTEINS IN EXERCISE

There is substantial evidence that glutamine is important for heat shock protein (HSP) generation in both *in vitro* and *in vivo* studies, for example, to help prevent atrophy of intestinal epithelial cells via HSP70 (Wischmeyer, 2002; Agostini and Biolo, 2009; Xue et al., 2011). Fehrenbach and Neiss (1998) suggested a protective effect of HSPs in leucocytes in athletes after endurance exercise. More recently, it was demonstrated first that glutamine supplementation decreased exercise-induced intestinal permeability and reduced nuclear factor kappa B activity in peripheral blood mononuclear cells, and second, that both these anti-inflammatory actions of glutamine could be mediated through activation of HSP70 and the heat shock response (Zuhl et al., 2014).

The circulating concentration of HSP72 increases after exercise. Furthermore, extracellular HSP72 stimulates cytokine activity, the "chaperokine" capacity of HSP72 (Asea et al., 2005). As it is known that glutaminase is present on the secretory granules of human neutrophils (Castell et al., 2004), it may be possible that glutamine effects on the heat shock response might induce changes in neutrophil function. Indeed, some studies have shown that HSP is responsible for facilitating neutrophil activity (Ortega et al., 2006; Hinchado et al., 2012).

23.5   PLASMA CONCENTRATION OF GLUTAMINE IN EXERCISE

The normal resting, fasting plasma concentration of glutamine (p[Gln]) in humans is 500–600 µM. In the authors' experience, most athletes have a slightly higher resting p[Gln] of 600–700 µM. Hiscock and Mackinnon (1998) found a considerable variation in resting, fasting p[Gln] in different sports: cyclists had the highest levels, while the lowest levels were observed in power lifters and swimmers. It is worth mentioning that not all studies give comparable values, since there is variation between the types of assay used and the results produced (see Section 23.7). However, the most commonly reported plasma concentrations are those shown above.

In 1976, Brodan et al. observed amino acid changes during 20-min cycling bouts, including increases in plasma alanine and p[Gln]. The likelihood is that this was a result of glutamine being released rapidly into the circulation from skeletal muscle during short-term exercise. It is well established that the p[Gln] is increased in athletes after short-term exercise (Poortmans et al., 1974; Maughan and Gleeson, 1988; Parry-Billings et al., 1992b). However, in athletes after prolonged, exhaustive exercise such as a full marathon, the p[Gln] can be decreased by as much as 20%–25% (Decombaz et al., 1979; Parry-Billings et al., 1992; Castell et al., 1996). This biphasic response of the p[Gln] to exercise was first reported by Poortmans et al. (1974) and Decombaz et al. (1979). Walsh et al. (1998) observed a decrease in p[Gln] 5 h after repeated bouts of cycling for 1 h. Similar decreases have been observed after other bouts of prolonged, exhaustive exercise.

In elite athletes in training camp at moderate altitude (Bailey et al., 2000) there was a more marked decrease in p[Gln] in those who had the highest incidence of, and the most severe, URI symptoms. A similar situation was observed in marines undertaking mountain winter training, which involved collecting samples before and after 1 month's intensive training in winter at altitudes up to 12,000 feet (Castell et al. 2010). A novel finding was that glutamine decreased by 12%–19% in fasting samples taken early in the morning, suggesting a cumulative effect of prolonged stress and fatigue, despite a few hours rest and recuperation overnight. Early morning samples taken from a small number (n = 7) of elite triathletes at the end of the season also showed a decrease in p[Gln] just prior to a marked increase in URTI and fatigue diagnosed by the team doctor. These decreases are similar to those observed within an hour or two of the recovery period after prolonged, exhaustive exercise, which is when most studies have normally obtained p[Gln] measurements. Thus, it is interesting to observe, as mentioned above, the similarity of athletes studied in training camp at moderate altitude (Bailey et al., 2000) to individuals with the highest illness scores in the mountain winter training study at a much higher altitude (Castell et al., 2010), who also tended to have the greatest decrease in p[Gln]. This might suggest a low resilience to stress in individuals in these groups.

If one reason for a decrease in p[Gln] is that glutamine is taken up by certain cells soon after the immune system is challenged, then glutamine availability might become a problem when the rate of release of glutamine from muscle slows down. In a study from the first author's group, Hiscock et al. (2002) measured intracellular Gln in peripheral blood mononucleocytes before, and at three different time points after 2 h cycling ergometry (Figure 23.1). There was a significant decrease in p[Gln] within 10 min after exercise. However, within 30 min the intracellular glutamine of peripheral blood mononucleocytes increased by 109% from baseline. The data indicate that glutamine availability was good at that stage and that it was clearly being removed from the circulation and being taken up by the cells. This intracellular acquisition of glutamine may be a major factor in the marked decrease in p[Gln] observed after strenuous exercise in many studies.

23.6   GLUTAMINE AS A MARKER OF EXERCISE-INDUCED IMMUNODEPRESSION AND ILLNESS

The post-exercise decrease in p[Gln] often tends to be concomitant with a decrease in circulating lymphocyte numbers, after a transient initial increase as part of the well-known leucocytosis observed after exhaustive exercise. Immune cell function is also decreased at this stage, both in

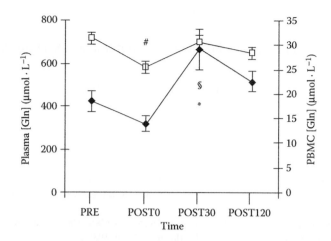

FIGURE 23.1 Comparison of p[Gln] (open squares) and PBMC[Gln] (filled diamonds) in response to 120 min cycling ergometry at 50% VO_{2peak} (mean ± SEM). #Significant difference in p[Gln] from PRE to POST0 ($p = 0.014$). §Significant difference in PBMC[Gln] from POST0 to POST30 ($p = 0.003$). *Significant difference in PBMC[Gln] from PRE to POST30 ($p = 0.022$). (Reproduced with kind permission from Hiscock, N., R. Morgan, G. Davidson et al. 2002. *J. Physiol.* 539P: 54P.)

lymphocytes and, for example, natural killer cell numbers and function which are depressed for up to 48 h after endurance exercise. Rohde et al. (1996) observed a marked decrease in p[Gln] in triathletes at 2 h after prolonged exercise, which was paralleled by changes in lymphokine activated killer cell activities. A decrease in p[Gln] in 18 marathon runners coincided with increases in acute phase markers such as IL-6 and complement C5a (Castell and Newsholme, 1998) and an increased incidence of URI. In a study on 58 marines undergoing mountain winter training, a significant decrease in p[Gln] occurred after 4 weeks' training and coincided with a high incidence of URI (Castell et al., 2010).

Fasting, resting p[Gln] was low (close to 500 µM) in athletes with unexplained underperformance syndrome (UPS; Parry-Billings et al., 1992; Rowbottom et al., 1997), formerly known as overtraining. UPS athletes are prone to a relatively high incidence of minor illnesses, as well as fatigue.

In a study on muscle glutamine, though glutamine did not change immediately post-exercise, a 30%–35% decrease in glutamine was observed in Type I and II muscle fibers in humans 2 h after resistance exercise (Blomstrand and Essen-Gustavsson, 2009). Interestingly, this decrease was concomitant with a decrease in plasma glutamate, which was emphasized by the authors as being an important intermediate in muscle energy metabolism in fibers.

23.7 INTERACTION OF PLASMA GLUTAMINE WITH GLUTAMATE

It has been proposed that the plasma concentration ratio of glutamine to glutamate (p[Gln/Glu]) might act as a marker of training tolerance in athletes undergoing heavy training (Smith and Norris, 2000). The authors observed a low glutamine/glutamate ratio of <3.58 in athletes whom they classified as being overtrained/underperforming, as opposed to well-trained, healthy athletes, who had a p[Gln/Glu] ratio of >5.88. Interestingly, this ratio was previously investigated in a clinical situation in the late 1980s (Ollenschlager et al., 1989) as a potential indicator of increased disease severity. Glutamate is a by-product of glutamine metabolism, and thus an increase in plasma glutamate is likely to be concomitant with increased glutamine utilization during stress such as disease cachexia or endurance exercise. Indeed, such observations were made in some samples from cardiopulmonary bypass patients (Powell et al., 1994). The conclusion by Ollenschlager et al. (1989) was that

TABLE 23.1

Plasma Concentration (μmol/L) of Glutamine and Glutamate in Samples Before and After a Marathon

	Glutamine	Glutamate	Gln/Glu
Pre-exercise	571	62	9.21
15 min post-exercise	462**	62	7.45
1 h post-exercise	421**	55	7.65
16 h post-exercise	555	63	8.81

Source: Reproduced from Castell, L.M. 2003. Glutamine supplementation *in vitro* and *in vivo*, in exercise and in immunodepression. *Sports Med.* 33: 323–345 with permission of Adis, a Wolters Kluwer business (copyright Adis Data information BV 2003. All rights reserved.)

Notes: Significance between pre- and post-exercise means is denoted by **$p < 0.001$. Assays were carried out enzymatically (glutamine, Windmueller and Spaeth, 1974; glutamate, Lund, 1980).

"valid information with respect to the progress of an individual [patient] cannot be obtained by the determination of plasma glutamate" and thus the p[Gln/Glu] ratio.

The first author saw no change in p[Glu] in marathon runners after a race compared with before exercise (Table 23.1), although there was a strongly significant decrease in p[Gln], thus in this study the ratio was dependent on p[Gln] (Castell, 2003). Nevertheless, studies in 2003 (Halson et al., 2003) and 2007 (Coutts et al., 2007) appear to support the notion of the ratio being a potential marker for overtraining. The present, first author's, work using the individual assays rather than the combined one (Lund, 1980; see below) used by Smith and Norris, did find some indication of the ratio as a potential marker of unexplained underperformance (unpublished observations). However, it is possible that inconsistent data might make this ratio a marker which may not always be reliable.

Different glutamine assays can produce different data, and it is unwise to compare the absolute values of one research group with another unless they have used identical assays. For the enzymatic assays, using either asparaginase (Windmueller and Spaeth, 1974) or glutaminase (Lund, 1980) to start the reaction which converts glutamine to glutamate and NH_4^+, the "normal" resting value (given that there is a good deal of individual variation) of p[Gln] is about 600 μM. Other assays can produce much higher (e.g., a bioassay using *Escherichia coli*) or lower values (e.g., high-performance liquid chromatography or HPLC) where glutamine values may be affected by poor resolution of coeluting amino acids.

23.8 GLUTAMINE SUPPLEMENTATION IN ATHLETES

About 50% of dietary glutamine is utilized by the intestine (Windmueller and Spaeth, 1974). Nevertheless, the provision of 0.1 g/kg of free glutamine as a bolus drink after an overnight fast, resulted in a twofold increase in the p[Gln] within 30 min in humans, remaining slightly elevated at 120 min (Castell and Newsholme, 1998). Another method of glutamine supplementation is via a dipepetide, for example, L-alanyl-glutamine, which tends to be more stable than free glutamine.

There are several published studies that have reported a decrease in the incidence of illness (particularly URI) in endurance athletes when glutamine or glutamine precursors (branched chain amino acids or BCAA) were provided after, or during training leading up to, an event. Castell and Newsholme (1997) observed a decrease in the self-reported incidence of illness (43%) in 150 marathon runners taking 5 g glutamine versus placebo after a race. Bassit et al. (2000) observed a similar decrease in triathletes supplemented for 1 month with BCAA compared with a placebo group. The BCAA maintained the p[Gln] (see also Cruzat et al., 2014) and the authors considered that this maintenance enabled an increased production of the cytokines IL-1, IL-2, tumor necrosis factor-α, and interferon-γ. The exercise-induced increase in plasma IL-6 has been well documented: augmentation of this response after 2 h cycling was shown to be due to glutamine or glutamine-enriched protein supplementation (Hiscock et al., 2003). *In vitro* studies (Yaqoob and Calder, 1998) have demonstrated a small increase in the production of T-lymphocyte derived cytokines (IL-1α, IL-6, and IL-10) in the presence of 1 mM glutamine.

Circulating numbers of neutrophils returned more rapidly to normal levels 16 h after a marathon in runners who had received glutamine supplementation versus placebo (Castell and Newsholme, 1997). In rats, Lagrahna et al. (2005) found that glutamine supplementation protected against exercise-induced changes in neutrophil function and against apoptosis.

Athletes undertaking a high volume of training, for example, rowers, endurance runners, are expending high calories and will therefore need to consume a higher volume of food and fluid to meet this need than a less active individual doing a lower volume of work. This will have implications for the gastrointestinal system and gut-associated lymphoid system (GALT) and glutamine is likely to play a role in this.

It is well established that some dietary amino acids such as glutamine, glutamate, and arginine are essential for the optimization of intestinal immune functions and GALT (Ruth and Field, 2013). The authors suggest that studies on supplementation of a mixed protein diet with single amino acids targeting specific GALT functions would be most beneficial. This may well be applicable to exercise-induced immunological impairment.

Marshall (1998) suggested the possibility that the gut might trigger an exercise-induced inflammatory response. Strenuous exercise may have a deleterious effect on glutamine synthesis in the gut, possibly via inhibition of glutamine synthetase (DeMarco et al., 1999). This would therefore reduce the availability of glutamine which might lead to increased gut atrophy (Platell et al., 1993), and possibly to increased permeability and hence bacterial translocation. This might also lead to a decrease in glutamine availability for rapidly dividing intestinal cells such as enterocytes, colonocytes, and lymphocytes. Thus, it is possible that glutamine supplementation might improve the digestive and defence mechanisms of the intestine (Castell et al., 1994; Dai et al., 2013; Wang et al., 2014). Certainly, in clinical situations, several studies have reported beneficial effects of glutamine on the gastrointestinal tract (see elsewhere in this book).

Nosaka et al. (2006) gave a supplement containing 12 amino acids during the recovery period and found an attenuation of both muscle soreness and damage, as well as lowered creatinine kinase. A similar mixture containing 12 amino acids improved training efficiency in athletes (Ohtani et al., 2006). BCAA are precursors for glutamine: Negro et al. (2008) provided BCAA to athletes and observed that p[Gln] was increased and muscle recovery helped. However, with all multi-ingredient supplement studies, it is difficult to ascertain precisely which component might be responsible for the changes observed.

Candow et al. (2001) found no effect of glutamine supplementation during 6 weeks of resistance training on muscle performance or protein degradation, nor on body composition in young adults at the end of the training period. No changes were found in glutamine levels in recreational bodybuilders who supplemented with whey isolate or casein (both known sources of glutamine) during 10 weeks of training (Cribb et al., 2006). For further discussion about the effects of glutamine and body building, readers are advised to look at the glutamine review by Castell (2003).

Koo et al. (2014) offered some support for glutamine and BCAA supplementation helping to enhance immune function in juvenile rowers training at maximal intensity. However, their numbers were too small ($n = 5$) to be convincing. Sasaki et al. (2012) gave glutamine to 26 male judoists versus placebo for 2 weeks and suggested that the glutamine supplementation contributed to preventing neutrophil function suppression: unfortunately they failed to measure plasma glutamine and also gave only 3 g/day. Kephart et al. (2016) observed that the neutrophil response was blunted in cyclists after 10 weeks of BCAA supplementation. Krieger et al. (2004) undertook a study in which they provided chronic glutamine supplementation (0.1 g/kg body weight four times daily) during 9 days of interval training. Glutamine increased nasal but not salivary IgA flow rate.

Several exercise studies using glutamine supplementation have found no, or limited, effects on specific aspects of immune function (e.g., Rohde et al., 1998a,b; Krzywkowski et al., 2001a). Some of the effects on the immune system observed are reduced neutrocytosis (Krzywkowski et al., 2001b) and increased circulating IL-6 (Hiscock et al., 2003). The former adds weight to the notion that there is a link between p[Gln] and neutrophils (Castell, 2003), and the latter might prove beneficial if IL-6 really does act as an anti-inflammatory cytokine (Petersen and Pedersen, 2006).

It is necessary to investigate whether other aspects of exercise-induced immunodepression might be altered by glutamine supplementation. The elimination of immunodepression would allow more effective training and thus improved performance in athletes. Increased availability of glutamine may result in decreased inflammation: it has also been suggested that it might lead to consequent health benefits associated with increased training (Agostini and Biolo, 2010).

23.9   GLUTAMINE SAFETY

Glutamine has a very good safety record with no side effects reported even at quite high doses (Garlick, 2001; Wernerman, 2008) (see Chapter 16). For example, 28 g/day has been well tolerated for 14 days in healthy humans (Gleeson, 2008). Nevertheless, there is little point in healthy individuals consuming more than 0.2 g/kg bodyweight per day. Apart from any other considerations, excessive doses will simply not be absorbed but will be excreted. Glutamine is also not a banned substance under the prohibitions of the World Anti-Doping Association. It is worth mentioning that glutamine is linked with glutathione, an important antioxidant: glutathione will feature in the Chapter 1. Readers may be interested to know that both glutamine and glutathione are discussed in the recent book *Nutritional Supplements in Sport, Exercise and Health: An A–Z Guide* (Castell et al., 2015).

23.10   CONCLUSIONS

Despite a good rationale for glutamine feeding based on sound biochemical investigation, laboratory-based studies have proved disappointing in terms of providing a direct enhancement of immune function due to glutamine feeding. However, data on the effects of glutamine supplementation in exercise on neutrophil function have become increasingly interesting, and further investigation in humans should prove to be useful. There is evidence that glutamine or a glutamine precursor can lessen the incidence of exercise-induced URI. In addition, a marked decrease in p[Gln] acts as a marker for fatigue, apparent immunodepression, and increased incidence of minor illnesses. Thus, a decrease in p[Gln] may indicate decreased well-being and immunocompetence in particular in the individual who is potentially vulnerable to opportunistic infections.

It remains to be deduced whether other aspects of immune function, as yet unstudied, may respond more effectively to the provision of glutamine before or after prolonged, exhaustive exercise.

23.11   DEDICATION

This chapter is dedicated to the memory of Professor Eric A. Newsholme who initiated a novel research in the glutamine field, particularly in the contexts of muscle, immune and gut function, nutritional support, and exercise performance. His broad-minded principle "You cannot prove or disprove a hypothesis: you can only add to the evidence for or against it" is particularly appropriate.

REFERENCES

Agostini, F. and G. Biolo. 2010. Effect of physical activity on glutamine metabolism. *Curr. Opin. Clin. Nutr. Metabol. Care* 13: 58–64.

Ardawi, M.S.M. and E.A. Newsholme. 1983. Glutamine metabolism in lymphocytes of the rat. *Biochem. J.* 212: 835–842.

Ardawi, M.S.M. and E.A. Newsholme. 1985. Metabolism in lymphocytes and its importance in the immune response. *Essays Biochem.* 21: 1–44.

Asea, A. 2005. Stress proteins and initiation of immune response: Chaperokine activity of HSP72. *Ex. Immunol. Rev.* 11: 34–45.

Awad, S., K.C.H. Fearon, I.A. Macdonald, and D.N. Lobo. 2010. A randomized, cross-over study of the metabolic and hormonal responses following two pre-operative conditioning drinks. *Nutrition* 27: 938–942.

Bailey, D.M., L.M. Castell, E.A. Newsholme, and B. Davies. 2000. Modulatory role of exposure time to environmental hypoxia during physical exercise: Implications for glutamine metabolism and exercise performance. *Brit. J. Sports Med.* 34: 210–212.

Bassit, R.A., L.A. Sawada, R.F.P. Bacurau, F. Navarro, and L.F.B.P. Costa Rosa. 2000. The effect of BCAA supplementation upon the immune response of triathletes. *Med. Sci. Sports Ex.* 32: 1214–1219.

Bergstrom, J., P. Furst, L.O. Noree, and E. Vinnars. 1974. Intracellular free amino acid concentration in human muscle tissue. *J. Appl. Physiol.* 36: 693–697.

Blomstrand, E. and B. Essen-Gustavsson. 2008. Changes in amino acid concentration in plasma and type I and type II fibres during resistance exercise and recovery in human subjects. *Amino Acids* 37: 629–636.

Brodan, V., E. Kuhn, J. Pechar, and D. Tomkova. 1976. Changes of free amino acids in plasma of healthy subjects induced by physical exercise. *Eur. J. Appl. Physiol.* 35: 69–77.

Candow, D.G., P.D. Chilibeck, D.G. Burke, K.S. Davison, and T. Smith-Palmer. 2001. Effect of glutamine supplementation combined with resistance training in young adults. *Eur. J. Appl. Physiol.* 86: 142–149.

Casey, J.M. and E.C. Dick. 1990. Acute respiratory infections. In: Casey et al. (Eds.). *Winter Sports Medicine*, pp.112–128. Philadelphia: F.A. Davis Co.

Castell, L.M. 2003. Glutamine supplementation *in vitro* and *in vivo*, in exercise and in immunodepression. *Sports Med.* 33: 323–345.

Castell, L.M., D. Atchley, N. Bravo, D. Niemeyer, A. Reyes, and P. Bradshaw. 1999. Effects of eight weeks of training and exhaustive exercise on some aspects of the immune system. *Int. J. Sports Med.* 21 (Suppl 1): Abst S85.

Castell, L.M., S.J. Bevan, P. Calder, and E.A. Newsholme. 1994. The role of glutamine in the immune system and in intestinal function in catabolic states. *Amino Acids* 7: 231–244.

Castell, L.M. and E.A. Newsholme. 1997. The effects of oral glutamine supplementation upon athletes after prolonged, exhaustive exercise. *Nutrition* 13: 738–742.

Castell, L.M. and E.A. Newsholme. 1998. Glutamine and the effects of exhaustive exercise upon the immune response. *Canad. J. Physiol. Pharmacol.* 76: 524–532.

Castell, L.M., P. Newsholme, and E.A. Newsholme. 2011. Glutamine. BJSM reviews: A-Z of nutritional supplements: Dietary supplements, sports nutrition and ergogenic aids for health and performance Part 18. *Brit. J. Sports Med.* 45: 230–232.

Castell, L.M., J. Poortmans, and E.A. Newsholme. 1996. Does glutamine have a role in reducing infections in athletes? *Eur. J. Appl. Physiol.* 73: 488–491.

Castell, L.M., S.J. Stear, and L.M. Burke (Eds.). 2015. *Nutritional Supplements in Sport, Exercise and Health: An A-Z Guide.* Abingdon, Oxon: Routledge.

Castell, L.M., D. Thake, and W. Ensign. 2010. Biochemical markers of possible immunodepression in military training in harsh environments. *Military Med.* 175: 158–165.

Castell, L.M., C. Vance, R. Abbott, J. Marquez, and P. Eggleton. 2004. Granule localization of glutaminase in human neutrophils and the consequence of glutamine utilization for neutrophil activity. *J. Biol. Chem.* 279: 13305–13310.

Cersosimo, E., P. Williams, B. Hoxworth, W. Lacy, and N. Abumrad. 1986. Glutamine blocks lipolysis and ketogenesis of fasting. *Am. J. Physiol.* 250: 248–252.

Coutts, A.J., P. Reaburn, T.J. Piva, and G.J. Rowsell. 2007. Monitoring for overreaching in rugby league players. *Eur. J. Appl. Physiol.* 99: 313–324.

Cribb, P.J., A.D. Williams, M.F. Carey and A. Hayes. 2006. The effect of whey isolate and resistance training on strength, body composition, and plasma glutamine. *Int. J. Sport Nutr. Exerc. Metab.* 16: 494–509.

Cruzat, V.F., M.M. Rogero, and J. Tirapegui. 2010. Effects of supplementation of free glutamine and the dipeptide alanyl-glutamine on parameters of muscle damage and inflammation in rats submitted to prolonged exercise. *Cell Biochem. Function* 28: 24–30.

Dai, Z.L., X.L. Li, J. Zhang, G. Wu, and W.Y. Zhu. 2013. L-glutamine regulates amino acid utilization by intestinal bacteria. *Amino Acids* 45: 501–512.

De Beaux, A.C., M.G. O'Riordan, J.A. Ross, L. Jodozi, D.C. Carter, and K.C. Fearon. 1998. Glutamine-supplemented total parenteral nutrition decreases blood mononuclear cell IL-8 release in severe acute pancreatitis. *Nutrition* 14: 261–265.

Decombaz, J., P. Reinhardt, K. Anantharaman, G. von Glutz, and J.R. Poortmans. 1979. Biochemical changes in a 100 km run: Free amino acids, urea and creatinine. *Eur. J. Appl. Physiol.* 41: 61–72.

DeMarco, V., K. Dyess, D. Strauss, C.M. West, and J. Neu. 1999. Inhibition of glutamine synthetase decreases proliferation of cultured rat intestinal epithelial cells. *J. Nutr.* 129: 57–62.

Elia, M., S. Wood, K. Khan, and E. Pullicino. 1990. Ketone body metabolism in lean male adults during short-term starvation, with particular reference to forearm muscle metabolism. *Clin. Sci.* 78: 579.

Fehrenbach, E. and A. Neiss. 1999. Role of heat shock proteins in the exercise response. *Exerc. Immunol. Rev.* 5: 57–77.

Furukawa, S., H. Saito, K. Fukatsu, Y. Hashiguchi, T. Inaba, M.T. Lin, T. Inoue, I. Han, T. Matsuda, and T. Muto. 1997. Glutamine-enhanced bacterial killing by neutrophils from postoperative patients. *Nutrition* 13: 863–869.

Garlick, P.J. 2001. Assessment of the safety of glutamine and other amino acids. *J. Nutr.* 131: 2556S–2561S.

Gleeson, M. 2008. Dosing and efficiency of glutamine supplementation in human exercise and sport training. *J. Nutr.* 13: 2045S–2049S.

Gohil, K., C. Viguie, W.C. Stanley, G.A. Brooks, and L. Packer. 1988. Blood glutathione oxidation during human exercise. *J. Appl. Physiol.* 64: 115–119.

Gwaltney, J.M., Jr, P. Moskalski, and J.O. Hendley. 1978. Hand-to-hand transmission of rhinovirus colds. *Ann. Intern. Med.* 88: 463–467.

Halson, S.L., G.I. Lancaster, A.E. Jeukendrup, and M. Gleeson. 2003. Immunological responses to over-reaching in cyclists. *Med. Sci. Sport Ex.* 35: 854–861.

Hinchado, M.D., E. Giralod, and E. Ortega. 2012. Adenoreceptors are involved in the stimulation of neu-trophils by exercise-induced circulating concentrations of HSP72: cAMP as a potential "intracellular danger signal". *J. Cell Physiol.* 227: 604–608.

Hiscock, N., R. Morgan, G. Davidson et al. 2002. Peripheral blood mononuclear cell glutamine concentration and *in vitro* proliferation in response to an acute, exercise-induced decrease in plasma glutamine con-centration in man. *J. Physiol.* 539P: 54P.

Hiscock, N., E.W. Petersen, and K. Krzywkowski et al. 2003. Glutamine supplementation further enhances exercise-induced plasma IL6. *J. Appl. Physiol.* 95: 145–148.

Horig, H., G.C. Spagnoli, L. Filgueira, R. Babst, H. Gallati, F. Harder, A. Juretic, and M. Heberer. 1993. Exogenous glutamine requirement is confined to late events of T cell activation. *J. Cell. Biochem.* 53: 343–351.

Iwashita, S., P. Williams, K. Jabhour et al. 2005. Impact of glutamine supplementation on glucose homeostasis during and after exercise. *J. Appl. Physiol.* 99: 1858–1865.

Kemeny, M.E. and M. Schedlowski. 2007. Understanding the interaction between psychosocial stress and immune-related diseases. *Brain Behav. Immunol.* 21: 1009–1018.

Kephart, W.C., T.D. Wachs, R. MacThompson et al. 2016. Ten weeks of branched-chain amino acid supple-mentation improves select performance and immunological variables in trained cyclists. *Amino Acids* 48: 779–789.

Koo, G.H., J. Woo, S. Kang, and K.O. Shin. 2014. Effects of supplementation with BCAA and L-glutamine on blood fatigue factors and cytokines in juvenile athletes submitted to maximal intensity rowing perfor-mance. *J. Phys. Ther. Sci.* 26: 1241–1246.

Krebs, H.A. 1980. Glutamine in the animal body. *Glutamine: Metabolism, Enzymology and Regulation.* Mora, J. and Palacios, R. (Eds.). New York: Academic Press, pp. 319–329.

Krieger, J.W., M. Crowe, and S.E. Blank. 2004. Chronic glutamine supplementation increased nasal but not salivary IgA during 9 days of interval training. *J. Appl. Physiol.* 97: 585–591.

Krzywkowski, K., E.W. Petersen, K. Ostrowski, J.H. Kristensen, J. Boza, and B.K. Pedersen. 2001a. Effect of glutamine supplementation on exercise-induced changes in lymphocyte function. *Am. J. Physiol. Cell Physiol.* 281: C1259–C1265.

Krzywkowski, K., E.W. Petersen, K. Ostrowski et al. 2001b. Effect of glutamine and protein supplementation on exercise-induced decreases in salivary IgA. *J. Appl. Physiol.* 91: 832–838.

Lacey, J.M. and D. Wilmore. 1990. Is glutamine a conditionally essential amino acid? *Nutr. Rev.* 48: 297–309.

Lagranha, C.J., T.M. de Lima, S.M. Senna, S.Q. Doi, R. Curi, and T.C. Pithon-Curi. 2005. The effect of glu-tamine supplementation on the function of neutrophils from exercised rats. *Cell Biochem. Funct.* 23: 101–107.

Lund, P. 1974. Determination with glutaminase and glutamate dehydrogenase. *Methods of Enzymatic Analysis.* Bergmeyer, H.U. (Ed.). Vol. 4. Verlag Chemie: Academic Press, pp. 1719–1722.

Marshall, J.C. 1998. The gut as a potential trigger of exercise-induced inflammatory responses. *Can. J. Physiol. Pharmacol.* 76: 479–484.

Maughan, R.J. and M. Gleeson. 1988. Influence of a 36 h fast followed by refeeding with glucose, glycerol or placebo on metabolism and performance during prolonged exercise. *Eur. J. Appl. Physiol.* 57: 570–576.

Murphy, C. and P. Newsholme. 1999. Macrophage-mediated lysis of a beta-cell line, TNF-alpha release from BCG-activated murine macrophages and interleukin-8 release from human monocytes are dependent on extracellular glutamine concentration and glutamine metabolism. *Clin. Sci.* 96: 89–97.

Negro, M., S. Giardina, B. Marzani, and F. Marzatico. 2008. BCAA supplementation does not enhance athletic performance but affects muscle recovery. *J. Sports Med. Phys. Fitness.* 48: 347–351.

Newsholme, E.A. and L.M. Castell. 2000. Amino acids, fatigue and immunodepression in exercise. In: *Nutrition in Sport IOC Encyclopaedia of Sport.* Maughan, R. J. (Ed.) Chapter 11. Oxford: Blackwell Science.

Newsholme, E.A., P. Newsholme, R. Curi, D.E. Challoner, and M. Ardawi. 1988. A role for muscle in the immune system and its importance in surgery, trauma, sepsis and burns. *Nutrition* 4: 261–268.

Newsholme, E.A. and M. Parry-Billings. 1990. Properties of glutamine release from muscle and its importance for the immune system. *J. Parent. Ent. Nutrition* 14: 63–67S.

Newsholme, P., K. Bender, A. Kiely, and L. Brennan. 2007. Amino acid metabolism, insulin secretion and diabetes. *Biochem. Soc. Trans.* 35: 1180–1186.

Newsholme, P., C. Gaudel, and N.H. McClenaghan. 2009. Nutrient regulation of insulin secretion and beta cell functional integrity. Advances in Experimental Biology and Medicine Book 'The Islets of Langerhans'. *Adv Exp Med Biol.* 654: 91–114.

Nieman, D. 1994. Exercise, upper respiratory tract infection and the immune system. *Med. Sci. Sports Ex.* 26: 128–139.

Nieman, D., L.M. Johanssen, J.W. Lee, and K. Arabtzis. 1990. Infectious episodes before and after the Los Angeles marathon. *J. Sports Med. Phys. Fitness* 30: 289–296.

Nosaka, K., P. Sacco, and K. Mawatari. 2006. Effects of amino acid supplementation on muscle soreness and damage. *Inj. J. Sport Nutr. Exerc. Metab.* 16: 620–635.

Ogle, C.K., J.D. Ogle, J.-X. Mao et al. 1994. Effect of glutamine on phagocytosis and bacterial killing by normal and pediatric burn patient neutrophils. *J. Parent Ent. Nutr.* 18: 128–133.

Ohtani, M., M. Sugita, and K. Maruyama. 2006. Amino acid mixture improves training efficiency in athletes. *J Nutrition* 136: 538–543S.

Ortega, E., E. Giraldo, and M.D. Hinchado. 2006. Role of Hsp72 and norepinephrine in the moderate exercise-induced stimulation of neutrophil/s' microbicide capacity. *Eur. J. Appl. Physiol.* 98: 250–255.

Parry-Billings, M., E. Blomstrand, N. McAndrew, and E.A. Newsholme. 1990a. A communicational link between skeletal muscle, brain, and cells of the immune system. *Int. J. Sports Med.* 11: S122–S128.

Parry-Billings, M., R. Budgett, Y. Koutedakis et al. 1992. Plasma amino acid concentrations in the overtraining syndrome: Possible effects on the immune system. *Med. Sci. Sports Ex.* 24: 1353–1358.

Parry-Billings, M., J. Evans, P.C. Calder, and E.A. Newsholme. 1990b. Does glutamine contribute to immunosuppression? *Lancet* 336: 523.

Petersen, A.M. and B.K. Pedersen. 2006. The role of IL-6 in mediating the anti-inflammatory effects of exercise. *J. Physiol. Pharm.* 57: 43–51.

Platell, C., R. McCauley, R. McCulloch, and J. Hall. 1993. The influence of parenteral glutamine and branched-chain amino acids on total parenteral nutrition-induced atrophy of the gut. *J. Parent. Ent. Nutr.* 17: 348–354.

Poortmans, J.R., G. Siest, M.M. Galteau, and O. Houot. 1974. Distribution of plasma amino acids in humans during submaximal prolonged exercise. *Eur. J. Appl. Physiol.* 32: 143–147.

Rennie, M.J., R.H.T. Edwards, S. Krywawych, C.T.M. Davies, D. Halliday, J.C. Waterlow, and D.J. Millward. 1981. Effect of exercise on protein turnover in man. *Clin. Sci.* 61: 627–639.

Robson, P.J., A.K. Blannin, N.P. Walsh, L.M. Castell, and M. Gleeson. 1999. Effects of exercise intensity, duration and recovery on *in vitro* neutrophil function in male athletes. *Int. J. Sports Med.* 20: 128–135.

Rohde, T., S. Asp, D.A. MacLean, and B.K. Pedersen. 1998a. Competitive sustained exercise in humans, lymphokine activated killer cell activity, and glutamine—An intervention study. *Eur. J. Appl. Physiol.* 78: 448–453.

Rohde, T., D.A. MacLean, A. Hartkopp, and B.K. Pedersen. 1996. The immune system and serum glutamine during a triathlon *Eur. J. Appl. Physiol.* 74: 428–434.

Rohde, T., D.A. MacLean, and B.K. Pedersen. 1998b. Effect of glutamine supplementation on changes in the immune system induced by repeated exercise. *Med. Sci. Sports. Exerc.* 30:856–862.

Rose, W.C. 1938. The nutritive significance of the amino acids. *Physiol. Rev.* 18: 109–136.

Rowbottom, D.G., D. Keast, and A.R. Morton. 1996. The emerging role of glutamine as an indicator of exercise stress and overtraining. *Sports Med.* 21: 80–97.

Ruth, M.R. and C.J. Field. 2013. The immune modifying effects of amino acids on gut-associated lymphoid tissue. *J. Animal Sci. Biotechnol.* 4: 27.

Sasaki, E., T. Umeda, I. Takahashi, K. Arata, Y. Yamamoto, M. Tanabe, K. Oyamada, E. Hashizume, and S. Nakaji. 2012. Effect of glutamine supplementation on neutrophil function in male judoists. *Luminescence* 28: 442–449.

Spence, L., W.J. Brown, D.B. Pyne, M.D. Nissen, T.P. Sloots, J.G. McCormack, A.S. Locke, and P.A. Fricker. 2007. Incidence, etiology and symptomatology of upper respiratory illness in elite athletes. *Med. Sci. Sports Ex.* 39: 577–586.

Vinnars, E., J. Bergstrom, and P. Furst. 1975. Influence of the postoperative state on the intracellular free amino acids in human muscle tissue. *Ann. Surg.* 182: 665–671.

Walsh, N.P., A.K. Blannin, A.M. Clark, L. Cook, P.J. Robson, and M. Gleeson. 1998. The effects of high-intensity intermittent exercise on the plasma concentrations of glutamine and organic acids. *Eur. J. Appl. Physiol.* 77: 434–438.

Wang, X., J.F. Pierre, A.F. Heneghan, R.A. Busch, and K.A. Kudsk. 2014. Glutamine improves innate immunity and prevents bacterial enteroinvasion during parenteral nutrition. *J. Parent Ent. Nutr.* EPub

Weidner, T.G. 1994. Literature review: Upper respiratory tract illness and sport and exercise. *Int. J. Sports Med.* 15: 1–9.

Welbourne, T., M. Weber, and N. Bank. 1972. The effect of glutamine administration on urinary ammonium excretion in normal subjects and patients with renal disease. *J. Clin. Invest.* 51: 1852–1860.

Wernerman, J. 2008. Role of glutamine in critically ill patients. *Curr. Opinion Anaesthesiol.* 21: 155–159.

Windmueller, H.G. and A.E. Spaeth. 1994. Uptake and metabolism of glutamine by the small intestine. *J. Biol. Chem.* 249: 5070–5079.

Wischmeyer, P.E., M.W. Musch, M.B. Madonna, R. Thisted, and E.B. Chang. 1997. Glutamine protects intestinal epithelial cells: role of inducible HSP70. *Am. J. Physiol.* 272: G879–G884.

Yaqoob, P. and P.C. Calder. 1998. Cytokine production by human peripheral blood mononuclear cells: Differential sensitivity to glutamine availability. *Cytokine* 10: 790–794.

Zuhl, M.N., K.R. Lanphere, L. Kravitz, C.M. Mermier, S. Schneider, K. Dokladny, and P.L. Moseley. 2014. Effects of oral glutamine supplementation on exercise-induced gastrointestinal permeability and tight junction protein expression. *J. Appl. Physiol.* 116: 183–191.

Section X

Glutamine and Aging

24 Glutamine Metabolism in Old Age

Dominique Meynial-Denis

CONTENTS

24.1 INTRODUCTION

There have been many extensive studies of glutamine, in particular that of Souba (1991), who wrote a full review of glutamine as a key substrate for the splanchnic bed in the whole body, and that of Ziegler et al. (2003), who described the role of glutamine as a specific nutrient in gastrointestinal research (adaptation, mucosal repair, and barrier function). Kalhan and Bier (2008) made a recent notable addition to the field in their review of the kinetics of glutamine and its relation to whole-body protein turnover in the neonate and adults. In contrast, to our knowledge, there are no data on aging. For this reason, the focus of this review will be specifically dedicated to the role of glutamine in aging.

Glutamine is a nonessential amino acid (NEAA) but becomes a conditionally essential amino acid in catabolic states because of the body's inability to synthesize sufficient amounts of glutamine during stress (Lacey and Wilmore 1990; Smith 1990; Bode 2001; Biolo et al. 2005). In other words, plasma levels of glutamine are insufficient to meet increased demands. Low concentrations of glutamine in plasma reflect reduced stores in muscle and this reduced availability of glutamine in the catabolic state seems to correlate with increased morbidity and mortality. Aging, which is characterized by reduced physical activity due mainly to the inevitable age-related loss of muscle mass or to skeletal muscle atrophy, a condition referred to as sarcopenia (Giresi et al. 2005; Solerte et al. 2008; Rosca et al. 2009; Cruz-Jentoft et al. 2010; Johnson et al. 2011; Bonaldo and Sandri 2013; Wall and van Loon 2013; Boirie et al. 2014; Paddon-Jones and Leidy 2014), may be related to a "physiological" catabolic state. Consequently, it is important to discuss the role of glutamine during sarcopenia because glutamine synthesis can be depressed in skeletal muscle owing to the muscle loss that occurs with aging.

In this review, our aim is to present current data on glutamine metabolism regulation, with particular reference to animal data, to have a better understanding of the cell mechanisms involved, and specifically to determine what we know about glutamine nutrition (needs and utilization); animal data are extended to old people while bearing in mind that, as reported by Welle (1999), the metabolism rate is faster in rats than in humans. Consequently, the reader's attention is drawn to the potential role of glutamine nutrition in aging, especially the relevance of glutamine supply for well-being and longevity.

24.2 PHYSIOLOGICAL IMPORTANCE AND BIOCHEMISTRY OF GLUTAMINE

Only the enzymes responsible for the synthesis and the degradation of glutamine in the cell are mentioned here.

Two principal enzymes regulate intracellular glutamine metabolism (Souba 1991). The enzyme glutaminase catalyzes the hydrolysis of glutamine to glutamate while glutamine synthetase (GS) catalyzes the synthesis of glutamine from glutamate and ammonia. Replicating cells, such as enterocytes, lymphocytes, endothelial cells, and tumor cells, tend to be avid glutamine consumers and in general have far greater amounts of glutaminase than GS. Skeletal muscle and lung, which synthesize and release net amounts of glutamine into the bloodstream, have substantial amounts of GS. The liver possesses both enzymes because it can switch from net glutamine utilization to net production, depending on physiological and nutritional conditions.

The data in this review essentially concern skeletal muscle, liver, gut, and other rapidly dividing cells.

24.3 OVERVIEW OF MOLECULAR AND CELLULAR ASPECTS OF GLUTAMINE METABOLISM IN BOTH MAMMALS AND HUMANS

Glutamine is the most abundant free amino acid in the body and is nutritionally classified among the nonessential amino acids (NEAA) such as glutamate, proline, glycine, and arginine (Wu et al. 2013). It plays a regulatory role in several cell-specific processes including metabolism, for example, nitrogen shuttle taking up excess ammonia and forming urea, oxidative fuel for rapidly dividing cells, such as in the gut and the immune system, gluconeogenic precursor, and lipogenic precursor, cell integrity (apoptosis, cell proliferation), protein synthesis, and degradation, contractile protein mass, redox potential, respiratory burst, insulin resistance, insulin secretion, and extracellular matrix synthesis. All these properties are illustrated and detailed in the sections 24.3.1, 24.3.2, 24.3.3 and 24.3.4. Glutamine has been shown to regulate the expression of many genes related to metabolism (see Sections 24.3.3 and 24.3.4) to activate several proteins. For example, it enhances the general transcription factor Sp1 as well as other transcription factors (C/EBP [Cytosine-Cytosine-Adenosine-Adenosine-Thymidine/Enhancer Binding Proteins], FXR/RXR [Farnesoid X Receptor/Retinoid X Receptor]) and regulates intracellular signaling pathways such as the mammalian target of rapamycin (mTOR) pathway (see Sections 24.3.3 and

24.4.1). Glutamine may also have a role in signal transduction, cell defense and repair, neurotransmission, and immunity. Thus, the function of glutamine goes beyond that of a simple metabolic fuel or protein precursor as previously assumed. We attempted to identify some of the common mechanisms underlying the regulation of glutamine-dependent cellular functions in both mammals and humans (Curi et al. 2005, 2007). Glutamine has important functions in both nutrition and health despite being classified among the NEAA. It should be taken into consideration in the concept of an "ideal protein" in which essential amino acids (EAA) and NEAA have to be included in order to improve protein accretion, food efficiency, growth, and health in animals and humans (Wu et al. 2013).

24.3.1 EFFECT OF GLUTAMINE STARVATION ON CELL SURVIVAL AND APOPTOSIS

The consequences of glutamine deprivation on cellular survival and gene expression have constructed a new paradigm for this amino acid, namely that limited extracellular glutamine supplies modulate stress and apoptotic responses. Under these conditions, plasma glutamine levels decline and as a result, the cells suffer from glutamine starvation. Apoptotic signaling mechanisms involved in the response to glutamine deprivation are cell type specific. New findings indicate that glutamine availability is strongly related to the induction of apoptosis and that glutamine works both as a nutrient and as a signaling molecule, acting directly or indirectly on the pathways leading to programmed cell death (Fuchs and Bode 2006). In addition, glutamine-starving cells show a reduced expression of the 70,000 M(r) heat shock protein, which is an important factor for cell survival (Oehler and Roth 2003). Consequently, glutamine-utilizing cells possess molecular mechanisms to detect the availability of glutamine and to respond specifically to changes in extracellular glutamine concentration (Oehler and Roth 2003).

24.3.2 REGULATIVE POTENTIAL OF GLUTAMINE: RELATION TO GLUTATHIONE METABOLISM

In animal studies, Roth demonstrated that administration of glutamine increases tissue concentration of reduced glutathione (Roth 2008). Glutamine (via glutamate), cysteine, and glycine are the precursor amino acids for glutathione, which is present within the cell in a reduced (GSH) and an oxidized form (GSSG). The ratio of GSH–GSSG is the most important regulator of the cellular redox potential. Thus, glutamine in its free or dipeptide forms influences this potential by enhancing all the more in catabolic states (Obled et al. 2002; Petry et al. 2015), the formation of glutathione, the major endogenous antioxidant in mammalian cells, which protects against oxidative injury and cell death (Mates et al. 2008).

24.3.3 GLUTAMINE SIGNALING IN THE INTESTINE

Glutamine is an essential nutrient for the small intestine, is a signal to enhance cell survival in the intestine, inhibits apoptosis in intestinal cells, is necessary for tight junction stabilization, and has anti-inflammatory effects in the intestine (decrease in proinflammatory IL-6 and IL-8 production, enhancement of anti-inflammatory IL-10, and reduction of NF-κB protein expression) (Rhoads and Wu 2009). Hence, glutamine plays a key role in the metabolism of rapidly dividing cells, including enterocytes and lymphocytes, which may contribute to its beneficial clinical effects. Gut mucosal homeostasis is achieved through a balance between cell proliferation and apoptosis. Whereas glutamine upregulates antiapoptotic proteins and downregulates proapoptotic proteins in T cells, glutamine prevents apoptosis in rat epithelial cell lines from gut mucosa, and glutamine starvation induces apoptosis through caspase activation (Deniel et al. 2007; Larson et al. 2007). In brief, glutamine may play a role in the gut-protected effect by inhibiting apoptosis via downregulation of the transcription factor Sp3, by contributing to cell survival during physiologic stress by induction of autophagy, by modulating intestinal barrier function under basal and inflammatory condition, or by demonstrating its anti-inflammatory effect via induction of nuclear degradation of the NF-κB p65 subunit (Beaufrère et al. 2014; Sakiyama et al. 2009).

Glutamine is a key regulator for amino acid controlled cell growth through the mTOR signaling pathway in rat intestinal epithelial cells (Naomoto et al. 2005; Deniel et al. 2007; Rhoads and Wu 2009; Brasse-Lagnel et al. 2010; Xi et al. 2011; Yao et al. 2012). Amino acids are important signaling regulators, especially for p70 S6 kinase (p70^{S6k}) and eIF-4E binding protein 1 (4E-BP1) via mTOR, which have two structurally and functionally distinct complexes termed mTORC1 and mTORC2 (mTORC1 is activated by nutrients [amino acids], growth factors, and cellular energy; mTORC2 is activated by growth factors alone). The mTOR pathway that regulates major cellular functions (growth and proliferation) plays a role in health and disease as well as in aging (Roth 2007; Dazert and Hall 2011; Laplante and Sabatini 2012; Mizunuma et al. 2014). Glutamine inhibits the activation of p70^{S6k} and phosphorylation of 4E-BP1 induced by arginine and leucine in rat intestinal epithelial cells. In contrast, in the fed state of healthy conditions, enteral proteins but not glutamine increased protein synthesis via an mTOR independent pathway in humans (Coeffier et al. 2013). Nakajo et al. have proposed a new concept for the biological role of phosphorylation of mTOR and intestinal cell growth: the signal induced by glutamine may stimulate cellular proliferation and increase cell number whereas leucine or arginine induces the signal for cell growth (increase in cell size) in rat intestinal epithelial cells. Glutamine suppresses only mTOR signaling for cell growth, and therefore it is considered as an EAA for cell culture (Nakajo et al. 2005). The intracellular signaling pathways involved in controlling intestinal glutamine transport during acidosis have been studied in Caco-2 cells, a model of human enterocytes. Metabolic acidosis stimulates glutamine transport via signaling pathways that lead to transcription of the glutamine transporter gene and to intestinal glutamine absorption (Epler et al. 2003).

24.3.4   GLUTAMINE SIGNALING IN THE LIVER

As in the intestine, glutamine has a direct regulatory potential in autophagic proteolysis of the liver due to a lysosomotropic toxicity of ammonia derived from glutamine degradation. Indeed, in most visceral tissues, the autophagic pathway is responsible for the bulk of proteolysis and is most sensitive to amino acid regulation (Kalhan and Edmison 2007). Glutamine, like leucine, tyrosine, phenylalanine, proline, methionine, tryptophan, and histidine, has a direct regulatory potential in the liver via amino receptor/sensor for their recognition at the plasma membrane and subsequent intracellular signaling (Kadowaki and Kanazawa 2003). Moreover, glutamine stimulates a number of metabolic pathways of the intermediary metabolism in the liver. For example, glutamine activates phosphoenolpyruvate in the liver and increases the phosphorylation state of p70^{S6K}, which is a key enzyme in liver protein synthesis. Glutamine is known to induce cell swelling and to mediate the inhibition of autophagic proteolysis; glutamine's antiproteolytic effect may be mediated through osmotic swelling and the p38^{MAPK} pathway (Haussinger and Schliess 2007).

24.4   IMPACT OF AGING ON THE REGULATION OF GLUTAMINE METABOLISM

Aging is defined as the progressive changes that occur after maturity in various organs, leading to a decrease in their functional ability and possible alterations in metabolic pathways. Because protein ingestion is crucial for the maintenance of a variety of body functions, the requirements of protein in the elderly are a major factor in maintaining skeletal muscle mass: the amount of protein ingested that induces maximal muscle protein synthesis must be higher in elderly than in young individuals in order to combat the anabolic resistance of the elderly (Young 1990; Evans 2010; Dideriksen et al. 2013; Pedersen and Cederholm 2014).

Dysregulation of autophagy (Bergamini et al. 2004; Codogno and Meijer 2010) contributes notably to aging. Autophagy, a lysosomal process involved in the maintenance of cellular homeostasis, is inhibited by the insulin–amino acid–mTOR signaling pathway that controls both protein synthesis and longevity (see Section 24.4.1). Autophagy declines and insulin resistance can develop during aging (Fujita et al. 2009). Thus, autophagy can provide protection against aging and cell death. Indeed, the best way to increase autophagy *in vivo* is by restricting calorie intake, which is in favor of longevity during aging. Moreover, glutamine inhibits autophagy and regulates cell growth. The role of glutamine metabolism in autophagy is related to the activation by leucine of mTOR, which is an activator of glutaminolysis (Duran and Hall 2012; Duran et al. 2012).

Aging is also characterized by protein wasting (see the following paragraph on glutamine and protein turnover in skeletal muscle with aging), and glutamine, which is the most abundant amino acid in the blood, may be a hallmark of catabolic states. Indeed, a low concentration of glutamine in plasma reflects reduced stores in muscle and this reduced availability of glutamine in the catabolic state seems to correlate with increased morbidity and mortality (Boelens et al. 2001). Moreover, in catabolic states, glutamine may be replenished by supplementation of BCAA. BCAA, especially leucine, stimulate protein synthesis, inhibit proteolysis (in cell culture and animals), and promote glutamine synthesis. Depletion of plasma glutamine may worsen BCAA and protein (Darmaun et al. 1998; Kimball and Jefferson 2002; Le Bacquer et al. 2007). When the "glutamine trap" (for example, phenylbutyrate) is used to deplete plasma glutamine, skeletal muscle glutamine is not depleted regardless of the age of rats, and muscle GS is not increased (Meynial-Denis et al. 2005). Despite this, there are few documented data in the literature on the role of glutamine in aging.

24.4.1 Is Glutamine the Cornerstone on the Protein Turnover in Skeletal Muscle with Aging?

The potential regulatory effect of glutamine in aging bears on the development and treatment of age-related muscle loss and strength loss (sarcopenia). There is a progressive decrease in lean body mass with aging and consequently in total body protein, due largely to a loss of skeletal muscle protein (Munro 1982; Young 1990). Sarcopenia is a highly significant public health problem. These changes in skeletal muscle are largely attributed to various molecular mediators affecting fiber size, mitochondrial homeostasis, and apoptosis and highlighting the mTORC1 pathway as a key therapeutic target to prevent sarcopenia (Fry et al. 2011; Dillon 2013; Sakuma et al. 2015; Sandri et al. 2013; Schiaffino et al. 2013). Indeed, in skeletal muscle, the activation of mTORC1 is involved in the regulation of protein synthesis and controls skeletal muscle mass (Sakuma et al. 2015). This progressive loss of skeletal muscle with aging is attributed to a disruption in the regulation of the skeletal muscle in protein turnover (Mosoni et al. 1993) and may be considered as a "physiological" catabolic state. For this reason, the role of protein and amino acids, notably glutamine as dietary supplementation could be used in fighting against muscle atrophy during aging.

However, dietary supplementation with proteins/amino acids seems inefficient in limiting the atrophy processes, and neither leucine (Koopman et al. 2008; Magne et al. 2013) nor glutamine (Mignon et al. 2007a), for example, improves the loss of skeletal muscle. Protein supplementation increased muscle mass gain only during resistance-type exercise training in elderly people (Tieland et al. 2012; Evans et al. 2013). During a 5-week exercise program, cysteine-rich whey protein increased lean body mass and decreased fat mass in comparison with a control diet but the authors made no mention of the effect on skeletal muscle mass per se (Droge 2005). Thus, neither glutamine nor EAAs such as leucine can be used to fight against sarcopenia; the increase in protein synthesis is not sufficient to increase muscle mass (Table 24.1).

Glutamine deficiency, which stimulates cell apoptosis, may stimulate sarcopenia thereby triggering a low inflammatory process (Roth 2007). Moreover, aging is known to induce a dysregulation of immune and inflammation functions that may affect protein synthesis rates in lymphoid tissues and plasma proteins (Papet et al. 2003). Aging has been also described as a condition characterized

TABLE 24.1

Recent Data on the Role of Glutamine and Other Amino Acids in Protein Turnover in Skeletal Muscle with Aging

Supplementation	Physical Activity	Whole-Body Improvement/ Preservation Muscle Functionality	Fat Body Mass	Lean Body Mass	Skeletal Muscle Atrophy
Leucine-rich whey protein or leucine alone or EAA	No or bed rest	Yes	Decrease	Increase	No efficient change
Glutamine	No	Yes	–	–	No change
Protein supplementation (2 × 15 g)	24-Week progressive resistance exercise	Yes	–	Increase	No
Cysteine-rich whey protein	5-Week exercise program	Yes	Decrease	Increase	No change

Source: For Leucine supplementation, data are from Casperson, S.L. et al. 2012. Leucine supplementation chronically improves muscle protein synthesis in older adults consuming the RDA for protein. *Clin. Nutr.* 31: 512–519; Dillon, E.L. et al. 2009. Amino acid supplementation increases lean body mass, basal muscle protein synthesis, and insulin-like growth factor-I expression in older women. *J Clin. Endocrinol. Metab.* 94: 1630–1637; Koopman, R. et al. 2008. Co-ingestion of leucine with protein does not further augment post-exercise muscle protein synthesis rates in elderly men. *Br. J. Nutr.* 99: 571–580; Magne, H. et al. 2013. Nutritional strategies to counteract muscle atrophy caused by disuse and to improve recovery. *Nutr. Res. Rev.* 26: 149–165; Walker, D.K. et al. 2011. Exercise, amino acids, and aging in the control of human muscle protein synthesis. *Med. Sci. Sports. Exerc.* 43: 2249–2258. For Glutamine, data are from Mignon, M. et al. 2007a. Does long-term intermittent treatment with glutamine improve the well-being of fed and fasted very old rats? *JPEN J. Parenter. Enteral Nutr.* 31: 456–462. For protein supplementation, data are from Tieland, M. et al. 2012. Protein supplementation increases muscle mass gain during prolonged resistance-type exercise training in frail elderly people: A randomized, double-blind, placebo-controlled trial. *J. Am. Med. Dir. Assoc.* 13: 713–719. For cysteine-rich whey protein, data are from Droge, W. 2005. Oxidative stress and ageing: Is ageing a cysteine deficiency syndrome? *Philos. Trans. R. Soc. Lond. B Biol. Sci.* 360(1464): 2355–2372.

by anabolic resistance to nutrients, especially amino acids, which impairs muscle protein synthesis and contributes to muscle wasting. This statement is illustrated by results of Table 24.1. Under inflammatory conditions, BCAA and notably leucine can be transaminated to glutamate in order to increase glutamine synthesis, which is a substrate highly consumed by inflammatory cells such as macrophages (Nicastro et al. 2012). But in old rats, muscle glutamine production and release are reduced in relation to the increased splanchnic sequestration of leucine and reduced renal and intestinal glutamine uptake to maintain whole-body glutamine homeostasis (Jourdan et al. 2013). However, glutamine depletion has a role in the low-grade inflammation and in sarcopenia observed with aging.

24.4.2 EFFECT OF AGING ON THE GLUTAMINE METABOLISM IN THE WHOLE BODY

A link can be made between aging and physical inactivity (experimental bed rest in healthy volunteers) since, as previously reported, inactivity contributes to sarcopenia (Biolo 2013). Physical activity generally decreases with age. Physical inactivity (Tessari 2000) reduces whole-body glutamine availability due to downregulated *de novo* synthesis and, more generally, due to anabolic resistance (Agostini and Biolo 2010). This alteration also results in decreased cytosolic ratios of glutamine/branched chain amino acid (leucine, valine, isoleucine) and glutamine/aromatic amino acid (tyrosine, phenylalanine). These changes in the profiles of free amino acids may be caused by sedentary lifestyle, nutrition, and immobilization, as commonly observed in the aging process (Stuerenburg et al. 2006). However, in very old rats aged 25 months (here female rats, whose mean life expectancy is ~27 months, with a maximum life span of 32 months), aging does not induce changes in either plasma or muscle glutamine concentrations (0.59 ± 0.13 vs. 0.55 ± 0.15 mM in plasma and 3.21 ± 0.60 vs. 3.18 ± 0.85 µmol/g in muscle) (Mignon et al. 2007a). Advanced age in rats corresponds to an age of about 75–80 years in humans. Glutamine deficiency in bed rest in humans also alters monocyte/macrophage activity, decreases the formation of heat shock proteins, stimulates cell apoptosis, and shifts the cellular redox potential by altering glutathione synthesis in lymphocytes. However, glutamine is able to preserve hepatic glutathione after hepatic injury (Roth 2008) as measured in the liver of very old female rats (Beaufrère et al. 2014).

24.4.3 IMPACT OF AGING ON GLUTAMINE SYNTHESIS IN SKELETAL MUSCLE: STUDY *IN VIVO* BY ^{13}C SRM

Skeletal muscle is the principal organ of the synthesis of glutamine, which is exported to other tissues such as the liver, gut, and immune cells according to the requirements of the cell. These requirements are dependent on age, as evidenced by the increase of GS activity with aging, reported below. Under normal healthy conditions, GS activity measured in skeletal muscle is enhanced in female and male rats of advanced age (about 25–27 months) compared with 8–22-month-old rats. In contrast, very old age (29–32 months), which corresponds to >85-year-old humans, including centenarians, is associated with significant muscle wasting, and most of the female rats had sustained basal "adult" GS activity, suggesting that these survivors may be physiologically younger than their age would indicate (Pinel et al. 2006). GS in muscle is a longevity-related gene and increases with caloric restriction in mice (Chiba et al. 2009). Because GS activity increases with fasting whatever the age of animals (Mezzarobba et al. 2003), we compared glutamine synthesis directly in skeletal muscle from 2-[13C] acetate by magnetic resonance spectroscopy (MRS) in fasted 25-month-old female Wistar rats and adult rats (8 months) (Mezzarobba et al., unpublished data). In old rats, glutamine and glutamate were undetectable in muscle *in vivo* but were detected in muscle extract at the end of the experiment (Figure 24.1). Consequently, flows of glutamine and glutamate through skeletal muscle were too quick to be detected by MRS *in vivo*. A metabolic schema is given in Figure 24.2.

24.4.4 IMPACT OF AGING ON GS IN SKELETAL MUSCLE: STUDY *IN VITRO* BY BIOCHEMISTRY

GS, which is a glucocorticoid-induced enzyme and has a key role in glutamine synthesis, is preserved with aging in skeletal muscle but not in smooth muscle such as the heart (Meynial-Denis et al. 1996). In contrast, other steroids such as sex steroids (progesterone, estradiol) do not affect GS activity in either the muscle or the heart irrespective of the age of animals. However, aged female rats maintain the possibility to secrete sex steroids. Although progesterone level was similar in adult and aged rats, estradiol was slightly but significantly lower in aged than in adult rats. Heart GS activity, which has an adrenal-dependent sensitivity and is not regulated by glucocorticoids, is dependent on mineralocorticoid hormones (aldosterone) (Verdier et al. 2002). An acute depletion of plasma glutamine does not modify the upregulation of muscle GS activity in response to fasting in either adult or aged rats (Meynial-Denis et al. 2005). In old rats, there is increased GS activity (in 25- to 27-month-old female and 24- to 27-month-old male rats, which are very old animals since mortality at this age is about 60%), suggesting a greater need for Gln. In some very old female rats, low GS activity may be associated with longevity or reflect a limitation in Gln production due to extremely advanced age per se (Pinel et al. 2006).

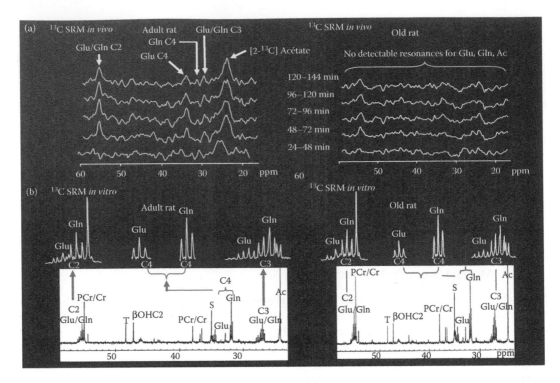

FIGURE 24.1 (a) ¹³C spectroscopy by resonance magnetic (SRM) skeletal muscle from adult (8 months) and old (25 months) rats: Kinetics of *in vivo* spectra between 24 and 144 min of [2-¹³C] acetate perfusion. (b) *In vitro* spectrum at the end of [2-¹³C] acetate perfusion. (From Mezzarobba, Meynial-Denis, and Renou, unpublished data.)

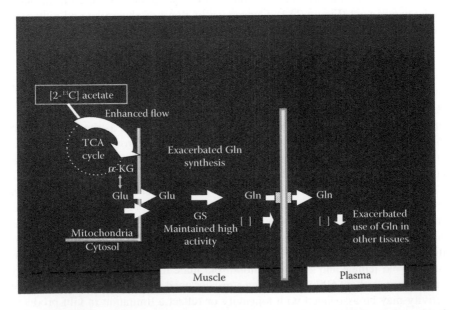

FIGURE 24.2 Hypothesis of glutamine and glutamate fluxes through the skeletal muscle to the plasma.

24.4.5 IMPACT OF AGING ON GLUTAMINE SYNTHESIS IN THE LIVER

The liver plays an important part in glutamine homeostasis and has a particular role in nitrogen salvage, and urea and glutamine metabolism (Brosnan et al. 1994; Curthoys and Watford 1995; Lopez et al. 1998; Watford et al. 2002; Gebhardt et al. 2007). It has the ability to both degrade glutamine and synthesize glutamine because the enzymes responsible, which are located in different hepatocyte populations, are simultaneously active. In the liver acinus (functional unit of the liver), ureagenesis and GA (L-glutamine amidohydrolase; EC 3.5.1.2) activity are predominantly localized in the periportal area, whereas GS (L-glutamate: ammonia ligase, ADP; EC 6.3.1.2) activity is exclusively found in a small perivenous hepatocyte population (~7% of all hepatocytes of an acinus). The pericentral expression pattern of GS in the liver is due to the upstream region of this enzyme (Lie-Venema et al. 1995). Because ammonium ions at low concentration are effectively removed by GS, but not by urea synthesis, both pathways contribute to ammonia detoxification in the liver acinus. The liver may switch from net glutamine utilization to net production, depending on physiological and nutritional conditions. For this reason, it is interesting to study the regulation of glutamine metabolism during aging. Although a large proportion of proteases (to which GS belongs) is known to be oxidatively modified with aging in the liver and neutral or alkaline proteolytic activity is maintained during aging, native GS remains active. Indeed, Sahakian demonstrated that hepatocyte GS decreased by 40%–50% between 3 and 26 months of age irrespective of gender (Sahakian et al. 1995). By contrast, we reported that, in fed male Wistar rats, liver GS remained constant whatever the age of animals (2–24 months) (Figure 24.3). Moreover, GA slightly and continuously increases with age (2–24 months) to become significantly different at 24 months (Figure 24.3) (Mouchard et al. 2008). Spindler demonstrated that, in contrast to our results, GA which is a key enzyme in liver nitrogen disposal, increased in caloric-restricted aged mice (Spindler 2001). This author also reported that GS decreased by about 40% in these conditions, which is in good agreement with our findings. It is noteworthy that our data showed that GA significantly increased only at 24 months in male Wistar rats; but at this age, 50% of them died (Pinel et al. 2006).

24.4.6 IMPACT OF AGING ON GLUTAMINE SYNTHESIS IN THE GUT

Glutamine may play a role in the gut-protective effect. Schlafen 3 is known as being a negative regulator of proliferation and decreases by 8- to 10-fold in the colonic mucosa of aged rats (Patel et al. 2009), and so it would be interesting to study the effect of glutamine on the Schlafen 3 gene. Glutamine also contributes to suppressing the tricarboxylic acid cycle as an oxidative and synthetic pathway with aging in jejunal epithelial cells (Fleming and Kight 1994).

In healthy humans, approximately 10%–15% of glutamine taken up by the intestines is converted to citrulline (Curis et al. 2005; Crenn et al. 2011). Quantitatively, glutamine is considered as a major precursor for intestinal citrulline release (Fujita and Yanaga 2007; van de Poll et al. 2007a,b). The intestines consume glutamine at a rate that is dependent on glutamine supply. There is a good relation between the amount of metabolically active gut tissue and gut and body citrulline production (Crenn et al. 2008; Deutz 2008; Rutten et al. 2006).

It would be interesting to know if the regulation of glutamine metabolism is the same during aging. We, therefore, studied the production of citrulline from glutamine in the gut in old female rats; glutamine was used as long-term intermittent supplement to evaluate the state of the gastrointestinal tract with advanced age (see Section 24.3.3) (Beaufrère et al. 2014).

Glutamine *de novo* synthesis plays a major role in the maintenance of intracellular glutamine pools in Caco-2 cells. In this model, glutamine availability affects the rates of protein synthesis. Caco-2 cells represent a model of human intestine enterocytes because the cell line is of human origin and originally derives from a colon carcinoma, and the cells undergo enterocytic differentiation *in vitro* and share many characteristics of normal human enterocytes. Glutamine deprivation in

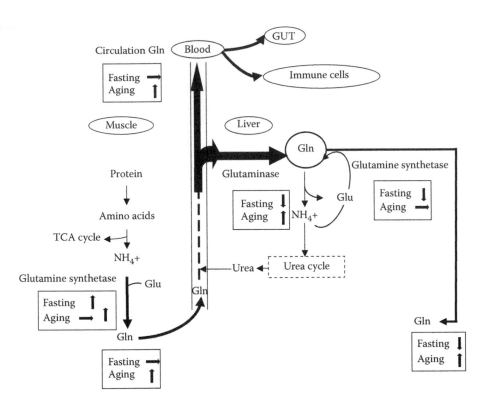

FIGURE 24.3 Effect of advanced age on interorgan glutamine flow between muscle, blood, and liver from Wistar rats. Glutamine orientation toward the gut and immune cells was not studied. Young rats were aged 2 months and very old rats 27 months. Muscle is the principal organ of glutamine synthesis. Glutamine was released from muscle into the blood. The liver uptakes glutamine and metabolizes it in urea, which is released into the blood. (Adapted from Mouchard, M.L. et al. 2008. *e-SPEN* 3:309–315; Pinel, C. et al. 2006. *Nutrition* 22:778–785; Meynial-Denis, D. et al. 2005. *Clin. Nut.* 24:398–406; and Mezzarobba, V. et al. 2003. *Clin. Nut.* 22:569–575.)

Caco-2 cells is obtained either by maintaining the cell in a glutamine-free medium or by using an inhibitor of GS, methionine sulfoximine (Le Bacquer et al. 2001).

In brief, recent studies highlighted a critical role for glutamine, which has been traditionally considered as an NEAA, in activating the mammalian target of rapamycin cell signaling in enterocytes. In catabolic states, glutamine has been reported to enhance intestinal and whole-body growth, to promote enterocyte proliferation and survival, and to regulate intestinal barrier function (Wang et al. 2015). Thus, glutamine holds great promise in protecting the gut from atrophy and injury in mammals and in humans during aging.

24.4.7 Impact of Aging on Glutamine Metabolism at the Cellular Level

Senescence-associated changes in the metabolic phenotype of human endothelial cells are related to glutaminolysis, which is an important target for *in vitro* induction of senescence. Indeed, a prerequisite of glutaminolysis is the overexpression of glutaminase, the first enzyme within the glutaminolytic pathway. Cell proliferation was found to correlate with glutaminase overexpression. Thus, premature senescence of human endothelial cells is induced by the inhibition of glutaminase (demonstrated by the use of a glutaminase inhibitor as 6-diaso-5-oxo-L-norleucine) (Unterluggauer et al. 2008). Senescence and apoptosis act as parallel pathways by which severely damaged cells are eliminated by the innate immune system from the body (Hornsby

2010). Programmed cell death pathways are promising targets for interventions in aging and aging-related diseases. But to inhibit them, muscle atrophy must be prevented with aging (Shen and Tower 2009).

24.5 IMPACT OF GLUTAMINE SUPPLEMENTATION IN OLD AGE

Can glutamine supplementation have an effect on age-related muscle wasting, on immunity, and, consequently, play a role in intestinal activity? In other words, can glutamine contribute to the well-being or the longevity of the elderly?

24.5.1 RATS

24.5.1.1 Short Supplementation

Glutamine was added to drinking water for 7 consecutive days each month (20% of dietary protein) after 5-day fasting to determine whether GS enhancement induced by fasting disappeared with glutamine supply irrespective of the age of the animal. This process was associated with refeeding. We compared the effect of glutamine supplementation with alanine and glycine supplementation. Only glutamine supplementation was able to significantly decrease the GS activity in the skeletal muscle of very old rats (27 months old), whereas supplementation with other amino acids decreased upregulated GS activity in adult rats (Mignon et al. 2007b).

24.5.1.2 Supplementation during 5 Months

Supplementation was the same as that given previously but lasted 5 months; this is an intermittent oral supplementation during 5 months (7 consecutive days each month). Long-term treatment with glutamine (started before advanced age was reached) had positive effects on very old rats (in good agreement with Neu (Neu et al. 2002)): (1) it prevented the loss of body weight, (2) it did not prevent the inevitable sarcopenia regardless of nutrition state (inefficient in modifying the rates of protein turnover), and (3) it only decreased upregulated GS activity of very old rats in the fed state. Glutamine requirements in the rat whole body may be satisfied in the fed state but would not be during catabolic states (fasting) with advanced age. Glutamine may also have an essentially beneficial role for the gut, maintaining both intestine integrity and intestinal immune function (Mignon et al. 2007a).

24.5.1.3 Long-Term Supplementation

24.5.1.3.1 Muscle

Supplementation was the same as above but was given for 50% of the rats' lifetime. GS activity increased in skeletal muscle with aging in very old fed and fasted animals. The enhancement of GS activity (1.5- to 2-fold) in 25- to 27-month-old rats may be a consequence of aging-induced stress (Mignon et al. 2007a). This is the case if glutamine supplementation is not interrupted before the study begins. Long-term treatment with glutamine before advanced age but discontinued 15 days before rat sacrifice is effective in increasing plasma glutamine to recover basal adult value and in maintaining plasma glutamine in very old rats, but has no long-lasting effect on the GS activity of skeletal muscle with advanced age (Meynial-Denis et al. 2013).

24.5.1.3.2 Intestine

Glutamine was added to the drinking water of very old (27 months) female rats for 10 months of their life span for 7 consecutive days a month (20% of dietary protein-average of the 10 glutamine treatments, 0.8 ± 0.1 g/rat/day) (Beaufrère et al. 2014).

Long-term treatment with glutamine initiated before advanced age maintains rat body weight and has a beneficial effect on the enterocytes by increasing gut mass, improving the villus height of mucosa, and thereby preventing the gut atrophy encountered in advanced age. The intact ability of enterocytes from very old rats—by preservation of mucosa enzyme activities for citrulline synthesis in the gut (Crenn et al.) (Crenn et al. 2008)—to continuously metabolize glutamine into citrulline allowed us, for the first time, to use citrulline as a noninvasive marker of intestinal atrophy induced by advanced age.

Further investigations would be warranted to explore the effect of very old age on this glutamine–citrulline interrelation *in vivo* in the gut in humans. The widely documented occurrence of intestinal atrophy with advanced age (reduction in the jejunal surface area) is a real public health issue, which may contribute to the frailty syndrome (Beaufrère et al. 2014).

24.5.2 HUMANS

Although the beneficial effects of glutamine supplementation were evidenced as early as 1990, few data were reported on healthy humans (Lowe et al. 1990; Smith 1990). Healthy elderly subjects account for a very small part of the general population and are of interest only to nutritional researchers and not to medical doctors. The interest of medical researchers in glutamine supplementation is as a means of improving patient health. Medical doctors study humans with an illness, whereas nutritional scientists place greater emphasis on prevention. The aging of the population will become an important societal question as the number of very old people increases worldwide.

The interest in glutamine has been altered in the last century because this amino acid does not fight against the muscle wasting during diseases or sarcopenia with aging. For this reason, only few data on healthy elderly are now reported in the literature. Nevertheless, glutamine is of continuing interest in medical research because of its potential role in the improvement of the well-being of ill humans (see the review of Boelens et al. 2001) (Boelens et al. 2001). Gut function in both healthy and ill old humans is incompletely understood and needs to be more fully investigated. To our knowledge, there exists only one published report on collagen synthesis after supplementation containing glutamine (Williams et al. 2002).

24.6 SUMMARY AND CONCLUSIONS

Glutamine, which was extensively reviewed in the last century, is a key substrate for the splanchnic bed in the whole body and a specific nutrient in gastrointestinal research. A marked decrease in plasma glutamine concentration has recently been observed in neonates and adults during acute illness and stress. Although acute studies in newborns have shown the benefits of parenteral and enteral supplementation of glutamine (by decreasing proteolysis and activating the immune system), clinical trials have not demonstrated prolonged advantages such as reduction in mortality and risk of infections in adults. In addition, glutamine is not able to fight against muscle wasting during disease or sarcopenia with aging. Oral glutamine supplementation initiated before advanced age in rats increases gut mass, improves the villus height of mucosa, and thereby prevents the gut atrophy encountered in advanced age. Enterocytes from very old rats continuously metabolize glutamine into citrulline, which allowed us, for the first time, to use citrulline as a noninvasive marker of intestinal atrophy induced by advanced age.

Preventive nutrition should be developed in France and other countries to maintain well-being and good health as long as possible in humans. This is particularly important with aging. Glutamine added to classical amino acid nutritional supplementation may contribute to the preservation of the gut by decreasing villus atrophy and maintaining gut function. Glutamine may therefore constitute an essential factor in the well-being and good health of very old people. In short, this review demonstrates that the function of glutamine goes beyond that of a simple metabolic fuel or protein precursor as previously assumed; it is both a nutrient and a signaling molecule.

REFERENCES

Agostini, F. and G. Biolo. 2010. Effect of physical activity on glutamine metabolism. *Curr. Opin. Clin. Nutr. Metab. Care* 13(1):58–64.

Beaufrère, A.M., N. Neveux, P. Patureau Mirand et al. 2014. Long-term intermittent glutamine supplementation repairs intestinal damage (structure and functional mass) with advanced age: Assessment with plasma citrulline in a rodent model. *J. Nutr. Health Aging* 18:814–819.

Bergamini, E., G. Cavallini, A. Donati, and Z. Gori. 2004. The role of macroautophagy in the ageing process, anti-ageing intervention and age-associated diseases. *Int. J. Biochem. Cell Biol.* 36(12): 2392–404.

Biolo, G. 2013. Protein metabolism and requirements. *World Rev. Nutr. Diet* 105:12–20.

Biolo, G., F. Zorat, R. Antonione, and B. Ciocchi. 2005. Muscle glutamine depletion in the intensive care unit. *Int. J. Biochem. Cell Biol.* 37(10):2169–79.

Bode, B. P. 2001. Recent molecular advances in mammalian glutamine transport. *J. Nutr.* 131(9 Suppl):2475S–85S; discussion 2486S–7S.

Boelens, P. G., R. J. Nijveldt, A. P. Houdijk, S. Meijer, and P. A. van Leeuwen. 2001. Glutamine alimentation in catabolic state. *J. Nutr.* 131(9 Suppl):2569S–77S; discussion 2590S.

Boirie, Y., B. Morio, E. Caumon, and N. J. Cano. 2014. Nutrition and protein energy homeostasis in elderly. *Mech. Ageing Dev.* 136–137:76–84.

Bonaldo, P. and M. Sandri. 2013. Cellular and molecular mechanisms of muscle atrophy. *Dis. Model. Mech.* 6(1):25–39.

Brasse-Lagnel, C. G., A. M. Lavoinne, and A. S. Husson. 2010. Amino acid regulation of mammalian gene expression in the intestine. *Biochimie* 92 (7):729–35.

Brosnan, J. T., H. S. Ewart, S. A. Squires, S. H. Day, Z. Kovacevic, and M. E. Brosnan. 1994. Hormonal and Dietary Control of Hepatic Glutamine Catabolism. In *Hormonal and Dietary Control of Hepatic Glutamine Catabolism*, edited by A. Tizianello, G. Baverel, H. Endou, A. C. Schoolwerth, and D. J. O'Donovan: Karger.

Casperson, S.L., Sheffield-Moore, M., Hewlings, S.J. et al. 2012. Leucine supplementation chronically improves muscle protein synthesis in older adults consuming the RDA for protein. *Clin Nutr* 31: 512–519.

Chiba, T., Y. Kamei, T. Shimizu et al. 2009. Overexpression of FOXO1 in skeletal muscle does not alter longevity in mice. *Mech. Ageing Dev.* 130(7):420–8.

Codogno, P. and A. J. Meijer. 2010. Autophagy: A potential link between obesity and insulin resistance. *Cell Metab.* 11(6):449–51.

Coeffier, M., S. Claeyssens, C. Bole-Feysot et al. 2013. Enteral delivery of proteins stimulates protein synthesis in human duodenal mucosa in the fed state through a mammalian target of rapamycin-independent pathway. *Am. J. Clin. Nutr.* 97(2):286–94.

Crenn, P., M. Hanachi, N. Neveux, and L. Cynober. 2011. [Circulating citrulline levels: A biomarker for intestinal functionality assessment]. *Ann. Biol. Clin. (Paris)* 69(5):513–21.

Crenn, P., B. Messing, and L. Cynober. 2008. Citrulline as a biomarker of intestinal failure due to enterocyte mass reduction. *Clin. Nutr.* 27(3):328–39.

Cruz-Jentoft, A. J., J. P. Baeyens, J. M. Bauer et al. 2010. Sarcopenia: European consensus on definition and diagnosis: Report of the European Working Group on Sarcopenia in Older People. *Age Ageing* 39(4):412–23.

Curi, R., C. J. Lagranha, S. Q. Doi et al. 2005. Molecular mechanisms of glutamine action. *J. Cell. Physiol.* 204(2):392–401.

Curi, R., P. Newsholme, J. Procopio, C. Lagranha, R. Gorjao, and T. C. Pithon-Curi. 2007. Glutamine, gene expression, and cell function. *Front. Biosci.* 12:344–57.

Curis, E., I. Nicolis, C. Moinard et al. 2005. Almost all about citrulline in mammals. *Amino Acids* 29(3):177–205.

Curthoys, N. P. and M. Watford. 1995. Regulation of glutaminase activity and glutamine metabolism. *Annu. Rev. Nutr.* 15:133–59.

Darmaun, D., S. Welch, A. Rini, B. K. Sager, A. Altomare, and M. W. Haymond. 1998. Phenylbutyrate-induced glutamine depletion in humans: Effect on leucine metabolism. *Am. J. Physiol. Endocrinol. Metab.* 274(37(5)):E801-07.

Dazert, E. and M. N. Hall. 2011. mTOR signaling in disease. *Curr. Opin. Cell Biol.* 23(6):744–55.

Deniel, N., R. Marion-Letellier, R. Charlionet et al. 2007. Glutamine regulates the human epithelial intestinal HCT-8 cell proteome under apoptotic conditions. *Mol. Cell Proteom.* 6(10):16711679.

Deniel, N. , R. Marion-Letellier, R. Charlionet, F. Tron, J. Leprince, H. Vaudry, P. Ducrotté, P. Déchelotte, and S. Thébault. 2007. Glutamine regulates the human epithelial intestinal HCT-8 cell proteome under apoptotic conditions. *Mol. Cell Proteom.* 6(10):1671–9.

Deutz, N. E. P. 2008. The 2007 ESPEN Sir David Cuthbertson Lecture: Amino acids between and within organs. The glutamate-glutamine-citrulline-arginine pathway. *Clin. Nutr.* 27(3):321–7.

Dideriksen, K., S. Reitelseder, and L. Holm. 2013. Influence of amino acids, dietary protein, and physical activity on muscle mass development in humans. *Nutrients* 5(3):852–76.

Dillon, E. L. 2013. Nutritionally essential amino acids and metabolic signaling in aging. *Amino Acids* 45(3):431–41.

Dillon, E.L., Sheffield-Moore, M., Paddon-Jones, D. et al. 2009. Amino acid supplementation increases lean body mass, basal muscle protein synthesis, and insulin-like growth factor-I expression in older women. *J. Clin. Endocrinol. Metab.* 94:1630–1637.

Droge, W. 2005. Oxidative stress and ageing: Is ageing a cysteine deficiency syndrome? *Philos. Trans. R. Soc. Lond. B Biol. Sci.* 360(1464):2355–72.

Duran, R. V. and M. N. Hall. 2012. Glutaminolysis feeds mTORC1. *Cell Cycle* 11(22):4107–8.

Duran, R. V., W. Oppliger, A. M. Robitaille et al. 2012. Glutaminolysis activates Rag-mTORC1 signaling. *Mol. Cell* 47(3):349–58.

Epler, M. J., W. W. Souba, Q. Meng et al. 2003. Metabolic acidosis stimulates intestinal glutamine absorption. *J. Gastrointest. Surg.* 7(8):1045–52.

Evans, W. J. 2010. Skeletal Muscle Loss: Cachexia, Sarcopenia, and Inactivity. *Am. J. Clin. Nutr.* 91(4):1123S–7S.

Evans, W. J., V. Boccardi, and G. Paolisso. 2013. Perspective: Dietary protein needs of elderly people: Protein supplementation as an effective strategy to counteract sarcopenia. *J. Am. Med. Dir. Assoc.* 14(1):67–9.

Fleming, S. E. and C. E. Kight. 1994. The TCA cycle as an oxidative and synthetic pathway is suppressed with aging in jejunal epithelial cells. *Canad. J. Physiol. Pharmacol.* 72(3):266–74.

Fry, C. S., M. J. Drummond, E. L. Glynn et al. 2011. Aging impairs contraction-induced human skeletal muscle mTORC1 signaling and protein synthesis. *Skelet. Muscle* 1–(1):11.

Fuchs, B. C. and B. P. Bode. 2006. Stressing out over survival: Glutamine as an apoptotic modulator. *J. Surg. Res.* 131–(1):26–40.

Fujita, S., E. L. Glynn, K. L. Timmerman, B. B. Rasmussen, and E. Volpi. 2009. Supraphysiological Hyperinsulinaemia Is Necessary to Stimulate Skeletal Muscle Protein Anabolism in Older Adults: Evidence of a True Age-Related Insulin Resistance of Muscle Protein Metabolism. *Diabetologia* 52(9):1889–98.

Fujita, T. and K. Yanaga. 2007. Association between glutamine extraction and release of citrulline and glycine by the human small intestine. *Life Sci.* 80(20):1846–50.

Gebhardt, R., A. Baldysiak-Figiel, V. Krugel, E. Ueberham, and F. Gaunitz. 2007. Hepatocellular expression of glutamine synthetase: An indicator of morphogen actions as master regulators of zonation in adult liver. *Progr. Histochem. Cytochem.* 41(4):201–66.

Giresi, P. G., E. J. Stevenson, J. Theilhaber et al. 2005. Identification of a molecular signature of sarcopenia. *Physiol. Genom.* 21(2):253–63.

Haussinger, D. and F. Schliess. 2007. Glutamine metabolism and signaling in the liver. *Front. Biosci.* 12:371–91.

Hornsby, P. J. 2010. Senescence and life span. *Pflugers Arch. Eur. J. Physiol.* 459(2):291–9.

Johnson, M. A., J. T. Dwyer, G. L. Jensen et al. 2011. Challenges and new opportunities for clinical nutrition interventions in the aged. *J. Nutr.* 141(3):535–41.

Jourdan, M., N. E. Deutz, L. Cynober, and C. Aussel. 2013. Consequences of age-related splanchnic sequestration of leucine on interorgan glutamine metabolism in old rats. *J. Appl. Physiol. (1985)* 115(2):229–34.

Kadowaki, M. and T. Kanazawa. 2003. Amino acids as regulators of proteolysis. *J. Nutr.* 133(6):2052S–6S.

Kalhan, S. C. and D. M. Bier. 2008. Protein and amino acid metabolism in the human newborn. *Annu. Rev. Nutr.* 28:389–410.

Kalhan, S. C. and J. M. Edmison. 2007. Effect of intravenous amino acids on protein kinetics in preterm infants. *Curr. Opin. Clin. Nutr. Metab. Care* 10 (1):69–74.

Kimball, S. R. and L. S. Jefferson. 2002. Control of protein synthesis by amino acid availability. *Curr. Opin. Clin. Nutr. Metab. Care* 5 (1):63–7.

Koopman, R., L. B. Verdijk, M. Beelen et al. 2008. Co-ingestion of leucine with protein does not further augment post-exercise muscle protein synthesis rates in elderly men. *Br. J. Nutr.* 99 (3):571–80.

Lacey, J. M. and D. W. Wilmore. 1990. Is glutamine a conditionally essential amino acid? *Nutr. Rev.* 48 (8):297–309.

Laplante, M. and D. M. Sabatini. 2012. mTOR signaling in growth control and disease. *Cell* 149 (2):274–93.

Larson, S. D., J. Li, D. H. Chung, and B. M. Evers. 2007. Molecular mechanisms contributing to glutamine-mediated intestinal cell survival. *Am. J. Physiol. Gastrointest. Liver Physiol.* 293(6):G1262–71.

Le Bacquer, O., N. Mauras, S. Welch, M. Haymond, and D. Darmaun. 2007. Acute depletion of plasma glutamine increases leucine oxidation in prednisone-treated humans. *Clin. Nutr.* 26(2):231–8.

Le Bacquer, O., H. Nazih, H. Blottiere, D. Meynial Denis, C. Laboisse, and D. Darmaun. 2001. Effects of
glutamine deprivation on protein synthesis in a model of human enterocytes in culture. *Am. J. Physiol.
Gastrointest. Liver Physiol.* 281(6):G1340–G1347.

Lie-Venema, H., W. T. Labruyère, M. A. Van Roon et al. 1995. The spatio-temporal control of the expression
of glutamine synthetase in the liver is mediated by its 5'-enhancer. *J. Biol. Chem.* 270 (47):28251–6.

Lopez, H. W., C. Moundras, C. Morand, C. Demigné, and C. Rémésy. 1998. Opposite fluxes of glutamine
and alanine in the splanchnic area are an efficient mechanism for nitrogen sparing in rats. *J. Nutr.*
128(9):1487–94.

Lowe, D. K., K. Benfell, R. J. Smith et al. 1990. Safety of glutamine-enriched parenteral nutrient solutions in
humans. *Am. J. Clin. Nutr.* 52(6):1101–6.

Magne, H., I. Savary-Auzeloux, D. Remond, and D. Dardevet. 2013. Nutritional strategies to counteract muscle atrophy caused by disuse and to improve recovery. *Nutr. Res. Rev.* 26(2):149–65.

Mates, J. M., J. A. Segura, F. J. Alonso, and J. Marquez. 2008. Intracellular redox status and oxidative stress:
Implications for cell proliferation, apoptosis, and carcinogenesis. *Arch. Toxicol.* 82(5):273–99.

Meynial-Denis, D., A.M. Beaufrere, M. Mignon, and P. Patureau Mirand. 2013. Effect of intermittent glutamine supplementation on skeletal muscle is not long-lasting in very old rats. *J. Nutr. Health Aging*
17:876–79.

Meynial-Denis, D., M. Mignon, A. Miri et al. 1996. Glutamine synthetase induction by glucocorticoids is
preserved in skeletal muscle of aged rats. *Am. J. Physiol. Endocrinol. Metab.* 271(34 (6)):E1061–6.

Meynial-Denis, D., L. Verdier, M. Mignon, J. N. Leclerc, G. Bayle, and D. Darmaun. 2005. Does acute glutamine depletion enhance the response of glutamine synthesis to fasting in muscle in adult and old rats?
Clin. Nutr. 24:398–406.

Mezzarobba, V., A. Torrent, I. Leydier et al. 2003. The role of adrenal hormones in the response of glutamine
synthetase to fasting in adult and old rats. *Clin. Nutr.* 22(6):569–75.

Mignon, M., A. M. Beaufrere, L. Combaret, and D. Meynial-Denis. 2007a. Does long-term intermittent treatment with glutamine improve the well-being of fed and fasted very old rats? *J. Parent. Enteral Nutr.*
31(6):456–62.

Mignon, M., L. Leveque, E. Bonnel, and D. Meynial-Denis. 2007b. Does glutamine supplementation decrease
the response of muscle glutamine synthesis to fasting in muscle in adult and very old rats? *J. Parent.
Enteral Nutr.* 31:26–31.

Mizunuma, M., E. Neumann-Haefelin, N. Moroz, Y. Li, and T. K. Blackwell. 2014. mTORC2-SGK-1 acts in
two environmentally responsive pathways with opposing effects on longevity. *Aging Cell* 13(5):869–78.

Mosoni, L., P. Patureau Mirand, M. L. Houlier, and M. Arnal. 1993. Age-related changes in protein synthesis
measured *in vivo* in rat liver and gastrocnemius muscle. *Mech. Ageing Dev.* 68(1–3):209–20.

Mouchard, M. L., S. Bes, M. Mignon, and D. Meynial-Denis. 2008. Fasting up-regulates muscle glutamine
synthetase while it down-regulates liver glutamine synthetase in male rats during aging. *e-SPEN*
3:309–15.

Munro, H. N. 1982. Adaptation of body protein metabolism in adult and aging man. *Clin. Nutr.* 1(2):95–108.

Nakajo, T., T. Yamatsuji, H. Ban et al. 2005. Glutamine is a key regulator for amino acid-controlled cell
growth through the mTOR signaling pathway in rat intestinal epithelial cells. *Biochem. Biophys. Res.
Commun.* 326(1):174–80.

Naomoto, Y., T. Yamatsuji, K. Shigemitsu et al. 2005. Rational role of amino acids in intestinal epithelial cells
(Review). *Int. J. Mol. Med.* 16(2):201–4.

Neu, J., V. DeMarco, and N. Li. 2002. Glutamine: Clinical applications and mechanisms of action. *Curr. Opin.
Clin. Nutr. Metab. Care* 5(1):69–75.

Nicastro, H., C. R. da Luz, D. F. Chaves et al. 2012. Does branched-chain amino acids supplementation modulate skeletal muscle remodeling through inflammation modulation? Possible mechanisms of action.
J. Nutr. Metab. 2012:136937.

Obled, C., I. Papet, and D. Breuillé. 2002. Metabolic bases of amino acid requirements in acute diseases. *Curr.
Opin. Clin. Nutr. Metab. Care* 5:189–97.

Oehler, R. and E. Roth. 2003. Regulative capacity of glutamine. *Curr. Opin. Clin. Nutr. Metab. Care*
6(3):277–82.

Paddon-Jones, D. and H. Leidy. 2014. Dietary protein and muscle in older persons. *Curr. Opin. Clin. Nutr.
Metab. Care* 17(1):5–11.

Papet, I., D. Dardevet, C. Sornet et al. 2003. Acute phase protein levels and thymus, spleen and plasma protein
synthesis rates differ in adult and old rats. *J. Nutr.* 133(1):215–9.

Patel, B. B., Y. Yu, J. Du et al. 2009. Schlafen 3, a novel gene, regulates colonic mucosal growth during aging. *Am. J. Physiol. Gastrointest. Liver Physiol.* 296(4):G955–G962.

Pedersen, A. N. and T. Cederholm. 2014. Health effects of protein intake in healthy elderly populations: A systematic literature review. *Food Nutr. Res.* 58.

Petry, E. R., V. F. Cruzat, T. G. Heck, P. I. Homem de Bittencourt, Jr., and J. Tirapegui. 2015. L-Glutamine Supplementations Enhance Liver Glutamine-Glutathione Axis and Heat Shock Factor-1 Expression in Endurance-Exercise Trained Rats. *Int. J. Sport Nutr. Exerc. Metab* 25(2):188–97.

Pinel, C., V. Coxam, M. Mignon et al. 2006. Alterations in glutamine synthetase activity in rat skeletal muscle are associated with advanced age. *Nutrition* 22(7–8):778–85.

Rhoads, M. J. and G. Wu. 2009. Glutamine, arginine, and leucine signaling in the intestine. *Amino Acids* 37(1):111–22.

Rosca, M. G., H. Lemieux, and C. L. Hoppel. 2009. Mitochondria in the Elderly: Is Acetylcarnitine a Rejuvenator? *Adv. Drug Deliv. Rev.* 61(14):1332–42.

Roth, E. 2007. Immune and cell modulation by amino acids. *Clin. Nutr.* 26(5):535–44.

Roth, E. 2008. Nonnutritive effects of glutamine. *J. Nutr.* 138(10):2025S–2031S.

Rutten, E. P., M. P. Engelen, E. F. Wouters, A. M. Schols, and N. E. Deutz. 2006. Metabolic effects of glutamine and glutamate ingestion in healthy subjects and in persons with Chronic obstructive pulmonary disease. *Am. J. Clin. Nutr.* 83(1):115–23.

Sahakian, J. A., L. I. Szweda, B. Friguet, K. Kitani, and R. L. Levine. 1995. Aging of the liver: Proteolysis of oxidatively modified glutamine synthetase. *Arch. Biochem. Biophys.* 318(2):411–7.

Sakiyama, T., M. W. Musch, M. J. Ropeleski, H. Tsubouchi, and E. B. Chang. 2009. Glutamine increases autophagy under Basal and stressed conditions in intestinal epithelial cells. *Gastroenterology* 136(3):924–32.

Sakuma, K., W. Aoi, and A. Yamaguchi. 2015. Current understanding of sarcopenia: Possible candidates modulating muscle mass. *Pflugers Arch.* 467(2):213–29. doi: 10.1007/s00424-014-1527-x. Epub 2014 May 7.

Sakuma, K., W. Aoi, and A. Yamaguchi. 2014. The intriguing regulators of muscle mass in sarcopenia and muscular dystrophy. *Front. Aging Neurosci.* 6:230.

Sandri, M., L. Barberi, A. Y. Bijlsma et al. 2013. Signalling pathways regulating muscle mass in ageing skeletal muscle: The role of the IGF1-Akt-mTOR-FoxO pathway. *Biogerontology* 14(3):303–23.

Schiaffino, S., K. A. Dyar, S. Ciciliot, B. Blaauw, and M. Sandri. 2013. Mechanisms regulating skeletal muscle growth and atrophy. *FEBS J.* 280(17):4294–314.

Shen, J. and J. Tower. 2009. Programmed cell death and apoptosis in aging and life span regulation. *Discov. Med.* 8(43):223–6.

Smith, R. J. 1990. Glutamine metabolism and its physiologic importance. *J. Parent. Enteral Nutr.* 14(4):40S–4S.

Solerte, S. B., C. Gazzaruso, R. Bonacasa et al. 2008. Nutritional supplements with oral amino acid mixtures increases whole-body lean mass and insulin sensitivity in elderly subjects with sarcopenia. *Am. J. Cardiol.* 101 (11A):69E–77E.

Souba, W. W. 1991. Glutamine: A key substrate for the splanchnic bed. *Annu. Rev. Nutr.* 11:285–308.

Spindler, S. R. 2001. Calorie restriction enhances the expression of key metabolic enzymes associated with protein renewal during aging. *Ann. New York Acad. Sci.* 928:296–304.

Stuerenburg, H. J., B. Stangneth, and B. G. Schoser. 2006. Age related profiles of free amino acids in human skeletal muscle. *Neuroendocrinol. Lett.* 27 (1–2):133–6.

Tessari, P. 2000. Changes in protein, carbohydrate, and fat metabolism with aging: Possible role of insulin. *Nutr. Rev.* 58 (1):11–9.

Tieland, M., M. L. Dirks, N. van der Zwaluw et al. 2012. Protein supplementation increases muscle mass gain during prolonged resistance-type exercise training in frail elderly people: A randomized, double-blind, placebo-controlled trial. *J. Am. Med. Dir. Assoc.* 13 (8):713–9.

Unterluggauer, H., S. Mazurek, B. Lener et al. 2008. Premature senescence of human endothelial cells induced by inhibition of glutaminase. *Biogerontology* 9(4):247–59.

van De Poll, M. C. G., M. P. C. Siroen, P. A. M. Van Leeuwen et al. 2007a. Interorgan amino acid exchange in humans: Consequences for arginine and citrulline metabolism. *Am. J. Clin. Nutr.* 85(1):167–72.

van de Poll, M. C., G. C. Ligthart-Melis, P. G. Boelens, N. E. Deutz, P. A. van Leeuwen, and C. H. Dejong. 2007b. Intestinal and hepatic metabolism of glutamine and citrulline in humans. *J. Physiol.* 581(Pt 2):819–27.

Verdier, L., Y. Boirie, S. Van Drieessche, M. Mignon, R. J. Begue, and D. Meynial Denis. 2002. Do sex steroids regulate glutamine synthesis with age? *Am. J. Physiol. Endocrinol. Metab.* 282(1):E215–21.

Wall, B. T. and L. J. van Loon. 2013. Nutritional strategies to attenuate muscle disuse atrophy. *Nutr. Rev.* 71(4):195–208.

Walker, D.K., Dickinson, J.M., Timmerman, K.L. et al. 2011. Exercise, amino acids, and aging in the control of human muscle protein synthesis. *Med. Sci. Sports Exerc.* 43:2249–2258.

Wang, B., G. Wu, Z. Zhou et al. 2015. Glutamine and intestinal barrier function. *Amino Acids* 47(10):2143–54.

Watford, M., V. Chellaraj, A. Ismat, P. Brown, and P. Raman. 2002. Hepatic glutamine metabolism. *Nutrition* 18(4):301–3.

Welle, S. 1999. In *Human Protein Metabolism*: Springer Verlag, New York. Original edition, Biochemistry & Biophysics.

Williams, J. Z., N. Abumrad, and A. Barbul. 2002. Effect of a specialized amino acid mixture on human collagen deposition. *Ann. Surg.* 236(3):369–74; discussion 374–5.

Wu, G., Z. Wu, Z. Dai et al. 2013. Dietary requirements of "nutritionally non-essential amino acids" by animals and humans. *Amino Acids* 44(4):1107–13.

Xi, P., Z. Jiang, C. Zheng, Y. Lin, and G. Wu. 2011. Regulation of protein metabolism by glutamine: Implications for nutrition and health. *Front. Biosci. (Landmark Ed)* 16:578–97.

Yao, K., Y. Yin, X. Li et al. 2012. Alpha-ketoglutarate inhibits glutamine degradation and enhances protein synthesis in intestinal porcine epithelial cells. *Amino Acids* 42(6):2491–500.

Young, V. R. 1990. Protein and amino acid metabolism with reference to aging and the elderly. *Prog. Clin. Biol. Res.* 1990;326:279–300.

Young, V. R. 1990. Amino acids and proteins in relation to the nutrition of elderly people. *Age Ageing* 19(4):S10–24.

Ziegler, T. R., M. E. Evans, C. Fernandez-Estivariz, and D. P. Jones. 2003. Trophic and cytoprotective nutrition for intestinal adaptation, mucosal repair, and barrier function. *Ann. Rev. Nutr.* 23:229–61.

Section XI

Conclusion

25 Sum Up and Future Research

Dominique Meynial-Denis

CONTENTS

This book presents the different functions of glutamine (Gln) in animals and humans. Glutamine's functions go beyond that of a simple metabolic fuel or protein precursor; Gln is both a nutrient and a signaling molecule.

25.1 SUM UP

25.1.1 BASICS OF GLUTAMINE METABOLISM

In Chapter 1, Cruzat and Newsholme present the different aspects of Gln biochemistry and metabolism. The importance of Gln for whole-body health and the increasing interest in nutritional supplementation are underlined. In humans, Gln supplementation may not prevent inflammation, damage, and disease, or even enhance performance but could help the recovery of cells under severe catabolic conditions.

25.1.2 NEW DATA ON THE BIOCHEMISTRY OF GLUTAMINE

In Chapter 2, Lamers et al. report new data on glutamine synthetase (GS) regulation in the small intestine and colon. This enzyme, responsible for synthesis of Gln in muscle or in liver, is also present in the intestine. The importance of goblet cells in GS expression and the role of GS expression on intestinal cell proliferation (by using GS-deficient mice) are emphasized.

In an overview of the interorgan metabolism of Gln, Curthoys describes the regulation of enzymes involved in Gln metabolism: glutaminases (GAs) for the catabolism and GS for the synthesis (Chapter 3).

25.1.3 MOLECULAR AND CELLULAR ASPECTS OF GLUTAMINE METABOLISM

Cruzat et al. report the importance of Gln to insulin secretion, insulin action, and glycemic control in Chapter 4. Gln increases insulin sensitivity (notably by reducing oxidative stress and inflammation) and has a hypoglycemic effect.

Gln supplementation can be useful in insulin resistance induced by some catabolic states such as type 2 diabetes mellitus, severe exercise, burns, trauma, surgery, sepsis and fasting, including perioperative fasting.

Gebhardt discusses the signaling role of Gln in autophagy (Chapter 5). Gln is a potent regulator of this process via mammalian target of rapamycin (mTOR) and glutaminolysis. This effect is strongly dependent on cell type and physiological conditions. Moreover, autophagy is an emerging concept in aging and an increase in autophagy *in vivo* can favor longevity.

Gebhardt and his collaborators describes the regulation of hepatic Gln and ammonia metabolism by morphogens (Chapter 6). They underlines the importance of liver zonation in the consumption or in the production of Gln by the liver. A full understanding of how morphogenic signaling controls liver zonation may reveal new therapeutic targets and open up avenues for the design of new drugs to modulate morphogenic signaling and, consequently, to fight against liver diseases.

25.1.4   GLUTAMINE, THE BRAIN, AND NEUROLOGICAL DISEASES

In Chapter 7, Albrecht et al. focus on the roles of Gln in neurotransmission. Gln has a function specific to the nervous system and abnormalities of its metabolism are central to the pathogenesis of selected central nervous system diseases. Three diseases are approached in this chapter: hepatic encephalopathy (HE), epilepsy, and brain tumors. More precisely, this chapter shows how impairments of the "Gln/Glu-gamma aminobutyric acid (GABA) cycle" are related to these pathological conditions. It demonstrates how the enzymes glutamine synthetase (GS) and glutaminase (GA) that are highly active in astrocytes as well as their inhibitors can be used to draw perspectives for therapies in neurological diseases. The basis of these therapies is on correcting the tissue Gln imbalance and more precisely to prevent the excess of Gln and ammonia in astrocytes, which contributes to brain tissue swelling.

The chapter of Butterworth and Bemeur (Chapter 8) is focused on acute liver failure and the consequences of this pathology on the central nervous system (CNS). Liver failure leads to increased plasma and brain concentrations of ammonia and its detoxification produces Gln, inducing HE. This chapter demonstrates that Gln is a key player in the pathogenesis of CNS complications of liver failure. Although GS, GA, glutamine transaminase, and astrocytic Gln transporter SNAT5 are involved in the severity of HE and are probably future therapeutic targets, no strategy to prevent or cure this pathology has so far been developed.

In Chapter 9, Chassain et al. deal with Parkinson's disease (PD), a common neurodegenerative disorder that affects the human population worldwide. Alterations in the metabolism of the cerebral neurotransmitter GABA and its precursors, Gln and Glu, may be involved in the pathophysiology of PD. Magnetic resonance spectroscopy has been used to detect changes in Glu and Gln concentrations in the striatum. This original method is an exciting opportunity to improve the mechanistic understanding of this pathology. The metabolite profile obtained could be used both for early diagnosis and to monitor therapeutic responsiveness.

25.1.5   GLUTAMINE AND THE INTESTINAL TRACT

Blachier et al. present in Chapter 10 the metabolic and physiological effects of Gln on the intestine in healthy situations and in several disease states in which the integrity of the intestinal mucosa is impaired. The obtained data underline that Gln is highly metabolized in the small and large intestinal mucosa. These results demonstrate that Gln supplementation is beneficial for the recovery of intestinal mucosal integrity and protects against the bacterial translocation seen in animal models of intestinal inflammation, mucosal healing, and endotoxemia. The efficiency of such supplementation remains to be demonstrated in human studies.

The chapter of Rhoads et al. (Chapter 11) is on the role of Gln as a general facilitator of gut absorption and repair. The chapter underlines that Gln no longer enjoys the prominence it had in the late twentieth century but still remains in widespread use in cases of critical illness, particularly in gastrointestinal injury, in which Gln stimulates mucosal recovery.

Xue and Wischmeyer give a good explanation of the therapeutic potential of Gln in *in vitro* and *in vivo* inflammatory bowel disease (IBD) models (Chapter 12). They underline that the emerging conception of administering Gln as a "therapeutic nutrient" warrants more experimental and clinical trials in the settings of IBD. Indeed, basic questions on how to administer this nutrient in a clinically relevant and effective paradigm, which have been defined in conditions such as critical illness, still remain poorly answered in IBD settings.

25.1.6 GLUTAMINE AND THE CATABOLIC STATE

25.1.6.1 Part I: Role of Glutamine in Critical Illness

25.1.6.1.1 Section A: During Childhood

Neu et al. report the effects of Gln supplementation in infants and critically ill children in Chapter 13. However, because there are few data available concerning childhood, the effect of Gln supplementation is largely unknown.

25.1.6.1.2 Section B: From Adulthood

Jahoor et al. report the role of Gln supplementation in critical illness in adults in Chapter 14. It is difficult to draw conclusions on the rationale and the efficiency of Gln supplementation because critically ill patients are very heterogeneous (e.g., they may be Gln deficient or have high baseline Gln concentrations).

Abumrad et al. show that Gln supplementation does not benefit all patient populations with critical illness (Chapter 15). Specific lessons have to be drawn from the REDOXS (Reducing Deaths due to Oxidative Stress) trial: it is important to carefully assess whether the patients have renal and hepatic dysfunctions or obesity or multiorgan system failure.

Smedberg and Wernerman give a good description of the clinical endpoints of Gln supplementation in critical illness in Chapter 16. They demonstrate that the use of Gln supplementation should not be discriminated in critically ill patients but for this to be efficient this depends on the low intracellular concentration of Gln in skeletal muscle. In brief, the need for Gln supplementation is related to hypoglutaminemia.

Coeffier and Dechelotte give a good explanation of the likely beneficial effects of Gln supplementation in critical illness by describing the mechanisms of action: modulation or inflammatory, immune and oxidative responses, induction of heat shock proteins, and improvement of glucose homeostasis by decrease of insulin resistance (Chapter 17).

In Chapter 18, Garibotto et al. describe chronic metabolic acidosis and renal injury. The reduced availability of Gln to the kidney may hinder the body's response in acidosis. Moreover, Gln supplementation may play a role in acute kidney injury (AKI). AKI is a complication of sepsis. These authors explain that there are benefits of Gln supplementation when the Gln level is low. However, Gln may become harmful for patients with critical illness and renal failure.

25.1.6.2 Part II: Role of Glutamine in Cancer

In Chapter 19, Bode reports data on the transport of Gln and its application in human cancer. New data are presented for developing effective tools to target deranged Gln biology in the diagnosis, treatment, and management of cancer in the twenty-first century. More precisely, this author focuses on Gln transporters and their potential roles in supporting the "tumor metabolome." He shows how some Gln transporters that activate mTOR signaling and are both a target for the oncogene c-myc and a driver of growth for cancer cells, GAC, and some mutants of *isocitrate dehydrogenase* have emerged as the most promising targets for the development of cancer detection tools and therapies.

Imaging Gln metabolism is a major challenge in cancer biology to monitor and understand cancer metabolism *in vivo* with the aim of improving diagnosis and, perhaps, therapy. Meynial-Denis and Renou report in Chapter 20 that Gln is a marker of tumor growth and division and that there is a relation between oncogene expression and the activity of the enzyme GA. It may be possible to use hyperpolarized [5-^{13}C] Gln (improvement in sensitivity of ^{13}C MRS by a factor of 10,000 via DNP preparation) to assess the effect of tumor treatment with cytostatic drugs.

25.1.7 GLUTAMINE, IMMUNITY, AND EXERCISE

Marino and Calder focus (Chapter 21) on Gln and the immune system in their chapter. First, immunity (innate, acquired, and that associated with the gut) and the function of cells of the immune system are clearly explained. The metabolic roles of Gln in immune cells, its mechanism of action, and its importance in animal models and humans are developed. In brief, Gln is used at a higher rate by cells of the immune system but is not fully oxidized. Gln is converted to a number of metabolites involved in signaling, biosynthesis, immune cell turnover, and function, and in both the protection and preservation of cells and tissues. Gln also plays a role in the upregulation of HSP70 in states in which the plasma level of Gln is lowered such as critical illness, septic shock, trauma, and severe burns. Hence, the demand for Gln may exceed the supply.

Rogero and Dos Santos focus (Chapter 22) on the main advances in the study of Gln, nutrition, and immune response during physical exercise in rats and humans. The physiological functions of Gln and its importance to the immune system are discussed. Then, these authors explain how nutrition and Gln can modulate the immune response during acute and chronic exercise.

Castell and Redgrave illustrate the role of Gln in exercise-induced immunodepression in humans in Chapter 23. This chapter underlines very well how a decrease in plasma Gln could indicate both a decrease in immunocompetence and an increased risk of infection after exercise and how the effect of Gln supplementation in exercise on neutrophil function should be studied in humans.

25.1.8 GLUTAMINE AND AGING

Meynial-Denis reports data on the impact of Gln on the well-being of aged rats in Chapter 24. Gln is a key substrate for the splanchnic bed and a specific nutrient in gastrointestinal research with aging. In addition, Gln is not able to prevent muscle wasting during sarcopenia. Oral Gln supplementation initiated before advanced age in rats increases gut mass, improves the villus height of mucosa, and thereby prevents the gut atrophy encountered in advanced age. Enterocytes from very old rats continuously metabolize Gln into citrulline, which allowed, for the first time, to use citrulline as a noninvasive marker of intestinal atrophy induced by advanced age.

25.2 FUTURE DIRECTIONS

These future directions are related with the prolific roles of Gln in metabolism and associated pleiotropic cellular effects.

Role of Gln due to its metabolism:

- Gln generally increases insulin sensitivity (notably by reducing oxidative stress and inflammation) and has a hypoglycemic effect. This property deserves to be studied in aging, which is a state of insulin resistance.
- Gln has a regulatory role in autophagy, which is an emerging concept in aging. Its effect depends on the type of cells. Moreover, an increase in autophagy *in vivo* can favor longevity. Consequently, it may be interesting to study the effect of Gln on autophagy during aging.

- The signaling of hepatic Gln and ammonia metabolism by morphogens explains the liver zonation and the consumption or the production of Gln by the liver. This specificity of Gln metabolism in the liver should be studied further in the future.
- Gln has a role in preventing exercise-induced immunosuppression and improving performance. Indeed, a decrease in plasma Gln may indicate decreased well-being and immunocompetence, in particular, in the individual who is potentially vulnerable to opportunistic infections.

Role of Gln due to its high levels in some tissues (brain, liver, etc.)

- Gln has a function specific to the nervous system and abnormalities of its metabolism are central to the pathogenesis of CNS diseases: for example, HE, epilepsy, and brain tumors. Thus, a high concentration of Gln in the brain may be toxic.
- Another disease, ALF, leads to increased plasma and brain concentrations of ammonia and its detoxification produces Gln, inducing HE. It may be interesting to study the toxicity of the accumulation of Gln in the brain.
- Higher concentrations of Glu, Gln, and GABA are also observed in the striatum of animal models of PD and explain this brain disease. It may be interesting to know more on the role of Gln in the production of GABA in the case of the PD, a common neurodegenerative disorder that affects the human population worldwide.

Role of Gln as a "conditionally essential" amino acid and interest of Gln supplementation in severe catabolic states as Type 2 diabetes mellitus, severe exercise, burns, trauma, surgery, sepsis and fasting, including perioperative fasting, etc.: Gln supplementation repletes low pools of Gln in plasma and in some tissues. Gln improves glycemic control and increases insulin sensitivity by various mechanisms including reduced oxidative stress and inflammation, which can interfere with insulin signaling. The limits of Gln supplementation are associated with toxicity in patients with renal or hepatic failure (increase of uremia) and may lead to death.

The impact of Gln in critical illness and the soundness of its supplementation have been studied a lot up to now:

- To use Gln supplementation only if there is hypoglutaminemia in critically ill humans
- To make sure that there is no renal or hepatic failure before use of Gln supplementation

In contrast, the role of Gln as a "therapeutic nutrient" to improve mucosal recovery in the human intestine deserves to be more studied in IBD. Moreover, because Gln improves both insulin sensitivity and the recovery of gut cells, Gln may be used in humans during aging. This application of Gln has not been used up to now, it may contribute to maintain the well-being and the good health in humans provided that the kidneys and liver function well.

Promising role of Gln in cancer biology:

Gln may contribute to resolve a major challenge of the twenty-first century: to better monitor and understand cancer metabolism *in vivo* with a goal of improved diagnosis and perhaps therapy. As seen in all rapidly proliferating cells, Gln is used at a high rate in cancer cells and inhibiting Gln uptake or metabolism could be an effective anticancer strategy.

Index

Printed and bound by CPI Group (UK) Ltd, Croydon, CR0 4YY

17/10/2024

01775698-0008